APPLICATIONS OF SOCIAL SCIENCE
TO CLINICAL MEDICINE AND HEALTH POLICY

Applications of

TO CLINICAL

HEALTH

Sponsored by the Medical Sociology Section of the
American Sociological Association

Social Science
MEDICINE AND
POLICY

Edited by Linda H. Aiken
and David Mechanic

Rutgers University Press   *New Brunswick, New Jersey*

Library of Congress Cataloging-in-Publication Data
Main entry under title:

Applications of social science to clinical medicine
  and health policy.

  Sponsored by the Medical Sociology Section of the
American Sociological Association.
  1. Social medicine. 2. Medical policy—Social
aspects. 3. Social medicine—United States. 4. Medical
policy—Social aspects—United States. I. Aiken,
Linda H. II. Mechanic, David, 1936–   . III. American
Sociological Association. Medical Sociology Section.
[DNLM: 1. Health Policy. 2. Social Medicine.
3. Sociology, Medical. WA 31 A652]
RA418.A69   1986   362.1'042   85–26251

ISBN 0–8135–1148–8
ISBN 0–8135–1149–6 (pbk.)

Contents

Acknowledgments

The Medical Sociology Section of the American Sociological Association initiated this volume. As editors we undertook the project because we believe that the contributions of the social sciences to clinical medicine and health policy are not well understood or appreciated by many medical educators and practitioners, or by policymakers in various levels of government. It was our goal to clarify the uses of social science research, to provide illustrations of how the social sciences have influenced our thinking about health care issues, and to underscore some promising and relevant areas of research for the future.

An editorial advisory committee appointed by the Council of the Medical Sociology Section provided valuable assistance in the selection of topics and contributors for the volume. The advisory committee consisted of John Colombotos, Constance Nathanson, Catherine Riessman, and Irving Zola. William d'Antonio, the executive officer of the American Sociological Association, was immensely helpful in implementing the project.

We would like to express our appreciation to the contributors, who undertook the very difficult task of translating the significance of their areas of scholarly work for a broader audience than they usually address. We are particularly grateful to Katherine Parker and Eileen Gnecco for managing the manuscript.

This project was made possible by a grant to the American Sociological Association from The Robert Wood Johnson Foundation.

Linda H. Aiken
David Mechanic

APPLICATIONS OF SOCIAL SCIENCE
TO CLINICAL MEDICINE AND HEALTH POLICY

Chapter 1

Social Science, Medicine, and Health Policy

David Mechanic and
Linda H. Aiken

Social science has a long history relevant to understanding the conditions promoting health and disease, the medical care process, and the issues of social responsibility for the poor, sick, and disabled. Many of these concerns can be traced to Edwin Chadwick and the public health movement early in the nineteenth century, the insights of Rudolf Virchow more than one hundred years ago concerning the complexity of disease causation and its relationship to social and economic conditions, and the early epidemiologists in Britain and the United States—Farr, Snow, Goldberger—who established the scientific basis for the study of disease in populations which now constitutes the core science of community medicine. As late as twenty years ago, however, a serious scholar in health could follow and master the world social science literature relevant to this vast arena without great difficulty.

In the past twenty years there has been an extraordinary growth of basic, applied, and evaluative research in the social sciences, addressing the following concerns: the broad determinants of health and disease; social and behavioral processes affecting the etiology, course, and outcome of pathology; the economic, social, and professional organization of the health services and how they function; the interplay between values, technology, economics, and patient care; the processes of interaction between patients and health practitioners; the way people care for their health, identify illness, seek help, and respond to the health care system; and numerous others. These areas have engaged the interest and efforts of social and behavioral scientists, epidemiologists, public health and health services research investigators, and many physicians and nurses who in their broad experience cannot help but notice how much their influence on patients depends on factors ordinarily seen as outside their professional preparation.

Medical care, and the behavioral determinants of health, have also increasingly engaged the attention of public-policy makers at every level. Health is an essential priority of every society, and in all developed countries health care needs increasingly are financed and regulated by public authorities. These authorities look to the social science community for basic information on trends in sickness and mortality, unmet needs for access to medical care and particular treatments, and cost-effective ways of dealing with major health problems that cause pain and disability and the loss of effective functioning. Policymakers are not scientists and cannot make decisions outside the political contexts in which they function, but they seek from the research community basic information and guidance that allows them to choose between feasible options in more informed ways. Policy decisions are now examined in more sophisticated terms than ever before and use in significant ways the perspectives, analytic techniques, and information that the social and behavioral sciences increasingly make available. The framing of policy issues, the examination of alternatives, and the modes of reaching policy determinations are implicitly, if not overtly, influenced by the broad range of studies and analyses that social scientists do.

It is not surprising that investigators of health and health services often feel their insights and data neglected because no one-to-one relationship exists between the flow of new knowledge and public policy or clinical application. The use of many of the insights achieved require translation relative to the prevailing social definitions, economic and political processes, and professional routines that in the aggregate shape health care responses and provision of necessary services. Much of social science knowledge is too abstract, too uncertain, and too qualified to serve the practitioner or policymaker in a way that can be applied immediately. More often than not such insights and data inform the practitioners' thinking, their view of the problem, and the options they consider. The results of social science may on occasion be useful immediately, but more often they percolate at the perimeters of policy-making and clinical activity, and are used when they fit a particular context or agenda. In the longer range, the work we do becomes common currency—what many come to define as "common sense"— and implicitly affects the public media, government issue papers, and the processes of professional education and patient care. In our society, almost all educated people think and work in a way influenced by the social sciences, although many are unaware of how they came to think about problems in this way.

The contributions of social science can be characterized in many ways, and no single book can provide more than a sample of illustrations. We have divided the turf in five ways that we think capture both the levels of social science efforts and the substantive use of the results. In the early years of medical sociology, it was common to differentiate between the sociology of medicine and the sociology in medicine. The former distinction concerned the use of medicine as an arena to study important social processes, such as stratification, professional socialization, and politics, with no particular concern with arriving at insights useful to practitioners. Sociology in medicine, in contrast, involved research that was structured more to serve medical care needs than to promote new basic knowledge. In retrospect, the distinction is too simple, and we increasingly have learned that the interplay between theory and practice improves both. The clinically motivated study of practical problems often sharpens theoretical thinking and brings it closer to reality; good theory suggests dimensions of the applied problem that enriches its investigation and comprehension.

Nevertheless, the styles of social science, the level at which issues are addressed, and the specific purposes of an investigation shape the result. Thus, the organization of the book takes such considerations into account. We emphasize that the distinctions are somewhat artificial, and at times misleading, but they also provide a useful coherence in communicating our objectives. In Part I, the chapters address broad issues and social forces such as the interplay between values, science, technology,

and social structure; social stratification affecting health such as the influence of social class; and other macro issues involving political science perspectives, the changing organization of the hospital and the profession of medicine, and new forms of medical organization. In this section we seek a broader understanding of the complex ways that states of health and health care organization arise from ongoing social processes.

Part II focuses on what we have learned about the three most significant contributors to mortality and morbidity, and preventive and treatment implications. It also discusses how social science techniques are used to measure and assess the state of health in the United States, how we reliably determine the effects of our health interventions, and how we identify factors that increase vulnerability to disease.

Part III focuses on crucial stages in the life cycle relevant to health, seeking to identify points of fruitful policy intervention. Included here is a discussion of contraception and childbearing; the determinants of infant mortality and prospects for prevention; the causes, consequences, and potential remedies for teenage childbearing; and the dilemmas created by a rapidly aging population for the organization and financing of health and social services. Part IV, on prevention and caring, illustrates some of the important social processes that affect vulnerability to illness and the outcomes of patient-practitioner relationships.

Part V addresses a variety of current concerns about the organization, financing, and provision of medical care services. The health care industry, now involving almost 11 percent of our GNP and expenditures of more than a billion dollars a day, has become a central focus of public concern. Rapidly mounting costs, the introduction of new technologies, the changing number and mix of health professionals, the growing population of the elderly, and the rapid entry of for-profit companies, all contribute to the perception of a major national issue and challenge. Health care in the United States is in ferment and on the threshold of significant change. We anticipate that the discussions here will contribute to helping the practitioner understand the influences that have brought us to where we are and the direction in which we might be going.

The study of health issues and health care policy engaged only a small number of social scientists just a few decades ago. Health care is now a major area of specialization for thousands of social scientists, economists, and public health analysts. There are well over a thousand medical sociologists alone, comprising the largest specialized section of the American Sociological Association.

As the current health care debate develops, it is appropriate to look back over the past couple of decades and assess what this large research effort among social scientists has contributed to improving the care of patients and resolving health policy issues. What new perspectives, insights, knowledge, and approaches have the social sciences contributed to resolving existing and impending medical care issues relevant to the management of the individual patient

and to the organization of the system as a whole?

In organizing this book, we selected some of the most outstanding social science and health services researchers to assess the relevance and contribution of their fields of study. In each case, we asked contributors to focus on major applications and existing implications for policy and clinical care and not on comprehensive literature reviews or summaries of the state of the field. Our objective is to stimulate and to give the reader an appreciation of the diversity of this very rich arena. Thus this book is more an introduction for further study than an effort to tell it all. We would hope, for example, that, after reading Newhouse's discussion of major experiments in health, many readers will be motivated to explore some of the experimental reports themselves, with their richness of detail and elegance of method.

One major contribution implied by much of the volume, but not explicitly expressed, is the way social and behavioral science has sensitized the sophisticated policymaker, clinician, and even layperson to assess evidence more critically and in a more sophisticated way. The quality of information we have on the determinants of health, and the functioning of our health services, has improved substantially over the years. The rigor of analysis, the sophistication of statistical methods, and the definition and use of appropriate control and comparison groups is a remarkable achievement that has not only added to the value of research results but also has contributed to the educated public's tough-mindedness about public policy issues. In the last twenty years the public has become a more sophisticated consumer of information, giving clinicians and policymakers increased incentive to review the facts carefully and present their decisions to consumers in more meaningful ways.

Perhaps the most significant contribution of the social sciences has been the many ways in which their research has affected how intelligent laypersons, as well as decision makers in varying settings, conceive of and conceptualize their worlds. These mind-sets have powerful influences on how issues are conceptualized and managed. Mind-sets, of course, are influenced by many historical, social, and cultural forces. In medical care, gains in science and technology, and many of the impressive results achieved, have shaped the thinking of the public as well as scientists and health professionals. The belief in the technologic imperative is not simply a physician value. Biomedical science and technology has captured the imaginations of almost all of us and are powerful forces that give high-technology medicine much of its momentum and credibility.

Recognition of the transformation of disease in developed nations, and many underdeveloped nations as well, is commonplace but nevertheless of the greatest importance. It is difficult for a young mother of today to appreciate the apprehension and panic associated with such previously common diseases as dysentery, typhoid, diphtheria, and scarlet fever. Serious illness and mortality from the common infectious diseases have virtually disappeared, and the main causes of suffering, incapacity, and death are typically chronic conditions that develop over a lifetime and often only show their effects in later life. There are, of course, such important exceptions as mental disorders and neoplasms that occur throughout the life span, and other threats to health and life induced by violence, risk taking, substance abuse, and a variety of noxious life-styles. But, increasingly, the burden of illness and the challenges of care are in the chronic disease arena.

The science and technology of cure is well developed, and increasingly being fined-tuned by advances in knowledge and their implementation, but the science and technology of prevention and maintenance of function is still in a very early stage. We know far too little about how to prevent disease, and we apply even the little we know rather poorly as many of our contributors point out. Too few children are successfully immunized; many mothers and babies still receive inadequate prenatal, infant, and child care; and contraceptive failure continues to be a pressing social problem. Too many children's life chances are truncated early on by inadequate parenting, poor schooling, early pregnancy and dependency, and a succession of influences that are transmitted from one to another generation. Thousands of mentally ill live on the streets, suffering not only from their incapacitating conditions but also from our failure to mobilize technologies of care within our means. Increasing numbers of elderly and their loved ones live pitiful lives in efforts to avoid nursing homes, but help only becomes available if the sick elderly patient is institutionalized. These, of course, are not simple or easily solved problems, but they suggest the enormity and importance of the effort to develop the technologies of caring and their financing, which are increasingly relevant in an aging society and among persons with irreversible chronic disease.

What, then, do we mean by the technology of caring, and how can it be enhanced by basic science in the social and behavioral disciplines? A particularly intriguing finding in studies of the chronically ill is the great variability in levels of functioning among persons with comparable physical impairment. While some develop profound social disabilities and may even exhibit total social incapacitation, others resume normal activities and obligations with limited decrement. If we think of some element of disability intrinsic to the patients' physical limitations as the primary disability, we then discover considerable variability in secondary disabilities resulting from variation in the patient's management and social environment. How we deal with chronic illness may either inhibit or exacerbate these additional incapacities.

The goal of the technology of caring is to manage illness to promote effective functioning and minimize unnecessary dependence. The components of this technology include but are not limited to educating patients appropriately about the nature of their conditions, teaching skills that allow them to manage their most troublesome symptoms, encouraging realistic independence and providing appropriate social support, teaching new coping skills to relace lost functioning, managing the medical regimen to insure least interference with continued normal functioning, and so on. Medical care for the elderly and for those with chronic disease requires considerable attention to the means of promoting a high quality of function. Such means are of many kinds, ranging from careful needs assessment and targeted teaching specific to decrements in performance to new technical devices that allow persons with sensory and mobility limitations to continue participating in their homes and communities. The technology of care and promoting function is not the soft underbelly of medical practice as some believe but a momentous challenge to health professionals to contribute their varied skills to improve the quality of life of the chronically ill.

Changes in patterns of illness, in the demography of the population, and in the organization of medical care make the contributions of social and behavioral science more important than ever before. New patterns of morbidity not only call on clinicians for long-term commitments to sustaining and enhancing function but also stimulate the search for risk factors to identify potential ways of preventing and ameliorating the development and course of disease processes. This demands not only keen efforts in clinical and analytic epidemiology but the development of strategies to prevent harmful patterns of behavior. Where prevention fails, and it often does, the goal is to identify adverse patterns of response early and change their course through skillful interventions and wise social policies.

The framework we use to think about illness and its treatment is undergoing fundamental change not only because of the escalation of medical care costs but also because of the fuzziness of boundaries between medicine and other sectors of our social life and major changes in values, life-styles, household structures, and the paradigms of health. The boundaries of medicine, and the roles of health practitioners, are in flux. Medicine increasingly involves itself with screening of asymptomatic populations, deviant behavior, fertility and infertility, developmental processes, and changes associated with aging over the life cycle. The boundaries between medicine and other aspects of our personal lives are permeable: while the medicalization of many aspects of life is increasing, other areas such as homosexuality and some handicaps have been substantially demedicalized. But in the aggregate these boundaries are clearly expanding, with physicians intimately involved in activities ranging from defining life itself to the anticipation of nuclear war and its consequences. Increasingly we will have difficulty differentiating medicine in the gray areas—where it blends with social services, community organization, and our systems of social entitlement, legal process, and social control. Many believe the physician's job has become too large not only for society but for the mental health and vitality of the physician as well.

The ferment in medical care organization requires more than ever before the tools of sophisticated policy analysis in assessing the costs and effectiveness of alternative financial and organizational arrangements, the effect of incentives on the behavior of patients and physicians, and the increasingly difficult ethical issues that arise from new science and technologies and the changing organization of care. Advances in biotechnology and computers, the perfection of transplantation and controls over immune processes—to suggest some examples among many—pose exciting but difficult challenges for the future. It seems clear that society must face more concretely than ever before the issue of allocation and must choose more narrowly among competing options. Such choices will not only require more detailed and accurate information and more refined decision making but also better forums for assessment of technology and evaluating options in a way seen by the general public as unbiased and equitable. In this context of more open discussion of limitations and trade-offs, policy analysis and social science research become essential.

The potentialities of technology and reality of fiscal constraints raise troublesome value questions at the core of ethics. As constraints increase, will our society attempt to achieve an equitable balance between need and the allocation of medical resources, or will we follow policies that enlarge the gaps in access and care between the affluent and the poor? Will we continue our efforts to insure all Americans access to basic health care coverage in relation to need, or will we, under the pressure of cost restraints and growing deficits, allow our support for public medical institutions to erode and increasingly limit eligibility in programs like Medicaid, designed to promote greater equity in medical care?

With the growth of new forms of medical organization and reimbursement, the incentives affecting administrators, doctors, other health professionals, and patients will be altered significantly. Physicians, traditionally agents and advocates for patients, will increasingly take on managerial roles that require them to balance more consciously the needs of the patient against the needs of an organization and its financing capacity to meet patient needs in the aggregate. Various theories suggest hypotheses about what to expect as payment of health professionals shifts from fee-for-service to salary and when reimbursement of organizations is based on capitation or global budgeting as compared with actual cost. But large gaps always exist between theory and reality, and much work must be done to understand how changing incentives modify behavior and how they affect access, quality of care, and the promotion of health.

If the past tells us anything about the future, inevitably we will confront surprising consequences of new social arrangements, some of which are perverse in relation to our basic goals. This requires that we have good data systems in place, that we have the capacity to monitor the performance of the system, and that we maintain mechanisms for corrective feedback and continued fine-tuning of our means to achieve valued objectives. Knowledge, technology, and new organizational arrangements all require far more complex interdependencies than have characterized medical care in the past. Teamwork is no longer rhetoric about desired objectives but a reality in carrying out the technical procedures in caring for the more seriously ill hospital patient who requires a greater complexity and intensity of care, and the growing numbers of patients in the community who depend on the successful coordination of medical, nursing, and social services, and rehabilitation approaches allied with other maintenance services. Whether in the hospital or the community, this teamwork will require more cooperation, coordination, and leadership. We will continue to need sophisticated research and analyses of alternative approaches for integrating the special skills of each of the professional groups and service occupations involved. These are not easy tasks; medical care may fail as easily as a result of ineffective communication or fragmentation of services as it does from an inaccurate diagnosis or the failure to provide essential follow-up care.

Values affecting health and health care are changing in the nation, and more effort than ever before will be devoted to issues of health maintenance and health promotion. Ironically, as we increasingly recognize the importance of social supports for health and effective functioning, these supports themselves are undergoing significant transformations. Both the changing age distribution, with growing numbers of the very old, and significant changes in household structure overall will increase the need for well-organized care plans and challenge the effectiveness of our health care and social services systems.

Between 1960 and 1983, one-parent households grew by 175 percent, one-person households by 173 percent, and households made up of unmarried couples by 331 percent. Single parents living with their children—mostly separated or divorced women, many with inadequate incomes—now constitute one of every ten households. Older women prevail among single-person households. These changes have significance for how we organize our medical and rehabilitation services. We well know that many services can be delivered efficiently on an outpatient basis when strong family supports are available. Home dialysis for patients with chronic kidney disease and non-hospital-based hospice services are considerably less expensive than hospital-based alternatives, but each depends not only on appropriate economic incentives but also on the availability of a capable and committed caretaker who can assume a great deal of responsibility in the caring process. Whether we consider these examples, or home care alternatives for the frail elderly or chronically ill patient, household structure, female participation in the labor force, or many other social trends, they are all crucial considerations in sound policy formulation.

In the final analysis, our most important goal in health care is to prevent disease and incapacity or delay them as long as humanly possible. Much of this effort depends on behavioral research that better identifies the determinants of risks and the ways to change life-styles and individual and group behaviors in constructive ways. Once the patient becomes ill and requires care, the largest challenge is not making the diagnosis and prescribing appropriate treatment, however important, but motivating and supporting the patient to accept and implement medication and life-style regimens that help limit incapacity and promote continued function. This job is difficult and often tedious, but the best diagnosis is worth nothing if there is a failure to follow through.

The foregoing suggests the inevitability of the growing importance of policy analysis and social science research. In almost every aspect of identifying disease, understanding precursors, implementing effective treatment, and controlling risk, behavioral research is central. In organizing to identify the burdens of ill health and provide an efficient and effective response, the role of social science and policy analysis is an essential ingredient. The challenge is formidable, and our knowledge and tools are still relatively paltry. By examining where we have been, the progress we have made, and the gaps in our knowledge that continue to exist, we hope this book can help set the stage for enhanced contributions in coming decades.

Part I

Social Contexts of Health Care and Health Policy

Chapter 2

Medicine, Science, and Technology

Renée C. Fox

The impact of medical science and technology on our health and illness, our life and death, has become a central preoccupation in American society since the 1960s. Continual discussion about the consequences and implications of the biological and therapeutic "revolution" that modern Western medicine has undergone pervades many spheres of our private, professional, and public activities. Certain biomedical advances are major foci of this ongoing discussion. Principal among them are the entrance of microbiology into the cosmos of the cell and its ultrastructures; the discovery of the double helical structure of deoxyribonucleic acid (DNA), and the deciphering of the genetic code; the development of life-support systems and intensive care units; the evolution of machines (such as computed tomography [CAT] and positron emission tomography [PET] scanners), that can look and hear into the deepest and smallest recesses of the body; the ability to operate on the human heart; the transplantation of live and cadaveric organs from one individual to another; the invention and deployment of the artificial kidney and the artificial heart; the use of powerful psychotropic, anticancer, and immunosuppressive drugs; the emerging possibilities of *in vitro* fertilization; and the prospects of genetic engineering.

A curious mixture of historical awareness and unawareness pervades the ongoing discussion of biomedical revolution. Although it is explicitly concentrated on a series of recent medical scientific and technological developments that have occurred since World War II, the discussion about these advances often proceeds as if they, and the diagnostic, therapeutic, and preventive armamentarium of medicine into which they fit, were centuries rather than four decades old. The chagrin frequently expressed over our medicine's failure to make more progress with the chief life-threatening illnesses that currently afflict us—cardiovascular disease and cancer; the cultural surprise exhibited over the appearance of a new, infectious disease like acquired immunodeficiency syndrome (AIDS); and the propensity to call some 12,900 reported cases of this syndrome an epidemic (Curran et al. 1985)—all suggest a kind of medical historical obliviousness. It ignores the fact that before the discovery of sulfa drugs and antibiotics in the 1930s and 1940s, infectious diseases were commonplace and rampant in our society, and that our medicine could do little for most illnesses of any sort, other than diagnose them, vigilantly follow their course, treat them with hands-on nursing care, and try to anticipate their outcome (Beeson 1980; Thomas 1983, 19–50).

The at-once historical and ahistorical commentary on medical science and technology and on what they have wrought is laced through with ambivalence. On the one hand the commentary is impressed with the knowledge and competence achieved in medicine. It is enthusiastic about the scientific and therapeutic "breakthroughs" periodically announced in professional journals and the media. It is expectant about biomedical progress still to come. On the other hand it is apprehensive about the biouncertainty that these medical advances entail—concerned about the

hard-to-predict risk and error, hazard and harm that can ensue from the energetic, manipulative, invasive ways that we bring science and technology to bear on sickness and health. It is harshly critical of the impersonal, relentless technicity of biomedicine. It attributes serious ethical as well as dangerous biological side effects to our medicine, especially to the scientific and technological developments around which so much of the talk about biomedical revolution turns. Alongside these feelings about the beneficial and injurious power of medicine are equally strong sentiments about its inadequacies: the limitations of what it has been able to do for our health and illness, the length and quality of our lives, our well-being, our pain and suffering, and the conditions surrounding our death. Public health measures and changes in life-style, it is often asserted, are more responsible for whatever progress we have made in preventing disease, promoting health, and prolonging life than is biomedicine, with its fixation on aggressive, ex post facto, scientific and technological means of treating illness.

What does this social and cultural ambivalence toward biomedicine represent? In part, it is a reflection of how complex and, in many respects, how contradictory the effects of the scientific and technical transformation of medicine have been. To some extent, it is indicative of a crisis of risen expectations that biomedical progress has helped to create: a crisis accompanied and augmented by the sociohistorical tendency, already noted, to "forget" how recent and prolific that progress has been. On deeper levels, the ambivalence is a paradoxical response to a process of change that is more than medical.

The biomedical revolution is part of a much larger social and cultural revolution. It is imbedded in a period of our national history and of the West when unusually massive, profound, and rapid change has challenged our established institutional and organizational structures and shaken our cultural assumptions, calling into question many of our basic concepts, values, and beliefs, and our overarching worldview. Biomedical advance has contributed to this social and cultural ferment. It has also been influenced by this ferment in ways that not only affect the social systems within which biomedical research and therapy are conducted, but also penetrate the scientific content of medicine and color its technical vocabulary. It seems more than coincidental, for example, that at a time when our society is grappling with a variety of issues pertaining to individualism, individuality, personhood, and the relationship of self to others (Fox and Willis 1983), the medical immunological approach to organ transplantation and the problem of graft reaction is intently focused on how the recipient is able to "recognize" grafted tissue as "not-self," using "individuality markers" to do so.

In this period of disorienting change, medicine (its science and technology, achievements and failures, uncertainties and limitations, promises and dangers, and its bearing on the human condition) has become an important symbolic center in our society. It is a projective screen, a metaphorical language, and a kind of code for the cultural questions we are asking and for our societal worry and perplexity in the face of them.

Chronic Illness

There is a wide array of phenomena associated with medical scientific and technological advance through which we are experiencing and pondering such "collective conscience" issues. The medical progress we have made in preventing, detecting, treating, and managing disease, and in sustaining and lengthening life, has altered the sociomedical landscape. Chronic rather than acute illnesses now prevail. Foremost among them are certain medical conditions—cancer, diseases of the heart, disorders of the brain and mind—that have great figurative as well as statistical significance. They affect organs and domains of the body that are anatomically and symbolically integral to our personhood. They are malignant, often insidious bearers of suffering and disability. They can be skillfully overseen, may occasionally abate or be arrested, and are sometimes cured; but by and large, these are illnesses that are incrementally progressive. The battery of drugs, surgical procedures, and mechanical devices that are used for their continuous, long-term care have multiple side effects whose cumulative implications are only beginning to be discerned. Chronic diseases are also harbingers of the physical form in which most of us will die our eventual deaths. They are medical incarnations, then, of what we still do not know, understand, and control in our advanced modern, scientifically sophisticated, technologically ingenious society; of the stubborn persistence of disease; and of our ultimate, mysterious mortality.

The societal impact of chronic illness and of the cultural messages it carries is enhanced because a sizeable proportion of our population (especially in older age groups) is living with these disorders. Never before in history have there been so many people with chronic health problems, wending their way through daily life as best they can, and medical science and treatment enable them to do; or so many individuals in later stages of enduring illnesses receiving prolonged, in-hospital and nursing home care for them. Those who are not personally touched by chronic disease are nonetheless constantly reminded of its presence by its sheer incidence, by its steady, prominent coverage by the media, by the medical predicaments of relatives, friends, and colleagues, and by the underlying awareness that their own freedom from such illness is temporary.

Critical Care and Sustaining Life

Out of the convergence of all that we are medically able and unable to do for chronic illness, a stream of tragic cases has been engendered that represent some of the most basic and awesome problems of life and death, meaning and decision that are now before us. These are cases like that of

William F. Bartling, a seventy-year-old man, in very poor health for six years, suffering from five chronic, usually fatal diseases (emphysema, arteriosclerosis, a malignant lung tumor, chronic respiratory failure, and an abdominal aneurysm), who was sustained on a life-support system in the intensive care unit of a hospital for six months, and who asked to be disconnected from the respirator. Bartling died on November 6, 1984, just twenty-three hours before his request was heard by a California appellate court that, on December 27, 1984, ruled in favor of what was deemed his constitutional right to refuse treatment. That a person of Bartling's advanced age, afflicted with such a plethora of lethal diseases, survived for the length of time he did is a consequence of the powerful medical technology we have developed and the unremitting expertise with which we wield it. The fact that in a case of this sort, the decision to forego life-sustaining treatment was made by a postmortem court ruling rather than by the patient himself, his family, or the medical professionals caring for him, and that this case is only one of the many related cases that appear regularly in the courts, is indicative of our societal unsureness about what is the right medical and moral thing to do under such circumstances and what is the right way to reach this decision. Through the dramaturgic attention that they have been given by the media, a number of such identified cases have become something akin to societal morality plays, publicly enacting our collective conflicts and anguish over the ethical and existential dilemmas that have been generated by the capacity of our medical scientific technology to maintain life and our strong cultural commitment to be vigorous and tenacious in our efforts to do so.

The Intensive Care Nursery

At the other end of the spectrum of life and age from William Bartling are the infants around whom our medical science and technology have built neonatal intensive care units (NICUs). These infants are at great risk because they were born very prematurely, are of very low birth weight, had their vital functions severely compromised due to perinatal adversity, or are suffering from congenital abnormalities (genetic, environmental, or unknown in origin), such as heart and neural defects associated with or independent of conditions like Down's syndrome or spina bifida. The special, high-technology, intensive nursing, pastel-colored, spaceshiplike (Rostain 1985) hospital units in which this group of infants live out their first days, weeks, and sometimes months, connected to machines (mechanical ventilators, radiant warmers, oxygen monitors, arterial catheters, intravenous feeding apparatus, among them) were recently established—in the 1960s, when neonatology also emerged as a pediatrics speciality. Many of the quarter million infants born prematurely, and with serious birth defects in the United States each year are now cared for in some seventy-five hundred NICU crib-beds, in approximately six hundred hospitals. Twenty, or even ten years ago, a sizeable number of these infants would not have survived. With the passage of every new year, these units make further progress in pushing back the limits of survival and of biological viability. It is now possible to keep an infant who is only in its twenty-fourth week of gestation, and who weighs as little as five hundred grams (scarcely more than one pound) alive in such an NICU.

We do not yet know the long-term consequences of the efforts and achievements of NICUs: how the infants treated in NICUs will develop, what kinds of health characteristics and illnesses they will have, or what the physical and intellectual, psychological and social qualities of their lives will be. The development of NICUs is so recent that it is only now becoming possible to do follow-up studies of the first cohorts of infants who received this type of intensive care. In a gross, clinical way, however, we do know that many of the infants who survive and leave the hospital do so with permanent physical and/or mental impairments, with continuing susceptibility to neuro-developmental and respiratory problems and to relatively serious, protracted illnesses, and with an ongoing need for specialized care of many kinds. Some of their medical difficulties are side effects of the very lifesaving measures that were taken on their behalf (for example, the blindness and scarred tracheas that may result from the use of mechanical ventilators for premature infants).

The dilemma To treat or not to treat? and the question What *are* we doing? hover over NICUs. These problems are as newborn as the units themselves, their infant patients, and the medical technological ability to save such infants from death. Questions about starting, stopping, and foregoing treatment are present in adult ICUs, too, but the NICU situation has added significance and greater pathos because it is associated with the powerful cultural meaning with which our society endows birth, babies, and parenthood. In basic, wrenchingly personified ways, the NICU's tiny patients and their parents represent helpless, innocent, suffering, striving, not-yet-lived human life, and the expectant human family.

This situation is apparent in the intensely emotional, highly polarized reactions to what have come to be known as the Baby Doe cases that have erupted onto the public scene in the past few years. These are cases in which, out of a process of consultation between medical professionals and parents, the decision has been made to withhold some medical or surgical treatment vital to maintaining the life of an infant. The Baby Doe–type cases that have received the most public attention entail two kinds of medical conditions, and treatment options, that epitomize tragic dilemmas. Usually, they have involved infants afflicted either with Down's syndrome or spina bifida, who have both correctable life-threatening defects, such as a blocked intestinal tract, a congenital heart problem, or an open spinal column that can be repaired surgically, and permanent, irreparable handicaps, such as mental retardation, paralysis, or incontinence, that do not jeopardize the infant's survival. Under these circumstances, a decision has been made not to treat a particular infant's remediable life-threatening condition.

Around such Baby Does, highly publicized court cases have occurred; newspapers, magazines, and television have developed extensive coverage; and political and religious as well as medical and ethical controversy has arisen. Over the past three years, no less than the president of the United States, the Department of Health and Human Services (DHHS), the Office of the U.S. Surgeon General, the Justice Department, a number of states and federal courts in different jurisdictions, the House of Representatives and the Senate of the U.S. Congress, numerous organizations of medical professionals (among them, the American Academy of Pediatrics, the American College of Obstetrics and Gynecology, the American College of Physicians, the American Medical Association, the American Hospital Association, and the American Nurses Association), voluntary organizations representing handicapped persons (such as the American Coalition of Citizens with Disabilities, the Association for Retarded Citizens, the Association for the Severely Handicapped, the Disability Rights Education and Defense Fund, and the Spina Bifida Association), individuals and groups of a religion-oriented, right-to-life suasion, and those with civil libertarian commitments have all been involved in the process by which successive versions of federal regulations, called

"Baby Doe rules," have been formulated, hotly debated, applied, and altered. Initiated by Pres. Ronald Reagan himself in 1983, these federal regulations extend rulings prohibiting discrimination against handicapped persons, and concerning child abuse prevention and treatment, to disabled infants with life-threatening conditions under care in NICUs. At the present writing (January 1985), all the NICUs of this country fall under the surveillance and jurisdiction arrangements that have been put into place by the rules on health care for handicapped newborns published by DHHS in December 1984 and by a bill passed by the U.S. Congress in October 1984. DHHS rule requires a sign to be posted in the NICU declaring that "nourishment and medically beneficial treatment (as determined with respect for reasonable medical judgments) should not be withheld from handicapped infants solely on the basis of their present or anticipated mental or physical impairments." This sign must also list two sets of telephone numbers for reporting suspected violations: those of a hospital review committee and of state child protection agencies. The congressional bill includes the "withholding of medically indicated treatment from disabled infants with life-threatening conditions" under child abuse and neglect, and, in common with the DHHS rules, states that "no heroic measures are required" if treatment would be "virtually futile in terms of the survival of the infant."

Although the foregoing are considered to be "final" regulations, it is highly unlikely that they are. They have certainly not resolved the maelstrom of questions that surround Baby Does. If anything, they may have added to the societal turbulence over a whole chain of interrelated issues: the irreducibly moral nature of the judgments that enter into decisions about whether treatments are "futile" or of potential medical benefit; the difficulties of making predictions about an infant's prognosis, and the life he or she might lead, particularly in light of the rapid medical technological progress that continues to be made in caring for these infants and the psychosocial, ethical, and existential considerations that such forecasting entails; widely divergent beliefs and interpretations of the meaning of life and death, health and handicap, childhood and parenthood, and the family and its relationships; and the issue of how best to protect the interests of handicapped children, while respecting what the courts have called "the most private and precious responsibility invested in parents for the care and nurture of their children" and parents' associated right to decide on the medical treatment they deem best for their child. What is more, the way that the executive, legislative, and judicial branches of our government have involved themselves with Baby Doe—related questions has raised another set of problems, fundamental to our Constitution and to the nature of our societal community. In a society like ours, with its underlying principles of pluralism and separation of church and state, should our polity be so actively and authoritatively intervening in Baby Doe matters that are as religious and metaphysical as they are medical and moral—taking an official stance and translating that position into rules and statutes that are binding on us all?

In sharp contrast to all the furor over the justifiability of nontreatment decisions in the NICU, very little attention has been paid to the implications of the fact that a disproportionately high number of extremely premature infants of very low birth weight, with severe congenital abnormalities, cared for in NICUs, are babies born to greatly disadvantaged mothers. The women who are at the highest risk for having such infants are poor, nonwhite, single teenagers, underweight and badly nourished, poorly educated, unemployed, who smoke, drink, and are prone to drug abuse, with a history of frequent, closely spaced pregnancies, and who may also be victims of the physical and psychological violence that so often occurs in their milieu. By and large, the public, professional, and private groups that are morally concerned about Baby Does and their life-sustaining treatment are disinclined to regard as *ethical* problems the deprived social conditions out of which many of these infants and their mothers come. And these groups are only weakly motivated, if at all, to recommend and initiate medical, public health, and social action programs that might reduce the likelihood of infants being born in this state and might improve their life chances after birth. Furthermore, the energy that has been devoted to insuring that infants receive life-maintaining care in the NICU far outweighs the interest and activity that

have been devoted to developing and funding services that can help families provide the specialized, emotionally and financially expensive care that many of the infants who graduate from NICUs will need for the rest of their lives.

The Elderly

Not only newborn infants at risk have experienced an impressive increase in survival in recent years. A very rapid decline in old-age mortality has also occurred in our society. "The U.S. Census Bureau's 1971 projection anticipated a life expectancy of 72.2 years in the year 2000. But already by 1982, life expectancy was 74.5 years, having increased more than twice as much in 10 years as it was expected to increase in 30" (Preston 1984, 435). The factors contributing to this change in the death rate and longevity of elderly people are complex. Primary among them are the medical, scientific, and technological progress that has occurred during the past twenty years in treating chronic illness and maintaining life, the intensive efforts that have been made to provide and increase access to medical services for the elderly, through Medicare and Medicaid, and the development of geriatric medicine and treatment programs.

Between 1960 and 1982, the number of persons in our population aged sixty-five and over grew 54 percent, while the number of children younger than fifteen years of age fell by 7 percent. The decline was due mainly to the drop in birthrate that followed the immediately post–World War II baby boom (Preston 1984, 435). The reduced birthrate is partly a consequence of the deep-structure changes in gender roles, and marriage and family patterns, that have taken place since the 1960s. The birthrate is also integrally connected to biomedicine through its dependency on the development and use of contraceptive drugs and devices, and of methods of abortion. As a consequence of these two converging processes—a significant decrease in the number of children and a rapid increase in the number of elderly—the age structure of the United States has been altered (with an abruptness, to a degree, and in a direction that were not even anticipated by demographers).

Societal responses to these major demographic changes have been admixed. There is much dolorous talk and writing about the number of elderly people in our society who are alone (including shelterless "bag ladies" and "vent men"), with meager financial resources, in frail health, disabled, mentally as well as physically afflicted, with dreaded conditions like Alzheimer's disease, for whom nursing homes are the only recourse. In sharp contrast to this melancholy portrait of the state of the elderly, many references are made to their individual vigor and collective influence. Stories about the robustness, lucidity, and continuing accomplishments of older people abound. There is increasing mention, too, of the political significance of persons over sixty-five years of age, through their active participation in voluntary associations that promote the interests of the elderly, and by virtue of their high rate of voter turnout in local and national elections. This bifurcated image of older Americans reflects different facets of their actual social situation. It also suggests the existence of deeply ambivalent feelings in the American population toward the elderly. Intermingled with palpable concern about what it is like to be an older person in our society, there is a considerable amount of more veiled ressentiment about the growing salience and importance of the elderly and the sizeable resources being allocated to them. This ressentiment is present, for example, in some of the commentaries that note the improvement during the past two decades of the social, economic, political, and medical conditions for older people while deploring the deterioration of these conditions for children. It is implied that this situation exists because, both advertently and inadvertently, we have chosen to favor our old at the expense of our young. A questionable notion about allocation of scarce resources underlies such an assumption; namely, if we distributed less of these resources to the elderly, we would necessarily provide more of them to children.

Contradictions around the Human Life Cycle

Birth, infancy, childhood, old age: it is interesting how many of the direct and indirect consequences of the evolution of modern medicine, its science and technology, plunge us into matters of the human life cycle, particularly its beginning and its end. It is around these essences and phases of what it is to be born, live, and die as a human person that our deepest cultural conflict and confusion are being expressed. At one and the same time in our society, we have organized "right to life" movements, and also "right to death" movements concerned with making our medicine- and technology-surrounded deaths more dignified and humane (Fox 1981). We have used legal means both to liberalize access to abortion and to insist that the NICUs of our country do everything possible to sustain the lives of premature infants who are close to the developmental age of previable fetuses, eligible for abortion. Through the relatively new field of perinatal medicine, we are making progress in our capacity to correct certain structural defects and metabolic disorders of fetuses in utero. In addition, we are developing innovative treatments for infertility: various forms of artificial insemination and *in vitro* fertilization. These activities, and the commitments underlying them, are so fraught with contradiction that we are having great societal difficulty in finding a way to reconcile them, or even to make cultural sense of them.

Twelve years after the landmark *Roe v. Wade* decision of the U.S. Supreme Court, which constitutionally supported a woman's right to decide whether to terminate her pregnancy, our society is more embattled than ever over the issue of abortion. Confrontations between so-called prolife and prochoice groups have escalated, as have incidents of violence associated with them. Yet for all this militancy, irresolution about the "rightness" or "wrongness" of abortion, and the consequences of its being legal or banned, seems to have grown. Close to 40 percent of the 757 adults who were polled this January by the Gallup Organization for *Newsweek* magazine answered yes to the question Do you ever wonder whether your own position on abortion is right or not? Affirmative answers were equally distributed between respondents who support abortion and those who oppose it ("America's Abortion Dilemma" 1984).

New Treatments for Infertility and the Concept of the Family

Our struggles over issues surrounding abortion, life-sustaining treatment, remedies for infertility, and the well-being of old persons and children in our society make it clear that we are having problems with our concept of the family as well. Profound disagreements over the value that we attach to the family, and over our beliefs about the rights and responsibilities that should be invested in it, have surfaced. Around the development of artificial insemination by donor (AID), egg donation, and surrogate pregnancy, questions basic to our very definition of a family have arisen. We have only begun to wrestle with our divergent ideas and strong sentiments about how we ought to think and feel about a family unit made up of a wife and a husband, and a child who was conceived and born through "artificial" methods (i.e., fertilization of the egg of the child's genetic mother with semen from a man who is not her husband, or in vitro fertilization, followed by implantation of the embryo in the uterus of a woman not genetically related to it). Are these acts inherently adulterous, no matter what the motivation and the quality of consent of the participants may be? Who is this child, biologically, socially, emotionally, and legally? Who are the child's parents? Is the family in which the child is raised "natural" and "right"? If we as a society were more sure about what we consider the core elements of family and of human kinship, other than biological relatedness, we might find these questions less enigmatic.

Hospitalization and Dehospitalization

All the medical phenomena thus far discussed occur in a system heavily oriented to the hospital as a locus of inpatient and outpatient care as well as a locus of the medical technologies extensively used to diagnose and treat illnesses, and nonillness conditions like pregnancy and infertility. This hospital centeredness coexists with the efforts since the 1960s to "dehospitalize"—efforts made by the women's, consumer health, holistic medicine, and alternative therapy movements, and increasingly by government bodies concerned with health and medical care. To a significant degree, this organized trend away from the hospital has been propelled by a social reaction to what is felt to be the domineering role of doctors, machines, and invasive procedures in hospital medicine, its crushing impersonality, its harmful physical and psychological side effects, its elaborate bureaucracy, and its high costs. An intricate push-pull relationship currently exists between these countervailing hospitalization-dehospitalization patterns. Nowhere is this relationship more starkly and troublingly apparent than in the sphere of the medical care of mental illness. What is usually termed "deinstitutionalization" has been a major movement in psychiatry since the mid-1950s. It has been estimated that over the course of some twenty-five years, from 1955 to 1980, the number of chronically mentally ill patients in large state hospitals has decreased from 559,000 to 138,000 (Gudeman and Shore 1984, 832). The development and use of psychotropic drugs to treat the symptoms of mental disorders, the growing philosophical and ideological conviction about the importance of freeing as many people as possible from the incarcerating control of "total institutions" like mental hospitals, the political advocacy to achieve this goal, and the economic incentives for extra hospital care provided by federal programs have all contributed to the decrease. However enlightened deinstitutionalization may be in some respects, and whatever benefit may be afforded certain categories of mentally ill persons to be released from a hospital-enclosed world, it has also had highly visible, disturbing consequences. During the same period that the patient populations of state hospitals have declined, the admission rates to these same hospitals have grown and accelerated. To a significant degree, this statistic is the result of readmissions of patients who are being hospitalized for shorter periods but who are more often rehospitalized than in the past. Not only has this "revolving door" phenomenon developed, but many of the unhospitalized persons with serious, chronic, mental disorders are not receiving the extensive, continuing medical and psychiatric care, housing, and vocational and social support services necessary for them to live some semblance of a normal life in the "outside world." Very sick and disabled persons, with flagrant symptoms and behavioral signs of their mental illness, make up a sizeable number of the homeless people who now live on the streets of our cities. The public distress and fear that their presence and predicament evoke have contributed to the romanticization, heard in some quarters, of the assets and accomplishments of mental hospitals and to serious talk about a policy shift in the direction of at least partially restoring these hospitals to the role they formerly played in sheltering, caring for, and treating mentally ill patients.

Cost and Cost Containment

The issues of hospitalization-dehospitalization, then, like the others we have explored, are surrounded by oscillating social attitudes that con-

flict and waver. The same kind of ambivalence also characterizes our societal outlook on the sharply rising costs of our science- and technology-driven medical care. Concern about these costs is one of the most prominent and consistent themes that runs through our perennial discussion of health, illness, and medicine. Despite the numerous measures that have been taken, nationally and locally, to reduce and slow down medical care costs, we have not made much progress in doing so. Nor have we arrived at a workable consensus about what the best and most right way to deal with this problem might be. The feelings and views of the American public about controlling medical costs are so split that commentators have ventured to call them "schizophrenic." National public opinion polls indicate, for example, that although most Americans are very troubled by the rising costs of hospitalization and visits to a physician, and although they are discontent with our system of care taken as a whole, they believe that our society is spending too little rather than too much on health and medical care. By and large, they are satisfied with the care that they personally receive (Blendon and Altman 1984).

Still, on a more general value level, cost containment has come to be seen not just as a pragmatically desirable condition but also as a moral virtue in the face of scarce resources, competition for them, and their adequate and equitable distribution. Particularly expensive and scarce advanced medical scientific technologies, such as intensive and critical care, organ transplants, and mechanical organs like the artificial kidney and heart, have become strategic foci of cost-containment / allocation-of-scarce-resources reflection and debate. The state of our economy during the past fifteen years, with its worrisome combination of slowdown and retrenchment, inflation and indebtedness, underlies these considerations; the language in which they are being deliberated is heavily economic in content and tone. How we ought to spend resources for medical care is a question infrequently raised. Saving is emphasized, advocated, and held up as exemplary. Only occasionally are public statements made about the good that can come from spending and the harm that may result from cutting back costs (Blendon and Rogers 1983).

Transplantation and Allocation of Organs

We are using a medical economic framework and vocabulary to talk to each other about essentially moral and religious questions: Who shall live, when not all can live? What are the value and meaning of sustaining life through extraordinary medical treatments in some of the circumstances in which we do so? And what are the nonmaterial costs that these treatments entail for patients, families, and medical professionals?

Nowhere is this framework more apparent than in the field of organ transplantation. Although the surgery, hospitalization, medication, and care that transplantation involves are expensive, the basic scarce resources

without which this procedure could never take place are other than financial. They are human organs, live or cadaveric, that become available for implantation in patients with end-stage diseases because human donors and/or their families were willing to give parts of themselves to others.

From its inception in the mid-1950s, clinical organ transplantation has been defined and experienced as a gift, at whose center lie overpowering questions of who shall give and who shall receive these supreme gifts of self and life and how, if ever, they can be reciprocated. Fundamental and transcendental issues concerning our individuality and individualism, our interconnectedness and interchangeability with others, our sense of community and society, and our relationship to dimensions of self and other, life and death that are "more than human," have all been called into play by our medical-surgical ability to transplant organs from one human body to another. The biological concomitants of this act (particularly our body's immunological capacity to "recognize" grafted tissues as "not-self," and its propensity to "reject" them), combined with the psychological, social, and spiritual meanings of transplantation, have endowed it with allegorical cultural significance.

As the range and number of organs that we can transplant have expanded, our public discourse about transplantation has intensified and become more focused on what is felt to be the insufficient supply of organs that our voluntary donation system makes available. Ethical debate is increasingly pitched on a societal level. And like so many other value- and belief-laden medical issues we are discussing these days, this debate is likely to be phrased in economics-influenced, need/supply, scarcity, procurement, allocation/distribution, cost/benefit, market terms. This is the current outer language for the inner questions that are at the core of the transplantation of organs. The "economization" of these questions does not alter their essence (Fox, Swazey, and Cameron 1984, 58):

> What obligations do we have to ourselves as individuals, to the various members of our family, to our close friends, colleagues and acquaintances? And beyond these relationships, what are our obligations to the countless persons in our daily social life, and in our society, whom we do not know? Should we be able to give ourselves to mere acquaintances or strangers in life and death, as we do to our families and intimate friends? Who is my brother, sister, mother, father, child? Who is my friend, and who is my stranger? How are we related to one another? Where does our individuality end, and our interconnection and solidarity begin?

Genetics and Genetic Engineering

The same kinds of thematic questions have emerged around the scientific findings of the "new biology" and their applied, biomedical implications. The field of molecular genetics is an especially striking case in point. In the eyes of both scientists and nonscientists, the fundamental knowledge of genes and their encoding, and the techniques to splice and engineer genes, are "special"—full of exceptional promise and danger, and of high relevance to the "continuous dialogue between the possible and the actual" (Jacob 1982) which the most powerful forms of scientific questing and "tinkering" entail. This outlook on genetics is based on the conviction, as cultural as it is scientific, that the cell and its microcomponents —above all the genes—are the constituent elements of life. Whether in future centuries and other civilizations they will still be seen as such, we cannot predict. But in the here and now of our knowledge and understanding, we believe them to be. Because we do, we accord them a special status, comparable only to atoms and their subcomponents in the physical universe. But partly because of the associations that we make between genes—the deepest levels of living matter, the evolution of life in all forms, and the building blocks of our very humanness—we react to genes and their manipulation with a kind of awe that is different from our sense of atoms. To be sure, we are mindful of the destructive potential in atoms and genes alike if they are handled incompetently, maliciously, or even too innocently by humankind. But it is only the thought of genetic manipulation that evokes something like primal dread and a shuddering sense of metaphysical danger over the mixed beings, hybrid monsters, and Frankensteinian creatures that our hubris-ridden interventions could produce.

Because of the relationship that we posit between genes and the "logic of life" (Jacob 1973), advances in genetics have evoked questions concerning our primary conceptions of what and who we are, singly and collectively; how we are distinct from and related to one another, and to other living beings; how mutable and fixed we are; where we come from and where we are going; what we can be said to possess (including our own bodies, its structures, organs, and secretions); and what we can transmit, give, and leave to one another, and to the planet on which we reside.[1]

Bioethics

Around the biomedical developments and the value and belief issues that we have reviewed, a field of inquiry and action has developed known as "bioethics." I have written at length, elsewhere (Fox 1974, 1976; Fox and Swazey 1984), about the origins of bioethics, its chief intellectual and professional participants, its research and policy activities, its publications, and its overall ethos. A few aspects of my sociological perspective on the phenomenon of bioethics have bearing on the analysis of the cultural and societal import of the interrelationship between medicine, science, and technology with which this chapter has been concerned.

Bioethics emerged in the late 1960s in the United States, during a period that was marked not only by explosive developments in medical science and technology but also by social and cultural upheaval that extended far beyond biology and medicine. During the past fifteen years, the field of bioethics and the phenomena that it treats have grown in private, professional, and public importance. Much of our individual, personal reflection is now devoted to bioethical questions. Our medical institutions (hospitals, research institutes, health agencies, medical and nursing schools), our classrooms, media, courts, legislatures, and other government agencies are pervaded by collective awareness of bioethical issues and organized attempts to grapple with them. The full-time professional role of "bioethicist" has emerged. Bioethicists of various disciplinary backgrounds (chiefly philosophers and jurists, and to a lesser extent, physicians and religionists) are constantly asked to give expert opinions and consultant advice in all the contexts where bioethical reflection and debate are ensuing.

The range of matters in which bioethics is involved is not confined to ethics. Bioethics is also concerned with moral questions, including those that lie at the heart of society and culture, and of religion. As time has passed and the field has unfolded, bioethics has dealt increasingly with issues concerning life and death and personhood, at the beginning and the end of the human life cycle.

From the outset, the conceptual framework of bioethics has been marked by tension between the weighty, often overriding emphasis it has placed on individualism—individual rights, autonomy, and self-determination—and the emphasis it has accorded to the social dimensions of our moral life: our caring interdependence with and responsibility for one another that bioethics refers to as "beneficence" and "community." Over the past year, admonitions about a too-singular insistence on autonomy as a moral good have begun to appear in bioethical discussion, along with occasional affirmations about the importance of "building a mature medical ethics that can handle social as well as individual ethical questions" (Veatch 1984, 40). These types of statements have been made in connection with scarce-resources problems, which have become a more dominant bioethical concern. They were also major motifs at the (June 1984) symposium "Autonomy, Paternalism, and Community," with which the Hastings Center, one of the pioneering organizations in bioethics, chose to celebrate its fifteenth anniversary (*Hastings Center Report* 1984). Whether these are signs that the central conflict between individual and social good that has characterized bioethics is beginning to be resolved, in the direction of an ethic that is turning more social, remains to be seen.

Conclusion

Around the revolutionary scientific and technological developments that have taken place in modern Western medicine since World War II, and in their application to the delivery of care, deep, far-reaching change has occurred, which has been felt in every sector of American society and by every group in its population. The relationship between this biomedical

and social change is complex. Biology and medicine have been as much affected by the change our society has been undergoing as they have been precipitants of it. They have also become important, empirical, and symbolic foci of our efforts to decipher and deal with the implications of the engulfing process of change that we have been experiencing.

It is not only the scope and velocity of this biomedical and social change that have been responsible for its extraordinary impact. Many of its concomitants suggest that it has touched and shaken ideas, values, and beliefs fundamental to our historical and cultural tradition, our worldview, and our conception of our place within it. Taken as a whole, the biomedical issues explored in this chapter have to do with nothing less than societal problems of definition, origin, identity, direction, and meaning—problems that we seem to be having about such elemental matters as our conceptions of life and death, body and mind, self and other, person and human, baby and child, aging and elderly, parent and family, rights and responsibilities, autonomy and reciprocity, solidarity and community. Medicine and its science and technology have given us a common voice and vocabulary to publicly discuss these basic components of personal and social existence. But despite our shared language, a penumbra of uncertainty and confusion, contradiction and conflict, ambivalence and anxiety surrounds our deliberations. We are having great difficulty achieving moral and social consensus about these issues or finding practical solutions to them to which we are mutually willing to consent, whether we privately agree with them or not. Our tendency to dichotomize the individual and the social, and to think in more individual than social terms about ethics and morality, has made this all the harder.

We persist in calling this range of issues "medical ethical," and lately, "medical economic" as well. In fact, the questions that confront us are more, and other, than that. They are also moral, social, religious, metaphysical, and epistemological; they are deeply and encompassingly related to the foundations, the cohesion, and the orientation of our society and culture. Defining these matters as primarily medical, ethical, and economic may make them feel less overwhelming and more amenable to logical analysis and technical solution. But, in the end, the definition masks that what we are grappling with are not just problems of right and wrong, and of dollars and cents pertaining to medicine, but also larger questions about who we are, what we stand for, and where we are going as a total society.

Note

1. The foregoing discussion of molecular genetics and genetic engineering is excerpted from the remarks I prepared for my participation in a roundtable discussion titled "The Genetic Revolution," which was part of a colloquium "Recherche Médicale, Santé, Société," held in Paris on October 27–28, 1984, at the Sorbonne, in celebration of the twentieth anniversary of the Institut National de la Santé et de la Recherche Médicale.

References

America's abortion dilemma. 1984. *Newsweek,* January 14, pp. 20–29.

Beeson, P. B. 1980. Changes in medical therapy during the past half century. *Medicine* 59:79–99.

Blendon, R. J., and D. E. Altman. 1984. Public attitudes about health-care costs: A lesson in national schizophrenia. *New England Journal of Medicine* 311:613–616.

Blendon, R. J., and D. E. Rogers. 1983. Cutting medical care costs: *Primum non nocere. Journal of the American Medical Association* 250:1880–1885.

Curran, J. W., W. M. Morgan, A. M. Hardy, H. W. Jaffe, W. W. Darrow, and W. R. Dowdle. 1985. The epidemiology of AIDS: Current status and future prospects. *Science* 229:1352–1357.

Fox, R. C. 1974. Ethical and existential developments in contemporaneous American medicine: Their implications for culture and society. *Milbank Memorial Fund Quarterly: Health and Society* 52:445–483.

_____. 1976. Advanced medical technology: Social and ethical implications. *Annual Review of Sociology* 2:231–268.

_____. 1981. The sting of death in American society. *Social Service Review* 55:42–59.

Fox, R. C., and J. P. Swazey. 1984. Medical morality is not bioethics: Medical ethics in China and the United States. *Perspectives in Biology and Medicine* 27:336–360.

Fox, R. C., J. P. Swazey, and E. M. Cameron. 1984. Social and ethical problems in the treatment of end-stage renal disease patients. In *Controversies in Nephrology and Hypertension*, ed. R. G. Narins, pp. 45–70. New York: Churchill Livingstone.

Fox, R. C., and D. P. Willis. 1983. Personhood, medicine, and American society. *Milbank Memorial Fund Quarterly: Health and Society* 61:127–147.

Gudeman, J. E., and M. F. Shore. 1984. Beyond deinstitutionalization: A new class of facilities for the mentally ill. *New England Journal of Medicine* 311:832–836.

Hastings Center Report. 1984. A selection of the papers presented at the fifteenth anniversary symposium, "Autonomy, Paternalism, and Community." 14:5.

Jacob, F. 1973. *The logic of life: A history of heredity*. Trans. B. E. Spillman. New York: Pantheon Books.

_____. 1982. *The possible and the actual*. New York: Pantheon Books.

Preston, S. H. 1984. Children and the elderly: Divergent paths for America's dependents. *Demography* 21:435–457.

Rostain, A. L. 1985. Deciding to forego life-sustaining treatment in the intensive care nursery: A sociologic account. Children's Hospital of Philadelphia, University of Pennsylvania, Philadelphia. Typescript.

Thomas, L. 1983. *The youngest science: Notes of a medicine-watcher*. New York: Viking Press.

Veatch, R. M. 1984. Autonomy's temporary triumph. *Hastings Center Report* 14:38–40.

Chapter 3

Social Class, Health, and Illness

Diana B. Dutton

We are, in the United States somewhat uncomfortable with the notion of social class, and we are even more reluctant to believe that it influences matters as basic as the chance of a premature death or a life blighted by disability. In the early 1960s, the rediscovery of poverty amid plenty—and the devastating effects of poverty on health —helped launch the federal government's War on Poverty. Medicaid and Medicare were established to reduce economic barriers to health care, while Neighborhood Health Centers and other public programs tried to reduce geographic barriers. With increasing access, however, came rising medical costs and a new policy agenda; the dominant concerns shifted from equity to cost-effectiveness, and from increasing access to controlling medical costs.

Improved access led to some gains in health status, yet for most measures there is still a large gap between rich and poor. This persisting gap is given short shrift in the new policy agenda. Indeed, current cutbacks involve the very programs that have been most successful over the last two decades in improving access and reducing inequalities in health. The government contends that the most needy will not be affected. Some analysts question the continued importance of income per se as a determinant of health in our society. Others argue that medical care will not solve the health problems of the poor, whatever their causes. Such arguments belie a wealth of data on the relationship between social class and health and the factors responsible for that relationship.

This chapter describes socioeconomic differences in morbidity and mortality and various possible causes, including adverse environmental conditions, psychological stress, social alienation, unhealthy life-styles, and inadequate medical care. It reviews evidence that medical care has had an impact on health among the disadvantaged, focusing especially on the accomplishments of Neighborhood Health Centers in breaking the cycle of poverty and illness. The chapter concludes with a discussion of the likely impact of current policy trends on the poor and a brief sketch of a more equitable alternative. Throughout, my goal is not to provide an exhaustive review of these issues but rather to outline and illuminate the key elements of each point. Special attention is given to children since they are disproportionately involved in—and affected by—the problem of poverty. In a very real sense, moreover, the future well-being of any society depends on its children's health.

Social Class and Health

Whether social class is measured by income, education, or occupation, much the same picture emerges: those at the bottom have the highest rates of death and disease. Race is strongly correlated with social class; although two-thirds of the poor (people below the official poverty level) are white, almost half of all blacks are poor (Price 1984). The poor are heavily concentrated in the South, where public assistance is least adequate. Half of the poor are children

and young adults under age twenty-two. In 1983 one out of four children in America—and nearly one out of two black children—lived in poverty (Demkovitch 1984). During the last decade the proportion of poor children has increased steadily (Preston 1984).

The following sections describe inequalities in morbidity and mortality by income, education, and race. It should be noted that the relation between illness and income—unlike that between either race and illness or education and illness—involves a two-way effect: being poor often leads to worse health, and, in turn, worse health may also lead to diminished earning capacity and hence reduced income. We must bear in mind both effects when interpreting comparisons by income for working age adults. For children, however, and for comparisons involving race or prior educational attainment, inequalities may be attributed largely or entirely to the impact of relative deprivation on health. That comparisons by income, education, and race all tend to show roughly the same pattern, even for working age adults, suggests that gradients by income also reflect primarily the adverse effects of poverty on health rather than vice versa.

Mortality

The United States ranks sixteenth in the world in infant mortality, mainly due to high rates of infant mortality among the poor and minorities. Infant mortality rates are highest in the South, which has the lowest per capita personal income (U.S. Congress,

House of Representatives 1979). Data on infant mortality by family income are not routinely collected; the closest approximation is a comparison of poverty and nonpoverty areas of nineteen large cities in 1969–1971, in which infant mortality rates were 50 percent higher in the poverty areas (U.S. Department of Health, Education, and Welfare, Public Health Service 1977). Differentials by race are even more pronounced: nonwhite babies continue to die at roughly twice the rate of white babies, despite improvements for both (U.S. Congress, House of Representatives 1984b). This differential is not confined to any single cause but is reflected in all listed causes of death (U.S. Depart-

ment of Health, Education, and Welfare, Public Health Service 1979b). Moreover, it shows no signs of disappearing. Between 1950 and 1980, in fact, the overall decline in infant mortality was proportionately greater for whites than nonwhites (National Center for Health Statistics 1982).

The racial gap in mortality does not end with infants but continues on into adulthood. As seen in table 3.1, death rates for nonwhites are substantially greater than for whites in all age groups up to sixty-five, with a more than twofold difference in the thirty-five to forty-four year age group.[1] No recent national data on death rates by income are available, but a 1983 study in Maine found that

TABLE 3.1
Death Rates in the United States by Age and Race, 1980

| Age Group | Death Rate per 100,000 Population | | Ratio of Nonwhite/White |
	White	Nonwhite	
< 1 year	1,088	2,070	1.90
1–4	58	91	1.57
5–14	30	35	1.19
15–24	112	134	1.19
25–34	120	236	1.97
35–44	197	411	2.08
45–54	540	965	1.79
55–64	1,273	2,008	1.58
65–74	2,885	3,597	1.25
75–84	6,601	6,940	1.05
85 and over	15,915	12,674	.80

Source: National Center for Health Statistics 1982a, 16–18.

children in low-income families had a death rate over three times higher than that of other children (Maine Department of Human Services 1983). This finding is consistent with national data from the early 1960s. In a major epidemiological investigation, for example, Kitagawa and Hauser (1973) found that age-sex-race-adjusted mortality ratios in 1960 were from 31 to 105 percent higher among individuals with the least education compared to those for individuals with the most education. Mortality ratios by income generally followed a similar pattern, although differential mortality among working-age men was greater for income than for education, reflecting the impact of poor health in reducing the income of male wage earners. A study of the elderly in Massachusetts estimated that for every age group, the poor had a shorter active life expectancy than the nonpoor, with differences ranging from less than a year for the oldest group to 2.4 years for those aged sixty-five to sixty-nine (Katz et al. 1983).

Acute Conditions

Great strides have been made against infectious diseases in this century, but they are still a threat to many of the disadvantaged. Figure 3.1 shows trends in age-adjusted death rates from influenza and pneumonia (the fifth leading cause of death) for whites and nonwhites. Although the death rate for nonwhites has declined markedly since 1950, it was still 50 percent higher than for whites in 1975. The greatest reductions have occurred

since 1968, probably as a result of the improved medical care—earlier detection and better treatment—provided by Medicaid and other publicly funded programs.

The prevalence of acute conditions, as reported in national household interviews, is somewhat higher among upper- than lower-income individuals (U.S. Department of Health, Education, and Welfare, Health Resources Administration 1979). However, "acute conditions" are defined as those requiring medical attention or resulting in restricted activities; these requirements probably tend to reduce reporting among the poor, who may be less likely than the more affluent to seek care for a given illness because of limited income, and also less likely to forego wage-earning opportunities. Moreover, there is evidence that the affluent report relatively mild conditions, while the poor are more likely to report only more severe conditions (U.S. Department of Health, Education, and Welfare, Health Resources Administration 1979). Significantly higher rates of hospitalization as well as longer lengths of stay for the poor and minorities (table 3.2) are consistent with this interpretation, suggesting more severe illness, much of which may be acute. Differentials in children's hospitalization are even greater (U.S. Congress, House of Representatives 1979).

Certain infectious diseases appear to be more prevalent as well as more severe among the poor. In a diphtheria epidemic in San Antonio, Texas, poor and minority children suffered twelve times as much disease as children who were white and affluent

FIGURE 3.1

Age-adjusted death rates in the United States for influenza and pneumonia, by color, 1950–78.

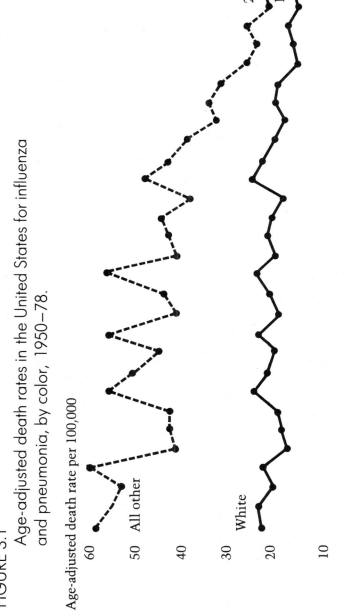

Age-adjusted death rate per 100,000

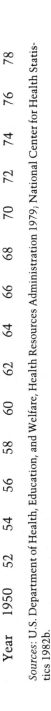

Sources: U.S. Department of Health, Education, and Welfare, Health Resources Administration 1979; National Center for Health Statistics 1982b.

TABLE 3.2
Hospitalization Rates in the United States by Income and Race, 1980

Family Income and Race	Discharges per 100 Persons per Year	Days per 100 Persons	Average Length of Stay
All persons	12.0	95.8	7.1
Income			
Under $7,000	15.8	145.8	8.4
$7,000 to $9,999	14.2	127.0	8.2
$10,000 to $14,999	12.0	96.0	6.9
$15,000 to $24,999	11.1	78.3	6.5
$25,000 or more	10.2	71.4	6.0
Race			
White	12.0	92.1	6.9
Nonwhite	13.0	136.6	9.2

Source: U.S. Department of Health and Human Services 1982.

(U.S. Congress, House of Representatives 1979). Tuberculosis has all but disappeared among the affluent but is still a serious problem for the poor and minorities, especially those living in urban poverty areas (U.S. Department of Health, Education, and Welfare Health Resources Administration 1979).

Chronic Illness and Disability

Chronic disease is sometimes thought of as the affliction of the well-to-do. But chronic illness now far outstrips acute illness in its disproportionate impact on the disadvantaged. For example, the prevalence of heart conditions, the leading cause of death, is over three times as high among low-income persons as among the most affluent (114 versus 35 per 1,000) (U.S. Department of Health, Education,

and Welfare, Health Resources Administration, 1979). Age-adjusted death rates from four of the five major causes of death—heart disease, cancer, stroke, and diabetes—were also higher among the disadvantaged. Arthritis, the leading cause of disability after heart disease, is twice as common among the poor; in 1977 the prevalence of activity-limiting arthritis was 39 per 1,000 for persons with incomes under $6,000, compared with 16 per 1,000 for the general population (Newacheck et al. 1980). Comparable prevalence differences are found across a wide range of chronic diseases (U.S. Department of Health, Education, and Welfare, Health Resources Administration 1979).

Restricted activity and other measures of disability reflect similar disparities. Restricted activity is more common among the poor than the nonpoor at all age levels, but the gap is greatest for persons aged forty-five to sixty-four; in 1980 poor people in this prime working-age category spent more than two months out of the year with restricted activity—more than four times as much time as those in the upper-income group (National Center for Health Statistics 1983b). There were comparable gradients in bed disability. Bed disability and restricted activity are good measures of the overall impact of health problems—their perceived severity as well as the resulting disruption of normal activities. Analyzing data from the 1977 National Health Interview Survey, Newacheck and colleagues (1980) found that about 75 percent of the gap in restricted activity and bed disability days between the poor and nonpoor was attributable to the greater prevalence and severity of activity-limiting chronic conditions among the poor.

Self-reported health status mirrors the same patterns, both for specific functional impairments and for global ratings of overall health. Nationally, the reported prevalence of most forms of impairment (including problems of speech, vision, and motor function) is two to ten times higher among the poor than the nonpoor (National Center for Health Statistics 1981c). More than three times as many low- as high-income people rate their health status as "fair or poor" (23 percent versus 7 percent in 1980), and there are similar differentials by education (U.S. Department of Health and Human Services 1982). Furthermore, both education and income exert an independent influence on perceived health: there are clear income gradients in self-rated health status at every educational level, and,

likewise, clear educational gradients in health status at every income level (National Center for Health Statistics 1983a).

For many measures, the health gap between rich and poor increases with age, reflecting the cumulative effects of a lifetime of impoverishment. Yet there are substantial disparities even among children. Based on a comprehensive review, Egbuono and Starfield (1982) concluded that poor children are more likely than others to become ill, to suffer adverse consequences from illness, and to die. They found that poor children had a higher prevalence of many specific disorders, including cytomegalic inclusion disease (the most common congenital infection), iron deficiency anemia, lead poisoning, hearing disorders, and poor vision, and almost twice as many bed disability days and four times as many hospital days as their more affluent peers. Poor children are also more than twice as likely to be reported by their parents as having chronic conditions and only "fair or poor" health; these parental ratings are confirmed in physicians' clinical examinations (National Center for Health Statistics 1973). Whatever it is about poverty that is detrimental to health apparently takes effect very early in life.

The Cycle of Poverty and Illness

There has been a longstanding debate about whether the worse health of lower socioeconomic groups should be attributed primarily to the material conditions of poverty and the biological and emotional stresses they create or to aspects of the life-style of the disadvantaged (e.g., cultural values and individual behavior). Economists such as Fuchs (1974) and Grossman (1975) argue that life-style factors are critical, and that education may affect life-style by making people more efficient producers of health and increasing their willingness to take action or delay gratification today for an expected return in the future. Empirically this debate has often revolved around whether income or education is more strongly related to illness. Although both appear to exert an independent influence on many illness measures (e.g., self-reported health status), the absence of a significant relation between income and illness independent of education is sometimes taken as support for the life-style interpretation. Such a finding may really mean that education and income are too highly correlated to distinguish their separate effects on health. In any case, their effects may not actually be "separate." In present society, people with more education tend to have higher incomes, and vice versa. Furthermore, over time, a change in one often produces a change in the other: when people get more education, they tend to earn more money; conversely, when people earn more money, they (or at least their offspring) frequently seek more education.

There is surely no single explanation for socioeconomic differentials in health. Figure 3.2 portrays various factors that appear to reinforce and perpetuate the cycle of poverty and illness. This section will describe some of the evidence for each of these different mechanisms.

Environmental Conditions

One of the most concrete problems faced by lower-social-class groups is adverse conditions in both home and work environments. Lower-status jobs tend to be more hazardous, menial, and physically taxing (Berman 1978) as well as less rewarding emotionally and economically. They involve more accidents, even within similar occupational groupings. For example, within each of the seventeen job categories listed by the Census Bureau, work-related accidents were more common among workers earning under $10,000 than among those earning $10,000 or more; for farm laborers, the difference was almost fourfold (National Center for Health Statistics 1980). There is even evidence suggesting that children of workers occupationally exposed to certain chemicals are more likely to have some types of malignant brain tumors (Starfield 1984).

Higher mortality levels in poor neighborhoods are well documented (Nagi and Stockwell 1973; Kitagawa and Hauser 1973; Jenkins 1983). Urban poverty areas are plagued by chemical and air pollution, noise, accidents, and crime. Air pollution has been linked to higher rates of respiratory disease and increased hospitalization (Carpenter et al. 1979; Whittemore 1981). National data show that lead poisoning is far more common among lower-income and minority children, probably because of

FIGURE 3.2
The cycle of poverty and
pathology.

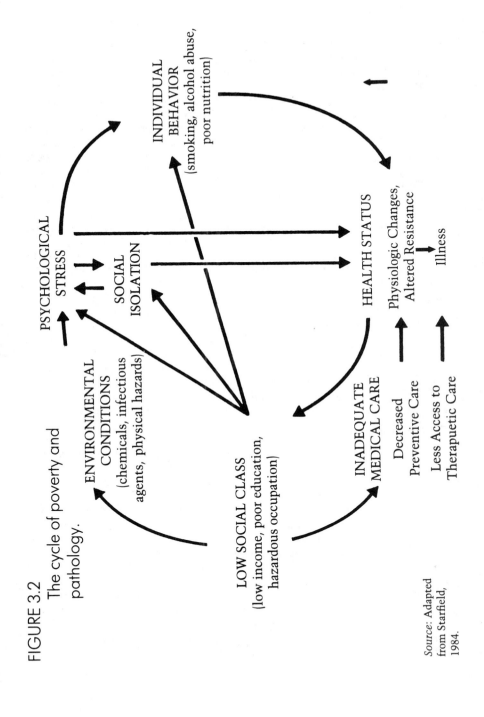

Source: Adapted
from Starfield,
1984.

their greater exposure to chips of lead-based paint, gasoline residues, and other environmental sources (Mahaffey et al. 1982). Exposure to constant noise produces physiological alterations suggesting generalized stress responses. Studies have shown that children living in noisy environments have blood pressure abnormalities and unusually high pulse rates as well as cognitive and behavioral problems; these effects did not appear to be attributable to other social factors, and some were not reversed when the noise abated (Starfield 1984).

Substandard housing conditions present various threats to health: rats and other vermin, poisons, fires, inadequate heat and plumbing, dangerous electrical wiring, trash, deteriorated structures, and crowding (Rainwater 1966). Research indicates that crowded housing leads to greater stress, less opportunity for rest and recuperation, and more susceptibility to infection, all of which may result in greater illness (Gove, Hughes, and Galle 1979).[2]

Psychological Stress and Social Isolation

Many of the physical and environmental conditions experienced by the poor probably also take a psychological and emotional toll on health. In an extensive review of environmental influences on health, Lindheim and Syme (1983) concluded that it is people's relative status in the social hierarchy—not their absolute position—that has the critical impact on health. They speculate that being "on

the bottom" of any hierarchy involves not only specific physical hardships but also stigmatization and humiliation in the eyes of the world and a damaging loss of self-esteem and perceived control over one's life.

Unemployment, for example, appears to have psychological and emotional consequences at least as serious as the financial problems caused by loss of income. People who are unemployed are more likely to report being unhappy and dissatisfied with life, to suffer from insomnia and headaches, and to increase smoking and drinking (Schlozman and Verba 1978). Recent data from Wisconsin show a clear relation between unemployment and child abuse. In the fifty-one counties where unemployment increased between 1981 and 1982, 69 percent reported an increase in child abuse; in the twenty-one counties where unemployment decreased, in contrast, 71 percent reported a decline in child abuse (Mills 1984). Time-series analyses of national macroeconomic data by Brenner (1977) and others have shown a correlation between the unemployment rate and trends in various stress-related destructive events, including mortality, suicide, homicide, and mental problems. While Brenner's conclusions and methods have been sharply challenged (Eyer 1977; LaPlante 1984), such trends are consistent with findings based on more reliable, microlevel data.

Social isolation is another potential source of psychological stress for lower socioeconomic groups. The importance of supportive social relationships was first demonstrated empirically in 1897 by Durkheim in his classic study of factors related to suicide. Cassel (1976) extended this notion to other health problems, noting that individuals without "meaningful social contacts" also tended to have higher rates of tuberculosis, schizophrenia, alcoholism, and accidents. Social isolation appears to be a special problem for the poor. In a nine-year study of mortality in Alameda County, California, Berkman and Syme (1979) found that the age-adjusted relative risk of the most isolated individuals was more than double that of the least isolated, independent of initial health status, medical care, personal health practices, and socioeconomic status. They concluded that social support—ties to family and the community—served as a buffer against disease.[3] This buffer was very unevenly distributed, however; Berkman and Syme's data indicate that lower-income individuals were much less likely than the more affluent to have a large number of social contacts. But lack of social support was apparently not the only explanation for the higher mortality rates of the poor; there were also socioeconomic gradients in mortality even *within* groups with high and low social contacts.

In light of the extraordinary consistency of social class gradients in morbidity and mortality, Syme and Berkman (1976) have suggested that a more general process of breakdown and vulnerability may be at work. Indeed, lowered resistance may heighten the effects of specific risk factors. In a study of 18,403 office-based civil servants in London, Marmot, Shipley, and Rose (1984) found threefold differences in mortality between men at the lowest and highest grades of employment, for all major causes of death. The authors attributed these remarkably consistent patterns to a combination of disease-specific factors along with a more general factor—related to the psychosocial stress experienced by lower-status workers—which increases susceptibility to all illness.

Exactly what causes increased susceptibility remains unclear, but psychosocial factors appear to play an important role. Stress and social isolation, for instance, appear to have a major influence on survival after heart attacks. Controlling for a number of prognostic indicators (including clinical variables), Ruberman et al. (1984) found that men who were socially isolated and who had a high degree of life stress had a risk of dying during the three years postattack more than four times as high as men with low levels of both stress and isolation. Education was also a risk factor, but mainly because men with low education tended to have high levels of stress and isolation; controlling for psychosocial factors largely eliminated educational gradients in mortality.

Individual Behavior

Some aspects of the life-style of the disadvantaged may also contribute to poor health. Alcohol consumption tends to be higher among lower socioeconomic groups (National Center for Health Statistics 1981b), as does cigarette smoking, at least for men (National Center for Health Statistics 1979).[4] Both may be seen as ways of coping with the stresses of relative deprivation. In addition, a more affluent life-style typically involves more leisure-time physical exercise and less obesity (Lambert et al. 1982). Yet these conventional risk factors do not appear to account for much of the health gap between rich and poor. In their study of London civil servants, Marmot, Shipley, and Rose (1984) still observed 50 to 100 percent differences in the relative risk of coronary heart disease mortality among men in different grades of employment, even after controlling for age, smoking levels, cholesterol, blood pressure, blood glucose, and height. Nor were these differences accounted for by leisure-time activity.

Poor and minority groups are also more likely to have an inferior diet. Data from the 1971–1975 National Health and Nutrition Examination Survey indicate that black children are consistently more likely to suffer from protein deficiency than white children. Likewise, about half of all low-income children under age four were below nutritional standards for vitamin A and C, a quarter were deficient in calcium, and 95 percent were deficient in iron (U.S. Department of Health, Education, and Welfare, Public Health Service 1979a). Eating habits are a likely cause; the daily diet of poor and minority children is much more likely to include candy, sweetened beverages, and salty snacks (Rice and Danchik 1979). Such habits may result not only from lack of proper dietary information but also from limited income and absence of parental supervision. Almost half of all children under six now living in poverty are members of female-headed households, and this number is projected to increase (U.S. Congress, House of Representatives 1983).

Poor eating habits are reflected in patterns of height and weight. The relation between weight and socioeconomic status varies according to sex; the heaviest females are those with the least education and income, while the heaviest males are those with the most education and income (National Center for Health Statistics 1981). Trends in height, on the other hand, are the same for both men and women; on average, adults with more education and income tend to be taller. Furthermore, height appears to be an independent predictor of longevity. In their study of London civil servants, Marmot, Shipley, and Rose (1984) found that short men had higher death rates from all causes than tall men, independent of grade of employment and other factors (as well as vice versa).

Inadequate Medical Care

The final link in the cycle of poverty and illness is inadequate medical care. Although utilization of services by disadvantaged groups has increased markedly over the last fifteen years (Robert Wood Johnson Foundation 1983), many inequalities remain. By a few measures—for example, hospitalization rates and annual number of physician visits—the poor now receive more care than the affluent. But such measures are misleading for they confound access with medical need; utilization is higher among the poor in large part because of their more prevalent and more severe illness (in fact, hospitalization rates are sometimes used as an indicator of illness severity). To determine whether the poor have adequate access to medical care, utilization must be measured in relation to the underlying level of illness, or medical need.

Measures that relate utilization to illness, such as the "use-disability ratio" (number of visits per one hundred disability days), indicate that the poor still receive significantly less care relative to illness than the rest of the population. Data from the 1978 National Health Interview Survey (NHIS) show, for example, that lower-income people had only about half as many physician vists per disability day as the affluent (Davis, Gold, and Makuc 1981).[5] Another way to take medical need into account is to compare individuals with a specified level of illness. Analyzing 1976–1978 NHIS data, Kleinman, Gold, and Makuc (1981) found income gradients within most age and race subgroups among people reporting fair or poor health status. Overall, the age-adjusted rate of physician visits for upper-income whites was about 35 percent higher than for poor whites, and more than 50 percent higher than for poor blacks.

Even without adjusting for medical need, the proportion of the population with at least one visit in the last year remains slightly higher among the white and affluent (Robert Wood Johnson Foundation 1983). This is a better measure of access than total physician visits since it indicates how many people were able to make initial contact with the medical system; follow-up visits, a major component

of total visits, are controlled largely by physicians rather than patients (Gertman 1974). And, despite higher illness levels, poor children receive less ambulatory care. In 1980 poor children under age five averaged 5.6 physician visits per year compared to an average of 7.5 visits for upper-income children (National Center for Statistics 1983c).

The adequacy of medical care depends not only on access and volume but also on the nature of the care provided. As Rogers (1980) testified before Congress:

Simply counting the number of visits people make to doctors each year is not sufficient. The term "physician visit" can mean many things. It can be a hurried visit to a "Medicaid mill" in which a patient is ping-ponged among a series of doctors, nurses and others to maximize reimbursement income. It can be hours spent waiting in a crowded, noisy hospital outpatient clinic or a few minutes with a doctor you've never seen before. At the other end of the scale—and far more desirable personally and medically—is the kind of visit you and I are accustomed to: seeing a doctor we know by name and who knows us and our families. Implicit in this relationship is the physician's assumption of personal responsibility for attending to an individual's medical care needs.

The poor tend to receive less preventive care—services that are viewed as "discretionary" regardless of their medical benefit. A third fewer low-income women receive prenatal care in the first trimester of pregnancy than high-income women (Aday, Anderson, and Fleming 1980). Likewise, four times as many low-income children as high-income children under seventeen had *never* had a routine physical examination in 1973 (20 percent versus less than 5 percent) (National Center for Health Statistics 1977). The consequences of undetected medical problems in children are potentially serious; regular health monitoring, especially during the early years of life, is widely recommended (Task Force Report 1976; Breslow and Somers 1977). Other clinically effective preventive services, including dental care, pap smears, breast exams, and childhood immunizations, are also less common among the disadvantaged (U.S. Department of Health and Human Services 1982; Davis, Gold, and Makuc 1981; Dutton 1981).

In part, these disparities stem from different patterns and sources of care; lower socioeconomic groups are much less likely to have a personal physician, or even a regular source of care. Nationally, three times as many low- as high-income children (18 percent versus 6 percent had no regular source of care in 1974 (Dutton 1981). When the poor and minorities do see a physician, they are more than twice as likely as others to have visits in hospital clinics rather than in doctors' offices or by telephone (U.S. Department of Health and Human Services 1982). In addition, various structural barriers make the process of obtaining care more difficult for the disadvantaged. National data show that twice as many low- as high-income persons travel more than a half-hour to reach their regular provider (12 percent versus 6 percent), and wait more than an hour to be seen (21 percent versus 9 percent) (Aday, Anderson, and Fleming 1980). And, despite Medicaid and other public programs, out-of-pocket medical expenses remain a much greater burden for the poor relative to income. Annual out-of-pocket medical expenses consumed 17 percent of income among people in the lowest income group in 1977 compared with less than 2 percent in the highest income group (National Medical Care Expenditure Survey 1984). Moreover, this disproportionate burden was borne by more than two-thirds of the poor. In 1984, there were nearly 39 million Americans, or 19 percent of the total population, without health insurance ("Uninsured Increase, Study Shows" 1984). Lack of insurance coverage has been shown to be associated with significantly lower rates of ambulatory care utilization (Davis and Rowland 1983).

There are, in short, a number of persisting inadequacies in the amount and types of medical care received by the disadvantaged, especially relative to medical need. But what is the evidence that such disparities lead to worse health?

Does Medical Care Matter?

Rising medical costs and mounting evidence of the importance of social and environmental determinants of health have led some observers to question the value of medical care. Critics such as Illich (1976) have called attention to the wide range of medical and social problems caused by medicine's highly professionalized, technological, and interventionist orientation. Might the poor be better off, skeptics have asked, with less access to care?

While obviously not all medical services are equally effective, there is substantial evidence that disadvantaged groups still go without basic forms of prevention and primary care that, when provided, yield real and measurable benefits to health (Starfield 1985; Brunswick 1984; Levine, Feldman, and Elinson 1983; Hadley 1982). One study which followed a group of California Medicaid recipients who lost their eligibility in 1982 showed that they had less access to ambulatory care and suffered significant deterioration of previously controlled hypertension and diabetes (Lurie et al. 1984). Preventive services have been particularly effective in counteracting prevailing patterns of illness. Periodic screening for breast cancer, for example, using mammography and palpation of the breast, was shown to eliminate the traditional racial differences in survival in a randomized trial of sixty-two thousand women in the Health Insurance Plan of New York. In the control group, which was not screened, nonwhite women with breast cancer had a lower five-year survival rate than white women, whereas there were no racial differences in survival among women who had been screened (Shapiro et al. 1982).

Childhood immunizations are an-

other effective form of disease prevention where needs are unmet. In California, about 40 percent of low-income children did not have the immunizations required to enter school in 1983 (Children's Research Institute of California 1984). Immunization rates for measles and rubella are lower in poverty areas, and the prevalence of infections correspondingly higher (U.S. Congress, House of Representatives 1979). Measles and mumps immunizations are highly cost-effective, with an estimated savings of $7 to $10 in medical and social expenses for every dollar spent on vaccination (Witte and Axnick 1975; Wiederman and Ambrosch 1979).

Public programs such as Maternal and Child Health (MCH), and Early Periodic Screening, Detection, and Treatment (EPSDT) have sought to fill some of these needs in urban and rural poverty areas by providing screening, immunizations, and a variety of other children's and maternity services. While evaluation has not been systematic, available data indicate that these programs have accomplished many of their goals (Davis and Schoen 1978). MCH services have been credited with higher levels of immunization among poor children and improved levels of hearing and vision (U.S. General Accounting Office 1979). The Alabama MCH program estimated savings of $5 to $10 in prevented illness for each $1 spent (National Health Law Program 1983). Evaluations of EPSDT in six state programs also showed cost-savings (Hiscock 1984). For example, a study of EPSDT in Pennsylvania found that children previously screened under EPSDT had almost 30 percent fewer abnormalities requiring care upon rescreening, and also significantly fewer abnormalities than a control group (Irwin and Conroy-Hughes 1982). A review by the Health Care Financing Administration of 150 studies on the effectiveness of preventive child health care concluded that the bulk of the evidence indicated preventive services did have a beneficial effect on health (Shadish 1981).

Many poor women do not receive appropriate prenatal care, another beneficial—and highly cost-effective —form of prevention. Although a few studies have not been able to demonstrate the benefits of prenatal care, the overwhelming majority indicate that prenatal care reduces the likelihood of low birth weight and other adverse outcomes, especially among high-risk women (Institute of Medicine 1985; Showstack, Budetti, and Minkler 1984; Norris and Williams 1984; Kessner et al. 1973; Eisner et al. 1979; Dott and Fort 1975; Donaldson and Billy 1984). Findings from a study by Levy, Wilkinson, and Marine (1971) of a three-year demonstration program that provided nurse-midwives to a disadvantaged population in rural California were particularly dramatic. During the program, prenatal care doubled and prematurity rates fell by 40 percent, with no significant changes in these measures in the surrounding areas; after its termination, both rates returned to roughly their earlier levels. Precisely how prenatal care yields these benefits, however, is not well understood.

A growing body of evidence also suggests that nutritional supplements provided through the federally funded Supplemental Food Program for Women, Infants, and Children (known as WIC) have been effective in improving pregnancy outcomes. While evaluation studies are subject to various methodological criticisms, the bulk of the evidence strongly suggests that WIC supplements decreased the risk of low birth weight, and perhaps also reduced neonatal mortality (U.S. General Accounting Office 1984; Kotelchuck et al. 1984). There is also evidence that nutritional supplements for newborns may affect subsequent cognitive and behavioral development. Hicks, Langham, and Tanenaka (1982) compared children in rural Louisiana who got WIC supplements during the perinatal period with their older siblings, who had not received nutritional supplements until after they were a year old. Some five to seven years later, the perinatally supplemented group showed significant enhancement on various intellectual and behavioral measures, including IQ, visual-motor synthesis, and school grade-point average, when compared with their siblings who had received the supplements later.[6]

Neighborhood Health Centers: Broadening the Definition of Medical Care

Traditional forms of disease prevention and primary care have clearly helped ameliorate some of the health problems of the poor. But they do nothing to attack the roots of those problems—the social, economic, and environmental conditions of poverty that compromise health and exacerbate illness. As long as these conditions exist, the vicious cycle of poverty and illness will continue.

Recognizing the limits of conventional medical approaches in dealing with the needs of the poor, Congress launched the Neighborhood Health Center Program in the mid-1960s to provide accessible and appropriate health care to the most disadvantaged urban and rural areas, where existing medical services were sparse and where health problems were caused or confounded by general deprivation. According to the original mandate, the new centers were "to assure that [health] services are made readily accessible to residents of such areas [of concentrated poverty], are furnished in a manner most responsive to their needs and with their participation, and whenever possible are combined with . . . arrangements for providing employment, education, social or other assistance needed by the families and individuals served" (quoted in Geiger 1984).

The most ambitious health centers sought to improve health not only through direct medical care but also through community organizing efforts designed to change basic social and economic circumstances. A good example is the center established in Mound Bayou, Mississippi, an extremely poor region in the Mississippi Delta. The challenge of poverty and illness in Mound Bayou was formidable. Sharecropping, once the area's major means of subsistence, had been made obsolete by mechanization. In the 1960s the vast majority of the area's predominantly black residents lived below poverty, in substandard housing, and without adequate water supply or waste removal. Rates of infant and maternal mortality were among the highest in the nation (Tokarz 1982; Geiger 1984).

To meet this challenge, Mound Bayou offered a broad array of social and environmental services in addition to basic clinical care. Environmental services included protected wells, water and sewage line construction, and home improvements such as screens and sanitary outhouses. Social services ranged from bus transportation to legal services, day care, and continuing education. The center responded to nutritional problems not only with prescriptions of food and emergency food programs but also by organizing a cooperative vegetable farm. As part of the center's "community health action" program, ten local health associations were created to foster social and economic development (Geiger 1984). The hope was to create self-sustaining initiatives that would ultimately enable the community to lift itself out of impoverishment.

Not all of Mound Bayou's pioneering programs have survived. With growing concern about cost control in the early 1970s, the federal government significantly narrowed the scope of reimbursable services in Neighborhood Health Centers nationally and instituted rigid standards of physician "productivity." Such constraints have tended to force community health centers toward a more traditional medical model. Nonetheless, Mound Bayou can claim credit for some notable achievements. The infant mortality rate dropped 40 percent in the first four years of the center's operation. Hundreds of townsfolk have better housing and sanitary water thanks to the environmental improvement campaigns. By 1984 the health center was seeing several hundred patients a day—mostly those with neither public nor private insurance—and had become the major employer in the community. Over one hundred people obtained post-secondary-school degrees, including thirteen M.D.s, as a result of health center–sponsored programs—in a community where the average adult education level had been four years of school. Many of these people, like the health center's medical director, returned to live and work in Mound Bayou.

The Community Health Center Program (as it is now called) has grown dramatically during the last two decades, surviving various political challenges and professional assaults; by 1982, 872 centers around the country served 4.2 million people, mostly the poor and minorities (Geiger 1984). On the whole, these centers appear to have been remarkably effective. They have made important inroads into problems of accessibility in underserved areas—although they still serve only a fraction of rural and inner-city residents without a regular private source of care (Davis and Schoen 1978). Evaluations have shown that the quality of medical care is equal to or better than that of traditional medical settings (Morehead, Donaldson, and Servall 1971; Sparer and Johnson 1971), and that center users have more appropriate and less costly patterns of utiliza-

tion: reduced hospitalization, fewer operations, and more ambulatory and preventive care (Reynolds 1976; Davis and Schoen 1978). In fact, evidence is accumulating that the total cost of care for center users is substantially lower than for control populations (Freeman, Kiecolt, and Allen 1982; Schwarz and Poppen 1982; Orso 1979; JRB Associates 1980). Even greater cost-savings might be realized under a broader definition of reimbursable services. Government programs are willing to pay $500 for the hospitalization of a child with severe infectious diarrhea because that is a "legitimate" medical expense, but refuse to pay $25 to dig a well or $75 to build an outhouse, which might have prevented the illness in the first place. Deciding where to draw the limits is not a simple matter, of course, but most would agree that present third-party reimbursement policies overemphasize curative medicine and underemphasize preventive care.

As well as saving money, Community Health Centers also appear to have had a positive effect on the health of the patients they serve. Studies have documented reductions in infant mortality of 25 to 40 percent in areas served by centers, with no change in surrounding areas (Anderson and Morgan 1973; Gold and Rosenberg 1974; Goldman and Grossman 1981). In Baltimore, low-income census tracts with comprehensive health centers[7] had a 60 percent reduction in the incidence of rheumatic fever over a ten-year period—a decrease attributed to early detection and treatment of streptococcal infections —whereas tracts without centers remained unchanged (Gordis 1973). And, as in Mound Bayou, many centers have led to improvements in the quality as well as quantity of life, with better housing, sanitation, and nutrition.

Understandably, of course, Community Health Centers have not solved all the health problems of the poor and underserved, nor have all centers been uniformly successful. Yet their overall record of accomplishments is still impressive. Not only have they made health care more widely available but they have also redrawn traditional medical boundaries. Starting from the premise that the primary determinants of health lie in the social order, they have attacked many different points in the cycle of poverty and illness, including nonmedical as well as medical factors. Some have sought to catalyze broader processes of human and economic development in their struggling communities. While this is not the only (and perhaps not even the most effective) way to achieve social change, in the end nonmedical aspects of the cycle of poverty and illness may hold the key to improvements in health.

Current Policy Trends: Impact on the Poor

The strengths of the Community Health Center model are notably absent from the current health policy agenda. Increasingly, people of all income levels are turning to hospital outpatient clinics and emergency rooms for regular care (Aday and Andersen 1983). Cost control has become the overriding goal of both the federal and state governments, leading to major contractions in most publicly funded health and social programs. Over the past three years, nearly every state has reduced the scope of Medicaid services, eligibility, or both (National Health Law Program 1984). An estimated 700,000 children lost their Medicaid coverage in 1982, as did 567,000 old people between 1981 and 1984 ("Health Care Found in 'Deterioration'" 1984). Many poor, elderly, and handicapped people depend on public programs to meet their basic medical needs and have gone without care or suffered financial hardship because of the new restrictions (Scott 1982). In some groups, as noted previously, deteriorating health status has been reported (Lurie et al. 1984). These cutbacks cannot help but exacerbate existing inequalities in health status and service utilization.

Federal funding for Community Health Centers has also been cut sharply, with revenue losses averaging 30 to 45 percent in 1982 (Brazda and Glenn 1984). As a result, 239 centers (28 percent of the total) have had to limit their services or close (National Health Law Program 1983). A study of five Community Health Centers in Boston revealed that budget cuts had led to a 14 percent decline in obstetrics visits and a 12 percent decline in pediatric visits; there was also a substantial increase in infant mortality (Feldman 1984). In view of the demonstrated health benefits of Community Health Centers and their record of substituting ambulatory and preventive care for hospitalization and other costly medical interventions, these cutbacks could well end up increasing total health care expenses for society.

Another trend in health policy that may boomerang is the growing emphasis in both Medicaid and Medicare on patient "cost sharing"—money paid out-of-pocket toward medical bills. Medicaid used to prohibit cost sharing; now the federal government has proposed mandatory copayments of $1 to $2 on all Medicaid-reimbursed hospital and physician visits. Cost sharing has also increased dramatically in the Medicare program. In 1965 a Medicare beneficiary paid the first $40 of a hospital stay; today, the deductible is $356 (Califano 1984).

The equity of imposing additional cost sharing on low-income groups is questionable since, as noted previously, they already spend 17 percent of their income on medical care compared to less than 2 percent by the well-to-do (National Medical Care Expenditure Survey 1984). But cost sharing for the poor may not make economic sense either. Low-income groups are disproportionately affected by even small copayments (Beck 1974; Dallek and Parks 1981).[8] When a $1.50 to $2.00 charge was imposed on physician visits in Saskatchewan, for example, the reduction in utilization among the aged and poor was three times that of the 6 percent reduction overall (Barer, Evans, and Stoddart 1979). If reduced ambulatory care eliminates needed services, it does not necessarily save money. In California's 1972 "copayment experiment," which imposed a $1 charge on certain Medicaid recipients, physician visits declined by 8 percent—

but hospitalization rose by 17 percent, resulting in a net increase in total program costs (Helms, Newhouse, and Phelps 1979).

Equally unsound, especially in the long run, are reductions in aid for needy children and pregnant women. Proposed cuts of $1.25 billion in the WIC program in fiscal 1985 would mean half a million fewer program participants (National Health Law Program 1984). Maternal and Child Health funds were cut 18 percent in 1981, leading to reductions in forty-four states in prenatal, delivery, and preventive services for pregnant women. Again, these cutbacks make no sense even in strictly economic terms. Savings in reduced prenatal visits are trivial compared with the costs associated with inadequate prenatal care: prematurity, mental retardation, and various developmental disorders. (In 1981, neonatal intensive care for a single premature infant averaged $60,000 to $100,000, and the costs of institutionalizing a mentally retarded person ran about $25,000 per year; Los Angeles County Health Alliance et al. 1982). The Department of Consumer Affairs in California has estimated the state could save approximately $66 million annually in neonatal intensive care costs if all women received adequate prenatal care (Dallek 1982). Another study found that for every dollar Medi-Cal reimbursed for prenatal care, the state would save $1.70 in reimbursements for newborn intensive care (Korenbrot 1984).

At the same time as poverty-related programs were being cut, poverty in the United States has been on the rise. Between 1980 and 1982, the number of poor children increased by 2 million (Price 1984). In 1983 the number of people living in poverty had risen to the highest level since 1965 (U.S. Department of Commerce, Bureau of the Census 1984). The gap between rich and poor has also been widening, reversing the gradual trend toward income equality that prevailed from the 1950s through the 1970s. Tax and benefit cuts enacted during 1983 further enlarged the gap: according to the Congressional Budget Office, families earning under $10,000 suffered a net loss of $390, while those earning over $80,000 enjoyed an overall gain of $8,270 (Demkovitch 1984). In a 1984 national survey, one out of every five adults reported that they could not always afford food for their families (Gallup 1984). With reduced funding for poverty-related programs, the swelling ranks of the poor warrant added concern.

Besides budget reductions and cost sharing, the other major cost-control strategy involves efforts to promote "competition" in the medical marketplace in hopes of altering cost-increasing incentives. This strategy may also prove detrimental to the poor. Proponents of competition contend that market forces can be harnessed through the use of prepaid contracts, or vouchers—that is, claims to a fixed annual amount of money—rather than through essentially open-ended reimbursement of specified services as in Medicaid. In a voucher system, "consumers" (patients) would select among insurance packages or health plans of varying costs. They would shop wisely for cost-effective care, it is argued, since

they would have to spend their own money for plans costing more than the voucher and could retain any savings from choosing a plan below the voucher (see, for example, Enthoven 1978). Providers, in turn, competing vigorously with each other for patient vouchers, would seek to minimize costs and maximize quality and efficiency.

Unfortunately, competitive incentives create a systematic bias against the disadvantaged. Because low-income groups tend to have problems that are more complex, serious, and harder to treat, caring for them tends to be more costly, and "competitive" providers have an incentive to direct their services toward groups with more tractable problems. This is not difficult to do: open-enrollment requirements can be timed to avoid unwanted enrollees, publicity can be aimed at affluent areas, and clinics can be located in places inconvenient for the poor (Dunham, Morone, and White 1982; Ricketts 1983). California's experience with competing prepaid health plans for the poor in the early 1970s was a case study of competitive incentives gone awry (Goldberg 1976).[9] Even without deliberate subversion, it is unclear that vouchers alone would attract health providers to underserved ghetto and rural areas. The Medicaid program offers open-ended reimbursement to providers and has still failed to overcome prevailing patterns of medical maldistribution.

If vouchers are too low, they create an even stronger bias against treating the poor. In most proposals, vouchers would *not* vary by factors such as income and race, and so would not reflect the disproportionate medical needs of disadvantaged groups. (And the poor are unlikely to be able to pay privately for services that exceed the voucher amount.) Moreover, economic pressures to reduce spending are likely to erode vouchers over time. If medical inflation continues to exceed general inflation, as many believe it will, a simple—and perhaps politically irresistible—way to control government expenditures would be to raise voucher levels at a rate below medical inflation, thus reducing real health benefits (Dunham, Morone, and White 1982). Indeed, if market advocates succeed in abolishing other regulatory mechanisms like certificate-of-need and rate review, cutting vouchers may be the only way to control government expenditures.

Conclusion

Illness, in this country as in most, is disproportionately concentrated in the lower social class. There is a large gap between those at the bottom of the socioeconomic ladder and those at the top in nearly every measure of morbidity and mortality. Some of this gap may still be due to inadequate medical care: despite the increased access provided by public entitlement programs, the poor still have lower rates of utilization among children, fewer services at all ages relative to illness levels, less preventive care, more reliance on hospital-based clinics, and greater financial and organizational barriers to access. But much of the gap undoubtedly stems from a variety of nonmedical factors, including a hazardous environment, unsafe and unrewarding work, poor nutrition, lack of social support, and, perhaps most important of all, the psychological and emotional stress of being poor and feeling powerless to do anything about it.

True efficiency in health care delivery requires matching services to needs. Health policy is currently moving in the opposite direction. Cutbacks in publicly funded programs and increased patient cost-sharing jeopardize previous gains in access and health status. Competitive strategies create incentives for providers to avoid caring for groups with the greatest needs, since their care is more costly and most cannot afford to pay privately for any extra services required. And all the while, the ranks of the poor are growing.

But medical care alone, even if equitably distributed, will not solve the health problems of the poor. Patterns of health care utilization in Britain's National Health Service have been considerably more equal than those in the United States for over three decades, yet a government study recently reported that social class differences in health are wider now than they were when the Health Service was established in 1948 (Gray 1982). The report attributed these differences not to the failings of the Health Service but rather to the range of other social inequalities that impinge, on health and called for a wide strategy of social policy measures to combat them.

It was precisely such a broad approach that Community Health Centers tried to take, of course. They directed their efforts not only at people but at social and environmental circumstances. In the final analysis, the short-run costs of this approach may be outweighed by long-run efficiencies; it is wasteful, and in fact futile, to treat people's ailments and then send them back into the same environment that made them sick.

To be efficient as well as effective, health care must remedy not only the consequences of poverty but must aid in efforts to change the underlying circumstances that perpetuate it. This is the most fundamental form of disease prevention, and perhaps ultimately the only truly effective one.

Notes

1. The reversal of this racial differential in the oldest age group is probably due to the older average age of whites aged eighty-five or more and also to the "natural selection" effect of the higher death rates among nonwhites in all of the younger age groups.

2. These effects have also been documented in laboratory studies. Particularly striking is an experiment by Riley 1975, in which environmental circumstances significantly affected the onset of illness in groups of genetically equivalent mice, all infected with a virus that produces mammary tumors. One group, exposed to "standard" laboratory conditions, developed the tumors when the mice were middle-aged; a group raised in more desirable conditions (quiet and spacious cages, a nocturnal schedule, and minimal disturbance) did not develop the tumors until the mice were near the end of their life span.

3. A recent analysis of chronic disease among Japanese men in Hawaii failed to show any significant protective effects of social support measures against the stresses of social mobility and sociocultural inconsistency (Reed, McGee, and Yano 1984). Unfortunately, no data on socioeconomic status were provided.

4. Smoking patterns among women differ depending on whether socioeconomic status is measured by education or income, and may be changing over time. In 1976 the proportion of women who smoked increased linearly with income, but exhibited a strong inverse U-shaped relationship with education (lowest proportion of smokers among the least and most educated women), (National Center for Health Statistics 1979, p. 22). Data for 1979 are available only by education and suggest a positive linear relation with education— higher rates of smoking among more educated women (National Center for Health Statistics 1981b, 15). For men, in contrast, the proportion who smoke is strongly inversely related to both income and education.

5. Using 1976 data from a different national sample with a different method of defining disability days, Aday, Anderson, and Fleming (1980) report a much smaller differential between the use-disability ratios of high- and low-income groups. However, for a variety of methodological reasons (Davis, Gold, and

Makuc 1981, 166; Dutton 1981, 372), results based on the National Health Interview Survey appear to be more reliable.

6. This study has also been criticized on methodological grounds, although all of the criticisms involve possible, rather than proven, problems (U.S. General Accounting Office 1984). Hence, the study findings cannot be dismissed without some indication as to whether the criticisms raised did in fact distort the results. Unfortunately, this investigation is the only one so far that has examined WIC's effects on children's subsequent mental development.

7. These centers were funded by the Children and Youth Program but resembled Neighborhood Health Centers in the comprehensiveness of the care provided.

8. Results from the Rand Health Insurance Experiment indicate that people of different income levels had a similar reduction in utilization in response to cost sharing that was proportionate to income (Newhouse et al. 1981). In the real world, unfortunately, most forms of cost sharing (including copayments and deductibles) are not proportionate to income but rather highly disproportionate. Furthermore, according to a subsequent Rand report, even income-related cost sharing was detrimental to the health of low-income people with high blood pressure (Brook et al. 1983).

9. California Prepaid Health Plans engaged in a variety of dubious marketing practices, including high-pressure door-to-door salesmen and misrepresentation of services, and some apparently took steps to screen out bad risks. While this experience is often attributed to bureaucratic mismanagement and other idiosyncratic factors, preliminary results from the Rand Health Insurance Experiment suggest that even "mainstream" prepaid plans do less well by the poor than do fee-for-service settings—perhaps because of similar cost-cutting incentives (John Ware, personal communication, February 10, 1986).

References

Aday, Lu Ann, and Ronald M. Andersen. 1983. *National trends in access to medical care: Where do we stand?* Paper presented at the American Public Health Association meeting in Dallas, Texas.

Aday, Lu Ann, Ronald M. Andersen, and Gretchen Fleming. 1980. *Health care in the U.S.: Equitable for whom?* Beverly Hills, Calif.: Sage.

Anderson, R. E., and S. Morgan. 1973. *Comprehensive health care: A southern view.* Atlanta: Southeast Regional Council.

Barer, M. L., Robert G. Evans, and Glenn L. Stoddart. 1979. *Controlling health care costs by direct charges to patients: Snare or delusion?* Toronto, Ontario: Ontario Economic Council.

Beck, R. G. 1974. The effect of copayment on the poor. *Journal of Human Resources* 9(1):129–142.

Berkman, Lisa F., and S. Leonard Syme. 1979. Social networks, host resistance, and mortality: A nine-year follow-up study of Alameda County residents. *American Journal of Epidemiology* 109(2):186–204.

Berman, Daniel M. 1978. *Death on the job: Occupational health and safety struggles in the U.S.* New York: Monthly Review Press.

Brazda, J. F., and K. Glenn. 1984. Block grant, part two: ADM and primary care. *Washington Perspectives*, July 16. McGraw-Hill.

Brenner, M. Harvey. 1977. Health costs and benefits of economic policy. *International Journal of Health Services* 7(4):581–623.

Breslow, Lester, and Anna Somers. 1977. The lifetime health-monitoring: A practical approach to preventive medicine. *New England Journal of Medicine* 296(11):601–608.

Brook, Robert H., John E. Ware, Jr., William H. Rogers, Emmett B. Keeler, Allyson R. Davies, Cathy A. Donald, George A. Goldberg, Kathleen N. Lohr, Patricia C. Masthay, Joseph P. Newhouse. 1983. Does free care improve adults' health? *New England Journal of Medicine* 309(23): 1426–1434.

Brunswick, Ann F. 1984. Effects of medical intervention in adolescence: A longitudinal study of urban black youth. *Youth and Society* 61(1):3–28.

Califano, Joseph A. 1984. U.S. must discipline health-care market. *New York Times*, May 6, p. E23.

Carpenter, Ben H., James R. Chromy, Walter D. Bach, D. A. LeSourd, and Donald G. Gillette. 1979. Health costs of air pollution: A study of hospitalization costs. *American Journal of Public Health* 69(12):1232–1241.

Cassel, John. 1976. The contribution of the social environment to host resistance. *American Journal of Epidemiology* 104(2):107–123.

Children's Research Institute of California. 1984. Capsule update. Sacramento, Calif.

Dallek, Geraldine. 1982. America's widening infant death gap. *Health & Medicine* (Summer/Fall):23–27.

Dallek, Geraldine, and Michael Parks. 1981. Cost-sharing revisited: Limiting medical care to the poor. *Clearing House Review*, March, pp. 1149–1158.

Davis, Karen, Marsha Gold, and Diane Makuc. 1981. Access to health care for the poor: Does the gap remain? *Annual Review of Public Health* 2:159–182.

Davis, Karen, and Diane Rowland. 1983. Uninsured and underserved: Inequities in health care in the United States. *Milbank Memorial Fund Quarterly: Health and Society* 61(2):149–176.

Davis, Karen, and Cathy Schoen. 1978. *Health and the War on Poverty: A ten-year appraisal.* Washington, D.C.: Brookings Institution.

Demkovich, Linda E. 1984. Fairness issue will be campaign test of Reagan's record on budget policies. *National Journal*, September 8, pp. 1648–1653.

Donaldson, Peter J., and John O. G. Billy. 1984. The impact of prenatal care on birth weight. *Medical Care* 22(2):177–188.

Dott, Andrew B., and Arthur T. Fort. 1975. The effect of availability and utilization of prenatal care and hospital services on infant mortality rates: Summary of the findings of the Louisiana Infant Mortality Study, part II. *American Journal of Obstetrics and Gynecology* 123(8):854–860.

Dunham, Andrew, James A. Morone, and William White. 1982. Restoring medical markets: Implications for the poor. *Journal of Health Politics, Policy, and Law* 7(2):488–501.

Dutton, Diana B. 1981. Children's health care: The myth of equal access. In *Better health for our children: A national strategy.* Report of the Select Panel for the Promotion of Child Health, DHHS (PHS) Publication No. 79-55071. Washington, D.C.: Government Printing Office.

Egbuonu, Lisa, and Barbara Starfield. 1982. Child health social status. *Pediatrics* 69(5):550–557.

Eisner, Victor, Joseph V. Brazie, Margaret W. Pratt, and Alfred C. Hexter. 1979. The risk of low birthweight. *American Journal of Public Health* 69(9): 887–893.

11 die after losing aid: U.S. found them fit to work. 1982. *San Francisco Chronicle*, Sept. 18, p. 4.

Enthoven, Alain. 1978. Consumer choice health plan. *New England Journal of Medicine* 298:650–658 (pt. 1) and 709–720 (pt. 2).

Eyer, Joseph. 1977. Does unemployment cause the death rate peak in each business cycle? A multifactor model of death rate change. *International Journal of Health Services* 7(4):625–662.

Feldman, Penny Hollander. 1984. Study of the impact of changes in health programs for the poor on primary care centers and local health departments. Final Report to the Robert Wood Johnson Foundation, Princeton, N.J.

Freeman, Howard E., K. Jill Kiecolt, and Harris M. Allen. 1982. Community health centers: An initiative of enduring utility. *Milbank Memorial Find Quarterly* 60(2):245–267.

Fuchs, Victor. 1974. *Who shall live?* New York: Basic Books.

Gallup, George. 1984. One of every 5 adults in U.S. can't always afford food. *San Francisco Chronicle*, March 19, p. 7.

Geiger, H. Jack. 1984. Community health centers: Health care as an instrument of social change. In *Reforming medicine: lessons of the last quarter century*, ed. Victor W. Sidel and Ruth Sidel. New York: Pantheon.

Gertman, P. M. 1974. Physicians as guiders of health services use. In *Incentives for health care*, ed. S. J. Mushkin, pp. 362–368. New York: Prodist.

Gold, M. R., and R. G. Rosenberg. 1974. The use of emergency room by the population of a neighborhood health center. *Health Services Reports.*

Goldberg, Victor. 1976. Some emerging problems of prepaid health plans in the Medi-Cal system. *Policy Analysis*, pp. 55–68.

Goldman, Fred, and Michael Grossman. 1981. The responsiveness and impacts of public health policy: The case of community health centers. Paper presented at the American Public Health Association Annual Meeting, Los Angeles, Calif., November 1–5.

Gordis, Leon. 1973. Effectiveness of comprehensive-care programs in preventing rheumatic fever. *New England Journal of Medicine* 289:331–335.

Gove, Walter R., M. Hughes, and O. R. Galle. 1979. Overcrowding in the home: An empirical investigation of its possible pathological consequences. *American Sociological Review* 44:59–80.

Gray, Alistar McIntosh. 1982. Inequalities in health, the Black report: A summary and comment. *International Journal of Health Services* 12(3):349–380.

Grossman, Michael. 1975. The correlation between health and schooling. In *Household production and consumption*, ed. Nestor E. Terleckyj. New York: Columbia University Press for the National Bureau of Economic Research.

Hadley, Jack. 1982. *More medical care, better health?* Washington, D.C.: Urban Institute Press.

Health care found in "deterioration." 1984. *San Francisco Chronicle*, Oct. 18, p. 14.

Helms, Jay, Joseph Newhouse, and Charles Phelps. 1979. Copayments and demand for medical care: The California Medicaid experience. *Bell Journal of Economics*.

Hicks, Lou E., Rose A. Langham, and Jean Takenaka. 1982. Cognitive and health measures following early nutritional supplementation: A sibling study. *American Journal of Public Health* 72(10):1110–1118.

Hiscock, W. McC. 1982. Prevention, primary care, and cost containment: The early and periodic screening, diagnosis, and treatment (EPSDT) programs. Internal memo, U.S. Department of Health and Human Services, March 23. Cited in Glenn Austin, Child health-care financing and competition, *New England Journal of Medicine* 311(17):1117–1120.

Illich, Ivan. 1976. *Medical nemesis: The expropriation of health.* New York: Pantheon Books.

Institute of Medicine. 1985. *The prevention of low birthweight.* Report of the Committee to Study the Prevention of Low Birthweight. Washington, D.C.: National Academy Press.

Irwin, Patrick H., and Rosemary Conroy-Hughes. 1982. EPSDT impact on health status: Estimates based on secondary analysis of administratively generated data. *Medical Care* 20(2):216–234.

Jenkins, C. D. 1983. Social enviornment and cancer mortality in men. *New England Journal of Medicine* 308(7):395–398.

JRB Associates, Inc. 1980. Final report for community health center cost-effectiveness evaluation.

Katz, Sidney, Lawrence B. Branch, Michael H. Branson, Joseph A. Papsidero, John C. Beck, and David S. Greer. 1983. Active life expectancy. *New England Journal of Medicine* 309(20):1218–1224.

Kessner, David M., James Singer, Carolyn E. Kalk, and Edward R. Schlesinger. 1973. *Infant death: An analysis by maternal risk and health care, con-*

trasts in health status. Vol. 1. Institute of Medicine. Washington, D.C.: National Academy of Science.

Kitagawa, Evelyn M., and Philip M. Hauser. 1973. *Differential mortality in the United States.* Cambridge: Harvard University Press.

Kleinman, Joel C., Marsha Gold, and Diane Makuc. 1981. Use of ambulatory medical care by the poor: Another look at equity. *Medical Care* 19(10): 1011–1029.

Korenbrot, Carol C. 1984. Risk reduction in pregnancies of low income women: Comprehensive prenatal care through the OB access project. *Mobius* 4(3):34–43.

Kotelchuck, Milton, Janet B. Schwartz, Marlene T. Anderka, and Karl S. Finison. 1984. WIC participation and pregnancy outcomes: Massachusetts statewide evaluation project. *American Journal of Public Health* 74(10): 1086–1092.

Lambert, Craig A., David R. Netherton, Lorenz J. Finison, James N. Hyde, and Sharon J. Spaight. 1982. Risk factors and life style: A statewide health-interview survey. *New England Journal of Medicine* 306(17):1048–1051.

LaPlante, Mitchell P. 1984. Is it unemployment or is it halibut? A review and re-analysis of the relationship of mortality and the business cycle. Paper presented at the seventy-ninth Annual Meeting of the American Sociological Association, San Antonio, Texas.

Levine, Sol, Jacob J. Feldman, and Jack Elinson. 1983. Does medical care do any good? In *Handbook of health, health care, health professions*, ed. David Mechanic. New York: Free Press.

Levy, Barry S., Frederick S. Wilkinson, and William M. Marine. 1971. Reducing neonatal mortality rate with nurse-midwives. *American Journal of Obstetrics and Gynecology* 109(1):50–58.

Lindheim, Roslyn, and S. Leonard Syme. 1983. Environments, people, and health. *Annual Review of the Public Health* 4:335–359.

Los Angeles County Health Alliance et al. 1982. Factual memorandum and argument in support of petition for rulemaking to declare prenatal care a public health service and establish standards for access to such care by low income women. Petition submitted to Beverly Myers, director of the State of Consumer Affairs, California.

Lurie, N., N. B. Ward, M. F. Shapiro, and R. H. Brook. 1984. Termination from Medi-Cal: Does it affect health? *New England Journal of Medicine* 311 (7):480–484.

Mahaffey, Kathryn R., Joseph L. Annest, Jean Roberts, and Robert S. Murphy. 1982. National estimates of blood lead levels: United States, 1976–1980. *New England Journal of Medicine* 307(10):573–579.

Maine Department of Human Services. 1983. *Children's deaths in Maine.* America's Children Project, Office of the Commissioner, Maine Department of Human Services, State House Station 11, Augusta, Maine.

Marmot, Michael G., M. J. Shipley, and Geoffrey Rose. 1984. Inequalities in death: Specific explanations of a general pattern? *Lancet* 1:1003–1006.

Mills, David. 1983. Statement in *Impact of unemployment on children and families*. Hearing before the Subcommittee on Labor Standards of the Committee on Education and Labor, House of Representatives, 98th Cong., 1st sess. Washington, D.C.: Government Printing Office.

Morehead, Mildred A., R. S. Donaldson, and M. R. Servall. 1971. Comparison between OEO's neighborhood health centers and other health care providers of ratings of the quality of health care. *American Journal of Public Health* 61:1294–1306.

Nagi, M. H., and E. G. Stockwell. 1973. Socioeconomic differentials in mortality by cause of death. *Public Health Reports* 88(5):449–456.

National Association of Neighborhood Health Centers, Inc. N.d.a. Issue paper: The effectiveness of community-based primary health care centers. Xerox copy. 1625 I Street, N.W.–Suite 420, Washington, D.C. 20006.

———. N.d.b. Issue paper: The efficiency of community-based primary health care centers. Xerox copy. 1625 I Street, N.W.–Suite 420, Washington, D.C. 20006.

National Center for Health Statistics. 1973. Examination and health history findings among children and youths 6–17 years, United States. Series 11, no. 129. Public Health Service.

———. 1977. Use of selected medical procedures associated with preventive care, United States, 1973. Series 10, no. 110. Public Health Service.

———. 1979. Use habits among adults of cigarettes, coffee, aspirin, and sleeping pills, United States, 1976. Series 10, no. 131. Public Health Service.

———. 1980. Selected health characteristics by occupation, United States, 1975–76. Series 10, no. 133. Public Health Service.

———. 1981a. Height and weight of adults ages 18–74 years by socioeconomic and geographic variables, United States, 1981. Series 11, no. 224. Public Health Service.

———. 1981b. Highlights from Wave I of the National Survey of Personal Health Practices and Consequences: United States, 1979. Series 15, no. 1. Public Health Service.

———. 1981c. Prevalence of selected impairments, United States, 1977. Series 10, no. 134. Public Health Service.

———. 1982a. Annual summary of births, deaths, marriages, and divorces: United States, 1981. Monthly vital statistics report. Vol. 30, no. 13. Public Health Service.

———. 1982b. Vital statistics of the United States, 1978. Vol. 2, part A. DHHS Publication No. (PHS) 83-1101. Public Health Service.

———. 1983a. Americans assess their health: United States, 1978. Series 10, no. 142. Public Health Service.

———. 1983b. Disability days: United States, 1980. Series 10, no. 143. Public Health Service.

———. 1983c. Physician visits: Volume and interval since last visit, United States, 1980. Series 10, no. 144. Public Health Service.

National Health Law Program. 1983. Hard facts: The administration's 1984 health budget. Los Angeles, Calif.

_____. 1984. In poor health: The administration's 1985 health budget. Los Angeles, Calif.

National Medical Care Expenditure Survey. 1984. Unpublished data provided by Dan Walden, National Center for Health Services Research, Hyattsville, Md.

Newacheck, Paul W., Lewis H. Butler, Aileen K. Harper, Dyan L. Piontkowski, and Patricia E. Franks. 1980. Income and illness. *Medical Care* 17(12): 1165–1176.

Newhouse, Joseph P., Willard G. Manning, Carl N. Morris, Larry L. Orr, Naihua Duan, Emmett B. Keeler, Arleen Leibowitz, Kent H. Marquis, M. Susan Marquis, Charles E. Phelps, and Robert H. Brook. 1981. Some interim results from a controlled trial of cost sharing in health insurance. *New England Journal of Medicine* 305(25):1501–1507.

Norris, Frank D., and Ronald L. Williams. 1984. Perinatal outcomes among medicaid recipients in California. *American Journal of Public Health* 74(10):1112–1117.

Orso, Camille L. 1979. Delivering ambulatory health care: The successful experience of an urban neighborhood health center. *Medical Care* 17(2):111–126.

Preston, Samuel H. 1984. Children and the elderly in the U.S. *Scientific American* 251(6):44–49.

Price, Deb. 1984. U.S. families face more poverty. *San Francisco Examiner and Chronicle*, March 11, p. A9.

Rainwater, Lee. 1966. Fear and the house-as-haven in the lower class. *Journal of the American Institute of Planning* 32:23–31.

Reed, Dwayne, Daniel McGee, and Katsuhiko Yano. 1984. Psychosocial processes and general susceptibility to chronic disease. *American Journal of Epidemiology* 119(3):356–370.

Reynolds, Roger A. 1976. Improving access to health care among the poor: The neighborhood health center experience. *Milbank Memorial Fund Quarterly: Health and Society* 54(1):47–82.

Rice, Dorothy, and Kathleen Danchik. 1979. Changing needs of children: Disease, disability, and access to care. Paper presented at Institute of Medicine Annual Meeting, Washington, D.C.

"Richer, poorer, truer." 1984. *New York Times*, August 8, p. 20E.

Ricketts, Tom. 1983. How to make the poor die elsewhere. *Washington Monthly*, February, p. 43.

Riley, Vernon. 1975. Mouse mammary tumors: Alteration of incidence as apparent function of stress. *Science* 189:465–467.

Robert Wood Johnson Foundation. 1983. Updated report on access to health care for the American people. Special Report No. 1. Princeton: R. W. Johnson Foundation.

Rogers, David E. 1980. Testimony before the Senate Subcommittee on Health and Scientific Research, Committee on Labor and Human Resources.

Ruberman, William, Eve Weinblatt, Judith D. Goldberg, and Banvir S. Chaud-hary. 1984. Psychosocial influences on mortality after myocardial infarc-tion. *New England Journal of Medicine* 311(9):552–559.

Schlozman, Kay L., and Sidney Verba. 1978. The new unemployment: Does it hurt? *Public Policy* 26(3):333–358.

Schwarz, Rachel, and Paul Poppen. 1982. *Measuring the impact of CHCs on pregnancy outcomes.* Final Report, Contract No. 240-81-0041. Health Re-sources and Services Administration. Rockville, Md.: Government Print-ing Office.

Scott, Austin. 1982. County's poor seen delaying visits to doctor. *Los Angeles Times,* Dec. 19, pt. 2, p. 1.

Shadish, William. 1981. Effectiveness of preventive child health care. Health Care Financing Administration. HSS Publication, HCFA Publication No. 03099. Washington, D.C.: Government Printing Office.

Shapiro, Sam, Wanda Venet, Philip Strax, Louis Venet, and Ruth Roeser. 1982. Prospects for eliminating racial differences in breast cancer survival rates. *American Journal of Public Health* 72(10):1142–1145.

Showstack, Jonathan A., Peter P. Budetti, and Donald Minkler. 1984. Factors associated with birthweight. An exploration of the roles of prenatal care and length of gestation. *American Journal of Public Health* 74(9):1003–1008.

Sparer, Gerald, and Joyce Johnson. 1971. Evaluation of OEO neighborhood health centers. *American Journal of Public Health* 61(May):931–942.

Starfield, Barbara. 1984. Social factors in child health. In *Ambulatory Pediat-rics III,* ed. Morris Green and Robert J. Haggerty, pp. 12–18. Philadelphia: W. B. Saunders.

_____. 1985. *Effectiveness of medical care: Validating clinical wisdom.* Baltimore: Md.: Johns Hopkins University Press.

Syme, S. Leonard, and Lisa F. Berkman. 1976. Social class, susceptibility, and sickness. *American Journal of Epidemiology* 104:1–8.

Task Force Report. 1976. Education and training of health manpower for pre-vention. In *Preventive Medicine USA.* New York: Prodist.

Tokarz, Wally. 1982. Controversy engulfs care project. *American Medical News,* February 12.

Uninsured increase, study shows. 1984. *Washington Report on Medicine and Health* 38:3.

U.S. Congress House of Representatives Committee on Interstate and Foreign Commerce. 1979. *Child Health Assurance Act of 1979.* Report No. 96-568. Washington, D.C.: Government Printing Office.

_____ Select Committee on Children, Youth, and Families. 1983. Demo-graphic and social trends: Implications for federal support of dependent-care services for children and the elderly. 98th Cong., 1st sess. Washing-ton, D.C.: Government Printing Office.

_____ 1984a. Children, youth, and families: 1983, a year-end report. 98th Cong., 2d sess. Washington, D.C.: Government Printing Office.

_____ 1984b. Infant mortality rates: Failure to close the black-white gap.

Subcommittee on Oversight. 98th Cong., 2d sess. Series no. 98-131. Washington, D.C.: Government Printing Office.

U.S. Department of Commerce. Bureau of the Census. 1984. Money income and poverty status of families and persons in the U.S., 1983. In *Current population reports*, p. 1. Series P-60, no. 145. Washington, D.C.: Government Printing Office.

U.S. Department of Health and Human Services. Public Health Service. 1982. *Health: United States, 1982.* National Center for Health Statistics. Hyattsville, Md.: Government Printing Office.

U.S. Department of Health, Education, and Welfare. Public Health Service. 1977. *Health of the disadvantaged: Chartbook.* DHEW Publication No. (HRA) 77-628. Office of Health Resources Opportunity. Hyattsville, Md.: Government Printing Office.

_____. 1979a. Dietary intake source data: U.S., 1971–74. DHEW Publication No. (PHS) 79-1221. Hyattsville, Md.: Government Printing Office.

_____. 1979b. *Healthy people: The surgeon general's report on health promotion and disease prevention, 1979.* DHEW Publication No. (PHS) 79-55071. Washington, D.C.: Government Printing Office.

_____. Health Resources Administration. 1979. *Health status of minorities and low-income groups.* DHEW Publication No. (HRA) 79-627. Washington, D.C.: Government Printing Office.

U.S. General Accounting Office. 1979. *Early childhood and family development programs improve the quality of life for low-income families.* Publication No. HRD-79-40. Washington, D.C.: Government Printing Office.

_____. 1984. WIC evaluations provide some favorable but no conclusive evidence on the effects expected for the special supplemental program for women, infants, and children. Report to the Senate Committee on Agriculture, Nutrition, and Forestry. GAO/PEMD-84-4. Washington, D.C.: Government Printing Office.

Whittemore, Alice S., 1981. Air pollution and respiratory disease. *Annual Review of Public Health* 2:397–429.

Wiederman, G., and F. Ambrosch. 1979. Costs and benefits of measles and mumps immunization in Austria. *Bulletin of the World Health Organization* 57(4):625–629.

Witte, J. J., and N. W. Axnick. 1975. The benefits from ten years of measles immunization in the U.S. *Public Health Reports* 90(30):205–207.

Chapter 4

The Medical Profession in Transition

Eliot Freidson

The past two decades have brought change to most professions in the United States, but the medical profession alone seems to be undergoing extensive changes. Some writers have characterized those changes as the decline of the medical profession (Burnham 1982), others as the "waning of professional sovereignty" (Starr 1978, 1982), and still others as "deprofessionalization" (Haug 1975) and "proletarianization" (McKinlay 1982). Elsewhere I have discussed those characterizations at length and criticized them as overgeneral, without any reasonably close relationship to the truly critical changes that have been taking place, and without the conceptual resources that allow adequate analysis of the consequences of change (Freidson 1985). Here I should like to identify the events that have precipitated changes in the environment of medical practice, the barriers that have channeled their implementation, and the consequences they are likely to have for the medical profession and its members over the next decade or so.

The Precipitating Factors of Change

Medicare and Medicaid legislation was the single most important factor of change for the health care system in the past two decades. These programs committed vast federal funds to pay for the health care of the elderly and the indigent, in the former case largely on the same permissive terms that private insurers had been paying for a large proportion of the working population. This commitment made the cost of health care more visible than it was in the past and politicized it, making it a topic for public consideration and debate and a subject for remedial legislation.

As we all know, a variety of other events were leading to an increase in health care costs. Continuous innovation in medical research and technique, fueled by new technology, led to the capacity to treat health problems that were previously treated far less expensively if treated at all. The new technology required increasingly larger sums of capital but at the same time, unlike many other kinds of technology, did not substitute for labor: health care remained labor intensive. Furthermore, labor costs themselves increased greatly when collective bargaining for previously low-paid hospital workers became legally possible, and in some areas fairly strong unions were formed. Of the professional workers in health care, nurses were especially conspicuous in unionizing. Labor costs were also increased by the trend toward licensing and certification among technically trained health occupations, many of which were developed to deal with the new health-care technology.

Even before Medicare and Medicaid legislation was enacted, a series of other events influenced the general climate of public opinion within which public discussion of health care takes place and by which it is politicized. The public's traditional ambivalence toward science in general and medicine in particular moved from fairly uncritical approval and trust to a considerably more qualified and concerned (but by no means wholly critical) attitude. In the 1960s, regulations were written requiring all research programs financed by the government to be reviewed in advance for their method of protecting the rights of "human subjects." During the 1970s, public preoccupation and debate grew, fed by the media, on the issue of the ethics of medical and other research involving human beings. At the same time concern for the pollution of the natural environment grew, as did concern for the safety of drugs and processed foods. Part and parcel of this shift in concern was a growth of suspicion about the competence and ethicality of physicians. Malpractice suits swelled, and the profession's reputation was damaged by publicity about the way its average income increased much faster than the rate of inflation during the years following passage of Medicare legislation.

More recently, the very success of advances in medical technique and medical technology added an additional increment of concern with the work of the doctor. Perhaps the Quinlan case can typify the issue—namely, that it had become possible to intervene medically into what was heretofore only natural uncontrolled processes leading to death, raising the question of the physician's role in the process. The successful movement to legalize and commercialize contraception and, later, abortion, and the women's movement, which pressed for the right of a woman to control her reproduction, also raised a host of ethical and legal questions. In all those issues the role of the physician was central, the lightning rod for unprecedented questioning. The abuse of medical authority was not so much the question as what authority a physician should have and what rights the patients and their families should have.

Most commentators have grievously exaggerated the consequences of this shift in the climate and focus of public opinion about health care. A recent, careful analysis of public opinion poll data has shown that there has indeed been a distinct decline in public confidence in American medicine. That decline is part and parcel of a decline of confidence in all American institutions, however. Compared to other American institutions, confidence remains highest of all in medicine (Lipset and Schneider 1983); polling data indicate that the vast majority of all Americans have been and remain satisfied with their health care (Health Insurance Association 1982). Neither medicine itself nor the health care institutions in which its members work are the objects of widespread and deep hostility or doubt, but they have become the objects of more questioning and challenge.

Another major phenomenon that has precipitated changes is rather difficult to characterize simply. I refer to the growth of an emphasis on competition, which stemmed from two distinct sources. If one can speak of the consumers' movement as a monolithic entity, some of its activities were concerned with gaining more stringent government regulation of the health industry so as to assure the safety and quality of its products and services. Others of its activities have been concerned with gaining for consumers more useful and complete information about the services and goods available to them, and providing them with better criteria for choice—a concern that has on occasion led to legislation. Another part of the consumer movement, however, has been in favor of decreasing government regulation and increasing competition among health care providers, partly by removing or tempering restrictions on practice posed by licensing laws and partly by reducing professional restraints on advertising prices, competitive bidding, and so forth. That "procompetitive" pressure also grew from an entirely different source—exponents of the nineteenth-century economic ideology of laissez-faire, who emphasize consumer activism in a free market. Understandably it came from representatives of industries that have been subject to government regulation, but it also came from economists, lawyers, political scientists, and policymakers.

Responses to Change

A variety of factors precipitated responses to subsequent events that have had an important impact on the traditional institutions of medicine. These factors include the following: continuous and unexpected rise in health care costs at the same time that financing became a public issue; an increasingly questioning attitude toward medicine and health care issues; and increased tendencies to challenge both government regulation and conventional methods of organizing and controlling the provision of health care.

It did not take many years after Medicare legislation for health care costs to be seen as out of control. Just a few years after the initial legislation there was political pressure to slow the rise. The initial target was primarily the largest source of expense—the hospital. The method of control developed by legislation was formal review. Each decision on the part of a physician to hospitalize a patient and, after hospitalization, the number of days the patient was hospitalized, was to be reviewed in light of the primary diagnosis by a medically constituted committee in the hospital. A series of subsequent legislative efforts tinkered with the organization, mode of operation, and sanctioning powers of such review committees, the general trend being toward greater standardization of the criteria by which medical decisions to hospitalize and treat patients are evaluated.

This development was very significant in that the principle of mandatory, formal review of medical decisions was established and given legitimacy. Some sort of collegial evaluation of physicians' decisions has probably always existed wherever they worked in proximity to each other, and most particularly in hospitals. The Joint Commission for the Accreditation of Hospitals has required for some time the existence of some form of committee to review facets of the medical care provided in hospital. In all teaching hospitals, furthermore, some form of supervision and evaluation is routinely exercised down the hierarchy of the medical

staff. But rules were not laid down to govern procedure from one institution to another, and records were neither complete nor consistent nor systematic. Nor were formal sanctions specified. At present, some observers have charged that the Peer Review Organizations (PRO, which is the latest in the series of changing review systems) do not function in a truly effective manner. However, they represent a sharp break with earlier times in that they constitute a formal system for the review of the propriety of physicians' decisions, which is much the same everywhere. Furthermore, the system, presently limited to hospitals, can be extended into ambulatory settings where most physicians now are subject solely to claims review.

In addition to those general utilization review mechanisms created in an effort to control the cost of care, a number of other, more specialized review groups have been constituted, primarily in hospitals, in response to public concern with the ethical, social, and medical issues created by the recent developments of sustaining life artificially, transplanting organs, implanting artificial organs, performing fetal surgery, and the like. In some cases, as in the Infant Care Review Committees created to monitor the life-support of deformed newborns, such formal review activity is mandated by governmental regulation, while in others it is voluntary. The PRO and other formal methods of reviewing medical decisions in hospitals do not exhaust movement toward closer surveillance, evaluation, and discipline over medical acts. In the past the disgruntled patient had recourse to the law of torts and the courts, where it was possible to sue a physician for malpractice and gain financial recompense. But financial penalties are one thing and losing one's very license to practice is quite another. Licensing boards and the disciplinary committees attached to them can revoke or suspend licenses. But when Derbyshire (1969) published his examination of the activities of such boards, he documented their lethargy. Political pressure, fed by well-publicized scandals, led to much greater activity since that time. Some states have passed "informer laws" that require physicians and others to report to the licensing authority the name of any physician they believe to have acted in a grossly negligent fashion. By 1983, when Derbyshire reported again on the activities of state agencies, the picture had changed considerably (Derbyshire 1983). Formal procedures for the systematic review and evaluation of both the ethical and technical quality of physicians' performance have been reinforced and extended, though their effectiveness should not be overestimated.

Taken together, it is appropriate to say that while many of those formal physician review enterprises had roots in past institutions, the emerging situation has been genuinely new for the profession. Where once a physician could bury his mistakes with no one the wiser, so private was his practice, where once judges denounced physicians for their "conspiracy of silence" in refusing to testify against colleagues being tried for malpractice, and where once the hospital was the physicians'

workshop where they were free to follow their own variable inclinations without serious interference, now a variety of groups review both the technical propriety of the everyday decisions of physicians and the moral acceptibility of their activities. Those groups, furthermore, are formally constituted, and thus are required to function in such a way as to keep systematic records and develop standardized procedures.

The imposition of formal review is one important step toward restructuring the milieu in which medicine is practiced. Another step stems from quite different sources that are more directly concerned with reducing the cost of health care in general and the level of physicians' charges in particular. Early in the 1970s federal legislation was passed to facilitate the formation of health maintenance organizations (HMOs) that could offer consumers prepaid service contracts —taking care of most of their needs for medical service and consultation in return for a fixed annual sum, instead of charging them or their insurers on a piece-rate or fee-for-service basis. HMOs are quite varied in form, some being loosely organized aggregates of physicians working in their own offices, others being partnerships among physicians working together, and still others being organizations with a staff of salaried physicians. What joins them all together, however, is the common condition of physicians entering into a contractual relationship with consumers and insuring organizations. In that contractual relationship, the physician has a formal obligation to provide specified services over a given period of time to eligible patients, which is quite different from the traditional fee-for-service relationship between physician and patient that was constrained by the barriers of a fee to be paid for each visit.

HMOs expanded considerably once federal legislation both neutralized state laws that handicapped their development and provided them with economic aid, but even now they cover less than 7 percent of the population. While they may be expected to grow further, in light of the varied forms of health insurance available, the persistent attraction of traditional forms of practice to many consumers, and the development of new, specialized forms of competitive ambulatory care, HMOs are unlikely to become the prototypical method of practice. But the contractual relationship with patients that they embody is likely to extend into other forms of practice and become more widespread than HMOs themselves. It can be extended into individual office practices by use of the recent "preferred provider" arrangements that are being explored by insurance organizations, hospitals, and employers seeking to reduce their costs for providing health benefits to their employees. Insofar as the number of physicians has been growing in relation to the population, many more may be interested in salaried practice (Friedman 1983) than has been the case in the past, while others may be interested in entering into service contracts out of their own offices. Such contracts, like salaries, could assure both that they have patients and that they get paid.

With both public and private financing agencies seeking to reduce costs, service contracts can be attractive insofar as there is sufficient competition among physicians or groups of physicians to lead to economic terms that are desirable for insurers and patients. Until recently, such competition could only be muted and covert and was significantly handicapped by the codes of "ethics" of medical and other professional associations. A series of Supreme Court decisions in the 1970s, however, concerned specifically with law, pharmacy, and engineering, destroyed the barrier that organized professions have traditionally raised against overt price competition among their members and against advertising price and other features of their services. Aggressive antitrust enforcement on the part of the Federal Trade Commission, sustained by the courts on appeal in 1982, extended the requirement to medicine. Now, physicians and health care organizations are free to advertise both the prices and the character of their services within as yet uncertain limits of truth and propriety, and are free to participate publicly in competitive bidding for clients or contracts with clients.

Another competitor for clients and the public and private insurance funds that pay for much of their care has emerged in the growth of for-profit health care enterprises financed and owned by lay investors. Traditionally, such enterprises have been financed and owned by physicians— the proprietary hospital being the best-known example, though some medical groups or clinics may also be mentioned. Given the recent climate of opinion that emphasizes the virtues of free competition, deprecates the motives and competence of public agencies, raises questions about the disinterestedness of physicians and representatives of the traditional nonprofit, voluntary health care institutions, deplores the cost of care, and resists the generation of investment capital for hospitals through taxation, many stimuli for the expansion of private investment existed. Apart from hospitals and nursing homes, home care, kidney dialysis, "urgent" (or more precisely, casual) ambulatory care, and a variety of other services have grown up as for-profit enterprises, some owned by lay investors and some by physician-entrepreneurs.

Few of these for-profit enterprises would have been initiated if there were not some large, reliable "third party" to pay their charges either directly or by reimbursing the patients who paid out of pocket. Even more attractive to for-profit enterprises was that initially, before costs came to be considered intolerable, little constraint was placed on the sums that could be charged for health care services. Most recently, however, large employers who bear the cost of health care benefits for their employees, health insurance companies themselves, and state and federal authorities have reinforced efforts to restrict the rise in health care costs by placing ceilings or "caps" on what they will pay. It is much too early to tell whether or not the effort will succeed and what its concrete consequences will be for particular health care enterprises, but it seems certain to put competitive pressure on traditional medical practices in both the private consulting room and the hospital

floors. Many physicians are likely to be drawn into some contractual agreement with large organizations able to advertise effectively and otherwise attract insured patients, and to rationalize payment and administration so as to restrict their operating costs. Other physicians are likely to be drawn into salaried and otherwise rationalized and limited economic arrangements. And medical decisions in hospitals are likely to receive even closer scrutiny and critical evaluation in light of their implications for hospital income.

Constraints on Change

The changes that have been taking place seem to have revolutionary implications for the medical profession. Instead of being free to exercise their own clinical judgment, physicians become subject to systematic and formal review of their decisions by increasingly standardized criteria. Instead of being protected by their monopoly over practice, they are thrown into a highly competitive marketplace in which price cutting and advertising may make the difference between success and failure. Instead of administering the affairs of their own practices in their own way, they become drawn into and dependent upon a highly rationalized and bureaucratic system of purportedly efficient management practices drawn directly from large business enterprises. They become subject to economic pressures that they cannot deal with on their own terms, in their own way, not the least of which is produced by entering into formal contractual arrangements with a large and powerful organization. If we take these changes at face value, without qualification by the social and legal context within which they occur, and if we assume that the trend will continue at the same pace into the future, the position of the medical profession might very well be characterized appropriately as declining. Even the extreme characterization of proletarianization may be accurate.

However, none of the changes I have described is thus far free of some very basic constraints that for the moment preclude the assumption that they will realize to the full their intrinsic logic in the near future. The medical profession retains its basic, legally enforced monopoly over the key functions of health care and, the consumer movement notwithstanding, retains its basic "cultural authority." At its edges, competitors have made some inroads on medicine's monopoly, but every inroad has been carefully limited by law, providing no hint of the possibility that the basic monopoly of medicine is seriously threatened.

Nonetheless, a monopoly does not necessarily have the consequence of situating the profession so well in the marketplace that economic returns to its members are inevitably handsome. Indeed, given the new competitive arrangements designed to reduce costs it is quite likely that the American medical profession will finally join the other professions of the advanced industrial nations and like them suffer a decline in income, monopoly or no (Scitovsky 1966). But its

monopoly is more than a device to maximize income: it is also a device to control work. While the monopoly is no longer able to contain competition among its members, it is still able to control some of the terms and most of the conditions, content, and goals of health care. In antitrust actions, as Kissam (1980) has noted, the courts have typically limited themselves to economic issues, leaving technical or scientific issues in the custody of the profession itself. Physicians continue to be the key people with the sole authority to legitimately diagnose and carry out the treatment of health problems. They are the ones who officially certify illness, who can admit to and discharge from hospitals, and who direct and coordinate the specialized activities of the varied health care occupations that are part of the health care division of labor. Their strategic location in the health care system cannot fail to provide practitioners with a strong lever for continuing to control much of what goes on in health care, even though their economic position has weakened.

A series of legal and quasi-legal requirements and practices sustains the capacity of the profession to retain a strong if not wholly determinative position in the health care system. Some may be seen in the federal and state staffing regulations governing the licensing of health care institutions and the designation of eligibility for reimbursement by health financing agencies, as well as in state laws governing the "corporate practice of medicine." Others may be seen in the regulations and practices governing the composition and operation of the official boards or committees that review medical decisions in health care organizations or that review consumer complaints against individual physicians. In a variety of ways, those legal and quasi-legal customs require that only physicians supervise the work of other physicians, review it, and evaluate it. The criteria by which the technical work of physicians is judged must be established by physicians. And in the formal review bodies in which the ethical and social issues of medical work are considered, physicians routinely predominate over lay members.

Because of the physicians' strategic position in the operation of the health care system, and the lack of any evidence that their position is changing in any marked way, one can understand why hospitals remain concerned with being attractive to physicians who can fill their beds with well-insured patients. Indeed, it seems no accident that something of a trend has been observed recently to include members of the medical staff on the governing boards of hospitals (Noie, Shortell, and Morrisey 1983). This trend is a reversal of past practices, when the medical staff had direct access to governing boards (instead of being represented by the chief executive officer) but were not often members. Furthermore, whenever for-profit hospitals are organized, they are reported to go to great lengths to attract physicians to their staff, in some cases coopting them as shareholders who have a financial stake in the hospital's fortunes. Physicians have somewhat less leverage in ambulatory settings, but it is a frequent legal requirement that in health care

enterprises outside the hospital, the chief executive officer be a physician. In the case of laws governing professional corporations, most states require that none but the working professionals themselves can own shares, and that those shares cannot be transferred to lay persons. Thus, professional control over the evaluation of medical work is mandated, as is control over the administration of medical work.

The Consequences for the Medical Profession

I have noted a variety of important changes in the fiscal, administrative, and social environment of health care that on first glance appear to have devastating consequences for the medical profession. I then noted a number of circumstances connected with the legal and quasi-legal position of the profession that have not changed markedly from the past and that exercise important constraints on change. These constraints should not be considered barriers to change so much as devices that channel change. Taken together, the interaction between the changing environment of medical practice and the relatively unchanging legal position of the profession in the system seems to produce the continued strength of the profession as a corporate body, for members of the profession administer and perform the new functions of control pushed onto it by external forces. At the same time the profession becomes divided internally as the brunt of change is born by the everyday practitioner.

Consider the matter of the proliferation of formal groups or agencies charged with the official duty to review systematically the medical and ethical practices of working physicians. Those review groups subject everyday practitioners to unprecedented surveillance and evaluation, and are empowered to impose concrete economic sanctions, in some cases so severe a sanction as suspending the license to practice. The review groups are, however, staffed by members of the medical profession, and the standards remain in the hands of members of the medical profession. But at the same time, a division is created between those serving on such review groups as judges and those they judge.

Similarly, as the organization of many practices becomes more complex, those physicians serving in the legally mandated positions of supervisor, staff director, or chief executive officer become superordinates, and the practitioners subordinates. Remembering that physicians themselves have been active participants in the new, for-profit enterprises in health care, we may also assume that in a growing number of cases a cleavage will develop between physicians as owners or shareholders of health care businesses and other physicians as their employees and profit producers. Finally, the likelihood being that standards for evaluating technical practices will shift away from common usage toward standards established by academic researchers, the

division between authoritative experts and mere practitioners will also deepen and intensify.

The profession as a corporate body, then, remains in control of the basic processes of the health care system by having its own members serve in the supervisory and standard-setting positions demanded by the forces of change. By competing and innovating or collaborating as entrepreneurs in the marketplace, by assuming administrative responsibility for reviewing and guiding if not actually dictating the performance of practitioners in complex systems, and by formulating defensible technical standards by which the competence and conscientiousness of their performance can be judged, the profession remains in charge, but it also intensifies divisions within itself.

Division and formalization of function are being organized into specialized roles around which develop specialized career lines and from which emerge distinct, organized interests. Whereas physicians serving in administrative or managerial roles were relatively uncommon and inconspicuous in the past, the number of organizations requiring their services has increased and they seem on the way to emerging as a self-conscious segment within the profession. Indeed, an American College of Physician Executives was formed not long ago. Like deans of medical schools and directors or chief executive officers of hospitals, their concern is negotiating with and accommodating to the external forces on which the prosperity of their organization depends. This means striving to fulfill the demands for efficiency and accountability made by public and private financing agencies and sustained by political pressure and the climate of public opinion. To fulfill those demands requires maintaining working conditions to which practitioners are not accustomed and for which their preconceptions do not prepare them.

Coping with New Working Conditions

Rank and file physicians confront all those changes from a different vantage point than the physician executive. Like all workers, they need to develop methods of tempering the pressures of their work environment. Traditionally, physicians kept their own medical records however they chose, and in hospitals were notorious for their recalcitrance in making entries and keeping the record up to date. In addition, they considered themselves free to follow their own clinical judgment, willing to consider the advice of colleagues but ultimately making their own decisions. In a health care organization like a hospital or a clinic they were willing to concede the legitimacy of the authority of lay and professional administrators over such "housekeeping" issues as scheduling hours, assigning space, and providing equipment, supplies, and supportive personnel but insisted on their sole right to make their own individual diagnostic and therapeutic decisions (cf. Goss 1961). Their diagnostic and therapeutic decisions were in turn used to strengthen and legitimize their demands for space, time, equipment, supportive personnel, and the like. Once cost became a pressing concern, however, and formal methods of accountability and review instituted, the capacity of the practitioner to maintain past attitudes, values, and behaviors was seriously weakened and relations with those in administrative positons as well as with their colleagues were changed.

By and large, it is in ambulatory care settings where the greatest tension between practitioners and administrators is likely to develop because in such settings the workload is subject to wide fluctuation. Periodically—as during the "flu season" in regions with cold winters—practitioners will experience an extremely heavy workload and may receive little or no relief in the form of additional supportive personnel or physicians. As one study found (Freidson 1980, 55–85), practitioners may cope with this overload by refusing service, by cutting corners in their physical examinations, or—something facilitated by a prepaid service contract—by referring their patients to consultants or sending them out for tests or X rays after perfunctory examination. And certainly the records they keep—always a bone of contention between administrators and practitioners—will suffer. Each of those methods of coping with overload poses problems to the organization—possibly violating contractual agreements, raising its expenses, shifting the boundaries of the jurisdiction of primary practitioners and their consultants so as to lead to heavier use of consultants, and risking both legal and financial difficulty by virtue of inadequate records. Since all practitioners in ambulatory settings work in the nominal privacy of consulting rooms, and since all have a significant degree of discretion in their work in spite of formal review processes, administrative efforts to reduce or eliminate such methods of coping are unlikely to be fully successful. The tension between practitioner and administrator, therefore, is likely to be endemic, increasing in intensity during recurring periods of overload.

The service contract creates new problems with patients, which cannot be dealt with easily by traditional methods. With a service contract, physicians, or their practice organizations, agree to provide services to patients who themselves can realize the benefits of their insurance only if they consult those who have agreed to the contract. In the past, patients and physicians rarely had formal commitments to each other. If patients were dissatisfied and had other alternatives available, they could switch to them. By the same token, if physicians thought a patient too difficult to be worth dealing with and they could afford the loss of fees, they could use a variety of devices, including raising their fees arbitrarily, to encourage the patient to seek care elsewhere. In a contractual relationship, however, it is not easy for either practitioner or patient to withdraw without undesirable costs or inconvenience (cf. Freidson 1980, 41–54). They are both, in a sense, trapped by

the contract and must work out some way of coping with each other rather than merely avoiding each other. Neither is able to act as individuals in a free market, for the contract is likely to prevent the doctor from raising a fee barrier and to discourage the patient from seeking care from someone else because it would cost money out of pocket.

Not all patients will pose many problems, however. From members of the affluent middle class physicians should expect the fewest overt difficulties, for the middle class are likely to have very generous and flexible health benefits that allow many options. And even when not, members of the middle class are less likely to find out-of-pocket costs burdensome in light of their total income. (For a recent study of physicians in HMOs and an up-to-date bibliography of others, see Barr and Steinberg, in press.) From the poor and from blue- and white-collar workers physicians should also expect to meet few difficulties, particularly if the agency paying for the poor is passive and if the employed have no union that negotiates their benefits, educates them about their contractual rights, and intervenes on their behalf. It is primarily the large and growing group of college-educated, middle-income professional and technical workers— sometimes called the new middle class— that has the greatest potential for creating difficulties for physicians working under contract. They are well educated enough to consider themselves capable of understanding medical matters, well enough exposed to the media to consider themselves well informed about up-to-date diagnoses and treatments, and of high enough status to wish to be treated as equals. Furthermore, they are likely to have a fairly detailed understanding of their contractual rights and, being articulate as well as familiar with bureaucratic procedures, inclined to seek bureaucratic satisfaction from the insurer if they cannot get it from the physician. Their moderate income discourages them from the option of exiting and paying out of pocket. They have little choice but to stay and voice their complaints and desires within the system itself.

It would not be wise to exaggerate the number of such patients in everyday medical interactions, for most encounters are routine and most patients cooperative. But even a small proportion of patients who are troublesome to them can so color the quality of physicians' experience as to transform their perception of their practice as a whole and of the appropriate role to play in it. How physicians learn to cope with that minority of patients in contract practice has profound implications for the spirit in which service is provided to all and at least some implications for the substance and cost of services (cf. Freidson 1980, 86-98). It is possible for physicians to guide their methods of coping by employing the criteria of traditional "free" practice—resenting contractual constraints, manipulating what they can to their financial advantage, and seeking opportunities to leave the system to become independent entrepreneurs. (For a rare study of physician entrepreneurs, see Goldstein 1984a, 1984b.)

Physicians can also adopt a bureaucratic stance toward their patients and their work. In cases of doubt or challenge they would go by the book, provide patients with what they ask as a contractual entitlement no matter what their personal judgment or medical necessity or propriety. It is easier to dispense the benefit than to argue. A quite different and more desirable possibility is for physicians to adopt a purely professional stance of holding to their own medical judgment when the evidence supports it and refusing to satisfy inappropriate demands from patients while at the same time attempting to teach why they are inappropriate.

Which of those alternative ways of coping with work problems under the new conditions of contractual practice is adopted depends less on the particular variation in the contractual arrangement that is employed than on the way collegial relations in practice are organized and on the degree of financial stringency imposed on the system as a whole. The professional stance is time consuming and thus expensive in the short run. It is, furthermore, virtually impossible to adopt in times of overload and too vulnerable to official reproach if "quality" standards employed by official review bodies are narrow and mechanical. If the system becomes "efficient" enough that overload is endemic and standards precisely calculable, then those who cannot leave it to become entrepreneurs and managers are likely, as rank and file, to have no other way to cope than to adopt the techniques of the bureaucratic official, going by the book in dispensing contractual benefits and in making medical decisions that are subject to formal review.

The Organized Profession in Transition

In most discussions of professions such as medicine and law, the professions are characterized as divided primarily along specialty lines. Specialization has in fact been the major source of segmentation in medicine during most of this century (cf. Stevens 1971) Less conspicuous and, until recently, less important have been the divisions of function that organize the way professional practice is carried out, no matter what the specialty. When the bulk of practice was carried out as an individual enterprise on an uninsured fee-for-service basis, individual practitioners themselves carried out the functions of administration and review and individual clients were obliged themselves to undertake evaluative and sanctioning actions. In medicine today, however, even individual practitioners in their own offices are bound into reimbursement and review systems in which others become full-time specialists devoted to performing the functions of administration, evaluation, and sanctioning.

On both analytic and pragmatic grounds these growing divisions between the managers and the managed, the judges and the judged, the employers and the employees, and the standard-setters and the standard-

followers are emerging to be a good deal more important than specialty in the segmentation of the profession as a whole. They cut across all the specialties, and they represent the hierarchical organization of economic, administrative, and cognitive authority over everyday practice no matter what the specialty. Furthermore, their growth creates a far more serious challenge to the political strength of the organized profession than the growth of specialty associations created in the past. Organized medicine in the United States has already lost through antitrust action some of its capacity to control the economic behavior of its membership. It is also in danger of losing its political position as the most effective representative of the profession as a whole.

While some very illuminating studies of the American Bar have been conducted recently (e.g., Halliday 1982; Cappell and Halliday 1983), the activities of the American Medical Association (AMA) have not received detailed analysis for some time, and I am not in a position to do so here. It is my impression, however, that while the AMA remains fairly influential on matters of licensing and on technical or scientific issues, the organization has lost much of its influence on economic and social policy. Part of that loss no doubt reflects the general decline in public confidence as well as the rise in importance of other sources of influence that combine to overweigh that of the AMA.

Even though the AMA carries on important joint activities with the American Hospital Association (AHA) and the Association of American Medical Colleges (AAMC), the

AHA and AAMC seem to have more frequently taken different positions than the AMA on policy issues; at the same time the AHA and AAMC have become more influential than earlier. This also appears to be the case with at least some specialty associations and the associations representing medical scientists or researchers. Indeed, while many of the latter participate in those activities of the AMA involving the communication of research findings, their associations are more closely allied with the AAMC. The AAMC, after all, and the AHA, insofar as it speaks for teaching hospitals, represent the institutions in which medical researchers and academics work and upon which their fortunes depend.

If the analysis of this paper is accurate, we should expect the growth in size and influence of other health-related associations that represent the interests of the expanding, new, or renovated forms of organized practice—HMOs, urgent care centers, ambulatory surgical centers, and the like. As is the case for hospitals and medical schools, representation in such associations is institutional in character, embodied in the directors, deans, or chief executive officers responsible for the institution as a whole. Their orientation is toward overall policy in light of the larger political and economic environment that provides the legal and economic resources upon which the institution depends. The needs of the rank and file practitioners in their organization are only one and perhaps not the major factor they take into consideration in guiding their institution and protecting its interests. Theirs is a "macro" or policy-oriented perspective (cf. Scott 1982, 222), which is quite different from the "micro" or clinical practice perspective of rank and file practitioners trying to cope with everyday problems of work. And they control the allocation of resources that has a direct impact on the way everyday medical work can be carried out.

In the past, like all professional associations, the AMA has attempted to be an umbrella association, representing the entire medical profession. Naturally, this policy has meant that, on issues that are deeply controversial among significant segments of the profession, it has had the choice of being silent, temporizing, adopting a very vague position, or adopting one of the contending positions and risking the alienation of those of its members who espouse the other. This problem, of course, is common. But if the issues become too important to evade and if perspectives on them are so distinctly different as to polarize large numbers of members, then it becomes impossible to exercise influence over their resolution without alienating one of those major segments and even splitting the association.

Thus far the AMA has tempered the winds of change by successfully maintaining professional control over the administrative, review, and sanctioning functions connected with health care. But it has not yet faced the implications of that short-term success for the creation of stronger divisions among its membership that will threaten its unity. The distinct possibility is that, as an absolutely greater number of physicians are drawn into organized systems of practice and become a distinct rank and file that is subordinate to other physicians who are employers, administrators, reviewers, and standard-setters, the satisfaction of their needs may run head-on against the needs of the system as they are conceived by those speaking for it. If the AMA is not successful in gaining agreement on some balance between the two needs, it may very well suffer the historic fate of schoolteaching, which is now divided into a large association for the rank and file alone and separate associations for their colleagues who are researchers and administrators. Sometimes these organizations are joined together on policy issues and sometimes they are bitterly opposed. The outcome of efforts to accommodate these different and equally legitimate interests will affect not merely the future of the profession as such but, more important, the spirit and substance of the profoundly essential human service it provides to the public.

References

Barr, J. K., and M. K. Steinberg. In press. A physician role typology: Colleague and client dependence in an HMO. *Social Science and Medicine.*

Burnham, J. C. 1982. American medicine's golden age: What happened to it? *Science* 215:1474–1479.

Cappell, C. L., and T. C. Halliday. 1983. Professional projects of elite Chicago lawyers, 1950–1974. *American Bar Foundation Research Journal* 1983: 291–340.

Derbyshire, R. C. 1969. *Medical licensure and discipline in the United States.* Baltimore: Johns Hopkins University Press.

———. 1983. How effective is medical self-regulation? *Law and Human Behavior* 7:279–290.

Freidson, E. 1980. *Doctoring together.* Chicago: University of Chicago Press.

———. 1985. The reorganization of the medical profession. *Medical Care Review* 42, no. 1 (Spring).

Friedman, E. 1983. Declaration of interdependence. More and more physicians find salaried practice attractive. *Hospitals* 57:73–80.

Goldstein, M. S. 1984a. Abortion as a medical career choice: Entrepreneurs, community physicians, and others. *Journal of Health and Social Behavior* 25:211–229.

———. 1984b. Creating and controlling a medical market: Abortion in Los Angeles after liberalization. *Social Problems* 31:514–529.

Goss, M. E. W. 1961. Influence and authority among physicians in an outpatient clinic. *American Sociological Review* 26:39–50.

Halliday, T. C. 1982. The idiom of legalism in bar politics: Lawyers, McCarthyism, and the civil rights era. *American Bar Foundation Research Journal* 1982:911–988.

Haug, M. R. 1975. The deprofessionalization of everyone? *Sociological Focus* 8:197–213.

Health Insurance Association of America. 1982. Health and health insurance: The public's view. Winter.

Kissam, P. C. 1980. Antitrust law, the First Amendment, and professional self-regulation of technical quality. In *Regulating the professions*, ed. R. D. Blair and Stephen Rubin, pp. 143–183. Lexington, Mass.: Lexington Books.

Lipset, S. M., and W. Schneider. 1983. *The confidence gap.* New York: Free Press.

McKinlay, J. B. 1982. Toward the proletarianization of physicians. In *Professionals as workers: Mental labor in advanced capitalism*, ed. C. Derber, pp. 37–62. Boston: G. K. Hall.

Noie, N. E., S. M. Shortell, and M. A. Morrisey. 1983. A survey of hospital medical staffs. *Hospitals* 57:80–84, 91–94.

Scitovsky, T. 1966. An international comparison of the trend of professional earnings. *American Economic Review* 56:25–42.

Scott, W. R. 1982. Managing professional work: Three models of control for health organizations. *Health Services Research* 17:213–240.

Starr, P. 1978. Medicine and the waning of professional sovereignty. *Daedalus* 107:175–193.

_____. 1982. *The social transformation of American medicine.* New York: Basic Books.

Stevens, R. 1971. *American medicine and the public interest.* New Haven: Yale University Press.

Chapter 5

The Changing Hospital

Rosemary Stevens

While the hospital's role may be different in the future than in the past, the hospital remains a central medical and social institution. As part of one of the largest enterprises in the United States and part of an expanding industry, hospitals will remain important on the national political and economic scene. Meanwhile, hospital policy-making is fraught not only with the uneasiness that comes with any rapid social change but also with the difficulty of coping with the concurrent metamorphosis of the hospital's function, structure, and management, and the uncertainty as to how far—and in what ways—hospitals should be seen, in the U.S. context, as public services or businesses.

The U.S. community general hospital,[1] as most of us know it, is being transformed. Some of the services that have been most central to the hospital are being removed to free-standing surgical centers and other ambulatory facilities, where patients may be admitted and discharged the same day. Home care is now possible for procedures as diverse as parenteral nutrition, orthopedic traction, and kidney dialysis—all conditions where patients would most certainly have been treated in a hospital only a few years ago. After decades of growth, hospital inpatient admissions declined from 36.5 million in 1981 to 36.2 million in 1983 (American Hospital Association 1984b). Meanwhile hospitals are expanding their activities into areas as diverse as rehabilitation services, home care, and primary care facilities.

Financially, U.S. hospitals have become big business. The total expenses of community general hospitals more than doubled between 1977 and 1983, from $51.8 billion to $116.6 billion, with concomitant rises in Medicare, Medicaid, Blue Cross, and commerical hospital insurance rates.

The average American now spends over $500 a year on hospital care, largely through employer-employee payroll contributions for health insurance, supplemented by Social Security contributions and general tax payments. Community general hospitals are one of the nation's major employers: with payroll disbursements of $55.6 billion and the full-time equivalent of 3.1 million employees in 1983. Hospitals, collectively, are an ineluctable part of the national labor market as well as of health care policy-making. Their future is bound up with the future of the health insurance industry (itself a major enterprise); with decisions made by major businesses about the amount of money to be spent on health care benefits and how it should be spent; with the politics and availability of money for tax-supported programs such as Medicare, a mainstay of hospital financing for the 27 million Americans over the age of sixty-five; with national swings in mood about the nature of government entitlement programs and of programs for the poor, such as Medicaid; and with the buoyancy of the stock and bond markets, which affect, in turn, investor interest in profit-making hospitals and the availability of capital for hospitals throughout the system.

Hospitals are part of a major industry in other ways, too. Their ownership is diverse and they are aggressively competitive. U.S. hospitals are pluralistic in patterns of both ownership (control) and funding (third-party reimbursement). Of the 5,843 hospitals classified by the American Hospital Association as "non-federal, short-term general and other special hospitals" in 1983—the basic U.S. community hospital—1,723 (29 percent) were owned by state and local government, 3,363 (58 percent) were organized as not-for-profit corporations, the so-called voluntary hospitals, and 757 (13 percent) were investor owned (for profit). One-third of all hospitals are now part of multi-institutional chains or systems (American Hospital Association 1984a). However, hospital ownership is rarely integrated at the local level. Usually each hospital competes for patients with its neighbors—and competes for the goodwill of local physicians, who bring in the patients to each institution.

U.S. hospitals also draw their revenues from diverse sources. One of the marks of the operational independence of these institutions is that the source of their revenues is not generally available, public information. However, some idea of the mix of income can be derived from the aggregate national figures for all types and ownerships of hospitals, governmental and nongovernmental, general, psychiatric, and other special institutions. The single largest proportion of total hospital expenditures (33 percent in 1982) is paid by a mix of private health insurance schemes, including Blue Cross, commercial health insurance, health maintenance organizations, and other special insurance arrangements. Next come federal payments through Medicare (27 percent). State-run Medicaid programs constituted 9 percent of total hospital expenditures in 1982, while an array of other federal and state programs provided a further 18 percent. Patients contributed 12 percent, as direct, out-of-pocket payments. Philanthropy and other gifts represented less than 2 percent (Gibson, Waldo, and Levit 1983, 12).

These patterns show the following: (1) that most hospital income (88 percent) flows through private and governmental third parties rather than is purchased directly by patients at the time of need; (2) that, because there are many such third parties, hospital income is not "unified" or controlled by any one outside agency; (3) that government agencies, collectively, have a substantial stake in hospital financing, providing more than half of total hospital budgets nationwide, although there is a reluctance to define hospitals as quasi-public agencies; and (4) that, despite the fact that the great majority of admissions to community hospitals are to not-for-profit, voluntary hospitals, many of which were founded as charitable institutions, charity in the form of philanthropy has virtually vanished from the American scene.

Because there is no centralized control of hospitals or effective centralized control of their budgets, U.S. community hospitals are subject to a much wider variety of environments and influences than are hospitals in countries with government-sponsored national health care schemes. As a result, the long-term implications of recent changes are difficult, if not impossible, to assess, while short-term change is under constant criticism and appraisal.

Recent changes in the power and money relationships affecting U.S. hospitals include the following: (1) the growth of formal hospital systems (i.e., the linking together of not-for-profit hospitals into regional and national chains and the growth of investor-owned hospital systems); (2) the development of contract management of profit-making, not-for-profit, and government hospitals by profit-making companies; (3) diversification of the hospital's functions into new or neglected areas (surgicenters, home care, medical office buildings, parking lots) and corporate restructuring to facilitate such changes; (4) substantial long-term borrowing of capital in the financial marketplace through bonds and bank loans; (5) major modification of the method through which hospitals are paid for services given to patients covered by the federal Medicare program—from a retrospective, cost-plus reimbursement system to a prospective payment system, based on expected costs of treatment in one of 468 diagnosis-related groups (DRGs); (6) widespread enthusiasm for marketplace and managerial ideologies, under which competition among hospitals is seen as a more desirable goal than cooperation among them or merging of facilities at the local level; and (7) a phenomenal growth of hospital "experts"—in the legal aspects of corporate restructuring, the accounting advantages of floating a $100 million bond issue, the marketing needs for developing a hospital's market share, and the systems implications, hardware and software, that optimize insurance reimbursement levels. Hospitals are going through a managerial revolution.

Managers are rising in importance on the grounds of a monopoly of financial and organizational expertise. Where hospitals (not for profit or investor owned) are part of multihospital systems, management links also occur through coordination and consultation with other organizations in the system, thus further extending the manager's role in comparison with the role of hospital trustees and hospital physicians. Trustees are finding themselves ill prepared to cope with the constant changes and arcane intricacies of hospital financing. Physicians, for whom the hospital was for many years the "doctor's workshop," are concerned about increasing institutional specification of what doctors do (expressed in the standards set for cost and length of stay by DRGs and by the developing, government-funded Peer Review Organizations) and their future influence on hospital operations. Thus the internal authority of the hospital, as well as its external environment, is marked by uncertainty and stress.

These trends in hospital function, structure, and authority, all largely products of the last decade, have mutually reinforcing, cumulative effects. The speed of change alone, coupled with rising hospital costs, would justify widespread unease about the future of hospitals, now being expressed within hospital communities, among third parties, in congressional debates, and in the national press. But unease also arises out of the inconsistencies and ambiguities of hospital development. U.S. hospitals can be seen, at one and the same time, as a story of enormous organizational success and of social failure; as a dynamic, expanding industry and as a social service that, at enormous cost, fails to provide appropriate care to millions of Americans: notably, to the estimated 33 million who are uninsured but also to those with chronic diseases who may need much more than the hospital can give.

But in part, the uncertainties infusing present policy debates reflect the fact that the countervailing social value of hospital care is difficult to measure and subject to conflicting interpretations. Does the sheer size of the figures spent on hospital care in the United States paint the humanitarian impulses of a generous society? Or reflect excess and waste? Do the amounts suggest the commitment to science, technology, and expertise that distinguishes more general aspects of twentieth-century American culture? Are the hospitals, perhaps, necessary as social icons, to inspire pride, or invention in other fields? Are the high costs the results of an expanding industry, the hospital industry, which has been able, to an extraordinary degree, to set its own financial targets and to develop its own markets? Or are hospitals to be seen in terms of social failure, providing expensive, acute care facilities for those with serious chronic diseases, while ignoring services for chronic disease prevention? That arguments can be made for all of these positions, and that to some extent each is true, attests to the many meanings *hospital* has acquired in twentieth-century America.

At times of rapid change history is perhaps the most relevant of the social sciences to understanding the form, values, characteristics, and constraints of complex systems. Indeed, because hospitals are particularly responsive to their cultural, political, and financial environments, there is probably more to learn about the present by explaining the American past than by comparing U.S. with foreign hospitals in the 1980s. The next sections, therefore, look selectively at the rapid changes in U.S. hospitals that have characterized the history of this industry in the twentieth century, and at notions of "community responsibility" in particular. The focus then moves to the interrelations, in terms of policy, between past and present.

The Past Is Prologue

While hospitals for the poor and sick have existed since ancient times, the modern hospital is, in historical terms, a relatively recent institution. If two factors can be said to define it, they are the presence of round-the-clock skilled nurses and the ability to undertake major surgery. Neither was a general feature of U.S. hospitals until at least the 1880s. The first professional nursing schools, based on Florence Nightingale's precepts, were established in 1873 at Bellevue Hospital in New York, the New Haven Hospital, and the Massachusetts General Hospital. Others followed rapidly in the next decade. Many, if not most, of the new hospitals springing up in the burgeoning towns and cities of the late nineteenth century were predicated from the beginning on the integral development of the nursing schools. Through changes in nursing alone the hospital was transformed from the often filthy, disorganized, and terrifying older institutions of the early 1870s into a monument to hope, science, and

efficiency (Rosenberg 1978; Stevens 1984). Total national expenditures on hospital operations for tax-supported and voluntary hospitals in 1903 were estimated as at least $28.2 million; of this amount, 43 percent came from patients, 8 percent from tax funds, and the remainder from charitable donations and endowments (U.S. Bureau of the Census 1905, 23). Already, then, American hospitals were mixed institutions, only partly charitable, increasingly selling their services for a fee. By the mid-1920s the middle class were using hospitals not only for serious surgery but also for obstetrics, tonsillectomies, and appendectomies.

Coincidentally and in connection, medical science was transformed through two concurrent movements between 1880 and 1914, with lasting effects to the present. The first was the professionalization of U.S. physicians, the second the discovery and acceptance of the germ theory, giving medicine the confidence that its major justification as a profession was its scientific base. By the late 1880s, when aseptic techniques were replacing antisepsis in the operating rooms and in the dressings given on the wards, the idea that disease was borne by specific microscopic organisms that could be identified, avoided, and destroyed and, more generally, that disease could be explained, was on the way to revolutionizing the intellectual outlook and practical applications of modern medicine. Surgeons began to wear white gowns in the 1880s. Nurses and other hospital staffs wore uniforms, suggesting not only cleanliness but specialized roles and organizational rituals. Beds were lined up with military precision, sheets folded into knife-edges. Even before World War I there were complaints that the needs of patients as individuals were being subsumed to the demands of hospital organization (Addams 1907), a process that would later be called "depersonalization." Patients, beneficiaries and prisoners of medical expertise, were expected to conform cooperatively and passively to the cultural expectations of the institution.

Surgery became—and has remained—the heart of the U.S. hospital, the most obvious evidence of medicine's success, and an emblem of twentieth-century American values: science, know-how, the willingness to take risks (on the part of both doctors and patients), decisiveness, organization, and invention. Samuel Gross, the famous Philadelphia surgeon, expressed the drama of surgery in the 1880s in words that could be applied to any decade since: "Progress stares us everywhere in the face. The surgical profession was never so busy as it is at the present moment; never so fruitful in great and beneficent results, or in bold and daring exploits. . . . Operative surgery challenges the respect and admiration of the world" (Gross 1883).

Because of the time period during which the American hospital developed as a modern institution—largely between 1870 and 1914—the hospital assumed an unusually important function as the embodiment of cultural aspirations. It served both as a modern and an ideal institution, symbolizing the wealth of the new and expanding U.S. cities, the order and glamour of science, the happy conjunction between humanitarianism and expertise in a society rife with money-making. It is not coincidental that U.S. hospitals have been among the most luxurious and costly structures ever built. A writer on the New York Hospital for *Harpers Magazine* in 1878 described its elevator, which was larger than those of a fashionable hotel, as so smooth in motion that it was like "a mechanical means of getting to heaven" ("Hospital Life in New York" 1878, 176).

Demonstration or "show," even conspicuous waste, became a lasting aspect of the U.S. hospital as symbol, one that has as yet received too little attention by social scientists, and one obvious cause of its increasing costs. That the modern U.S. hospital is a monument, symbolizing in its architecture and equipment more than its basic function, is apparent not only in the historical literature but in the lavish style of buildings erected even in time of depression (e.g., by the WPA in the 1930s). Another example can be drawn from the early 1960s, when there was enormous public concern about the poor hospital care available in run-down hospitals in inner-city areas. The solutions sought were for rebuilding and major renovating, rather than for the kind of "making do" in drafty basements that has been a continuing characteristic of the British scene. Today's hospitals, despite concern about the massive costs of hospital care, are among the most modern, high-technology, costly structures being built in modern America. They continue to speak, subtly, to an implied link between cost and expertise.

The hospital also came to symbolize medicine as a vehicle of precision and control. Mastery of diagnosis (understanding the causes and progression of disease) gives a comforting illusion of control to both doctors and patients, even where little effective treatment is available—and for most nonsurgical conditions there was little effective treatment, except good nursing techniques, until the advent of the sulfa drugs in the 1930s and the antibiotics after World War II. The promise of surgery and of specific remedies against infectious diseases, inherent in major discoveries before World War I, consolidated the image of the doctor as a hero fighting disease with twentieth-century tools. The increasing subdivision of medicine into specialties after World War I carried forward this image by placing the greatest emphasis, in terms of prestige and income, on the most heroic interventions. Thus neurosurgery carried greater prestige than psychiatry; radiotherapy than pediatrics.

As a projection of a profession whose archetypes were control, daring, and entrepreneurship, the twentieth-century U.S. hospital (in parallel with the medical schools) was always ill suited to deal with chronic diseases, where causes were multifactorial and medical success was often problematical, and with the collective realms of public health. Even before World War I, the hospital could be criticized for tending to view itself merely from the inside; that is, from the self-generated perceptions of its board of trustees and its physicians. It followed that the hospital did "not feel itself an intimate part of the social order; it stands forbiddingly isolated and aloof" (Goldstein 1907, 160–161). That the potential existed, in theory at least, for the hospital to provide health services to the whole population in a defined service district, to compile epidemiological statistics, to offer public health education and maternal and child welfare clinics, and to deal with the patient's family as well as with the patient would become a source of irritation to generations of disappointed critics.

The success and visibility of the hospital in providing acute, specialized care obscured its relatively limited role in the overall picture of health and disease. Nevertheless, the hospital could be described by the 1920s, as later, as an expression of pessimism, a "negative instrument of evolution," somewhat akin to refuse and sewage disposal, in that it dealt with problems of society rather than in positive solutions (Meyer 1919, 17). Social work departments were started in leading hospitals, following the example at the Massachusetts General Hospital in 1905, in the belief that such departments would help to eradicate the widely held notion that the hospital was an impersonal institution and to elucidate the social causes of disease (Cannon 1913). However, there were at least three reasons why social service failed to become the core of community health care efforts: (1) the concentration of social service work on the poor, who attended outpatient departments with such socially unappealing conditions as venereal diseases, unmarried motherhood, and tuberculosis; (2) the lack of fees for social work, making it dependent on charity and on cost shifting from the hospital's paying patients; and (3) the lack of power and the desire by social workers themselves to become a clinical profession, on the medical model, dealing with the psychosocial symptoms of individual patients rather than with community service needs.

Meanwhile, U.S. hospitals became successful at marketing acute services to paying patients. Public relations became an acceptable aspect of hospital management in the 1920s, with hospital fairs, radio spots, and even movies extolling the virtues of hospital care. Even in the depths of the depression of the 1930s—with enormous pressures put on local government hospitals, as the unemployed sought free medical care, together with the closing of hundreds of small institutions—the majority of income to the hospital industry came from patient fees. In not-for-profit hospitals, the standard bearers for hospital quality in the United States, 71 percent of hospital income in 1935 came from patients (Pennell, Mountin, and Pearson 1939, 22). The development of Blue Cross insurance schemes in the 1930s, commercial hospital insurance in the 1940s, and Medicare in the mid-1960s buttressed the idea of hospital care as acute services, while increasing hospital income. None of these schemes typically included out-of-hospital diagnosis, preventive services, education, or social services whereby hospitals could reach out to the community as comprehensive health care centers. There were thus no financial incentives to override the heroic, specialized medical model for hospital care.

U.S. Hospitals and Their Communities

Besides the emerging character of the U.S. hospital as an acute facility, thriving in a market for paying patients and orienting itself both to a broader vision of the medical profession and to a money = value nexus, the hospital acquired ascribed values whose properties were largely mythological—and not the less powerful, for that. One of the most potent of these values was (and is) the idea of "community." Nonfederal acute hospitals are termed "community hospitals" by the American Hospital Association, irrespective of their location, size, or level of care, and the term appears to be idiosyncratically American.

Two initial points can readily be made about the notion of the community hospital. First, since hospitals are not community *health* centers, the term has an ironic ambiguity right from the beginning. Second, the word *community*, like the word *voluntary* (long applied to not-for-profit hospitals) has emotive power in a much larger social and political context than the hospital field. Community flexibility stands in contrast to state or national standard-setting, voluntary activity against the implied rigidity of government intervention. In the United States, *community* suggests creative, local, private activities, such as volunteer fire departments, school boards, or the PTA; they are part of American cultural tradition. Part of the attachment of the word *community* to hospitals thus reflects vague assumptions of the public good. Yet, in three specific ways U.S. hospitals have traditionally had strong community affiliations. First, hospitals have traditionally served communities of interest within local power structures. Second, hospitals have been an important part of the hierarchical organization of the medical profession. Third, hospitals have provided centers for education, employment, and voluntary work for community residents. The combined effect of these patterns has been to define, further, the U.S. hospital as "American."

As major expressions of charitable, social, and economic interests, the hospitals that developed in the late-nineteenth and into the twentieth century reflected the segmentation of U.S. society into diverse ethnic, religious, and occupational groups, and into defined social classes. Hospitals were both a concrete expression of solidarity and a training ground for nurses and doctors in groups likely to be excluded from other institutions (notably, Jewish and black physicians and black nurses). Thus they represented both community successes and community failures. By 1920 the United States was dotted with hospitals run by hundreds of different private associations, including Roman Catholics, Lutherans, Methodists, Episcopalians, Southern Baptists, Jews, blacks, Swedes, and Germans, depending on the power structures of local populations. Philadelphia, for example, in 1923 had seventy-one hospitals, general and specialized (US Bureau of the Census 1925, 29); it now has seventy-two. Most were run by not-for-profit associations. Their varied social origins were apparent in

names such as Hospital of the University of Pennsylvania (for teaching), Jewish Hospital of Philadelphia, St. Mary's (Roman Catholic), Methodist Episcopal, Frederick Douglass (founded by the black community), and Lankenau (originally a German hospital, the name was changed because of World War I).

In many areas local governments developed hospitals out of their poorhouses for the indigent. These hospitals, like hospitals under not-for-profit auspices, ranged from tiny units of twenty-five beds or less to enormous barrackslike institutions. (Philadelphia General Hospital, run by the city, reported two thousand beds in the early 1920s.) Railroads, lumber companies, and occasionally other corporations built hospitals for their employees. For example, in the first decade of the century the Santa Fe Railroad, which ran from Chicago to Houston and Galveston, and from Santa Fe to San Francisco, could report emergency hospitals for accidents at all its major repair and service centers, supported by monthly contributions from employees (Going 1909, 117).

The federal government operated a string of hospitals in seaports and on the major rivers, to care for sick and injured merchant seamen; it also developed veterans hospitals after World War I, while army hospitals served U.S. camps and forts. Meanwhile, an uncounted army of physicians opened their own small hospitals to serve their paying patients, technically on a profit-making basis. In short, U.S. hospitals rose concurrently as diverse and multipurpose institutions, serving different clienteles, with different communities of interest and with a distinctive set of social meanings.

Reflecting patterns of social stratification and discrimination in their local communities, the new hospitals of the early twentieth century were rarely "community hospitals" in the sense of serving the entire population on an equal basis, even for inpatient care. The city and county hospitals, such as Philadelphia General, Bellevue or Kings County in New York, Cook County in Chicago, or San Francisco General, which developed from the old poorhouses, remained institutions primarily for the very poor. When governmental or voluntary hospitals accepted private patients, they were typically housed in separate buildings and in well-furnished private rooms rather than in wards. These patients ate better food, cooked in separate kitchens, and had less restricted visiting hours. Indigence continued to carry the heavy weight of social stigma, even as hospitals were medicalized around progressive scientific ideas.

Until well after World War II, major differences in the patterns of disease treated by public and not-for-profit city hospitals added to the sense of social distinctions. Cleveland City Hospital (with 785 beds) was excluded from a major survey of hospitals in Cleveland in the early 1920s because it treated large groups of patients with tuberculosis, alcoholism, venereal diseases, and contagious diseases. Patients with these illnesses were not accepted at any other hospital in the area (Cleveland Hospital Council 1920, 831). Cook County was criticized in the late 1930s, as it has been

since, for its poor physical surroundings, overcrowded waiting rooms, patients lying on stretchers in corridors, machinery that did not work, and shortages of even common equipment (Dowling 1982, 145). In short, American hospitals have never, as a group, served as egalitarian forces in the culture as a whole.

Mirroring the diversity of community structure across the United States, enormous variations continue to be found in the relative roles of tax-supported, voluntary, and profit-making hospitals from place to place. In a settled city like Philadelphia, class differences could be seen even between the poor patients admitted to the Pennsylvania Hospital ("respectable," "deserving" poor) and the city hospital, dumping ground for all the rest. However small governmental hospitals in counties where there was only one hospital probably always behaved similarly to not-for-profit or profit-making institutions in the same circumstances—taking in all social classes, with income from paying patients representing the great majority of their budgets. Such an observation suggests that control of the hospital may be less important as a distinguishing factor of U.S. institutions than segmentation of hospital services across diverse social groups. In short, the important variable, for social policy purposes, is not stratification by ownership but stratification by clientele, a direct reflection of "community."

In the 1980s, as in the 1950s and earlier, relatively homogeneous communities (e.g., in rural areas or suburbs) are likely to produce more homogeneous institutions, with less social distance between patients and between staff and patients than, for example, a major city teaching hospital which may attract two opposite kinds of patients, the relatively rich on its boards and committees and as private patients of leading physicians and the very poor, traditional recipients of charity care (see Burling, Lentz, and Wilson 1956). Such differences obviously shape differing institutional personalities and add to the diversity among hospitals in the United States. The differences have also been sharpened recently, at least in perception, by the location of investor-owned hospitals in relatively homogeneous (middle-class) areas, suggesting that ownership and social class are necessarily correlated, and by the lack of funding for indigent patients.

The passage of Medicare (for the elderly and disabled) and Medicaid (for the indigent) in 1965, in a brief period of egalitarianism, was to indicate that, at least for a short time, everyone, rich and poor, young and old, was to be given similar if not identical hospital treatment. But the power of community patterns, as well as cutbacks in Medicaid, were to prove such optimism unrealistic and short-lived. In retrospect, the egalitarian expectations for Medicaid appear as an aberration in a long history of class discrimination in hospital care in the United States. Financially tottering city and county hospitals remain the dumping ground for patients no one else will take.

The focus on competition and managerialism of the 1970s through the 1980s has added a new dimension to the diversity of hospital care across different communities and classes by sanctioning, on business grounds, the refusal of hospitals to serve patients who cannot pay (either directly or through insurance, Medicare, or Medicaid). For example, in Pensacola, Florida, the city turned over the management of its hospital to a profit-making organization in the 1970s, closed its emergency room, and opened a fee-paying ambulatory center instead. Hospitals can indeed be seen as community institutions, in the broadest sense, reflecting the patterns and priorities of the societies in which they are based—both at the local and national levels.

At the same time, the "community" for many hospital purposes has expanded beyond the local area, to national and state programs and national consensus-building. Physicians, through the American College of Surgeons, launched a major movement in 1917–1918 to "standardize" hospitals around national norms and expectations—the beginnings of hospital accreditation. As Blue Cross schemes developed after the 1930s into statewide programs, the definition of hospital care for reimbursement purposes was extended beyond the town or city. Statewide planning of hospital care was initiated at the time of the Hill-Burton Act (1946), stimulated by federal construction monies provided to the states under that program, and further developed through the federal health planning program in the 1960s and 1970s, and through state certificate-of-need legislation. Meanwhile, Medicare provided the force of national regulation and national expectations, while allowing for substantial local service variations. The diagnosis-related group (DRG) program can be seen as an extension of national standard-setting through attempts to define and standardize courses of hospital treatment across the United States, for Medicare patients at least.

The courts have also played a role in defining national community norms, whether through asserting hospitals' responsibility for the quality of their medical care, requiring racial desegregation, or providing definitions of life and death. In these examples, the term *community* can be seen as divisible into questions of community service, community control, and community consensus. However *community* remains a vague concept at best, a cherished aim with ambiguous meanings, something constantly to be sought but never to be fully achieved. Its strength lies, perhaps, in its idea that something should be done at the local level. In this sense the present development of local health care coalitions (of businesses, other groups, or some combination) can be seen as continuation of a traditional theme.

Meanwhile the development of competing hospital systems sets up new forms of segmentation of hospital service at the local level, threatening the idea of the hospital as part of its local community power structure, or structures. In addition, the visibility of groups other than boards of trustees, physicians, and administrators is changing the broader power structure of hospital care. Stockbrokers, fringe benefit managers, business leaders, self-help groups, and unions also have legitimate, often powerful roles to play in hospital de-

velopment. A forty-seven-day strike against thirty hospitals and fifteen nursing homes in New York City in the summer of 1984 affected 18,000 patients and 52,000 workers ("Hospital Walkout Ends" 1984). A single bond issue can lock a hospital into a pattern of fiscal operation for thirty years, whatever its pattern of ownership may be. The activity of major purchasers of stocks and bonds, including pension funds and insurance companies, affects the availability of capital for hospital development.

In these and other examples, there is a growing army of new "communities," that is, vested interests, with diverse purposes, in constant conflict. The idea of a hospital as the embodiment of medical expertise has given way to the exercise of monopoly power by numerous groups. Hospital management and planning become the outcome of a continuing process of bargaining, negotiation, and consensus building among differing points of view, both inside and outside the institution.

The relationship of the community of doctors to hospitals has also been marked by ambiguity. In comparison with hospitals in most other countries, U.S. physicians have had—and still largely have—a peculiar relationship to medicine's major institution. The typical U.S. physician remains in private, fee-for-service practice, working independently or as a member of a physician group. When the modern hospital developed in the United States, local fee-for-service practitioners volunteered their services in the hospitals, serving charity patients without charging them a fee. The medical profession became, in effect, a volunteer attending staff, since the doctors who admitted patients (and were thus crucial to the financial viability of the hospital with respect to admitting private paying patients) were not employees of the institution. Indeed, from the hospital's point of view, the physician could be seen as a guest of the institution. In contrast, to the physician the hospital was an extension of his or her private practice of medicine.

American hospitals have also developed in large part as "open staff" institutions, that is, with the expectation that all qualified physicians in a given field ought to have appointments on the attending staff of local institutions. The great majority of all physicians had some kind of hospital attachment by the late 1920s, a pattern that has continued since. Indeed, hospital affiliations have been necessary for many of the most specialized fields. The relationship between physicians and hospitals is sharply distinguished in the United States, for example, from the system in Britain where only salaried specialists typically have hospital affiliations. Although there has been a rapid increase in the number of salaried hospital physicians in U.S. hospitals in the last decade, the formal separation of doctors and hospitals largely continues, requiring new readjustments as hospitals become part of competing systems.

Past and Present

What emerges out of a review of U.S. hospital history is a set of culture-specific characteristics that mark the hospitals as American institutions. These include the segmentation and diversity of ownership of hospitals, the division between hospitals and the medical profession (a division echoed in the separate development of hospital insurance and medical insurance in the United States), the acceptance of social stratification of the patient population both among hospitals and within different institutions, the pervasiveness of the pay or commodity ethos in U.S. medicine, and the general expectation that the role of government is necessary but should be limited to filling in gaps in medical care (through programs such as Medicare or Medicaid) and in providing an atmosphere conducive to the development of services in the private sector.

More generally, the fundamental values attached to the hospital industry and its power structures — its communities of interest — are marked by ambiguity. Strauss and his colleagues observed, of a single hospital in the 1950s, that because its overall goals were unclear, goals were constantly being negotiated within the established orders of the institution (Strauss et al. 1963). It is useful, in the 1980s, to think of this process of goal negotiation as an intrinsic, continuing element of the national hospital system.

Over and above these general observations, three specific themes mark the continuation of hospital history from past to present. First, U.S. hospitals remain segmented in their interests, communities, and control. Second, decision making continues to be diversified — that is, diffused over communities of interest, ranging from the health professions to individual hospital boards, corporate headquarters, government programs, and major purchasers of hospital insurance. Third, American hospitals are expert at adapting very rapidly to explicit external incentives, usually financial incentives.

Where social needs are made explicit—for example, in civil rights legislation or the passage of Medicare—U.S. hospitals are socially responsive institutions. Where there is ambivalence or apathy—for example, in providing medical care to the homeless, uninsured, or indigent—hospitals look to other institutions (notably to government) to meet such needs, disclaiming the responsibility of being "public" institutions. In this respect, too, hospitals can be seen as socially responsive, that is, as reflecting the messages from the broader culture in which they are based. Lacking a unified hospital or health system, and lacking consensus about the appropriate philosophy for a U.S. welfare state, U.S. health policy is marked by skittishness and change.

In the absence of consensus, decisions about hospital policy have been left to the jockeying of influence among communities of interest. Part of the uneasiness about high costs and increased profit making in hospital care derives from a perceived need to develop national consensus about hospital policy without resorting either to a government-dominated health care system or to one dominated by a few massive corporations. A high-cost system is the trade-off for avoiding either of these two extremes. The present system allows for organizational experiment and di-

versity, for avoidance of draconic management decisions (the specter of "rationing") and overt limitations of care for middle-class Americans, and for accommodation of conflict among reasonable but opposing points of view. In this sense the hospital system can be described in terms of "constructive ambiguity."

To those struggling with their implications, rapid changes cry out for simple theories of explanation and simple solutions. DRGs became the solution to the rising cost of hospital care in the 1980s, just as Medicaid was the apparent answer, in the late 1960s, to bringing the poor into the "mainstream of medicine." Alternatively, the hospital system can be seen as analogous to the development of other industries—for example, consolidation of the manufacturing industry at the beginning of the twentieth century, which again followed the consolidation of the railroads. Under this model, hospitals are small firms that will inevitably move toward industrial consolidation (and that have, perhaps, been held back by the monopoly interests of the medical profession). However, such analogies beg the question of whether hospitals are legitimately "businesses," and, if so, what this definition means. How far hospital service is an appropriate comparison to manufacturing is another question that demands elucidation—indeed, whether any service industry can be appropriately compared to any manufacturing industry. The urge for simple explanations remains. Meanwhile, there are those who claim that profit making in health services is ethically wrong and socially dangerous; others are more concerned that medicine is rapidly being dominated by a "medical-industrial complex" in which the traditional rights of doctors and patients will be swamped by the coming of the monolithic "corporation" (Relman 1980; Starr 1982).

However, the search for simple theories and the "one best way" of doing things ignores the obvious, that organizational life in the late twentieth century is messy and complex. Decisions have to be made in a climate of conflict and negotiation, whether one is speaking of hospitals, factories, government, or schools—and hospitals, like other institutions, carry with them the burdens and potential of their history.

The history of hospitals in the United States in the twentieth century, at least up to the 1970s, assumed that hospital care is an unalloyed social good, that hospitals represented an expanding industry, ever more successful in what it was doing, and that this industry would create surpluses not deficits. Such premises have been critically tested in hospitals serving large numbers of poverty patients, notably local government hospitals in large cities and hospitals attached to medical schools. Instead, the premises have been carried over into the investor-owned hospital sector, which has become in many ways the logical outcome of a system that has assumed that hospital services are not social services (to be shared out, like public education, across the whole population) but services bought and sold in the marketplace. The implantation of the artificial heart is an American phenomenon: heroic medicine in a profit-making setting. There is—at least as yet—no new public health ethos on which consensus based on a social service role for U.S. hospitals could be developed—or that could be set against the prevailing profit-making ethos of the 1980s. It is this debate that is now taking place. Indeed, we may see, in the 1990s, a renewed social commitment to "mainstream medicine."

Meanwhile, the rise of investor-owned corporations and the rise of hospital systems since the mid-1970s have created new patterns of segmentation and diversity within the hospital industry. Beside the development of major investor-owned hospital chains, such as Hospital Corporation of America, the not-for-profit hospitals have banded together through mergers and, more widely, in mutually supportive alliances. The largest of the alliances, Voluntary Hospitals of America, serves 250 health care institutions, with combined revenues of $7 billion. Such systems provide hospitals with joint purchasing arrangements, the ability to raise capital, consultants, and expertise, joint ventures among hospitals and between hospitals and groups of physicians, and, not least, a vehicle for lobbying on the national scene.

In turn, the alliances provide policy challenges for hospitals not included in such groups, notably university and other teaching hospitals, municipal hospitals, and other government institutions. University teaching hospitals have set up their own voluntary alliance to stake their claims with respect to reimbursement for medical teaching, for the additional costs associated with teaching and with the superspecialized care given in university hospitals, and for the relatively large proportion of Medicaid patients these hospitals see. A challenge for the teaching hospitals, in general, is to maintain their credibility as educational institutions by continuing to stimulate clinical research in a market where there may be little financial incentive to do so.

Meanwhile, local government hospitals are under siege, financially and in terms of their social justification, and veterans hospitals are a focus for potential cutbacks. Logically, in a hospital system relying almost entirely on third-party reimbursement, the government-owned hospital is not strictly necessary—assuming that all members of the population are covered adequately by third-party payment mechanisms, private or governmental. Indeed, it can be argued that the type of ownership of any hospital (investor-owned, voluntary, governmental) is immaterial in a system controlled largely through third-party reimbursement. It follows (1) that national hospital policy will continue to be made most forcefully through the controls exerted on health insurance packages and hospital reimbursement practices and constraints; (2) that present concerns about investor ownership of hospitals may be overstated; and (3) that competition among different types of hospitals will be most effective where third-party reimbursement is standardized over hospitals of all types, for example, through increased national control over health insurance as a whole.

All of these observations assume that hospital insurance is available to the whole population—and in the 1980s this is clearly not the case. The need to provide hospital care to the uninsured and to provide adequate reimbursement for Medicaid patients are the single most important questions of hospital policy in the next decade. This is so, not merely on grounds of social conscience or humanitarianism. It is also essential for the continuation of the pluralistic, competitive structure of hospital care in the United States.

Without such measures the hospital industry will become more rapidly segmented and stratified by economic class, with investor-owned hospitals drawing a relatively prosperous clientele, voluntary hospitals behaving (as far as possible) the same way, and local government hospitals retrenching or becoming increasingly financially stressed, each type of hospital reluctant to deal with hospital care for the poorest members of the population, who may need such care the most. In the process all hospitals will lose face. For-profit hospitals run the risk of being labeled hard-hearted and self-serving. Voluntary hospitals lose whatever cachet still attaches to their historical role of public, charitable institutions. Government hospitals revert to their ancient almshouse functions.

In the short run a major challenge for the investor-owned chains is to demonstrate their public-spirited interests, through the establishment of "flagship" hospitals affiliated with major universities and through the development of community boards at the local level. A major challenge for the voluntary hospital chains is to demonstrate, at one and the same time, their management efficiency and competitiveness vis-à-vis investor-owned systems and to define what, if any, image they wish to project by being "voluntary" or "not-for-profit" institutions. Such hospitals have, so far, gone little further than to talk vaguely about a "special mission." Yet it is quite possible that voluntary hospitals, as a group, will find it to their advantage, in the future, to differentiate themselves more clearly in the political arena from profit-making institutions. If, for example, investment dollars are shifted from hospitals to other growth industries, with concurrent public disillusion with the ethos of profit making, voluntary hospitals can then claim their long, historical "public" role, irrespective of their present behavior as profit-making entities.

Because of the segmentation of control in the hospital industry, the diffusion of decision making, and the uncertainty as to future reimbursement methods, the future shape of the American hospital system is impossible to predict. Possible "futures" include a system of hospitals dominated by fifteen or twenty major national chains, for profit and not for profit; the general expansion of hospitals, through diversification, into health care conglomerates, offering a wide range of services, not necessarily on the same site; a sudden shift of investment out of profit-making hospitals, following a tightening of reimbursement levels and increased government regulation, with such hospitals reorganized as, or merged with, not-for-profit institutions; a shift in the general political rhetoric from "competition" to "cooperation," accompanied by stringent hospital planning at the local level; a general "sizing down" of the hospital industry, under pressure from private and public payers, with relatively more money going to preventive care, consumer education, treatment in doctors' offices, at home, and in other kinds of institutions; the introduction of a comprehensive national health insurance or health care system; or a continuation—even an exaggeration—of expansion and diversity, whereby large chains will co-exist with large individual hospitals and small-scale independent institutions and there will continue to be profit-making, voluntary, and government ownership, with shifting alliances among segments of the different groups. I think the latter is the most likely development.

The power of physicians vis-à-vis hospitals will probably increase in the next decades. Hospital medical staffs will become more highly organized in terms of management and policy decisions, through the establishment of full-time medical directors, executive committees, or inner circles of physicians who have major commitments to single institutions—for example, via hospital-based physician offices or joint, risk-sharing ventures. At the same time the division of physicians into competing groups, with different organizational affiliations, promises a growing conflict of interests within the profession.

The role of government agencies throughout the twentieth century has been to support the prosperity of private institutions rather than to develop government programs as an alternative endeavor. Although it has become clear that private organizations have interests that may not be compatible with national goals (including expanding markets, high overall costs, and the exclusion of those unable to pay), the overall philosophy is too entrenched for major change, absent a major national breakdown in hospital provision for middle-class Americans. U.S. government agencies will continue to exert their influence primarily through detailed regulation and standard setting. In the short term the poor will be taken care of in American hospitals through a mix of methods: through Medicaid, through special taxes for the poor in some states, through local coalitions of hospitals, through foundation efforts, and through continuing charity by those institutions that can afford it. In the long run only government, directly (through institutional subsidy or programs such as Medicaid) or indirectly (through regulation requiring charity care, or enabling legislation for shifts of funds and internal subsidies to care for the poor within private systems) can shoulder the costs for those who are otherwise unable to pay. Thus a balancing act between private and public financing will continue to be an intrinsic element of the U.S. system.

All systems have their strengths and weaknesses, and it is easier to point to weaknesses than strengths. However two final, general points need to be made about the in-built resilience of the U.S. system. The first is the constructive role of ambiguity, which allows for rapid adaptation and change in the hospital system and its power structures. The second is the dynamic force of the hospitals' many communities of interest, from local health care coalitions to new national lobbying groups. The institution known as a "hospital" may change radically in the next decades. Yet the hospital system has a long history of organizational success. Hospital policies will continue to be constantly renegotiated.

Acknowledgments

This paper, part of a larger study of the history of U.S. general hospitals in the twentieth century, is supported by the Commonwealth Fund, by research grant 5-ROI-LMO3849 from the National Library of Medicine, and—in academic year 1984–1985—by a Guggenheim Fellowship.

Note

1. By *community general hospital* I mean those hospitals included by the American Hospital Assocation under the term *nonfederal short-term general and other special*. Important changes are also taking place in psychiatric hospi-

tals and, to a lesser extent, in hospitals for rehabilitation services, but these are subjects outside the scope of this chapter.

References

Addams, J. 1907. The layman's view of hospital work among the poor. In *Transactions of the American Hospital Association*, pp. 57–63. Chicago: American Hospital Association.

American Hospital Association. 1984a. *Directory of multihospital systems.* 4th ed. Chicago: American Hospital Publishing.

———. 1984b. *Hospital statistics.* Data from the American Hospital Association 1983 Annual Survey. Chicago: American Hospital Association.

Burling, T., E. M. Lentz, and R. N. Wilson. 1956. The give and take in hospitals: A study of human organization in hospitals. New York: Putnam.

Cannon, I. 1913. *Social work in hospitals: A contribution to progressive medicine.* New York: Russell Sage Foundation.

Cleveland Hospital Council. 1920. *Cleveland hospital and health survey.* Cleveland: Cleveland Hospital Council.

Dowling, H. F. 1982. *City hospitals: The undercare of the underprivileged.* Cambridge: Harvard University Press.

Gibson, R. M., D. R. Waldo, and K. R. Levit. 1983. National health expenditures, 1982. *Health Care Financing Review* 5(1):1–31.

Going, C. B. 1909. *Methods of the Santa Fe: Efficiency in the manufacture of transportation.* New York: Reprinted from *Engineering Magazine.* March–July 1909.

Goldstein, S. 1907. The social function of the hospital. *Charities and the Commons* 18:160–166.

Gross, S. D. 1883. Address of Welcome. *Transactions of the American Surgical Association* 1: xxii.

Hospital Life in New York. 1878. *Harper's New Monthly Magazine*, pp. 171–189.

Hospital walkout ends as the union cites vote results. 1984. *New York Times,* August 29.

Meyer, E. C. 1919. Relative value of hospitals and dispensaries as public-health agencies and as fields of activity for the Rockefeller Foundation. New York: Rockefeller Foundation, International Health Board.

Pennell, E. H., J. W. Mountin, and K. Pearson. 1939. Business census of hospitals, 1935: General Report. Supplement No. 154 to the *Public Health Reports.* Public Health Service. Washington, D.C.: Government Printing Office.

Relman, A. 1980. The new medical-industrial complex. *New England Journal of Medicine* 303:963–970.

Rosenberg, C. 1978. Inward vision and outward glance: The shaping of the American hospital, 1880–1914. *Bulletin of the History of Medicine* 53: 346–395.

Starr, P. 1982. *The social transformation of American medicine.* New York: Basic Books.

Stevens, R. 1984. Sweet charity: State aid to hospitals in Pennsylvania, 1880–1910. *Bulletin of the History of Medicine* 58:287–314, 474–495.

Strauss, A., L. Schatzman, D. Ehrlich, R. Bucher, and M. Sabshin. 1963. The hospital and its negotiated order. In *The hospital in modern society*, ed. E. Freidson, pp. 147–169. London: Free Press.

U.S. Bureau of the Census. 1905. *Benevolent institutions, 1904.* Washington, D.C.: Government Printing Office.

———. 1925. *Hospitals and dispensaries, 1923.* Washington, D.C.: Government Printing Office.

Chapter 6

Two Views of a Changing Health Care System

Drew E. Altman

It is difficult to pick up a health care publication these days without reading about diagnosis-related groups and other new payment arrangements, the shifting of care from inpatient to ambulatory settings, the diversification of the hospital industry, and other important parameters of a changing health care delivery system. These developments are themselves products of broader forces that have been shaping the evolution of American health care—among them the aging of our population, advances in medical science and medical technology, substantial increases in the number of physicians, and a variety of increasingly aggressive efforts to control health care costs. Suffice it to say that in U.S. health care today there is a perception of rapid if not dramatic change and some considerable apprehension about the impact that change will have.

This perception is understandable. The changes that are occuring will have important implications for health professionals and health care institutions. The nature of hospital care and medical practice as well as individual institutional and personal futures are at stake. But how quickly and to what extent are these developments affecting the general public? Are they significantly altering the outcomes of our health system, and with what effects?

In thinking about this question, consider the analogy of the airline industry, another sector of our economy seemingly in a state of transformation. Since deregulation, the view from inside the airline industry must be one of very significant change. Airlines are going out of business; new carriers are entering the market; new products are being developed and sold; and prices, it would appear, are in a constant state of flux. Yet when viewed from the outside, only three factors are of major concern to most people. These are: Will air travel cost the customer more or will costs be reduced? Will Americans be able to get the services they want? And will there be any adverse impact on air traffic safety and on people's lives?

These, too, are the fundamental concerns most people will have about the changes now occurring in our health care system. What impact will they have on health care costs? Will people be able to get the health services they want and feel they need? Will there be any adverse impact on people's health? The answers to these questions are not merely of academic interest, they will be important to the way in which health policy unfolds in the coming years and to the impact change in our health care system has on different groups in our society.

Unless the many changes occurring in health care are perceived to significantly affect these major outcomes, most individuals and public and private leaders in our country will be prepared to be relatively neutral about them (Key 1961). As a result, decisions about the shape of our health care system in the future will be dominated by interest groups and experts with a direct stake in the outcome, principally those who pay for and those who provide health services (Truman 1951). Health policy, like, say, trade policy, will unfold primarily as a political contest between inside groups. The changes that occur, though vital to these inside groups, are likely to be incremental in nature —nowhere as significant, for example, as the passage of Medicare and Medicaid—and their societal impact hard to measure at any one point (Lindblom 1970). Moreover, major institutional and professional interest groups with expertise and organization are likely to dominate the policymaking process. Others—for example, low-income groups—will be heard less often and will have less impact (Dahl 1956). In contrast, if effects in these areas are perceived as major, the public, the media, and our highest political and private leaders will be regularly involved in the debate. Bigger changes in direction will be possible, and the policy process will be opened up to many more groups (Jones 1975).

Which of these scenarios best fits American health care today? Certainly, inside the health care field there is a perception of rapid and significant change. But another view is possible. What looks so dramatic to insiders may appear less significant to those without a personal, institutional, or professional stake in our health care system. Consider the perspective of a senior representative of the Office of the Speaker of the House when discussing the new Medicare DRG payment system. The Medicare DRGs have been widely heralded as the most significant change in health care finance in almost twenty years. "This year," he said, "I predict we will see further technical and regulatory changes and fixes similar to last year when we passed the DRGs." When asked how a hospital administrator's revolution could be viewed from the Speaker's chair as a technical fix, he elaborated. "You have to appreciate how we work and what our concerns are in the Congress. Less than twenty members really understand what DRGs are about. The others had no reason to learn because the lobbying groups were relatively quiet. These days, we deal with things in blocks and what we are principally concerned with are bottom-line deficit savings. Except for defense, we know that health care costs will continue to be the fastest rising item in the federal budget, despite the DRGs and other things. So where is the big change?"

To a health care person, these views may be hard to digest. It is indeed tempting to dismiss them as the casual remarks of one caught up in other issues and in the Washington scene. Yet they are actually quite consistent with the perspectives of others from "outside" the health care system who have systematically and objectively looked at such matters. For example, they are quite consistent with the thrust of what the social scientists have said about change in areas such as health.

One of the fundamental teachings of political science, for example, is that except in unusual circumstances, change in our country occurs very slowly and in small steps (Lindblom 1970). *Incrementalism* is the term of art. Only when we experience a major crisis or national problem, when there is consensus about what to do, and when the leadership emerges to harness these forces, do we see big swings in national policy. The passage of Social Security, the Civil Rights Act of 1964, Medicare and Medicaid, and the passage of landmark environmental legislation in 1970 are examples of this kind of sweeping policy change. But political scientists so lament the difficulties of achieving change of this magnitude in the domestic policy arena very often that Aaron Wildavsky has written of the United States's "two presidencies" — one in foreign policy, where it seems bolder moves can sometimes be made; and one in domestic policy, where what we mainly do is "muddle through" (Wildavsky 1966).

When we do somehow manage to enact major new policy or programs, the verdict from the social sciences is usually not very favorable. The literature on program implementation suggests that few programs work as planned. In fact, the conclusion of a major work on this topic is that even where new programs escape big problems, multiple little ones are likely to prove just as fatal (Pressman and Wildavsky 1973). Thus, seemingly major policy changes may have only minor impacts in practice. Likewise, much of the evaluative research on the impact of programs that are implemented suggest far less than their hoped-for effects.

Which perspective fits U.S. health care today? Are the changes occurring in our health care system truly fundamental or are they primarily an insider's concern? To answer these questions, let us focus on the major outcomes of a changing health care system, which will be of concern to most Americans—cost, access to health services, and the impact on people's health.

Costs

Current forecasts suggest that our health spending will continue to rise sharply over the next fifteen years. As a nation, we currently spend about $1 billion a day on health care; predictions are that we will spend $5 billion a day ($1.9 trillion per year and 14 percent of GNP) by the year 2000 (Blendon and Altman 1984, 613). Though recently the view that we are reversing these trends through DRGs and other measures appears to be gaining wide media play, such claims would seem to be exaggerated, or at a minimum premature. Between 1983 and 1984, annual growth in personal health spending did fall significantly, from 7 to 4.5 percent. But the 4.5 percent rate of increase in 1984 represented about the average real rate of increase over the last decade and did not approach the lowest rates of increase achieved between 1973 and 1974, and 1979 and 1980, of 2.5 and 2 percent respectively. Moreover, it would appear that success in reducing spending for hospital care is being offset substantially by spending in other areas. Real growth in hospital spending did fall to 2.5 percent in 1984 (approaching the low point for the decade of 2 percent in 1979), but real growth in all other health expenditures, including physician care, fell only slightly from the record levels for the decade set in 1983 of 7.5 per-

cent (Merrill 1985). Thus, there is little reason to conclude at this point that our spending will not continue to rise sharply as forecasted.

But if the forecasted numbers for health spending are alarming, they are not alarming in the same way to everyone. The problem of sharply rising health spending is mainly a concern for government, the largest single payer (now accounting for 42 percent of our health care bill), and also for U.S. business, which is becoming increasingly concerned about health care costs. If there is, in fact, a "crisis" in health care costs, it is primarily a payer's crisis, and primarily governmental.

What both government and business are worried about are their total expenditures for health care. For the federal government, the major federal expenditures for health—Medicare Part A (hospitals), Medicare Part B (physicians), and the federal share of Medicaid—represent the second, third, and fourth largest line items in the domestic federal budget and are among the fastest growing. The concern at the federal level is that these expenditures will crowd out other spending priorities, add to the deficit and impede economic growth, and increase the size of government, already viewed by the current administration as too large. For the states, the principal worry is with expenditures for Medicaid—for most states the second largest item in their budgets, and in recent years the fastest rising. Businesses' main concern is with the increasing percentage of the costs of operations that are claimed by employee health benefits. For most large companies, expenditures for health insurance represent the single largest payroll cost (between 6 and 8 percent of payroll) and the fastest rising (Sapolsky et al. 1981).

For state governments as well as business, however, concern for health spending is closely tied to the overall performance of the economy. Health spending is greatly heightened during periods of recession, when sharply rising health expenditures and declining tax revenues and profits make it much more difficult to balance a state budget or turn a profit. In addition, businesses facing stiff competition from foreign competitors with lower labor costs feel more threatened by rising health expenditures.

In sum, both government and business are primarily concerned about their increasing total outlays for health. Their efforts to slow the rate of increase in health spending, through DRGs, state rate setting, preferred provider organizations, health benefit redesign, and other strategies, have been the principal forces of change in the financing and organization of health services.

Coping with these changes is the inescapable concern today of health care professionals and health care institutions, the other major group of insiders worried about health care costs. From their vantage point, the changes that are occurring are indeed significant. For hospitals, for example, cost pressures and other factors point to continued declines in hospital days and hospital occupancy throughout the next decade (Institute for the Future 1983). Most hospitals (like many airlines) are doing well. In the aggregate, hospital financial mar-

gins have been increasing. But these trends will have a profound impact on the financial well-being, if not survival, of some hospitals. It will force others to expand outreach and referral efforts, to discount prices to maintain market shares, to join with other institutions in chains, and to enter into nonhealth ventures to enhance revenues and preserve access to capital. It may also force some to cut back on charity care.

Similarly, all signs point to a continuation of changes in how physicians practice. More physicians will practice in groups and on a salaried basis, and in ambulatory settings such as surgicenters and emergicenters. Some will search for new fields such as wellness or sports medicine. A more entrepreneurial subgroup will seek to establish their own high-tech businesses such as diagnostic imaging centers and the like. Cost reduction efforts will also have an impact on other segments of the medical marketplace. Hospital supply companies and the pharmaceutical industry are already reporting slumping sales as hospitals seek to cut their costs. Today, literally hundreds of trade journals report the latest permutations of these and similar developments, while researchers study their precise effects.

For physicians, perhaps even more important than the economic threat of efforts to control health spending is the perception that the traditional autonomy of the medical profession is being eroded. Medicare was passed, it should be recalled, only when agreement was reached on a pledge that government would not interfere with the practice of medicine. Now, with

DRGs, more aggressive utilization review, and other cost-containment strategies, there is a perception that government will increasingly influence medical practice. This perception appears to be strongly held, despite the limited success that cost-containment practices have met thus far.

However, in sharp contrast to the perspectives of payers, health care institutions, and health professionals, the public has a very different perspective on health care costs (and what to do about them). Unlike government and business, the average American is not terribly troubled by our increasing expenditures for health. In fact, even at a time when the public wants federal spending reduced, public opinion polls consistently show that most Americans favor more federal spending for health, not less. What bothers most Americans, instead, is the price they pay for a visit to a doctor or a hospital. They are also increasingly concerned about the share of their personal health care bill paid out of pocket (Blendon and Altman 1984).

Not only is the public's concern about health care costs different from that of the major payers, it is also less strongly held. According to the polls, the problem of health care costs does not rank among the top concerns for most Americans. In fact, Americans have never ranked health care costs among the top ten problems to be addressed by our nation (Blendon and Altman 1984). This view stands in sharp contrast to the intense public concern that normally precedes the passage of legislation signaling major new policy directions. For example,

prior to the passage in 1970 of the most significant federal environmental legislation in history, the Clean Air Act, reducing air and water pollution had become the number-two domestic priority (just behind reducing crime) identified in public opinion polls as requiring national action.

Even more important, whatever their concern about health care costs, most Americans are quite satisfied with their own current medical arrangements and do not want to change them—to reduce health spending or for any other reason—except by their own choice. In fact, between 75 and 85 percent report on various surveys that they are "completely satisfied" with their medical care. Thus, it is not surprising that Americans are extremely reluctant to accept any cost reduction efforts that would alter those arrangements to a significant degree, according to the polls (Blendon and Altman 1984).

What is the significance of these differences between insiders and the general public on health care costs? The broadest and most important implication is that despite the concern with rising health costs, we are extremely unlikely to see a consensus reached on any single "solution" to the health cost problem that would require significant change in how Americans get their health care. Instead, government and business will continue to chip away at health care costs through a variety of approaches. We will witness no clear victory for either of the two major strategies for controlling health costs—government regulation and marketplace competition.

Second, in the absence of any comprehensive strategy, government and business will continue to focus primarily on reducing their own health spending. This has been the pattern in recent years—for example, the federal DRGs apply only to Medicare. It has prompted fears of cost shifting to private patients, as well as of the erosion of the cross-subsidies for care to the poor and the very sick provided through private insurance. The latter would occur if business responds through preferred provider organizations and other means by attempting to eliminate the subsidies for such care that they have heretofore been willing to pay.

A third implication is that the major thrust of efforts to control health spending will be toward changing the way hospitals and doctors are paid and reducing levels of payment. This trend is already underway with DRGs, all-payer prospective rate-setting systems, preferred provider organizations, the expansion of prepayment. and so forth. Because they are not viewed by the average American as directly threatening his or her current medical arrangements, changing payment arrangements for providers is among the cost-containment strategies most acceptable to the general public. In fact, according to the polls, more than 60 percent of the American people favor government price controls for hospitals and doctors (Blendon and Altman 1984).

Politicians understand well that the withdrawal of covered benefits and eligibility, or significant increases in cost sharing are more likely to prove politically unpopular and to prompt resistance. Underscoring this point, in 1983, 28.7 percent of all health care expenditures were paid directly by patients, with the remainder paid by private insurance and government. Current estimates are that in 1990, 28 percent of our health care bill will be paid out of pocket by individuals. Hardly a major change, at least as a proportion of our overall health care bill (*Health Care Finance Review* 1984).

Other factors too will lead to an emphasis on financing strategies. It is widely accepted that financial incentives are important determinants of physician and hospital behavior and that fee-for-service and cost reimbursement are highly inflationary. Thus, there is an expectation that changing financing will produce big results. Moreover, a great many promising alternatives are not readily available to government and business. Of the many factors responsible for rising health care costs (inflation in the general economy, our aging population, the increasing sophistication of medical technology, etc.), changing payment is among the easiest and quickest routes for government and business to take.

If the struggle over health care costs is primarily a contest between groups with a direct economic, professional, or institutional concern, payers will have an advantage in this insiders' game because the health care industry is highly divided. The interest of doctors, hospitals, nursing homes, and the various subgroups within these categories are hardly the same. Either disinterested in one another's fights, or unwilling to use up political capital of their own, the various segments of the health care industry will seldom unite. The public, generally satisfied with medical care and more concerned with other issues, will take a back seat in this political process. Only those groups with a strong voice in Washington—principally the elderly and seldom the poor—will play a significant role, and even then only occasionally. Moreover, though still high relative to other professions and institutions, public faith and confidence in medicine has slipped significantly in recent years, adding to the advantage payers have (Blendon and Altman 1984).

In summary, cost containment efforts in health will have significant implications for government and business, and for doctors, nurses, hospitals, and other health care institutions. But in light of the general public's views and the signals they send to our elected officials, our efforts to control health care costs will likely continue to be piecemeal and incremental, falling short of sweeping solutions that would touch most Americans' lives and focusing mainly on reducing payments to health care institutions and doctors. This route may be inelegant and ideologically unsatisfying for some. For example, many advocates of competition or regulation may have a hard time reconciling themselves to a state like Massachusetts, which at the same time boasts an all-payer rate-setting system and the third highest HMO penetration in the nation. But, nevertheless, this route is the one we are most likely to follow.

Access to Health Services

Like health care costs, the issue of access to health care is now widely debated by health policy experts and health professionals. The dominant perception among these groups is that the nature of the health services Americans will have access to are changing dramatically, and also that access for some groups may be threatened.

With regard to the first point, there can be little debate. Over the past fifteen years, we have witnessed a significant growth of new or alternative forms of health care organizations. The number of Americans enrolled in HMOs, for example, has grown from 2.5 million in 1970 to 15 million today. HMO growth rates of 15 percent per year are expected to continue, led by the large multistate HMO firms. Ambulatory surgical centers and freestanding emergicenters are expected to experience even faster growth rates. Home health care services are projected to grow almost as fast ("1985" 1984). Increasingly, Americans will be getting their medical care and their surgery outside of hospital walls, and when they are admitted to a hospital, they will be staying fewer days.

Changes are also occurring in the physician and hospital communities. More than 22 percent of all physicians now practice in groups, compared with 10 percent in 1970 (American Medical Association 1984). By 1984, 83 percent of all hospitals were offering at least one alternative service, with home health care, occupational health, rehabilitation centers, birthing centers, and wellness centers showing the most growth ("Home Health Care" 1984). The growth of multihospital systems also continues apace. By 1982 one-third of all hospitals were owned, leased, or managed by a system. For-profit chains are also predicted to grow. For-profits operated about 8 percent of U.S. hospital beds in 1982. Projections are that this group will control 19 percent of all hospital beds by 1990 ("1985" 1984).

Clearly, Americans have more health care choices and options than ever before. But how pervasive have these changes really been to date? Though the face of U.S. health care is beginning to change, most Americans, it would appear, have thus far maintained their old patterns of care. According to a national survey conducted in 1982, for example, almost 90 percent of all Americans reported that their usual source of care was a physician whom they could name (Robert Wood Johnson Foundation 1983). In another survey, 60 percent reported that they were unwilling to break ties with their physician to be treated by a less costly group of physicians or at a clinic (Blendon and Altman 1984). (When patients do leave their physicians, the overwhelming reason given is dissatisfaction with the care they have received, rather than price; Harris and Associates 1985.) Finally, even though people will be using the hospital less for many procedures, current estimates are that the apportionment of our health care dollar will change relatively little by 1990. In 1983 hospitals received 42.7 percent and physicians 19.3 percent of our health care dollar. In 1990 they are projected to receive 45 percent and 18.8 percent respectively (*Health Care Finance Review* 1984). This is hardly suggestive of a truly revolutionary change in the role of the hospital in our health care system.

More important, however, these relatively small changes for most of us may mask bigger changes for some. For a minority of Americans —those without health insurance, and particulary the uninsured poor —the changes occurring in health care may portend significant access problems in the coming years. Studies show that persons without health insurance receive substantially less care than persons with it—for physician care 35 percent less, and for hospital care 48 percent less (Blendon, Altman, and Kilstein 1983). Unfortunately, at a time when we are making progress on most fronts in American medicine, the problem of access for the uninsured appears to be growing. In the process, the health access problem has become more one of financial than geographic access to care.

Between 1979 and 1984, the number of uninsured Americans increased by 22.3 percent, from 28.7 to 35.1 million persons (U.S. Department of Commerce, Bureau of the Census 1984). These 35 million persons make up a diverse group that includes those who are working and uninsured (57 percent), those who are unemployed and uninsured (26 percent), and those who are out of the workforce altogether (17 percent) (Blendon, Altman, and Kilstein 1983). Across these three categories, approximately one-third are children. These increases in the ranks of the uninsured are due to several factors, including a growth in the number of Americans living below the poverty line (from 12 to 17 percent during this period), growth in unemployment, and cutbacks in government insurance programs. Between 1976 and 1984, for example, the percentage of the poor and near poor covered by Medicaid dropped from 64 to 48 percent (U.S. Department of Commerce, Bureau of the Census, Health Care Financing Administration 1984).

This growth in the ranks of the uninsured might not be a major concern if our health care system were able to respond through increased "charity care" services. However, available data do not suggest that this increase has occurred. Between 1980 and 1982, for example, the number of poor persons without health insurance rose 21.9 percent. During this period, however, hospital charity care increased less than 3 percent, with almost all of the increase concentrated in public hospitals (Feder and Hadley 1983). Already beset by cost-containment pressures, the hospitals that have historically shouldered the burden of providing care to the uninsured—principally public hospitals and a small number of selected voluntary institutions—were unable or chose not to increase their level of effort to provide care to this group.

In sum, for most Americans access to health services continues to improve. Most still rely primarily on doctors and hospitals for their care, but new options increasingly are becoming available and are being used. But for persons without health insurance, and particularly the uninsured poor who cannot pay their own way, it does not appear that this progress is being sustained. Access to basic physician and hospital services appears to be deteriorating, while home care, HMOs, wellness centers, and the other new delivery options remain largely unaffordable. As cost containment and budget pressures increase, these problems are likely to remain, if not intensify.

Health Status

While some may debate the extent to which medical care is responsible, there is little doubt that Americans are living healthier lives. In general, the changes occurring in our health care system can be expected to contribute to continued improvements in health status nationally. Infant mortality rates are down. Death rates from stroke and heart disease have dropped significantly. Cancer survival rates are up. Neonatal intensive care units are saving lives. So too are transplants, new drugs, and other fruits of medical science—most, of course, at increased cost. In general, Americans are living healthier and longer lives.

Against this backdrop, the changes occurring in health care have raised several important concerns. One is that as technology becomes more powerful, we will have increasing difficulty with the ethical decisions of prolonging life, particularly for the very young and the very old. This problem can touch virtually everyone's lives. It will not be resolved easily or in one bold stroke.

Ironically, while we are concerned with overusing medical technology, we are also concerned that, because of increasing cost pressures, we will not have it available when we need it. Some medical professionals and health policy experts see a future when, as in England, we will ration technology based on its cost. Some suggest we will do so openly as an explicit policy decision made by major payers; others see rationing occurring through the invisible hand of the marketplace as institutions avoid providing very expensive care in an increasingly cost-conscious environment (Aaron and Schwartz 1983).

Taking a broad view of this issue, the prospect that the United States will ration lifesaving technology due to cost would seem to be small—at least for the majority of Americans who have health insurance. For one thing, unlike England, the United States is a relatively rich country. We are likely to go the route of Sweden (which recently performed its first heart transplant) and other developed nations, not England, always erring on the side of providing medical technology rather than withholding it. For another, Americans consistently want no less than the latest and the best that scientific progress has to offer. Public opinion studies show that Americans strongly favor the continued development of lifesaving technologies and new procedures such as organ transplantation. They place biomedical research highest among all research priorities (Blendon and Altman 1984). For their part, physicians want no less than do their patients. They are trained to do all that is possible to diagnose and treat illness and disease. In light of these public and professional views, politicians will have even more difficulty with the idea of rationing lifesaving technology to save money. Nor, finally, do we have available a "technology" for making rationing decisions, cost-benefit analysis still being an imperfect science valued primarily by its practitioners. In short, in the political and public arena we are likely to opt for technology much more often than against, despite the concerns now being voiced.

A third major health status concern prompted by the changes now occurring in U.S. health care is that moderate- and high-income Americans will benefit more from improvements in health status than will the poor. Today there are approximately 35 million Americans living below the government poverty standard. Studies show that they are at greater risk than others of being in poor health—more than two times greater for both poor adults and children. About half of the poor have no health insurance and thus experience the greatest difficulties obtaining access to care. As government and the private sector move to cut back their health spending, this latter group, the uninsured poor, would appear to be at greatest risk of suffering adverse health consequences. Recently, some small scale studies have begun to report just such findings (Lurie et al. 1984).

Conclusion

Physicians, nurses, hospital managers, government health officials, and corporate benefits officers see, today, a period of rapid if not unprecedented change. This is not surprising. In a $400 billion health care system, billion dollar savings for government and business, and for personal and institutional futures, can depend on only minor alterations of course. But for most Americans our health care system is changing only slowly and in relatively small ways.

Moreover, as in most other domestic policy areas, decisions about the future have been and will continue to be dominated by insiders with a direct stake in their outcome—by government and business, and by organized institutional and professional groups. The changes in our health care system likely to result will continue to be incremental in nature. No sweeping change is likely.

Much of this news would appear to be good. We may be beginning to get a handle on rising costs, but we will have to wait and see if the reductions in hospital spending achieved in 1984 are sustained and if these savings are lost as costs are shifted to other out-of-hospital expenditure areas. Although there may be big effects on health care institutions and health professionals which will need to be watched closely, change is occurring with only small effects on patients; most of these changes would appear to offer more options and the potential for improved access and health. In short, despite the changes, the sky is hardly falling in American health care. Yet, our optimism must be tempered by a major problem, one that, if current trends persist, is likely to get worse as everything else gets better. For a large group of Americans—people without health insurance, and particularly the uninsured poor—the changes occurring in American health care could add up to growing problems. For this group, always dependent on government programs and private cross-subsidies, some solution other than unplanned, incremental change will be needed.

References

Aaron, Henry, and William Schwartz. 1983. *The painful prescription.* Washington, D.C.: Brookings Institution.

American Medical Association. 1984. *Social economic characteristics of medical practice.* Chicago.

Blendon, R. J., and D. E. Altman. 1984. Public attitudes about health care costs: A lesson in national schizophrenia. *New England Journal of Medicine,* August 30.

Blendon, R. J., D. E. Altman, and S. M. Kilstein. 1983. Health insurance for the unemployed and uninsured. *National Journal,* May 28.

Dahl, Robert A. 1956. *A preface to democratic theory.* Chicago: University of Chicago Press.

Feder, Judith, and Jack Hadley. 1983. Cutbacks, recession, and care to the poor: Will the urban poor get hospital care? Washington, D.C.: Urban Institute.

Harris, Louis, and Associates. 1985. *USA Today,* January 31, p. 3D.

Health Care Finance Review. 1984. Vol. 6, no. 2 (Winter).

Home health care leads rising trend of new services. 1984. CEO Poll. *Modern Health Care* (December).

Institute for the Future. 1983. Hospital utilization to 1995. California.

Jones, Charles. 1975. *Clean air.* Pittsburgh, Pa.: University of Pittsburgh Press.

Key, V. O., Jr. 1961. *Public opinion and American democracy.* New York: Alfred A. Knopf.

Lindblom, Charles E. 1970. The science of muddling through. In *Readings in American political behavior,* ed. Raymond E. Wolfinger. Englewood Cliffs, N.J.: Prentice Hall.

Lurie, Nicole, Nancy B. Ward, Martin F. Shapiro, and Robert H. Brook. 1984. Termination from Medi-Cal: Does it affect health? *New England Journal of Medicine* 311, no. 7.

Merrill, Jeffrey C. 1985. Unpublished data, based on *U.S. industrial outlook.* U.S. Department of Commerce. Washington, D.C.

1985: The restructuring health industry. 1984. *Health Central* (March).

Pressman, Jeffrey, and Aaron Wildavsky. 1973. *Implementation.* Berkeley: University of California Press.

Robert Wood Johnson Foundation. 1983. Access to health care for the American people. Princeton: Robert Wood Johnson Foundation.

Sapolsky, H., A. Altman, R. Greene, and J. Moore. 1981. Corporate attitudes toward health care costs. *Milbank* 59, no. 4.

Truman, David B. 1951. *The governmental process.* New York: Alfred A. Knopf.

U.S. Department of Commerce. Bureau of the Census. 1984. *Current population survey.* Washington, D.C.: Government Printing Office.

———. Health Care Financing Administration. 1984. *Current population reports.* Series 3, no. 145, p. 60. Washington, D.C.: Government Printing Office.

Wildavsky, Aaron. 1966. The two presidencies. *Transaction,* December, pp. 7-14.

Chapter 7

Research and Policy Formulation

Karen Davis

The policy formulation process in the United States has become increasingly sophisticated in the last twenty years. At the federal level, cabinet departments have added policy units to direct policy formulation for cabinet secretaries; lower-level government officials heading agencies or bureaus have also added policy staffs. Domestic policy staffs of the president have been expanded to provide independent policy analysis and advice in the consideration of policy proposals emanating from cabinet officials. Congressional staff have increased in number and expertise, with major committees staffed by highly professional policy analysts. Major interest groups have added or expanded policy analysis units to provide the research support for lobbying activities.

This increasing support from the policy staff has resulted in greater emphasis on good analysis based on research, empirical evidence, and evaluation of experience with public programs. The level of debate over major policy issues has been elevated, and legislation, as a result, has become increasingly detailed. Policy decision makers have been able to make better choices, with explicit trade-offs among competing priorities, through introduction, for example, of the congressional budget resolution process.

The premium on good policy analysis has elevated the role of research in policy formulation. Yet many gaps remain to be bridged. The research community is rarely familiar with specific questions for which policy officials want answers: nor is it familiar with types of information or methods of presentation that could help policy officials make choices among alternatives. Nor is the research community typically familiar with the time schedule for decisions on major policy issues. Thus, research findings are not always presented in a timely fashion. These gaps occur in part because the policy community is action oriented and has little time to communicate to the research community its own processes, requirements, and points of intervention.

This chapter tries to bridge these gaps by indicating how research can contribute to policy formulation, outlining the policy-making process within the federal government, and describing the analytic framework used by policy analysts in presenting issues to decision makers for decision. It concludes with some recommendations for enhancing the role of research in policy formulation.

The Contribution of Research to Policy Formulation

Research can influence public policy in two ways: by identifying problems that require policy intervention to correct or by identifying appropriate solutions. More typically, research has been instrumental in raising policy officials' consciousness about the seriousness of a problem for which intervention is appropriate.

The mechanisms by which research has an influence on policy are varied. On occasion a single study or set of studies bear immediately on a policy issue under debate and swing

consideration of that issue. More typically, however, an accumulation of knowledge results through research so that research findings become part of the "common wisdom." Policy officials simply come to understand that there is a physician surplus, that health care costs are rising too rapidly, that smoking is bad for health, and so forth, without being explicitly aware of a particular study that helped create the body of evidence for that view.

Top policy officials become familiar with research in a variety of ways. Their own policy analysis staffs may distill important findings for them. Hearings with expert witnesses may bring important findings to their attention. Or policy officials may learn of them through popular media coverage. Many specific policy proposals, in fact, designed by individuals who are more directly familiar with research studies, originate at the staff level. These proposals may include regulations, budgetary allocations, or legislative proposals.

Examples of the influence of research on policy decisions are numerous. Expanded coverage of low-income pregnant women and children under the Medicaid program was included in the Budget Deficit Reduction Act of 1984. Despite the overall economic stringency and concern with the size of the deficit, and the fact that the bill itself consisted of proposals to reduce the deficit, this expenditure-increasing measure was included. It reflected research on the large numbers of uninsured low-income pregnant women and children, and the barriers to adequate health care faced by these groups. But it is unfair to say that the provision came about solely because research findings persuasively made the case. In 1982–1983 the American Public Health Association (APHA) adopted passage of such a provision as a key legislative priority and approached a key congressman, Rep. Henry Waxman (D.-Cal.), chairman of the House Health and Environment Subcommittee, and asked him to assume leadership in getting the measure enacted. The APHA, the Children's Defense Fund, the American Academy of Pediatrics, and other child advocate organizations worked closely with Congressman Waxman to develop a bill and to shepherd it through Congress. This development coincided with a growing awareness by Congress from media acounts that previous cutbacks in Medicaid and other public health programs were having an adverse impact on the poor. The president, eager to avoid charges of unfairness to the poor during a presidential election campaign, did not actively oppose the adoption of the measure in its final stages of consideration by Congress. Thus, a measure that grew out of research findings was enacted through a combination of forces.

Research has sometimes been a factor in halting consideration of legislative proposals. Support for expanded health coverage for the unemployed was high among congressional members during the deep recession of 1981 and 1982. A report minimizing the number of unemployed losing their health insurance coverage upon unemployment (since many had no insurance even prior to unemployment) undercut support for action on the measure (Wilensky and Berk 1982). This study coincided with a turnaround in the recession and decline in unemployment. Congressional interest in legislative action subsided as the magnitude of the problem was perceived to lessen. Interestingly, later research indicated that absence of health insurance coverage was a serious problem for the uninsured, that it led to difficulties in obtaining necessary health care (Robert Wood Johnson Foundation 1983). By this time, however, the issue was no longer under serious consideration. It seems likely, however, that the issue will surface in future years and that this accumulation of evidence will be drawn upon in future policy debates.

One of the most clear-cut examples of research influencing public policy was the research conducted on prepaid group practices. This research demonstrated that such organizations had markedly lower costs than the traditional health system—in large part because such practices had lower rates of hospitalization. The subsequent passage of the Health Maintenance Organization Act drew heavily upon this research.

Another more recent example is the introduction, under Medicare, of a prospective payment system for hospitals, based on the diagnosis-related-group method of patient case-mix classification. This proposal drew on almost ten years of research, conducted at Yale, on the classification of patients. This system was first adopted in the state of New Jersey and later formed the basis for the Medicare hospital payment system.

Interest groups have also become

more sophisticated about using research in their efforts to sway policy officials' decisions. One major example of the influence of interest groups concerns the containment of hospital costs. The American Hospital Association and the American Medical Association adamantly opposed the Carter hospital cost-containment bill of 1977 and 1979 which would have placed limits on payments to hospitals for care of all patients. Numerous data-based documents were prepared by these groups to show that the bill would have inequitable effects, be difficult to administer, and impede the development of new technology or quality care. The groups were particularly effective at demonstrating that without legislation they were moving voluntarily to curb rises in costs. Monthly notices reporting statistics heralding the restraint in hospital costs achieved in that month were sent to each member of Congress. The legislation was subsequently defeated in the House of Representatives in the fall of 1979, largely because of a belief that, without "heavy-handed bureaucratic" intervention, voluntary efforts by the hospital industry would be sufficient to curb rising costs.

With the defeat of this legislation, hospital costs accelerated rapidly (Davis 1981). Congressional hearings were held on "Whatever Happened to the Voluntary Effort?" The rapid increases were disastrous for public program outlays; Medicare expenditures alone shot up over 20 percent annually. In 1982 the disillusioned Congress moved to institute major limits on Medicare hospital payments under the Tax Equity and Fiscal Responsibility Act (TEFRA). These limits were virtually identical to those proposed in the Carter bill (with the exception that privately insured patients were excluded). Arguments by the hospital industry were disregarded. After the bill's passage, the American Hospital Association called for a change in the method of payment that would achieve the same level of savings already embodied in TEFRA but would put the entire system on a diagnostic-based prospective method of payment. Given that this change would be "budget neutral"—it would neither save nor cost the federal government money beyond that already achieved by the TEFRA provisions—and that it was supported by the hospital industry as a more rational way of allocating expenditures, it was readily approved by the president and the Congress.

While these examples highlight the importance of research, other factors affect the course of public policy formulation in the United States. Any given policy reflects to varying degrees the interplay among such factors as the following: research findings or evidence bearing on policy issues; political ideology or basic tenets of the political party in power; the personal experience of key policy officials; the influence of special interest groups that lobby on behalf of legislation or budgetary allocations; media attention; major events creating public concern; and broad economic, political, and social forces affecting public opinion and support for policy directions.

It is unrealistic in a democratic society to expect that any one force is capable of single-handedly shaping policy formulation. Under some presidents, ideology or political considerations may be relatively more important; under others, hard analyses regarding the benefits and costs of policy options may be given more weight. But regardless of the mix of influences, research can be a critically important factor, providing the facts and evidence that guide rational, informed decision-making.

Typically, a combination of forces comes together to change direction or establish a new policy—either through legislative action, budgetary allocations, or regulatory provisions. But research that is broadly defined to include a range of evidence bearing on the merits of policy alternatives is certainly a major contributing factor. With the increased scrutiny attending all proposals for change, rarely does that change occur without the necessary supporting evidence on its impact and cost.

The Policy-Making Process

Researchers wishing to have a greater impact on policy formulation need to be familiar with both the process and the analytic techniques that are brought to bear in policy formulation. Understanding the major actors in the policy process, the procedures followed, and the time schedule for action is extremely important.

At the federal level, policy formulation is driven by the president's budget and legislative submission in January of each year. Legislative or regulatory proposals may surface at other times, but the major proposals typically are outlined as part of the legislative-budgetary process.

Congress may initiate proposals. Usually, however, the president sets the policy agenda. That is, the president largely determines what issues are considered, even if the specific proposal enacted by Congress differs markedly from that proposed by the president. Therefore, if the president submits a major tax reform proposal, Congress will work on a tax reform bill that in the end may bear only the remotest resemblance to the bill put forward by the president. But the Congress works on tax reform, not welfare reform or Social Security benefit enhancements.

The president's budget, while announced in January, has its origins almost a year earlier. Individual agencies begin the previous spring to surface, analyze, and prepare supporting materials for legislative and budgetary proposals. By June, in most governmental agencies, the top cabinet officials will be engaged in the budgetary process. Policy staffs of the secretary will analyze proposals submitted by major agencies and prepare other alternatives for consideration by the secretary. The Office of Management and Budget may give some guidance to the cabinet officer on the total budget mark to be achieved by the department and on major proposals it wishes included in the department's submission to the president. The cabinet secretary may also receive direct guidance from the president or his aides on initiatives the president wishes developed.

By the end of the summer, the department's legislative and budgetary package will be transmitted to the Office of Management and Budget (OMB) for review. Analysts will go over the request in detail, and prepare analyses and alternative proposals for review by the director of OMB. By Thanksgiving, the director's decisions will be returned to the department for review. The secretary will decide which decisions to appeal, first to the director of the Office of Management and Budget, and in some cases to the president. Press accounts of preliminary decisions are common, as cabinet officials and other midlevel government program managers attempt to rally public opinion or special interest groups to place pressure on OMB or the president before final decisions are reached. This process within the executive branch culminates with announcement in January of the president's budget and legislative package.

Late in the fall, Congress typically adjourns for the remainder of the year. Congressional policy staffs begin to plan ahead for the coming year. As leaks regarding the president's forthcoming budget become commonplace, staff begin to analyze those proposals and prepare alternatives for consideration of congressional members. At this time many of the basic directions and positions that influential members will take in the upcoming year are set.

Once the president's budget and State of the Union address to the Congress are released, congressional review of the budget-legislative package begins in earnest. Under the Congressional Budget Act of 1974, Congress has established a process for agreeing on an overall budgetary ceil-ing, with specific allocations to functional areas such as defense or health. This budgetary ceiling is adopted each year in the form of a Congressional Budget Resolution. Then individual committees are charged with bringing to the floor of the House of Representatives and the Senate specific legislative measures or appropriations bills that will achieve these budgetary ceilings. This process forces Congress to set policy regarding the overall size and allocation of the federal budget and to make choices among alternative types of expenditures. It also requires that all entitlement legislation (e.g., changes to the Medicare and Medicaid programs) enacted by the Congress be carefully analyzed to ascertain its first-year and five-year budgetary impact.

By March 15 the Budget Committee must receive from each key committee a request regarding the proposed allocation and general proposals to achieve that allocation. Hearings are held on the president's budget to get executive branch analysis and rationale for the specific proposals. Other witnesses provide research findings or views of special interest groups on the president's proposals. By May 15 (or typically by June 30) Congress reaches agreement on the broad ceilings to be imposed and passes the Budget Resolution.

Implementation of the Budget Resolution may take the form of an Omnibus Reconciliation Act, that is, a bill containing all legislative proposals that are required to meet the budgetary ceilings for the year. Such an act may be passed by September, before the beginning of the federal government's fiscal year beginning October 1.

In any given year this process may break down. Since the Congressional Budget Act sets rules for Congress, Congress may decide to alter its rules. In some years no Budget Resolution is passed; in others the legislation to implement ceilings is not forthcoming or ceilings are exceeded. Yet Congress tends to take the process seriously and has developed a fairly strict timetable for consideration of major policy alternatives.

Major proposals may require consideration over a longer period of time, however. Typically, major bills would be introduced in the first year of a two-year congressional session. Hearings would be held on the legislation, followed by "mark-up" sessions where the specific sections of a bill are debated and modified. Subcommittees with jurisdiction over the legislation would first follow this process; later it would be repeated by a full committee.

In some cases jurisdiction is split between committees. For example, major health legislation typically is handled by two sets of subcommittees and committees in the House and the Senate. Thus, any major health legislative proposal must receive a majority of votes in as many as ten places: the House Health and Environment Subcommittee and its parent committee, the House Energy and Commerce Committee, the House Ways and Means Health Subcommittee and full committee, the House floor, the Senate Human Resources Health Subcommittee and full committee, the Senate Finance Health Subcommittee and full com-

mittee, and the Senate floor, plus approval by the House and Senate Rules Committee in order to take the legislation to the floor. House and Senate Appropriations committees must authorize spending under all nonentitlement programs, for example, most Public Health Service programs. Differing versions of the House and Senate bills must be compromised in conference. At various stages party leadership in the two houses of Congress may intervene to set directions or priorities for consideration.

This flurry of activity during a constrained period of time makes it difficult for policy staffs to turn to outside researchers for relevant information and for academic researchers to understand when some information of what type and in what form would be useful in the policy process.

The key point for influencing executive branch action is likely to be during the late spring or early summer months when departmental policy is being shaped and when staff of OMB are preparing for the fall budget review. Bringing ideas or research findings to the attention of key policy staffs during the April–June period could lead to receptivity for inclusion in the budgetary-legislative package and the supporting analysis.

The key point for influencing congressional action is likely to be during the somewhat quieter period in November and December when congressional staff members are eager for new ideas and information. But the early months when the president's budget is being considered are also crucial. Material presented at hearings can be helpful, although direct contact with congressional staff members and succinct pertinent information to key members of Congress can be even more effective.

Policy Analysis as an Analytic Technique

The particular environment in which policy is formulated has led to the evolution of a form of analysis quite different from that followed by academic researchers. Policy analysis is by nature condensed, with the most pertinent information presented in a clear, well-organized fashion so that those for whom time is an extraordinarily scarce commodity can quickly absorb the major points that are being made. Policy analysis is not concerned with new knowledge development, as research is, but with summarizing the best available information bearing on choices among policy alternatives. Information on the cost implications of policy alternatives is paramount, given the budgetary constraints within which both the executive branch and the legislative branch must operate. Nor is it possible to conclude that a decision cannot be made because not enough is known or that more research is needed, since in fact decisions must be made within a fixed time frame. In the absence of hard information, best guesses or informed judgment must be relied upon.

Policy Documents

Policy analysis can take several specific forms. In the executive branch the most common policy document is the decision memorandum. This memorandum sets forth the issue that the decision maker must decide, background on the way the issue is handled currently and problems with the present practice, options for change, analysis of these options according to fairly standard criteria, recommendations of policy advisers to the decision maker, and a "decision box" requesting the policy official's decision.

Within the legislative branch a similar document is prepared for subcommittee or committee "mark-up" sessions. This document, sometimes called a Blue Book, generally sets forth the major issues to be decided by the committee, the president's position on those issues, and alternative options prepared by the staff for consideration by the committee. If members of Congress have competing legislative proposals, provisions of these bills may be included in the analysis. The bill's cost or savings to the federal budget, or individual provisions of the bill, are set forth in the "mark-up" document. Once the committee has approved a bill, the staff prepare a committee report to accompany the bill to the floor of the House or Senate. This committee report sets forth the rationale and analysis supporting the specific bill approved by the committee.

The format of a decision memorandum, a mark-up document, or a committee print may vary depending upon the specific issue with which it deals. In general, however, policy analysis encompasses three steps: description of current practice, analysis of problems caused by current practice, and analysis of alternatives for changing current practice. Alternatives would be analyzed by criteria based on benefits or impact of the option, costs, administrative feasibility, and political support. Both quantitative and qualitative information on each of these criteria for each option would be distilled.

This format is designed to conserve the time of busy policy officials; at the same time it assures that action moves forward. The emphasis throughout is on what the decision maker needs to decide and on what he or she needs to know to make the decision. Even when policy analysis is in the form of a verbal presentation as opposed to a written decision document, it focuses on these central questions.

In this respect policy analysis has a very different orientation than research. A researcher starts with a hypothesis about relationships among or between different factors and then tests to see if empirical evidence supports or does not support that hypothesis. Results may be conclusive or inconclusive. Given the imperfections of data and the flaws even in controlled experiments, research usually must be replicated or applied in a variety of settings before the researcher can with conviction assert that the findings are valid. The researcher by nature tends to be tentative and to minimize the implications or significance of the findings.

The policy official must act even on the basis of imperfect or limited information. Further, to mobilize the necessary support for change the case must be presented in a clear and compelling fashion rather than carefully hedged. Thus, even the style of presentation with which the researcher is most comfortable is alien to the policy official.

Relationship of Policy Analysis to Cost-Benefit and Cost-Effectiveness Analysis

Policy analysis has been made more rigorous in recent years by building on some of the concepts embodied in cost-benefit and cost-effectiveness analysis. However, policy analysis differs from cost-benefit and cost-effectiveness analysis in that it relies on informed judgment to make decisions rather than on the analysis itself.

Under cost-benefit analysis (Klarman 1967), a public investment was viewed as beneficial if the discounted stream of benefits over time exceeded the discounted stream of costs. One type of public investment would be preferred over another if its ratio of benefits to costs was greater. Despite early enthusiasm for this method, it proved difficult to implement in practice. Quantifying and measuring benefits were frequently difficult, if not impossible. Further, important social objections were raised about measuring benefits strictly in economic terms. For example the future earning potential of individuals is not an appropriate valuation of lives saved because it discriminates against both the poor and the aged. Such discrimination was found to be socially unacceptable.

To meet some of these objections, cost-effectiveness analysis began to receive greater attention (Klarman 1982). Cost-effectiveness analysis attempts to compare alternative approaches for achieving the same objective. It ascertains which alternatives achieve a fixed outcome at the lowest cost and has much more limited scope than cost-benefit analysis. It does not attempt to compare public investments in health and housing, or in biomedical research and primary care services for pregnant women. Rather it limits itself to comparing public investments with the same objective, such as reducing infant mortality.

Both cost-benefit analysis and cost-effectiveness analysis have proven to be of limited helpfulness in assisting public policy decision-making. Instead, decisions are part of a political process, where competing priorities are weighed and judgments made on the basis of a politically determined social consensus. In the absence of quantitative measures of alternative policy strategies, political determinations fill the gap. In the United States, elected officials determine the priorities for public funding and resource allocation.

To assist with this political determination, public policy analysis utilizes many of the concepts of these earlier techniques. Rather than attempt to quantify all benefits and costs, policy analysis is concerned with defining policy decisions that need to be made, arraying the choices policymakers have for dealing with problems, and systematically analyzing those choices in terms of their benefits or impacts, costs, administrative feasibility, and political support. Both qualitative and quantitative information is summarized, and no attempt is made to force all information into dollar terms. Further,

policy analysis does not attempt to make decisions but to synthesize and distill both quantitative and qualitative information, which leads to informed debate and decision making by elected officials or their representatives. Policy analysis can never totally replace judgment because political and social considerations, as well as strictly economic considerations, need to be weighed.

Increasing the Contribution of Research to Policy Formulation: Some Recommendations

With the development of policy staffs to set forth major policy options and evidence bearing on these choices, policy officials are increasingly interested in using research findings in their decision making. However, a reorientation of the research community is required to make maximum use of this opportunity. While policy officials and staff should, themselves, initiate more outreach into the research community and make the effort to comb research reports for material relevant to include in policy documents, given the time demands this expectation seems unrealistic. Researchers must either personally bridge this gap, add to their research team someone whose responsibility is policy dissemination of the research, or work through an association or group whose responsibility is to fill this role.

Congress has developed some

mechanisms for translating research into policy-usable analysis. These mechanisms include the establishment of the Congressional Budget Office, the Office of Technology Assessment, the General Accounting Office, and the Congressional Research Service. All of these mechanisms conduct studies or pull relevant research information into policy reports to the congress. Researchers may find it useful to channel their findings to staff in these organizations.

Whatever mechanism is followed, several steps are required to bridge the gap between researchers and the policy community. Perhaps the most essential is that researchers focus on the policy decision makers principal questions: What does he or she need to decide? What choices are available? What does he or she need to know to decide among these choices?

Research can be helpful in answering each of these questions. Research that documents the dimensions of problems created by present policies—for example, rising health care costs, barriers to health care for the poor, adverse health consequences of inadequate health care, premature mortality from lack of attention to preventive measures—can be important in bringing an issue to the top of the policy agenda and thus shaping what the decision maker needs to decide. Similarly, research that generates new ideas on approaches or solutions can expand the range of policy options. Research that generates evidence on the effectiveness of different policy interventions, their impact on people, their administrative feasibility, and their costs can provide much of the essential information that the decision maker needs to make an informed choice.

Research on the cost or savings implications of alternatives is especially at a premium, given economic and budgetary constraints. Rarely does a policy have only beneficial impact; hard information on who gains and who loses, by how much, under different policy alternatives is also important in helping decision makers make trade-offs among competing priorities.

Familiarization with the policy process, timing of decisions, the types of information used, and the format of presentation is important to maximize use of research. The researcher should begin by asking who would be interested in his or her research—what governmental agency would be affected, what congressional committee would have jurisdiction over any policy recommendations emanating from the study, what interest groups or associations would have an interest.

The researcher should understand when in the time schedule policy staffs would be most accessible and open to new information and ideas. Know what issues will be considered when, and pay special attention to the budget-legislative cycle that occurs annually.

Reseachers must be willing to draw conclusions. Policy staff and officials want findings, not long involved explanations of methodology. And they want to know the implications of those findings for actions that need to be taken. Research so carefully hedged with caveats that policy staff do not know what to make of the study is of little value. Nothing frustrates policy officials more than statements that additional research is needed, especially when officials know they will have to act on the basis of what is known or the best available judgment.

Most important, some means must be found for getting this information to staff members without requiring them to read tomes of information written in a format quite dissimilar from their own work products. Dealing with key policy staff personally is critically important. It requires developing contacts with policy staff, working through professional associations that maintain such contacts, or finding forums, at which policy staff members will be present, for presenting ideas and research findings.

Popularization of research into media accounts, such as writing op-ed articles for major newspapers, issuing press releases on major studies, holding press conferences or press background meetings, and making oneself available to reporters, can also provide an avenue for making research more visible to policy officials.

Researchers should present work to policy staffs in a form that will be easy to grasp quickly. Using charts or other visual aids, material should be brief and to the point. Major "bullets" or facts that bear on problems or policy options should be set forth clearly and succinctly.

Researchers can understand which issues are relevant and which types of information go into shaping decisions on those issues by reading some policy documents—for example, departmental press releases on the budget, fact sheets and charts on major legislative proposals, internal decision memoranda on major issues, bills submitted or sponsors' fact sheets and press statements, hearings, lists of witnesses and testimony, committee mark-up documents, and congressional committee prints. Many publications are oriented toward digesting and synthesizing such information. For example, in the health area the weekly newsletter *Washington Report on Medicine and Health* published by McGraw-Hill is read avidly every Monday morning by health policy analysts and lobbyists eager to know the status of health policy issues currently on the policy agenda. Major interest groups maintain their own newsletters to keep members informed of action on issues relevant to them.

Finally, researchers could initiate experiences that would give them a greater awareness of policy issues and decision-making procedures. This initiation might include serving for a limited period in a policy office, which would help researchers develop contacts and attain a better understanding of the policy process and points of intervention. Alternatively, policy staff might be invited to visit research institutions and give seminars on issues they see as major ones for the upcoming period.

All of these steps require that researchers adopt a substantially different orientation than has been traditional. These steps take time and compete for the researcher's attention with other activities, such as publication, that may reap greater internal rewards.

Universities will need to rethink reward structures, giving greater credit to policy activities, or to establish positions for those whose function would be to bridge the gap between researchers and policy staffs. The social responsibility of the academic community extends beyond the generation of new knowledge to the translation of that knowledge into action beneficial to society. This reorientation is not to argue that universities encourage or reward advocacy based on ideology. But universities should encourage researchers to go beyond publication of research in scientific journals by translating their research into a form that will make it useful for policy officials. This form may include more popular writing in the news media or presentations before policy officials and staffs. Such activity is unlikely to be pursued, however, unless university promotion policies recognize congressional testimony, popular writing, and so forth as well as scientific journal publications.

Foundations and nongovernmental funding sources must be willing to support policy-related research that generates information on problems or policy options not popular within a given presidential administration and to support activities that will help bridge the gap between researchers and the policy community.

Finally, it must be recognized that multiple factors affect policy formulation. Even in the best of worlds, in a democratic society research is only one facet of a many-faceted decision-making process. Expectations must be realistic. But it is clear that policy decision-making today is vastly different than it was twenty years ago and that it will continue to change markedly in the future. Hopefully, these suggestions will help stimulate many of those in the research community to become more involved in the policy applications of their research and will help bring ever-increasing analytic soundness to the formulation of public policy.

References

Califano, J. A., Jr. 1981. *Governing America: An insider's report from the White House and the Cabinet.* New York: Simon and Schuster.

Davis, K. 1981. Recent trends in hospital costs: Failure of the voluntary effort. *Hearings before the U.S. House of Representatives, Committee on Energy and Commerce, Subcommittee on Health and the Environment*, pp. 202–213. Washington, D.C.: Government Printing Office.

Klarman, H. E. 1967. Present status of cost-benefit analysis in the health field. *American Journal of Public Health* 57 (November): 1948–1953.

———— 1982. The road to cost-effectiveness analysis. *Milbank Memorial Fund Quarterly: Health and Society* 60, no. 4 (Fall): 585–603.

Robert Wood Johnson Foundation. 1983. Report on access to health care for the American people. Updated. Special Report No. 1. Princeton: Robert Wood Johnson Foundation.

Wilensky, G., and M. Berk. 1982. Health care, the poor, and the role of Medicaid. *Health Affairs* 1, no. 4 (Fall): 93–100.

Part II

Major Medical Problems and Monitoring Health Outcomes

Chapter 8

Cardiovascular Disease

Adrian M. Ostfeld

lmost all the mortality that results from cardiovascular disease (CD), and most morbidity, is a result of high blood pressure (HBP) and stroke and coronary heart disease (CHD) (Havlik and Feinleib 1979). This chapter is limited to these three conditions. To relate social variables to CD is a threefold task. The first is to indicate how they affect incidence, mortality, and course of these conditions; the second is to consider how social factors have influenced the recent decline in the U.S. death rate of stroke and CHD; and the third is to indicate how social factors may affect cost control, prevention, and treatment of CD in the future.

First we require some background information (National Heart, Lung, and Blood Institute 1982). About 73 million Americans suffer from one or more of the several forms of CD. About 60 million have HBP, defined as a pressure equaling or exceeding 140/90 mmHg; 4.6 million have CHD, and more than 1.8 million have had a stroke. CD was responsible for approximately 1 million deaths in 1980 or just over half the deaths in that year. More than one-fifth of these deaths occurred in people under sixty-five. In 1978 CD accounted for about 595 million days of restricted activity, 172 million days spent in bed, and 44 million days of work loss. In 1979 CD caused 49 million days in short-stay hospitals and 50 million visits to physicians' offices. Four years earlier more than 177,000 workers with CD were allowed Social Security disability benefits. CD's cost to the U.S. economy is much the largest of any diagnostic group, an estimated $81.3 billion in 1979. Thirty billion dollars were spent on hospitals, nursing homes, drugs, and professional fees, and $50 billion of productivity was lost.

Risk Factors for CD

The major factors leading to HBP are obesity, lower socioeconomic status, black descent, older age, large alcohol intake, and use of oral contraceptives; other factors may include prolonged excessive vigilance/arousal and repression of hostility and guilt over its expression. A complex interaction between sodium, potassium, calcium and other inorganic substances in the diet (Stamler, Stamler, and Pullman 1967; Paul 1975; Page 1976; D'alonzo and Pell 1968; Langford 1983; Intersociety Commission for Heart Disease Resources, Atherosclerosis Study Group and Epidemiology Study Group 1970) may also contribute to increasing blood pressure.

The major risk factors for CHD are relatively higher levels of serum total cholesterol, cigarette smoking, and higher blood pressures (Intersociety Commission for Heart Disease Resources, Atherosclerosis Study Group and Epidemiology Study Group 1970; National Heart, Lung, and Blood Institute 1981; American Heart Association Steering Committee for Medical and Community Program 1980; Blackburn 1975; Shurtleff 1974; Keys 1975; European Society of Cardiology 1978). The relationship between CHD incidence and total serum cholesterol is present, is demonstrated in prospective studies, both within and between populations, is dose related, occurs in both sexes, and is independent of other risk factors (Stamler 1978; Kato et al. 1973; Westlund and Nicolaysen 1972; Epstein 1979). The conclusion that high serum cholesterol is a cause of CHD is further supported by the fact that cholesterol predominates in the fatty substances accumulated in arterial walls (Wissler 1974; Small 1977) and that experimental variation in serum cholesterol increases or lowers the amount of fat in arterial walls as one raises or lowers serum cholesterol (Armstrong 1976; Wissler and Vesselinovitch 1975).

Fractionation of total serum cholesterol into its components has revealed several lipid-protein complexes, among which are VLDL which is not important to the atherosclerotic process, LDL which enhances lipid deposition in the arterial wall, and HDL which inhibits atherosclerosis (Rhoads, Gulbrandsen, and Kagan 1976; Castelli et al. 1977b; Goldbourt and Medalie 1979; Workshop Report Epidemiological Section 1979).

Among the many determinants of serum cholesterol and its fractions are genes, hormones, physical activity, age, alcohol intake, and, possibly, behavior patterns ("Dietary Fat and Coronary Heart Disease" 1974; Grundy et al. 1982; Great Britain Committee on Medical Aspects of Food Policy, Subcommittee on Nutritional Surveillance 1974; Intersociety Commission for Heart Disease Resources, Atherosclerosis Study Group and Epidemiology Study Group 1974). No environmental factor has been shown to affect LDL and serum total cholesterol more strongly than the diet (Keys and Fidanza 1960; Glueck and Common 1978; Jackson et al. 1978). Serum cholesterol is lowered by weight reduction, unsaturated fat in the diet, dietary fiber, and vegetable protein; it is raised by excess calories, saturated fat, and cholesterol in the diet (Durington et al. 1977; Kay and Truswell 1980; Lewis et al. 1981). Alcohol raises HDL cholesterol (Henneken, Rosner, and Cole 1978; Castelli et al. 1977a), and it is interesting to note that France and Italy have among the highest alcohol intakes and lowest CHD death rates of any developed nations in the world (Havlik and Feinleib 1979).

No strong evidence shows that blood lipid levels affect the risk of stroke (Ostfeld, Shekelle, and Klawans 1974; Ostfeld 1980).

As would be expected, the criteria used for defining HBP determine the prevalence of the disease. If defined as 140/90 or more, about 60 million Americans or nearly one-third of the adult population have HBP (National Health Survey 1977). Of these, 75 percent will have mild HBP (a diastolic pressure of 90 to 104 mmHg). HBP is the major cause of the 500,000 strokes and 175,000 stroke deaths annually in the United States (Ostfeld 1980; Hypertension Detection and Follow-up Cooperative Group 1977; Borhani 1979) and is one of the major causes of the 1.5 million heart attacks and 567,000 heart attack deaths each year (Kannel 1975b). The risk of each major cardiovascular disease is directly related to blood pressure level, and even small elevations produce a substantial excess risk (Hypertension Detection and Follow-up Cooperative Group 1977; Kannel 1975b). Elevation of either the systolic or diastolic pressure, whether variable or fixed and whether measured under usual office conditions or after rest, increases the risk of stroke, heart failure, and CHD (Kannel, Sorlie, and

Gordon 1980; Kannel, Dawber, and McGee 1980; Ostfeld 1978).

Cigarette smoking is a direct cause of myocardial infarction and sudden death although it plays little or no role in inducing stroke (Ostfeld 1980). The evidence that cigarette smoking causes these disorders is strong and internally consistent, shows a graded relationship to exposure, is independent of other risk factors, prospectively predicts CHD in a wide variety of populations, and is buttressed by clinicopathological studies and experimental data in animals (Luce and Schweitzer 1978; Kannel 1981; Pooling Project Research Group 1978).

When diabetes mellitus is present, it doubles the CD death rate (Kannel and McGee 1979a). It has a greater detrimental effect in women but a lesser impact in persons past sixty (Epstein 1967; Kannel and McGee 1979b; Ostfeld 1980). Diabetes causes direct damage to heart muscle and increases the risk of stroke (Jarrett 1977; Rubler et al. 1972).

Although it is widely believed that regular physical activity at work or leisure is beneficial to the cardiovascular system, the evidence is not established beyond a reasonable doubt. Assessment of the relationship has been hampered by inadequate methods for assessing physical activity. There is some evidence that regular vigorous physical activity at work or leisure is beneficial (Morris et al. 1973; Paffenbarger, Wing, and Hyde 1978; Paffenbarger and Hale 1975), but Finnish lumbermen who perform strenuous work have the world's highest rate of myocardial infarction (Keys 1970). There are records of many deaths due to CHD among joggers and marathon runners (Noakes et al. 1979; Thompson et al. 1979). Throughout Rhode Island, from 1975 to 1980, joggers had seven times the CHD death rate while jogging than was estimated to be their rate while in a sedentary state (Thompson et al. 1982). Jogging may help prevent CHD, but it may also increase the risk of fatality while jogging. Finally, the evidence that exercise training improves the outlook for heart patients is not convincing (Frolicher 1981; Verani et al. 1981).

Marked overweight is associated with a high level of serum fats, higher blood pressure, and greater likelihood of diabetes—thereby contributing to the risk of CHD and stroke (Ashley and Kannel 1974; Rimm and White 1979; Montoye, Epstein, and Kjelsberg 1966).

Psychosocial Variables and CD

Although the risk-factor concept of CHD and stroke is firmly established, the risk factors described above do not by any means account for all the occurrence of CD in the United States and explain even less of the incidence in populations with less atherosclerosis. The most likely candidates for additional risk factors are psychosocial variables. Of course, psychosocial factors may influence CD rates in other ways as well.

Now let me blur the boundaries between what are called "social" and what are called "psychological" factors as they relate to CD. While I will emphasize social variables, personal-

ity, behavior and other psychological factors will not be excluded.

A consistent inverse relationship exists between socioeconomic status (SES) and blood pressure, cigarette smoking and total serum cholesterol (Syme, Oakes, and Friedman 1974; Keil, Sandifer, and Loadholt 1981; Keil, Tyroler, and Sandifer 1977), both in the United States and in other countries (Holme, Helgegard, and Hjermann 1976; Rose and Marmot 1981). Differences in levels of risk factors by SES do not explain all the excess morbidity and mortality among those with less schooling and less prestigious occupations. Perhaps inadequate medical care, lack of knowledge about health, and inadequate income are also involved. More research is needed here.

As with much of our knowledge of CHD, the available data on the previously mentioned relationships are derived from studies of white males. Much less information is available about women, blacks, and Hispanics, and we cannot assume that the relationships for the latter three groups are the same as for employed white males.

In the last fifteen years, a relationship between measures of status inconsistency, incongruity, and social mobility and CHD has been described. One of the more persistent and intriguing relationships involves educational attainment of husbands and wives. Shekelle, Ostfeld, and Paul (1969) found that men whose wives had more education than they had significantly higher risk of CHD than men whose education exceeded their wives'. Haynes, Eaker, and Feinleib (1982) noted that in the Framingham cohort, men whose wives had some college were 2.6 times more likely to get CHD than men whose wives had eight grades or less of schooling. Follow-up studies at Framingham (Haynes, Eaker, and Feinleib 1983; Eaker, Haynes, and Feinleib 1983) indicated that the effect of wives' education on CHD was limited to men whose wives worked outside the home and men whose working conditions were difficult. An interaction between Type A behavior and wives' educational and employment status was noted. The effects on CHD risk of Type A behavior were greater in men whose wives had some college and worked outside the home (Eaker, Haynes, and Feinleib 1983). The ways in which these social variables induce increased risk of CHD is not known, but the process may be mediated by psychological stress in the home and by feelings of insecurity and self-doubt among the husbands.

Chronic life situations and life events have been studied for their relationships to diseases including CD (Rahe and Lind 1971; Rahe and Passakivi 1971; Rissaner, Rowo, and Siltanen 1978). The variables that have received the most attention are major life change and the work environment (Sales and House 1971; Sharet and Salvevdy 1982). Among life changes that have been studied for their effects on CD are change in marital status, job loss, and residential change (Kasl and Cobb 1980; Kasl et al. 1980; Jacobs and Ostfeld 1977). Increasing rates of CD mortality have been identified among the widowed, the divorced, and the socioculturally and geographically mobile. Tyroler and Cassel (1964) observed an effect of urbanization on CHD mortality in rural residents of North Carolina. Syme, Hyman, and Enterline (1964), in a case-control study, noted an effect of sociocultural mobility on CD in rural and urban residents. Several migrant populations have been noted to develop increased risk of CHD and risk-factor levels as they move from traditional to western life-style. Westernization usually means changes in diet, work, cigarette and alcohol use, physical activity, and infectious disease susceptibility as well as changes in social roles, social networks and supports, and factors inducing and alleviating anxiety (Ostfeld and D'Atri 1977; Cabral, Gusman, and Estrada 1981; Marmot and Syme 1976; Fries 1976). It is not easy to tease apart the relationships and interactions between these life changes, but it needs to be done.

Measures of SES have repeatedly been good predictors of CD morbidity and mortality. But epidemiologists have tended to think about SES as a fixed background variable rather than viewing it in a dynamic sense. SES affects behavior, social supports, job and personal flexibility, knowledge of health, access to medical care and doctors' communications to patients. The effects of SES and gender on doctor-patient communication have been recently described by Waitzkin (1984). Physicians talk one way to nonphysician professional peers and quite another way to blue-collar workers. The information given, the detail with which it is given, possibilities of treatment and outcome, and advice on prevention are sometimes stated differently by the same physician to patients of differing gender and SES. More serious concern with how SES affects all these dynamic aspects of life and health is necessary.

Cassel (1976), Berkman and Syme (1979) and Blazer (1982) have suggested that lack of or disruption of social bonds to other people has increased the risk of disease. Study of social networks and social supports is a promising new direction. A recent conference on psychosocial variables in cardiovascular epidemiology (Ostfeld and Eaker 1985) has concluded that social supports may reduce the incidence and mortality of CD in one or more of at least four ways. They may facilitate getting good care, act directly to benefit care by providing payment for care and transportation to medical facilities, and enhance group norms of behavior that promote health, as in Mormons and Seventh-Day Adventists. Such supports may also influence the neuroendocrine systems to promote resistance to disease.

An extensive but somewhat inconsistent literature has reported associations between CHD and anxiety-neuroticism, life dissatisfaction, and the Type A behavior pattern (Jenkins 1971, 1976). There is some evidence that psychological variables prospectively characterizing persons who will develop varying types of CHD differ. Men who are going to develop angina pectoris score significantly higher on measures of hysteria and hypochondriasis than men going to develop either myocardial infarction or sudden death. Men who are going to die suddenly of CHD may show higher scores on a measure of depression than those going to develop

angina or infarction (Medalie et al. 1973; Lebovitz et al. 1967).

Recent observations have dealt with the relationship of CHD to Type A behavior, a manifest pattern characterized by time urgency and competitiveness, sometimes accompanied by generalized hostility. Earlier studies indicated that such behavior was predictive of CHD (Roseman, Brand, and Jenkins 1975; Haynes, Feinleib, and Kannel 1980), but recent studies have not confirmed the results (Shekelle et al. 1985; Multiple Risk Factor Intervention Trial 1982). Pathogenetic mechanisms for an independent effect of Type A have yet to be convincingly demonstrated (Shekelle, Hulley, and Neaton 1983). Problems in assessment of Type A are substantial. The behavior requires a social context to make it manifest. Essentially, many are Type A at work but few are Type A sitting by the fireplace fondling a pet dog. Several subsets of variables make up the total construct of Type A. And we do not understand the biological basis for Type A and its effects.

Natural History of CHD and the Technology of Diagnosis and Treatment

The natural history of CHD is substantially different in men than in women (Bengtsson 1973; Kannel et al. 1976; Gordon et al. 1978). In the Framingham cohort not a single premenopausal woman had a myocardial infarction or coronary death, a picture very different from that of men of comparable age. In men the most common first manifestation of CHD is myocardial infarction or sudden death. Angina pectoris is a much less common first manifestation. In women angina—the least threatening form of CHD—predominates, and myocardial infarction and sudden death as initial events are less common. In women angina has only a small effect on life expectancy; in men angina reduces life expectancy substantially. Prognosis after one heart attack does not differ by gender. The reasons for these male-female differences are unknown. Originally attributed to a protective effect of female hormones, the difference in male-female prognosis has a causation much more obscure (Kannel et al. 1976; Gordon et al. 1978).

The principal reason for sudden death in CHD is ventricular fibrillation, a rapid, irregular, and weak beat of the heart that cannot sustain life. Sudden death because of this abnormality is the only manifestation of CHD in about one-fifth of cases. The recurrence rate of this lethal cardiac rhythm is high, about 30 percent in the first year after the initial episode and nearly 50 percent by three years afterward. When ventricular fibrillation appears, resuscitative measures must be applied within four to six minutes to avoid brain injury. It is evident that current technology will not help those who develop this lethal rhythm outside the hospital.

Patients who survive long enough to reach the hospital are usually taken promptly to the coronary care unit (CCU). The essential role of the CCU is to prevent or treat all disease manifestations threatening life or increasing discomfort. Electrical instability of the heart that might lead to sudden death must receive primary attention. Dyspnea (hunger for air) and pain must be alleviated. Shock, heart failure, and rapid heart beat must be sought and promptly treated. Emotional reactions such as anxiety, denial, or depression must be monitored and treated. The technology enabling CCU personnel to perform these tasks includes electrocardiographic monitors, defibrillators and pacemakers to maintain the normal rhythm of the heart, respirators, blood gas analyzers, and a large number of medications.

Later in the CCU, patients are encouraged to shave and feed themselves, sit up, dangle feet, use a bedpan or commode, and walk very slowly. If the patient's course proceeds satisfactorily, plans are made with the patient and family for the initiation of a risk-factor reduction program, control of hypertension and diabetes, an individually planned program of intermittent physical activity, and a psychologic, social, and vocational evaluation. Patients with an uneventful course in the CCU are usually sent home after about two-and-one-half weeks, but rehabilitation must not stop there. Concern over the resumption of sexual activity can sometimes be alleviated by pointing out that such activity is not harmful to the heart and does not lead to a worsening of pain and disability. The return to work requires planning between the patient, the family, and the employer.

The rehabilitation of the stroke patient is a much more complex effort. Unlike cardiac rehabilitation, stroke rehabilitation takes months. Treatment of hypertension is essential. Among the problems in stroke patients that must be identified and treated are cognitive impairment, loss of speech and language, reduction in vision, urinary and fecal incontinence, and burning pain in the paralyzed area. Regimens have been developed by specialists in rehabilitation to attempt to deal with these disorders.

For those stroke patients with persistent muscular paralysis, returning to the home and the community requires careful evaluation by the physician, with the help of the social worker and psychologist. The status of the family and the home must likewise be assessed to determine the likelihood of further gain of function and promote an optimistic attitude. Patients who remain severely cognitively impaired or those with persistent urinary and fecal incontinence may need to enter nursing homes.

A large and dazzling array of new diagnostic and therapeutic technology for the heart and stroke patient has grown up in the last three decades and continues to proliferate. These methods are denoted as noninvasive and invasive.

Among the more widely used noninvasive methods for heart patients are echocardiography which utilizes reflected soundwaves to identify cardiac abnormalities, continuous recording of the electrocardiogram including electrocardiography during graded physical exercise, and myocardial imaging that makes use of specially prepared radioactive material that identifies dead muscle or muscle whose circulation is compromised. Invasive techniques include cardiac catheterization in which fine hollow tubes are inserted into an artery and then placed in various locations in the heart chambers and great vessels. Cardiac catheterization determines the output of the heart and pressures in heart chambers and great vessels and provides a good view of the structure and functions of the heart. Cardiac catheterization, usually accompanied by coronary angiography, is required to evaluate patients who may be candidates for coronary artery bypass surgery. Newer technology, including image intensifiers and cineangiography, has improved the quality of the assessment of heart function. These invasive procedures are not without risk. In cardiac catheterization the rate of serious complications is about 3 percent and of death about 0.3 percent (Sokolow and McElroy 1981).

This new technology has contributed to the widespread use of coronary artery bypass surgery to the point where about one hundred thousand of these surgical procedures are carried out each year. Done primarily to relieve the distress and disability of angina pectoris, these procedures are not always better than conservative treatment with medication. Only in disease of the left main coronary artery or extensive atherosclerosis in three sites in the coronary arteries does surgical treatment prolong life more than the use of drugs (Detre, Hultgren, and Rakaro 1977; Detre,

Murphy, and Hultgren 1977; Takaro et al. 1982).

A recent analysis of survival rates in those treated surgically or medically in the Veterans Administration Coronary Bypass Surgery Trial shows no difference in survival by surgical or medical treatment after eleven years of follow-up, except for those at high risk of dying (Veterans Administration Coronary Bypass Surgery Cooperative Study Group 1984).

The latter group, characterized by evidence of severe coronary atherosclerosis, badly impaired cardiac function, and ominous electrocardiographic pattern benefit somewhat more from surgery than from medical treatment. Risky, painful, and expensive surgery has a way of reanimating dormant social networks and mobilizing social supports. The contribution of these social factors to the benefit of surgery has not been examined.

In stroke newer noninvasive diagnostic methods are aiding in diagnosis and in planning treatment. These newer methods include computerized axial tomography and nuclear magnetic resonance spectroscopy.

These technological advances and the development of specialized coronary care units have produced new professional roles, an increasingly complex hierarchy of health care providers, and marked increases in patient expenses. These technologies and newer therapies, expensive and risky as they may be, are now considered as usual modes of diagnosis and treatment; not to use them is viewed by many to be unethical and unprofessional. The issue is further complicated by real doubts about the benefits of the new technology—a dilemma that will be examined later.

Reduction in Morbidity and Mortality in CHD and Stroke

After CHD mortality reached an epidemic peak in the United States in the early 1960s, it dropped 31 percent between 1963 and 1980 (Havlik and Feinleib 1979; National Heart, Lung, and Blood Institute 1982). The declines have been greater for those of middle age and less striking for older persons. However, declines are observed in all age, race, and sex groups and generally throughout the country. These declines have been larger in the United States than in any country in the world.

The reason for these improvements is not entirely clear. The major innovations in the hospital treatment of CHD are coronary artery bypass surgery whose limited benefits we have cited earlier (Detre, Murphy, and Hultgren 1977; Detre, Hultgren, and Takaro 1977; Takaro et al. 1982; Veterans Administration Coronary Bypass Surgery Cooperative Study Group 1984) and the Coronary Care Unit (CCU) for the management of acute myocardial infarction. But after about eighteen years of proliferation of CCUs, we have meager evidence except personal opinion that they are better than treatment elsewhere in the hospital or home. The only controlled clinical trials that have been done show no value of CCUs over treatment at other sites (Mather et al.

1971; Hill, Hampton, and Mitchell 1979). One analysis of data from a Canadian province likewise shows no benefits of CCUs (Morris et al. 1983), and a careful review of results from Maryland hospitals (Gordis, Noggar, and Tonaschia 1977) indicates that survival in the CCU is less than in other hospital sites. The Canadian data are particularly instructive because treatment in a CCU or regular hospital bed depended on where you lived and not on the presumed severity of the heart attack. One cannot, therefore, claim that CCUs do not perform as well as other treatment sites because they get the more severe cases. In a nine-year study of all sixty-three acute care hospitals in the Boston area (Goldman et al. 1982), overall mortality rates of acute myocardial infarction (AMI) declined while hospitaliztion rates and mortality rates of inpatients did not change. Out-of-hospital mortality rates declined, a clear indication that hospital treatment of AMI was not responsible for the drop in coronary mortality. Fatal AMI was prevented, not treated more effectively in the hospital. It is also important to note that the U.S. decline in coronary mortality began in 1964, well before the widespread use of coronary bypass surgery or increased use of cardiopulmonary resuscitation. Thus, there is no compelling reason to attribute the declining CHD death rate to modern technology.

Let us examine an alternative explanation. Death rates may be dropping because CHD is being prevented. If this were true, we should be able to identify three trends: (1) that CHD incidence in the United States is coming down; (2) that levels of CHD risk factors in the United States are coming down chronologically parallel with the decline in mortality and of a magnitude sufficient to be responsible for the decline; and (3) that in a country whose risk factor levels are increasing, coronary mortality rates are going up.

Some evidence indicates that coronary incidence is down in the United States. Among male employees of a large industry, the number of patients hospitalized for CHD dropped 18 percent within a decade. In a large medical care plan providing care for several hundred thousand people, hospitalization rates for heart attack fell 27 percent within six years (Havlik and Feinleib 1979).

What has happened to levels of risk factors? The percentage of male cigarette smokers has declined 25 percent between 1965 and 1978 (Walker 1977; U. S. Department of Agriculture 1976; Mass 1979). Surveys of American's eating patterns by the U.S. Department of Agriculture show an appreciable change in consumption particularly among younger and more affluent persons (Mass 1979; Rizek and Jackson 1980; Page and Friend 1978). Consumption of butter, lard, eggs, and other sources of saturated fat is reduced, and there has been an increase in the use of unsaturated oils of vegetable sources. Total cholesterol levels have come down, and the chief reason appears to be dietary change (Stamler 1981; Abraham, Johnson, and Carroll 1978). Blood pressure levels are lower now than they were a decade or two earlier (Castelli 1975; Rowland and

Roberts 1982). The proportion of hypertensives whose condition has been identified, treated, and controlled has increased from one in eight to one in two between 1970 and 1979 (National Heart, Lung, and Blood Institute 1982). The amount of decline of risk factors is sufficient to account for the decrease in mortality, and the chronological relationships support the view that the risk-factor declines are responsible (National Heart, Lung, and Blood Institute 1982). The amount of change in risk factors has been shown by epidemiologic multiple logistic estimates to be large enough to be responsible for the moderate decline in CHD mortality occurring in the last two decades.

If our hypothesis is correct, that a decline in risk factors nationwide has led to a decline in CHD mortality, it follows that a country whose risk-factor levels are rising will show an increase in CHD mortality. This rise is exactly what is occurring in the USSR (Cooper 1981; Dutton 1976). Mortality rates of CHD have been increasing there for the past decade. Cooper and Schatzkin (1982), analyzing data from Soviet sources as well as information from French and U.S. sources, calculate that tobacco consumption increased 60 percent in the USSR from 1960 to 1977. Now Soviet cigarette use is close to that in the United States and Europe (Johns Hopkins University 1979). Consumption of foods high in saturated fat and cholesterol has been increasing in the Soviet Union since the Second World War while consumpton of complex carbohydrates such as potatoes and grain has decreased (Organization for Eco-nomic Cooperation and Development 1979; Food and Agricultureal Organization 1977). Between 1965 and 1977 consumption of meat, eggs, and milk and milk products increased 39 percent, 80 percent, and 28 percent, respectively, in the Soviet Union (Organization for Economic Cooperation and Development 1979). Soviet population surveys based on representative community samples in Moscow and Leningrad indicated a prevalence of hypertension twice that found in U.S. groups when care was taken to assure identical methods of collecting data (Tyroler, Glasunov, and Deev 1979; Glasunov, Chazova, and Alexandrov 1980).

Impressive as has been the decline in U.S. CHD mortality, the fall in stroke mortality has been even greater. U.S. stroke death rates were cut almost in half in the decade 1970–1979. Improved detection, treatment, and control of HBP is the primary reason for the decline in stroke mortality (Ostfeld 1980).

Health Policy Change in the Public and Private Sectors

Let us review the history of events that were part of the cause for these U.S. declines in CHD and stroke mortality. In 1964 two important public health recommendations were made to Americans—the first surgeon general's report detailed the effects of smoking and the prudent diet of the

American Heart Association recommended reducing consumption of saturated fat and cholesterol in the diet (Walker 1977). In 1974 the Intersociety Commission for Heart Disease Resources (ICHD), in a report widely distributed to physicians, called for prevention as long-term national policy and provided clear and feasible recommendations to achieve dietary change (Intersociety Commission for Heart Disease Resources, Atherosclerosis Study Group and Epidemiology Study Group 1974, 15) and to control blood lipid levels, HBP, overweight, diabetes, and cigarette smoking. Similar recommendations were made the following year by the White House Conference on Food, Nutrition, and Health (1970) and the National Heart and Lung Institute Task Force on Arteriosclerosis (1971). The earlier attempts to reduce CD were largely directed to the health professions personnel.

emphasis on education of the public was added to that of professional education. In that year, the National High Blood Pressure Education Program was launched by the Secretary of Health, Education, and Welfare through NHLBI. The health consumer as well as nurses, dentists, physicians, pharmacists, and school health educators were reached through mass media, mailed educational material, and public demonstration programs. In the late 1970s, the Select Commission on Nutrition and Human Needs (1977) of the U.S. Senate made the public more aware of dietary prevention of CD. Through the 1970s the American Heart Association promoted public education and,

through its fifty-five affiliates and hundreds of chapters and divisions, screened at least 14 million Americans in their own communities for HBP and other risk factors (Ostfeld 1980). Seven statewide programs to reduce HBP-related morbidity and mortality through coordination of resources in the public and private sector were funded by NHLBI. In 1979 the American Diabetes Association joined with the American Dietetic Association (1976) to revise their recommendations on diet for diabetics by advocating a diet that would not only reduce diabetic complications but also reduce the risk of CD (Nuttal and Bruzell 1979). In the same year, the surgeon general issued a report entitled *Healthy People* (U.S. Department of Health, Education, and Welfare 1979) that strongly advocated styles of living that would maintain health and reduce the risk of a wide spectrum of diseases including CD. Additional recommendations dealing with diet followed from other national agencies.

Among many voluntary and governmental agencies and organizations of health providers and consumers, the near unanimity of public health policy on prevention of CD has been impressive. The near unanimity has been maintained for twenty years while national administrations have changed parties three times.

Earlier I referred to seven statewide high blood pressure control programs. Connecticut was one of those states. Because these programs emphasized prevention of CD and stroke through community-based coordination of resources, I will review very briefly the content and outcome of the program.

The Connecticut High Blood Pressure Program

In the period 1975–1982, the author and many colleagues developed and implemented a statewide high blood pressure control program throughout Connecticut. At its height in 1977–1982, the program was a cooperative venture of the Connecticut State Department of Health Services (SDHS), the American Heart Association, Connecticut affiliate (AHA), and the Department of Epidemiology and Public Health (EPH), Yale School of Medicine. SDHS was administratively and fiscally responsible for the program, and most of the funding was federal. The purposes of the program were to increase awareness of the disease, treatment, and control among persons in the state with HBP and to decrease hypertension-related mortality in the state, preferably by an amount greater than that occurring in the United States as a whole.

The protocol was straightforward. Baseline surveys of the prevalence of HBP and the awareness, treatment, and control status of persons with it were determined on statewide probability samples of households before and then three years after intense programmatic activity. The number of households surveyed each time was about 3,225, and participation rates were about 73 percent. The two samples, before and after, were independent. The survey questionnaire contained items dealing with sociodemographic data, history of medical conditions, sources of medical care, diet, knowledge about HBP, and other subjects. One method of evaluating the program was to compare the awareness, treatment, and control status in two independent samples, one taken before and one after three years of community program (D'Atri et al. 1981; Freeman et al. 1983; Freeman, Ostfeld, and Hellenbrand 1985).

In addition to obtaining these data from the consumers of health care, data on hypertension control activities of health providers and health provider organizations were obtained both before and after the three years of activity. Questionnaires, mailed to providers, were developed individually for each kind of health provider, whether individuals or agencies. The health professionals and agencies surveyed were either the universe or representative samples of the universe in Connecticut. Among those surveyed were physicians who treat hypertensive patients (internists, family practitioners, and cardiologists), dentists, pharmacists, acute care hospitals, local and district health departments, WIC nutrition programs, industries, public and proprietary nursing agencies, elderly housing projects, VD control programs, Red Cross chapters, Planned Parenthood, and other groups. The questionnaires asked these individuals and groups about specific practices that were related to HBP control. A few examples will clarify the aim and content of the questionnaires.

Physicians were asked what they did when a hypertensive patient missed an appointment. Multiple choice answers ranged from "doing nothing" to "sending a post card to the home with a reminder to make a new appointment." Red Cross chapters were asked, among other things, what they did when a potential blood donor had pressures too high to give blood. Response categories ranged from "merely telling them their pressure was too high to give blood" to "telling the person his blood pressure was too high, providing clear and simple educational materials and recommending they see their physicians." Proprietary nursing agencies were given a list of HBP control activities and asked which ones they carried out.

The change in HBP control activities occurring between 1978–1979 and 1982 was most interesting. In 1978–1979 less than one physician in five routinely contacted patients who missed an appointment. In 1983 the proportion who made patient contacts had doubled. In 1979, provision of literature and physician referral of potential donors with HBP was not done by any Red Cross chapter. By 1982, 65 percent of chapters in the state were providing educational materials and 29 percent were systematically referring to physicians. In 1978, 20 percent of proprietary nursing agencies had HBP screening programs and 75 percent referred hypertensives to sources of treatment. In 1982 these percentages had increased to 56 percent and 91 percent respectively. Although a dozen other groups and agencies also showed impressive changes in HBP control activities,

three kinds of groups did not. Groups unable or unwilling to change included small agencies with limited budgets, health departments without full-time directors, and organizations with loose regionalized structure.

A third evaluation of the program was conducted by monitoring age-adjusted mortality rates of CD and stroke. Our expectation was that if the Connecticut program were successful, mortality rates would decline more in Connecticut than in the United States during the period.

All three evaluation measures supported the inference that the program was successful. Awareness, treatment, and control of HBP increased significantly in most age-sex-race categories in the state in three years. As described earlier most health provider groups and organizations reported small to large improvements in HBP control activities.

A comparison of mortality rates in Connecticut and in the United States, shown in tables 8.1 and 8.2, is largely self-explanatory. Age-adjusted heart disease and stroke mortality rates were quite similar in the two areas in 1978; in a period when U.S. rates were falling, Connecticut's rates were coming down even more. The protective effect of treatment for high blood pressure begins almost immediately so it would be expected that morbidity and mortality would show effects promptly.

That the public and the health professions have been able to modify their behavior voluntarily to produce a substantial increase in HBP control is impressive. Equally impressive, in the community the state program was carried out largely independent of

TABLE 8.1

Age-Adjusted Heart Disease Mortality Rates per 100,000, 1978–1981 (1970 standard million)

	Connecticut	United States
1978	302.5	307.7
1979	291.4	300.5
1980	279.5	307.4
1981	267.4	291.6
Total rate of change	− 11.6%	− 5.2%

complex hospital-based technology. The most expensive equipment purchased by the program was mercury manometers for taking blood pressure. The total amount of money spent on community programs between 1974 and 1982 was about $1.7 million and for any one year never exceeded $420,000.

These results have great importance for the extreme increases in medical care costs in recent decades and indicate what can be done in the community with a modest budget, a dedicated staff, and a little imagination.

We have already indicated that the value of coronary care units and coronary bypass surgery is open to question. But even if hospital-based technology were better than it is, it could not deal with the problem of CHD and stroke. Only one of every five heart attacks is preceded by chronic angina. Two of every three CHD deaths occur suddenly outside the

TABLE 8.2

Age-Adjusted Stroke Mortality Rates per 100,000, 1978–1981 (1970 standard million)

	Connecticut	United States
1978	72.7	73.5
1979	63.9	69.0
1980	55.4	67.8
1981	52.1	62.1
Total rate of change	− 28.3%	− 15.5%

hospital. For one in five coronary events sudden death is the first, last and only manifestation. More than 90 percent of strokes are not preceded by early warning signs (Ostfeld 1980). Even those who are hospitalized for heart attack and survive have five times the risk of dying in the next five years when compared to the general population.

Our country is greatly concerned with rising hospital costs, but ironically, for the nation's number one killer these costs may well have little benefit. We are even beginning to think about a system of rationing this expensive technology, making it accessible to some and not to others. Certain vital questions arise. Why did the use of coronary care units and coronary bypass surgery grow so precipitously when there was little or no evidence supporting their widespread use? Why does their widespread use continue after we know that they are either of no benefit or of only limited help? The Food and Drug Administration is empowered to assure that new drugs are safe and effective before their general use. What is to protect the American public from expensive, painful hospitalizations, surgery, and use of new technology before their benefit and safety are evaluated?

The estimated annual national expenditures for doctors, hospitals, nursing homes, and drugs in treatment of CD were earlier said to be $31 billion. A comparable figure for stroke is about $3.3 billion (National Survey of Stroke 1981). How much would it cost nationwide each year to add a program such as the Connecticut High Blood Pressure Program to what is now being spent for disease

prevention? About $44 million. For intervention programs in which control of other risk factors such as smoking and high blood lipids would be pursued along with HBP control, the national annual bill might be $70 million in addition to current funding for prevention. These incremental funds amount to 0.2 percent of what is now spent for treatment.

What changes in professional orientation and national approach to disease are required to deal with the problem of CD and stroke? My recommendations are based principally on a document recently published (Kannel et al. 1984) and are organized around three questions: (1) What can physicians and other health professionals do to reduce CD and stroke incidence, mortality, and costs? (2) What can the public learn and do to reduce CD and stroke incidence, mortality, and costs? (3) What public health measures can be taken to reduce CD and stroke incidence, mortality, and costs?

Physician's Role

The identification of levels of risk factors is easily done in the office, is relatively inexpensive, and is extremely beneficial. Based on these levels evaluated individually and together, the physican can recommend a specific program to reduce the risk of CD.

The primary approach to management of an ominous blood lipid profile should focus on diet, weight control, and exercise. These measures are particularly important to the diabetic patient because attention to blood sugar levels alone is less likely to benefit the diabetic patient than control of risk factors for CHD. The detection and control of high blood pressure is a central objective in the prevention of CHD, stroke, and heart failure. While medications will usually be required, attention to weight control, increased physical activity, avoidance of heavy drinking, and concern for sodium, potassium, and calcium in the diet are part of the treatment of high blood pressure. Behavioral methods of lowering blood pressure have received a good deal of attention and may have value. However, they have been used in too few patients for too short a period of time to show whether they can replace medications for many hypertensives. Smoking cessation is extremely important to CD prevention and note should be made to patients that filter cigarettes offer no protection from CHD. Certain kinds of oral contraceptives increase the risk of several forms of CD and, when taken by cigarette smokers, are more likely to cause problems than in nonsmokers. Although the increased risk conferred by the pill is very small, the physician has the obligation to be alert to and prevent the possibility of harm. While proof of the benefits of increased physical activity in preventing CD does not exist, the potential benefits of exercise are substantial. Exercise may make weight control easier, increases HDL levels, may improve control of diabetes, and is said—although the author has never experienced it—to make people feel better. Attempts at psychosocial intervention such as amelioration of the Type

A behavior pattern may be beneficial, but more needs to be known before widespread application. Control of other risk factors in the Type A person is more likely to be beneficial than dealing with behavior alone.

Recommendations to the General Public

The promotion of a healthful lifestyle requires little sacrifice. A diet that will help prevent CD can be tasty and meet the nutritional needs of all segments of the population including pregnant and nursing women, children, adolescents, and old people. The key is to reduce total calories, red meat, total fat, saturated fat, and cholesterol in the diet and to increase consumption of fish, skinned fowl, whole grains, legumes, fruits, and vegetables.

In permitting the public to make these changes, the food industry, encouraged by the public and private sector, ought to make available more lean meats and processed meats as well as dairy products, frozen desserts, and baked goods low in saturated fats, cholesterol, and calories. Margarines, shortenings, mayonnaises, and salad oils low in saturated fat and cholesterol should be promoted more heavily. Because many meals are eaten outside the home, hotels, restaurants, and fast food chains ought to make available more healthful alternatives to their current offerings.

Discontinuing or, even better, not starting to smoke is critically important. So too is having blood pressure checked at least yearly if it reads less than 140/90 and more often if it reads above that level. These points must be constantly emphasized by voluntary health agencies.

The dairy industry should be encouraged to develop techniques for reducing cholesterol, saturated fat, and salt in milk and milk products, especially in cheeses, whose consumption is growing in the United States. The consumer of dairy foods and the voluntary health associations should press for changing standards of milk pricing. Wholesale pricing of dairy products is still based on butterfat content, a now outmoded practice dating from the days when butterfat content was determined to detect watering or skimming of milk. Nondairy cream substitutes often have high coconut oil content and hydrogenated vegetable oil. Such content raises serum cholesterol whereas peanut oil, corn oil, safflower oil, walnut oil, and others do not. A change in these nondairy cream substitutes is needed.

Public Health Measures

A wide variety of public health measures is available to reduce CD. First, antiquated and harmful laws and regulations should be repealed. A few examples will suffice. Unsaturated fat cannot be added to processed meats because the Food and Drug Administration (FDA), the U.S. Department of Agriculture (USDA), and some states and localities define this practice as adulteration. Although we have known for two decades that a high intake of saturated fat and cholesterol causes heart disease, the FDA has consistently refused to permit food advertising to claim that products low in cholesterol protect against CD. A study of the problem by the Concil of Foods and Nutrition of the American Medical Association has recommended such an action.

Tobacco contains many chemical compounds that greatly affect the human body. (What is a drug but a chemical compound that affects the human body!) The FDA ought to regulate tobacco use as it does the use of saccharin or cyclamates. One of the best investments in the health of Americans would be diversification of the cigarette industry into other products and support that would permit those now employed by the tobacco industry to gain employment in new fields. Current government giveaways to tobacco growers and exporters should be stopped.

Improvement in school lunch, food stamps, other supplementary food programs, and other federally administered food programs such as those in the armed forces and the Veterans Administration must be supported. If school health curricula are to promote healthful living, they should emphasize abstention from cigarettes, a prudent diet, and exercise that individuals can maintain on their own over a lifetime. Industries should be encouraged to make more healthful menus available to employees who eat there and to provide referral to antismoking agencies.

The voluntary health agencies should join with government to institute a nationwide antismoking campaign. Mass media education programs showing the dreadful effects of cigarettes should be implemented to redress the imbalance created by decades of intensive cigarette advertising. Because smoking usually begins in early adolescence, particular effort should be made to reduce smoking among adolescents by strict restraints on the advertising and sale of cigarettes.

Development of a comprehensive and sustained program of public and professional nutrition education should encourage Americans to modify their eating of all five major sources of fat in their diet: meat, dairy products, baked goods, eggs, and cooking and table fats.

The National High Blood Pressure Education Program and the Connecticut High Blood Pressure Program have demonstrated that physicians respond favorably to data indicating the value of CD risk-factor reduction and correspondingly help reduce their patients' risk of morbidity and mortality. Industry, pharmacists, local health departments, schools, nursing agencies, and others are willing to do more to prevent CD, provided they are convinced that what they are doing is beneficial to the American people.

If our people, our organizations, and our country want to make deep cuts in the death rate and in hospital care costs due to the leading cause of death in the United States, the methods are available to do so.

References

Abraham, S., C. L. Johnson, and M. D. Carroll. 1978. Total serum cholesterol levels of adults 18–74 years. In *Vital and health statistics data from National Health Survey, U.S., 1971–1974.* U.S. Department of Health, Education, and Welfare. Series 11, no. 5. Washington, D.C.: Government Printing Office.

American Diabetes Association, Inc., and American Dietetic Association. 1976. *Exchange lists for meal planning.* New York: American Diabetes Association, Inc.; Chicago: American Diabetic Association.

American Heart Association Steering Committee for Medical and Community Program. 1980. Risk factors and coronary disease: A statement for physicians. *Circulation* 62:455A–494A.

Armstrong, M. L. 1976. Regression of atherosclerosis. In *Atherosclerosis reviews,* ed. R. Paoletti and A. M. Gotto, Jr., vol. 1. New York: Raven Press.

Ashley, F. W., Jr., and W. B. Kannel. 1974. Relation of weight change to changes in atherogenic traits: The Framingham study. *Journal of Chronic Disease* 27:103.

Bengtsson, C. 1973. Ischemic heart disease in women: A study based on a randomized population sample of women and women with myocardial infarction. *Acta Medica Scandinavica* 5:1.

Berkman, L., and S. L. Syme. 1979. Social networks, host resistance, and mortality: A nine-year followup study of Alameda County residents. *American Journal of Epidemiology* 109:186.

Blazer, D. 1982. Social support and mortality in an all elderly community population. *American Journal of Epidemiology* 115:684.

Borhani, N. O. 1979. Mortality trends in hypertension, United States, 1950–1976. In *Proceedings of the conference on the decline in coronary heart disease mortality*, ed. R. J. Havlik and M. Feinleib. U.S. Department of Health Education and Welfare. NIH Publication No. 79-1610. Washington, D.C.: Government Printing Office.

Cabral, E. I., S. V. Gusman, and J. Estrada. 1981. Prevalence and severity of hypertension in individuals aged fifty years or over from urban and rural communities in the Philippines. In *Hypertension in the young and the old*, ed. G. Onesti and K. E. Kim. New York: Grune and Stratton.

Cassel, J. 1976. The contribution of the social environment to host resistance. *American Journal of Epidemiology* 104(2):107.

Castelli, W. P. 1975. The Framingham offspring study: Design and preliminary data. *Preventive Medicine* 4:518.

Castelli, W. P., J. T. Doyle, T. Gordon, C. Hames, M. Hjortland, S. B. Hulley, A. Kagan, and W. Zukel. 1977a. Alcohol and blood lipids . . . the cooperative lipoprotein phenotype program study. *Lancet* 2:153.

————. 1977b. HDL cholesterol and other lipids in coronary heart disease: The cooperative lipoprotein phenotyping study. *Circulation* 55:767.

Cooper, R. 1981. Rising death rates in the Soviet Union: The impact of coronary heart disease. *New England Journal of Medicine* 304:1259.

Cooper, R., and A. Schatzkin. 1982. Recent trends in coronary risk factors in the USSR: The impact of social policy on public health. Unpublished report, Department of Community Health, Northwestern University Medical School, Chicago.

D'alonzo, C. A., and S. Pell. 1968. Cardiovascular disease among problem drinkers. *Journal of Occupational Medicine* 10:344.

D'Atri, D. A., E. F. Fitzgerald, D. H. Freeman, J. N. Vitale, and A. M. Ostfeld. 1981. The Connecticut high blood pressure program: A program of public education and high blood pressure screening. *Preventive Medicine* 9:107.

Detre, K., H. Hultgren, and T. Takaro. 1977. Veterans Administration cooperative study of surgery for coronary arterial occlusive disease. *American Journal of Cardiology* 40:212.

Detre, K., M. L. Murphy, and H. Hultgren. 1977. Effect of coronary bypass surgery on longevity in high and low risk patients. Reports from the VA Cooperative Coronary Surgery Study. *Lancet* 2:1243.

Dietary fat and coronary heart disease: A review. 1974. *Medical Journal of Australia* 575:616, 633.

Durrington, P. N., C. H. Bolton, M. Hartog, R. Angelinetta, P. Emmel, and S. Furniss. 1977. The effect of a low cholesterol, high polyunsaturate diet on serum lipid levels, apolipoprotein B levels, and triglyceride fatty acid composition. *Atherosclerosis* 27:465.

Dutton, J., Jr. 1976. Changes in Soviet mortality patterns, 1959–1977. *Population and Development Review* 5:267.

Eaker, E. D., S. G. Haynes, and M. Feinleib. 1983. Spouse behavior and coronary heart disease in men: Prospective results from the Framingham Heart Study II: Modification of risk in Type A husbands according to the social and psychological status of their wives. *American Journal of Epidemiology* 118:23.

Epstein, F. H. 1967. Hyperglycemia: A risk factor in coronary disease. *Circulation* 36:606.

Epstein, F. H. 1979. Predicting, explaining, and preventing coronary heart disease: An epidemiologic view. *Modern Concepts of Cardiovascular Disease* 48:7–11.

European Society of Cardiology. 1978. *Preventing coronary heart disease: A guide for the practicing physician.* Assen, The Netherlands: Van Gorcum.

Food and Agricultural Organization. 1977. *Food balance sheets.*

Freeman, D. H., D. A. D'Atri, K. Hellenbrand, A. M. Ostfeld, E. Papke, K. Piorun, V. A. Richards, and A. Sardinas. 1983. The prevalence distribution of hypertension: Connecticut adults, 1978–1979. *Journal of Chronic Disease* 36:171.

Freeman, D. H., A. M. Ostfeld, K. Hellenbrand Richards, V. R. and Tracy, R. 1985. Changes in the prevalence distribution of hypertension, Connecticut adults, 1978–1979 to 1982. *Journal of Chronic Disease* 38(2):157–164.

Fries, E. D. 1976. Salt, volume, and the prevention of hypertension. *Circulation* 53:589.

Frolicher, V. 1981. Exercise and health (editorial). *American Journal of Medicine* 70:987.

Glasunov, I. S., A. A. Chazova, and R. Alexandrov. 1980. Further population studies on hypertension in the USSR. In *Hypertension in the USA and the USSR: Basic, clinical, and population research.* Second USA-USSR Joint Symposium, May 14–16, 1976, National Institutes of Health. Bethesda, Md.: Government Printing Office.

Glueck, C. J., and W. E. Common. 1978. The diet-coronary heart disease relationship reconnoitered. *American Journal of Clinical Nutrition* 31:727.

Goldbourt, V., and J. H. Medalie. 1979. High density lipoprotein cholesterol and incidence of coronary heart disease: The Israeli Ischemic Heart Disease Study. *American Journal of Epidemiology* 109:296.

Goldman, L., F. Cook, B. Hashimoto, S. Stone, J. Muller, and A. Loscalzo. 1982. Evidence that hospital care for acute myocardial infarction has not contributed to the decline in coronary mortality between 1973–1974 and 1978–1979. *Circulation* 65(5):936.

Gordis, L., L. Noggar, and J. Tonaschia. 1977. Pitfalls in evaluating the impact of coronary care units on mortality from myocardial infarction. *Johns Hopkins Medical Journal* 144:287.

Gordon T., W. B. Kannel, M. C. Hjortland, and P. M. McNamara. 1978. Menopause and coronary heart disease: The Framingham Study. *Annals of Internal Medicine* 89:157.

Great Britain Committee on Medical Aspects of Food Policy. Subcommittee on Nutritional Surveillance. 1974. *Diet and coronary heart disease: Reports on health and social subjects.* London: Her Majesty's Stationery Office.

Grundy, S. M., D. Bilheimer, N. Blackburn, W. V. Brown, P. O. Kwiterovich, F. Mathson, G. Schoenfeld, and W. N. Weidman. 1982. Rationale of the diet-heart statement of the American Heart Association. Report of Nutrition Committee. *Circulation* 65:839A.

Havlik, R. J., and M. Feinleib, eds. 1979. *Proceedings of the conference on the decline in coronary heart disease mortality.* U.S. Department of Health, Education, and Welfare, Public Health Service, National Institutes of Health. Washington, D.C.: Government Printing Office.

Haynes, S. G., E. Eaker, and M. Feinleib. 1982. Spouse behavior and CHD results from a 10-year followup study in Framingham. *American Heart Association CVD Epidemiology Newsletter* 21:22.

————. 1983. Spouse behavior and coronary heart disease in men: Prospective results from the Framingham Heart Study. Concordance of risk factors and the relationship of psychosocial status to coronary incidence. *American Journal of Epidemiology* 111:1.

Haynes, S. G., M. Feinleib, and W. B. Kannel. 1980. The relationship of psychosocial factors to coronary heart disease in the Framingham Study III: Eight year incidence of coronary heart disease. *American Journal of Epidemiology* 111:37.

Henneken, C. H., B. Rosner, and D. S. Cole. 1978. Daily alcohol consumption and coronary heart disease. *American Journal of Epidemiology* 107:196.

Hill, J. D., J. R. Hampton, and J. R. Mitchell. 1979. A randomized trial of home versus hospital management for patients with suspected myocardial infarction. *Lancet* 1:837.

Holme, I., A. Helgegard, and I. Hjermann. 1976. Coronary risk factors and socioeconomic status: The Oslo study. *Lancet* 2:1396.

Hypertension Detection and Follow-up Cooperative Group. 1977. The Hypertension Detection and Follow-up Program: A progress report. *Circulation Research* (supp. 1): I-106.

Intersociety Commission for Heart Disease Resources, Atherosclerosis Study Group and Epidemiology Study Group. 1970. Primary prevention of the atherosclerotic diseases. *Circulation* 42:A55–A87.

————. 1974. Primary Prevention of the Atherosclerotic Disease. In *Cardiovascular disease: Guidelines for prevention and care*, ed. I. S. Wright and D. T. Frederickson. Washington, D.C.: Government Printing Office.

Jackson, R. L., O. D. Taunton, J. D. Morrisett, and A. M. Gotto. 1978. The role of dietary polyunsaturated fat in lowering blood cholesterol in man. *Circulation Research* 42:447.

Jacobs, S., and A. M. Ostfeld. 1977. An epidemiological review of the mortality of bereavement. *Psychosomatic Medicine* 39(5):241.

Jarrett, J. 1977. Diabetes and the heart: Coronary heart diseases. *Clinical Endocrinology and Metabolism* 6:389.

Jenkins, C. D. 1976. Recent evidence supporting psychologic and social risk factors for coronary disease. *New England Journal of Medicine* 294:987–1033.

Johns Hopkins University. 1979. *Tobacco: Hazards to health and human reproduction.* Population Report Series L, no. 1. Baltimore, Md.: Hampton House.

Kannel, W. B. 1975a. *The natural history of myocardial infarction: The Framingham Study.* Leiden, The Netherlands: Leiden University Press.

———. 1975b. Role of blood pressure in cardiovascular disease: The Framingham Study. *Angiology* 26:1.

———. 1981. Update on the role of cigarette smoking in coronary artery disease. *American Heart Journal* 101:319.

Kannel. W. B., T. R. Dawber, and D. L. McGee. 1980. Perspectives on systolic hypertension: The Framingham Study. *Circulation* 61:1183.

Kannel, W. B., J. T. Doyle, A. M. Ostfeld, C. D. Jenkins, L. Kuller, R. N. Podell, and J. Stamler. 1984. Optimal resources for primary prevention of atherosclerotic disease. *Circulation* 70(1):157A–205A.

Kannel, W. B., M. C. Hjortland, P. M. McNamara, and T. Gordon. 1976. Menopause and risk of cardiovascular disease: The Framingham Study. *Archives of Internal Medicine* 85:447.

Kannel, W. B., and D. L. McGee. 1979a. Diabetes and cardiovascular risk factors: The Framingham Study. *Circulation* 59:8.

———. 1979b. Diabetes and glucose tolerance as risk factors for cardiovascular disease: The Framingham Study. *Diabetes Care* 2:120.

Kannel, W. B., P. Sorlie, and T. Gordon. 1980. Labile hypertension: A faulty concept? The Framingham Study. *Circulation* 61:1179.

Kannel, W. B., P. Sorlie, and P. M. McNamara. 1979. Prognosis after initial myocardial infarction: The Framingham Study. *American Journal of Cardiology* 44:53.

Kasl, S. V., and S. Cobb. 1980. The experience of losing a job: Some effects on cardiovascular functioning. *Psychotherapy and Psychosomatics* 34:88.

Kasl, S. V., A. M. Ostfeld, G. M. Broady, L. Snell, and A. C. Price. 1980. Effects of "involuntary" relocation on the health and behavior of the elderly. In *Second conference on the epidemiology of aging*, ed. S. G. Haynes and M. Feinleib. Publication No. 80-969 211. Washington, D.C.: Government Printing Office.

Kato, H., J. Tillotson, J. Z. Nichaman, G. G. Rhoads, and H. G. Hamilton. 1973. Epidemiologic studies of coronary heart disease and stroke in Japanese men living in Japan, Hawaii, and California: Serum lipids and diet. *American Journal of Epidemiology* 97:372.

Kay, R. M., and A. S. Truswell. 1980. Dietary fiber: Effects in plasma and total lipids. In *Medical aspects of dietary fiber*, ed. G. A. Spiller and R. M. Kay. New York: Plenum Publishing.

Keil, J. E., S. H. Sandifer, and C. B. Loadholt. 1981. Skin color and education effects on blood pressure. *American Journal of Public Health* 71:532.

Keil, J. E., H. A. Tyroler, and S. H. Sandifer. 1977. Hypertension: Effects of social class and racial admixture: The results of a cohort study in the black population of Charleston, South Carolina. *American Journal of Public Health* 67:634.

Keys, A. 1975. Coronary heart disease: The global picture. *Atherosclerosis* 22:149.

_____, ed. 1970. *Coronary heart disease in seven countries.* Monograph No. 29. American Heart Assn.

Keys, A., and T. Fidanza. 1960. Serum cholesterol and relative body weight of coronary patients in different populations. *Circulation* 22:1091.

Langford, A. G. 1983. Dietary potassium and hypertension: Epidemiologic data. *Annals of Internal Medicine* 98:770.

Lebovits, B. Z., R. B. Shekelle, A. M. Ostfeld, and O. Paul. 1967. Prospective and retrospective psychological studies of coronary heart disease. *Psychosomatic Medicine* 29:265.

Lewis, B., F. Hammett, M. B. Katon, R. M. Kay, I. Merka, A. Nobels, N. E. Miller, and A. V. Swan. 1981. Toward a lipid-coronary diet: Additive effect of changes in nutrient intake. *Lancet* 2:1310.

Luce, B. R., and S. O. Schweitzer. 1978. Smoking and alcohol abuse: A comparison of their economic consequences. *New England Journal of Medicine* 298:569.

Marmot, M. G., and S. L. Syme. 1976. Acculturation and coronary heart disease in Japanese-Americans. *American Journal of Epidemiology* 104:225.

Mass, A. J. 1979. Changes in cigarette smoking and current smoking practices among adults. National Center for Health Statistics. Advance Data No. 52. Washington, D.C.: Government Printing Office.

Mather, H. G., N. G. Pearson, D. B. Read, G. R. Stead, M. G. Thorne, S. Jones, C. J. Guerrier, C. D. Erant, P. M. McHugh, N. R. Chowdhury, M. H. Jofary, and T. J. Wallace. 1971. Acute myocardial infarction: Home and hospital treatment. *British Medical Journal* 3:334.

Medalie, H. H., M. Snyder, J. Green, H. N. Neufeld, V. Goldbourt, and E. Riss. 1973. Angina pectoris among 10,000 men: 5-year incidence and univariable analysis. *American Journal of Medicine* 55:583.

Montoye, H. J., F. H. Epstein, and M. O. Kjelsberg. 1966. Relationship between serum cholesterol and body fatness: An epidemiologic study. *American Journal of Clinical Nutrition* 18:397.

Morris A. L., V. Nernberg, N. P. Roos, P. Henteloff, and L. Roos. 1983. Acute myocardial infarction: Survey of urban and rural hospitals mortality. *American Heart Journal* 105:44.

Morris, J. N., S. P. Chase, C. Adam, C. Sivey, L. Epstein, and D. J. Sheehan. 1973. Vigorous exercise in leisure-time and the incidence of coronary heart disease. *Lancet* 1:333.

Multiple Risk Factor Intervention Trial. 1982. Risk factor changes and mortality results. *Journal of the American Medical Association* 248:1465.

National Health Survey. 1977. *Blood pressure levels of persons aged 6–74,*

United States, 1971–1974: Vital and health statistics. Data from National Health Survey, series 11, No. 203. U.S. Department of Health, Education, and Welfare. Washington, D.C.: Government Printing Office.

National Heart, Lung, and Blood Institute. 1981. *Arteriosclerosis.* Vol. 2. U.S. Department of Health and Human Services. NIH Publication No. 82-2035. Washington, D.C.: Government Printing Office.

———. 1982. *Heart and vascular diseases.* Vol. 2 Tenth report of the director. Washington, D.C.: Government Printing Office.

National Heart and Lung Institute Task Force on Arteriosclerosis. 1971. *Arteriosclerosis.* Vol. 1. U.S. Department of Health, Education, and Welfare, Public Health Service. Publication No. 72-137. Washington, D.C.: Government Printing Office.

National Survey of Stroke. 1981. *Stroke: A Journal of Cerebral Circulation Part II*, ed. F. D. Weinfeld (Supp. 1) I-1–I-91.

Noakes, T. D., L. N. Opie, A. G. Rose, P. H. Keynhan, N. S. Scheper, and B. Dawdeswell. 1979. Autopsy: Proved coronary atherosclerosis in marathon runner. *New England Journal of Medicine* 301:86.

Nuttal, F. Q., and D. Bruzell. 1979. Principles of nutrition and dietary recommendations for individuals with diabetes mellitis. Report of the American Diabetes Association. *Diabetes* 28:1027.

Organization for Economic Cooperation and Development. 1979. *Prospects for Soviet agricultural production in 1980 and 1985.* Paris.

Ostfeld, A. M. 1978. Elderly hypertensive patient. *Epidemiologic Review: N.Y. State Medical Journal* 78:1125.

———. 1980. A review of stroke epidemiology. *Epidemiologic Reviews* 2:136.

Ostfeld, A. M., and D. D'Atri. 1977. Rapid sociocultural change and high blood pressure. *Advances in Psychosomatic Medicine* 9:20.

Ostfeld, A. M., and E. Eaker. 1985. National heart, lung, and blood disease conference on psychosocial variables in epidemiologic studies of cardiovascular disease. *Atherosclerosis* (in press).

Ostfeld, A. M., R. B. Shekelle, and H. Klawans. 1974. Epidemiology of stroke in an elderly welfare population. *American Journal of Public Health* 64:450.

Paffenbarger, R. S., and W. E. Hale. 1975. Work activity and coronary artery mortality. *New England Journal of Medicine* 292:545.

Paffenbarger, R. S., A. L. Wing, and R. T. Hyde. 1978. Physical activity as an index of heart attack risk in college alumni. *American Journal of Epidemiology* 108:161.

Page, L. B. 1976. Epidemiologic evidence on the etiology of human hypertension and its possible prevention. *American Heart Journal* 91:527.

Page, L., and B. Friend. 1978. The changing United States diet. *Bioscience* 28:192.

Paul, O., ed. 1975. *Epidemiology and control of hypertension.* Chicago: Year Book Medicine.

Pooling Project Research Group. 1978. Relationship of blood pressure, serum cholesterol, smoking habit, relative weight and EGG to incidence of major coronary events: Final report of the Pooling Project. *Journal of Chronic Disease* 31:201.

Rahe, R. H., and E. Lind. 1971. Psychosocial factors and sudden cardiac death: A pilot study. *Journal of Psychosomatic Research* 15.

Rahe, R. H., and J. Passakivi. 1971. Psychosocial factors and myocardial infarction, II: An outpatient study in Sweden. *Journal of Psychosomatic Research* 15.

Rhoads, G. G., C. L. Gulbrandsen, and A. Kagan. 1976. Serum lipoproteins and coronary heart disease in a population study of Hawaii-Japanese men. *New England Journal of Medicine* 294:293.

Rimm, A. A., and P. L. White. 1979. Obesity: Its risks and hazards. In *Obesity in America*, ed. G. A. Bray. U.S. Department of Health, Education, and Welfare. Publication No. NIH 79-359. Washington, D.C.: Government Printing Office.

Rissaner, V., M. Rowo, and P. Siltanen. 1978. Premonitory symptons of stress factors preceding sudden death from ischemic heart disease. *Acta Medica Scandinavica* 1978:204.

Rizek, R. L., and E. M. Jackson. 1980. *Current food consumption practices and nutrient sources in the American diet.* Consumer Nutrition Center, Human Nutrition Science and Education Administration, U.S. Department of Agriculture. Hyattsville, Md.: Government Printing Office.

Rose, G., and M. G. Marmot. 1981. Social class and coronary heart disease. *British Heart Journal* 45:13.

Roseman, R. H., R. J. Brand, and C. D. Jenkins. 1975. Coronary heart disease in the Western Collaborative Group Study: Final followup of 8 1/2 years. *Journal of the American Medical Association* 233:872.

Rowland, R., and J. Roberts. 1982. Blood pressure levels and hypertension in persons ages 6–74 years: United States, 1976–1980. National Center for Health Statistics, Advance Data No. 84. Washington, D.C.: Government Printing Office.

Rubler, S., J. Dlugash, Y. Z. Yucoglu, T. Kumral, A. W. Branwood, and A. Grishman. 1972. New type of cardiomyopathy associated with diabetic glomerulosclerosis. *American Journal of Cardiology* 30:595.

Sales, S. M., and J. House. 1971. Job dissatisfaction as a possible risk factor in coronary heart disease. *Journal of Chronic Disease* 23:861.

Sharet, J., and Salvevdy, G. 1982. Occupational stress: Review and reappraisal. *Human Factors* 24:129.

Shekelle, R. B., S. B. Hulley, and J. Neaton. 1983. The Multiple Risk Factor Intervention Trial Behavior Pattern Study II: Type A behavior pattern and incidence of coronary heart disease. Typescript.

Shekelle, R. B., S. B. Hulley, J. D. Neaton, H. H. Billings, N. O. Borhani, T. A. Gerace, D. R. Jacobs, N. L. Lasser, M. D. Mittlemark, and J. Stamler. 1985. The MRFIT Behavioral Pattern Study II: Type A behavior and incidence of coronary heart disease. *American Journal of Epidemiology* 22:4, 559–570.

Shekelle, R. B., A. M. Ostfeld, and O. Paul. 1969. Social status and incidence of coronary heart disease. *Journal of Chronic Disease* 22:381.

Shurtleff, D. 1974. Some characteristics related to the incidence of cardiovascular disease and death: The Framingham Study, 18 year followup. In *An epidemiologic investigation of cardiovascular disease*, ed. W. B. Kannel and T. Gordon. U.S. Department of Health, Education, and Welfare, Public Health Service. Washington, D.C.: Government Printing Office.

Small, D. M. 1977. Cellular mechanisms for lipid deposition in arterial walls. *New England Journal of Medicine* 297:873.

Sokolow, M., and McElroy, M. D. 1981. *Clinical cardiology.* 3d ed. New York: Lange.

Sorlie, P. 1977. Cardiovascular disease and death following myocardial infarction and angina pectoris. In *The Framingham Study: An epidemiological investigation of cardiovascular disease*, ed. W. B. Kavarel and T. Gordon. Washington, D.C.: Government Printing Office.

Stamler, J. 1978. Lifestyles, major risk factors, proof and public policy. George Lyman Duff Memorial Lecture. *Circulation* 58:3–12.

———. 1981. Primary prevention of coronary heart disease: The last 20 years. *American Journal of Cardiology* 47:722.

Stamler, J., R. Stamler, and T. Pullman, eds. 1967. *Epidemiology of hypertension.* New York: Grune and Stratton.

Syme, S. L., M. M. Hyman, and P. E. Enterline. 1964. Some social and cultural factors associated with the occurrence of coronary heart disease. *Journal of Chronic Disease* 17:277.

Syme, S. L., T. W. Oakes, and G. D. Friedman. 1974. Social class and racial differences in blood pressure. *American Journal of Public Health* 64:619.

Takaro, T., H. Hultgren, K. Detre, and W. Peduzzi. 1982. The VA Cooperative Study of stable angina: Current status. *Circulation* 65:60.

Thompson, P. D., E. J. Funk, R. A. Carleton, and W. Q. Sturner. 1982. Incidence of death during jogging in Rhode Island from 1975 through 1980. *Journal of the American Medical Association* 247(18):2535.

Thompson, P. D., M. P. Stern, P. William, K. Duncan, W. L. Haskell, and P. D. Wood. 1979. Death during jogging or running. *Journal of the American Medical Association* 242:1265.

Tyroler, H. A., J. Cassel. 1964. Health consequences of culture change II: The effect of urbanization on coronary heart disease mortality in rural residents. *Journal of Chronic Disease* 17:167.

Tyroler, H. A., I. S. Glasunov, and A. D. Deev. 1979. A comparison of high blood pressure prevalence and treatment status in selected U.S. and USSR population. In *First joint US-USSR symposium on hypertension*, pp. 423–434. U.S. Department of Health, Education, and Welfare. Washington, D.C.: Government Printing Office.

U.S. Congress. Senate. Select Committee on Nutrition and Human Needs. 1977. *Dietary goals for the United States.* 2d ed. Washington, D.C.: Government Printing Office.

U.S. Department of Agriculture. 1976. *Agricultural statistics*. Washington, D.C.: Government Printing Office.

U.S. Department of Health, Education, and Welfare. 1979. *Healthy people*. Surgeon General's Report on Health Promotion and Disease Prevention, Publication No. 70-55071. Washington, D.C.: Government Printing Office.

————. 1973. *National conference on high blood pressure education*. Publication No. 73-486. Washington, D.C.: Government Printing Office.

Verani, M. S., G. H. Hartung, J. Hoepfel-Harris, D. E. Welton, C. M. Pratt, and R. R. Miller. 1981. Effects of excerise training on left ventricular performance and myocardial perfusion in patients with coronary artery disease. *American Journal of Cardiology* 47:797.

Veterans Administration Coronary Bypass Surgery Cooperative Study Group. 1984. Eleven-year survival in the Veterans Administration randomized trial of coronary bypass surgery for stable angina. *New England Journal of Medicine* 311(21):1333–1339.

Waitzkin, H. 1984. Doctor-patient communication: Clinical implications for social scientific research. *Journal of the American Medical Association* 252(17)2441–2446.

Walker, J. J. 1977. Changing United States life-style and declining vascular mortality: Cause or coincidence (editorial). *New England Journal of Medicine* 297(3):163.

Westlund, K., and R. Nicolaysen. 1972. Ten-year mortality and morbidity related to serum cholesterol: A followup of 3,751 men aged 40–49. *Scandinavian Journal Clinical and Laboratory Investigation* 30(supp. 127).

White House Conference on Food, Nutrition, and Health. 1970. *Final report*. Washington, D.C.: Government Printing Office.

Wissler, R. W. 1974. Development of the atherosclerotic plaque in the myocardium: In *Failure and infarction*, ed. E. Braunwald. New York: H. P. Publishing Co.

Wissler, R. W., and D. Vesselinovitch. 1975. Regression of atherosclerosis in experimental animals and man. *Deutsche Gesellschaft Innere Medizin* 81:857–862.

Workshop Report Epidemiological Section. 1979. Conference on the health effects of blood lipids: Optimal distribution for populations. *Preventive Medicine* 8:612.

Chapter 9

Cancer

*James Marshall and
Saxon Graham*

The sociological and behavioral sciences have played an increasing role in addressing the problem of cancer. The environment contributes in large part to the development of cancer, and the social behaviors of populations expose them to environments that may protect them against cancer or may enhance their risk. Along with studying social factors related to early diagnosis of cancer, efforts must be made to achieve more expeditious care, thus enhancing the likelihood of surviving cancer. Problems of rehabilitation also have important social and psychological dimensions. Measured in terms of avoidance of pain, economic expenditures, and loss to society of individuals in the prime of life, the study of behavior that could prevent cancer has great potential.

This chapter examines briefly the broad problem of cancer: its major role in mortality, its cost to individuals, families, and society at large, and the benefits derived from technological advances and therapy to date. This discussion emphasizes prevention and will examine, in a limited way, research that may help contribute to this goal.

Prevention can be facilitated by understanding the chain of events leading to cancer and learning how to interrupt the sequence. This task is complicated. Cancer is not one disease but many. Although many of the forty-odd types of cancer share some causative factors, it is equally likely that many have unique causative factors. Thus, while lung and colon cancer have some features in common, other factors in their etiologies are widely different: exposure to cigarette smoke or certain airborne industrial fumes increases the risk of lung cancer but apparently has no direct impact on the risk of colon cancer. The study of the epidemiology of these two diseases and the behaviors that expose individuals must be approached separately. Prevention is also difficult because changing human behavior is a formidable task.

Occurrence and Distribution

Incidence and Mortality

Because cancer is not, in general, a reportable disease, complete tabulations of its incidence are not readily available. Mortality statistics are more completely recorded, so incidence is often estimated from mortality. According to the American Cancer Society (1984), over 800,000 persons per year are diagnosed as having cancer. These statistics include 130,000 with cancer of the lung, 120,000 with cancer of the colon or rectum, and 110,000 women with cancer of the breast. It makes such abstract figures a bit more concrete to point out that, at this incidence rate, one in four individuals living today in the United States will, at some point, develop cancer.

Cancer mortality in the United States is approximately one-half the incidence. Some 430,000 persons per year die of cancer. This can be translated into a total yearly mortality rate of approximately 176 per 100,000 population. This total mortality includes 110,000 individuals dying of

cancer of the lung, 57,000 dying of cancer of the colon or rectum, and 37,000 women dying of cancer of the breast.

Age has an important bearing upon cancer risk. The bulk of cancer mortality occurs among the aged. Among those younger than fifteen, the rate is a little higher than 5 per 100,000 per year. Among those fifteen or older, the rate increases consistently, reaching a level of 1,446 per 100,000 among individuals aged eighty-five and over. Because of these marked age differences, it is important that any study of the determinants of cancer risk take careful account of the effects of age upon risk.

Cancer is clearly a major threat to health and life, but we must consider the threat in proportion to other major causes of death. The annual crude mortality rate for all causes of death combined is approximately 878 per 100,000 population per year. Of these 878 deaths, 323 or 38 percent are caused by heart disease, with 176, or approximately 20 percent, caused by cancer. Cerebral vascular diseases are responsible for some 10 percent of all deaths.

Changes in Incidence: The Cancer Epidemic

Both the popular press and the public have voiced considerable concern about a cancer "epidemic." Indeed, one frequently encounters speculation and concern about the causes of such an epidemic, while its actuality is rarely questioned. In fact, cancer mortality has increased. In 1950 the male and female rates of cancer mortality, respectively, were 172 and 145 per 100,000 population. By the late 1970's these annual rates had risen to 215 per 100,000 for men while dropping to 135 per 100,000 for women. Clearly, cancer has increased among males though not among females.

A small part of this increase is artifactual—a result of better diagnosis. Because of advances in diagnosis, fewer deaths are described as "natural" and more are attributed to cancer. There has also been a true increase in incidence. However, little of even the true increase in cancer among males would have occurred except for the cancers caused by smoking (American Cancer Society 1984). For example, the age-adjusted mortality rate for cancer of the colon and rectum remained at about 26 per 100,000 per year throughout the entire period. Stomach cancer mortality decreased for both men and women during this period—among men from 22 to 9 per 100,000 per year and among women from 12 to 4 per 100,000. Uterine cancer mortality dropped, from 20 to 9 per 100,000. Liver cancer mortality dropped among both men and women.

In contrast, a number of cancers, all subsequently found to be mainly associated with tobacco, increased in incidence. For example, pancreatic cancer mortality increased from 8 to 11 per 100,000 among men and from 5 to 7 per 100,000 among women. Cancer of the larynx and bladder increased in incidence. But the largest single source of increase in cancer mortality during this period was cancer of the lung. The annual lung cancer mortality rate increased from 26 to 70 per 100,000 among men and from 5 to 18 per 100,000 among women.

Recently, the increase in lung cancer mortality has been concentrated among women. Lung cancer mortality among women is almost as high now as colorectal cancer mortality. It has been projected that, within a few years, at the present rate of increase, more women will die each year of lung cancer than of breast cancer (American Cancer Society 1984). This unfortunate increase is believed largely due to the increase in smoking among women, which began in the early 1950s.

If male lung cancer mortality had remained constant at its 1950 level, if it had not increased by 44 per 100,000, there would have been no increase in the male cancer rate. Instead of increasing 43 per 100,000 (from 172 to 215), the rate would have actually declined from 172 to 171 per 100,000.

Consequences

Results for the Individual

Cancer is widely regarded as a threatening, dreadful affliction, perhaps because it is usually depicted as a disease that slowly but inexorably consumes its victim (Sontag 1978). And perhaps much of the present concern over hidden carcinogens in food, water, and air stems from the considerable fear that cancer commands. Popular fear of cancer is well founded; except for nonmelanoma skin cancer the disease is life threatening and generally painful over its course. It has been reported (Marshall, Burnett, and Brasure 1983) that the occurrence of cancer doubles the probability of suicide.

The degree of threat cancer imposes can be usefully described by reference to five-year relative survival rates. (Relative survival is the proportion of individuals diagnosed at a given point who are alive five years later, with adjustment for some dying of other causes.) With all cancers grouped, the relative five-year survival rate of cancer patients is 48 percent. Thus, with other threats to life taken into account, an individual's likelihood of being alive five years hence is approximately halved by his or her having developed cancer (U.S. Department of Health and Human Services 1983).

Relative survival is often used to operationally indicate that a cancer has been cured. To define cure in this way is necessary because it is impossible to medically document that a cancer has been completely eradicated. A procedure that fails to destroy or incapacitate even a few cancer cells may merely slow down the progress of the disease, so if the patient survives an extended perod of time, such as five years, it is reasonable to assume that the cancer was cured.

Necessary though it is, this operational definition can lead to confusion. A small percentage of the people who survive five years after cancer diagnosis and treatment have not in fact been cured; they will eventually die of their cancer. Thus, earlier diagnosis can lead to longer survival and an increased likelihood of surviving five years independent of whether the cancer was cured. Assume, for example, that an individual diagnosed with a cancer at a given stage could be expected, on the average, to survive k months. Development of a procedure for diagnosis three months earlier would expand that expectation to $k + 3$ months, even if the probability of cure is not altered. Because of this ambiguity, some epidemiologists have questioned whether the widely publicized claims about improvements in cancer survival are essentially artifacts of earlier diagnosis.

Clearly the potential for bias exists in operationalizing cure by survival, but most evidence suggests that earlier diagnosis does lead to improved survival (Jacques et al. 1981). Cancer discovered at earlier stages appears to be much more treatable than that discovered at later points in its clinical course.

The danger imposed by cancer varies considerably by the cancer's anatomic location (American Cancer Society 1984). The relative five-year survival of thyroid cancer patients is over 90 percent; unfortunately, only about 2 percent of all cancers originate in the thyroid. For a number of more common cancers, relative survival is at least 70 percent; these include cancer of the uterine corpus, urinary bladder, breast, and testis, malignant melanoma, and Hodgkin's disease.

Because of cervical screening, most cancer of the uterine cervix is now detected in early stages. Forty years ago, this cancer was deadly; the relative five-year survival of cervical cancer patients today is nearly 80 percent. On the other hand, cancer of the lung is such a virulent disease, and so likely to have spread to other organ systems by the time of diagnosis, that the five-year relative survival of those diagnosed with lung cancer is only 12 percent. The relative survival of esophageal cancer patients is about 5 percent. The relative probablility that patients diagnosed with cancer of the pancreas will be alive five years later is about 2 percent. However, the threat to life does not fully describe the dislocation caused by cancer.

Cancer generates a need for life-altering therapy, including any combination of conventional treatment protocols: surgery, radiation, and chemotherapy. The choice of treatment is generally regarded as a clinical matter determined by site, by what is believed to be most likely to succeed, and by what the patient is believed to be able to stand (Ackerman and del Regato 1970). Any of the therapies can be extremely disruptive and physically, socially, and financially very costly (Moss 1980).

There is no doubt that surgery greatly increases the probability of survival for people struggling with some forms of cancer; there is also no doubt that this increased survival probability is often costly. Surgery—the excising of the cancerous lesion and the removal of enough surrounding flesh to make spread of the lesion unlikely—is a crude, disheartening form of therapy. It often is disfiguring: a breast cancer patient may have to live with one breast, an oral cancer patient without a lower jaw. It can be demeaning: a colon cancer patient may have to use a plastic bag attached to his or her side as a repository for feces, the prostatic cancer patient may be left impotent, and the laryngeal cancer patient, to talk, will have to swallow air and belch words or phrases.

Ionizing radiation is effectively used to destroy tumor tissue. It also damages healthy tissues, so it can result in disfiguring burns near the region irradiated. Radiation can cause severe systemic illness: anorexia, nausea, general debilitation. Moreover, an individual may be successfully treated by radiation therapy for one cancer but then later experience another caused by the therapy.

Chemotherapy—the use as medication of toxic substances that kill cancererous tissue—has resulted in impressive improvement in cancer patient survival. But this improvement, too, is costly. In spite of its significant therapeutic value, chemotherapy's severe systemic effects can devastate an individual. It is not uncommon, in fact, for the course of chemotherapy to be changed because the therapy's side effects have become so severe that they are life threatening. Clearly, work and other aspects of social functioning can be severely disrupted by such treatment.

In short, in spite of its successes, a large proportion of cancer therapy is unsuccessful. Many therapies are disfiguring and incapacitating in major ways. The human devastation imposed by these diseases has not nearly been eliminated.

Tremendous variation exists in the

clinical course of the different cancers and in the forms of therapy that may be implemented. Nevertheless, cancer is financially a costly affliction. A hospital bed frequently costs in excess of $300 per day. According to the National Cancer Institute (U.S. Department of Health and Human Services 1983), an episode of hospitalization for a severely ill cancer patient can exceed $15,000; a cancer patient may experience several hospitalizations during the course of the disease. It was recently reported that, during the year before dying, the typical American cancer patient accumulated a medical care bill in excess of $22,000.

Societal Cost

An important societal cost of cancer is premature death and disability of hundreds of thousands of cancer patients yearly. This cost is added to the billions spent for treatment. Although a substantial proportion of the cost of treating cancer patients is assumed by state and national government or medical insurance plans, such costs are passed on to taxpayers and insurance subscribers. In 1983 the total direct cost of medical care for cancer was estimated to be approximately $11 billion (American Cancer Society 1984). This figure amounts to about 7 percent of the total short-stay hospital expenditures in any one year (Mettlin 1984). The indirect cost of cancer, however, is much higher. During the 1980s, lost wages, lost workers, and the premature liquidation of assets have each year amounted to over $20 billion.

Cancer Treatment: Technological Advance in Perspective

As already noted, the malignancy of cancer varies by the organ or system it affects. The considerable cancer research expenditures of National Institutes of Health have produced substantial improvement in the relative survival rates of individuals with many cancers. These improvements mostly involve cancers of the blood and the blood-forming or lymphatic organs. For patients with Hodgkin's disease, the five-year survival rate in 1960 was 40 percent; it is now approximately 70 percent. Patients with acute lymphocytic leukemia in 1960 had a 4 percent five-year relative survival rate; that rate now exceeds 40 percent. However, even the diseases for which improvements have been noted are still very dangerous. Note that the complement of relative survival is relative mortality. Thus, one-third of the patients with Hodgkin's disease will not, even if other causes of death are taken into account, survive five years after diagnosis. Among women diagnosed with cancer of the uterine corpus, relative survival is 88 percent; relative mortality is, therefore, 12 percent. For a number of cancers, relative survival is 70 percent; relative mortality induced by these diseases is, therefore, 30 percent. Advances in therapy have not nearly vitiated these cancers as threats to life. Moreover, these success stories of cancer therapy—for cancer of the blood and the blood-forming or lymphatic organs—comprise a relatively small portion of total incidence; in 1983 they involved only 8 percent of total cancer incidence.

With therapy for many other cancers, there has been less progress. There has been no progress against cancer of the pancreas. The five-year relative survival rate of patients with cancer of the lung increased from approximately 8 to 12 percent between 1960 and early 1980. Cancer of the colon and rectum generated a relative survival rate of approximately 41 percent in 1960, 50 percent by 1983 (American Cancer Society 1984).

A substantial proportion of the improvement in relative survival is a result of early detection, diagnosis, and treatment. Patients diagnosed with localized stomach cancer experience a 48 percent five-year survival rate; for those in whom the disease has spread, relative survival is only about 6 percent. Among patients with cancer of the colon, the five-year relative survival rates of those with localized and advanced disease are, respectively, 77 and 29 percent. Those few patients diagnosed with localized cancer of the lung experience a relatively promising 42 percent five-year survival, but for those diagnosed once the disease has spread, survival is about 4 percent. Patients diagnosed with localized cancer of the bladder can expect a 67 percent survival. Among those in whom the disease has spread, survival is about 12 percent.

The Importance of Prevention

Prevention of cancer is much preferred to therapy, and preventive measures can be developed if we understand something about cancer's causes. The resources allocated to animal studies and human epidemiological inquiries to further understand the etiology of the disease have been small compared with the sums spent on therapy and therapy research. Nevertheless, we already have at hand tools that could substantially reduce the incidence and mortality from cancer, perhaps by as much as one-third.

Measures for prevention can be devised following a number of strategies once the key etiologic events have been understood. If individuals of a particular genetic background have a higher risk of a certain type of cancer and if these individuals can be identified, perhaps by an understanding of the distribution of the same cancer in blood relatives, they can be alerted to get routine checkups for development of the cancer in question. Some of these cancers could be found early enough to allow successful therapy. Similarly, individuals in a specific occupation who behave so as to expose themselves to high risk for a given cancer can be warned about the dangers, and measures can be taken for early identification of such cancers. This approach has been called secondary prevention, but it is prevention only in a very limited way; it really enables physicians and their patients to find cancers early enough to make therapy more effective.

The most important use of knowledge of the etiologic chain of events is to devise means of limiting exposures that otherwise would eventuate in cancer. We know that smoking is responsible for almost all lung cancer; preventing lung cancer should be easy. We know that asbestos workers have a relatively low risk of lung cancer but that the risk among those who smoke is multiplied approximately eightyfold. The logical course is to induce asbestos workers not to smoke. Many of the factors that appear to be important in the genesis of cancer are behavioral (Graham and Reeder 1972).

Social Epidemiology of Cancer

Social Setting and Environment

A number of students in the field have asserted that cancer, as well as other diseases, is largely environmentally induced. Of course, the environment must act upon a biologically predisposed individual, and this biologic predisposition may have been brought about not only by intrauterine or postnatal assaults and the wear and tear of everyday life but also by genetic heritage. Social scientists too often neglect to consider the importance of genetic background. The environment, we are aware, is pro-

foundly influenced by culture and social structure. So are individuals as they carry out certain kinds of behaviors at different risk for disease. This behavior gives us clues about how we may identify persons at risk. If we can discern differences in risk associated with specific occupations, ethnic group membership, certain kinds of diets or habits such as smoking, drinking, or chewing betel nuts, we can begin to zero in on factors that may be associated in a causative fashion with risk of the disease. We can consider risk associated not only with specific individual behaviors but also with membership in social groups.

A number of categories of social relevance, such as socioeconomic status, race, ethnic relationships, religion, rural or urban residence, and occuptional membership, may enhance or reduce risk of certain cancers. These categories identify which groups at high risk should be studied further to ascertain the specific behaviors responsible for the disease.

Given the likelihood that the impact of social environment is indirect and mediated by specific exposures in the individual's environment, it makes sense to study all kinds of potentially relevant exposures. Among those receiving attention are environmental pollution, occupational exposure, irradiation, and various aspects of life-style, such as diet, smoking, sexual practices, usage of various medications, and exercise.

Environmental Pollution

Since the publicity surrounding the discovery of chemical contamination at Love Canal in New York, String-fellow Acid Pits in California, and Times Beach in Missouri, considerable attention has been focused on inadequate disposal of dangerous industrial chemicals. The realization that certain compounds produced by widely used industrial processes are dangerous carcinogens has engendered a great deal of alarm. Clearly, if people were exposed to such substances in sufficient quantity, they might suffer substantially increased cancer risk.

Indeed, there has been considerable effort to examine the effects of environmental pollution upon human populations, but documenting cause-effect links between environmental pollution and cancer risk is difficult. It has proven even more difficult to secure evidence regarding the magnitude of any risk that may be imposed. Little is known about the proportion of cancer that results from environmental pollution.

The methodologic problems that obscure possible relationships between environmental toxin exposures and cancer risk are immense. The number of potentially dangerous chemicals used in common industrial processes is mind-boggling. Additionally, many of the cancers suspected to stem from environmental exposures can also result from nonindustrial exposures; few if any cancers were recognized only after the advent of the industrial revolution. Most were first identified hundreds of years ago.

Moreover, assessing past exposure for epidemiologic purposes is difficult. How does one assess, for example, the total past air pollution exposure of an individual living in a specific location? The assessment of such exposure becomes even more elusive if the individual lived in one location and went to school or worked in another. It is possible that environmental pollution may simply potentiate the effects of other carcinogens. For example, Pike et al. (1975) and Vena (1982) have shown that the impact of cigarette smoking upon cancer risk is greater in urban than in rural areas. Individuals living in cities are exposed to more environmental toxins in addition to smoking than are individuals living in more rural areas; cigarette smoking may be more potent for individuals breathing polluted air.

The identification of pathogenic environmental exposures is difficult unless the effect is large and immediate. In the case of cancer, most exposures have involved relatively few people, ranging from a few hundred to a few thousand, whereas the incidence of cancer is measured as occurring in a few per hundred thousand population per year. Moreover cancer is believed to require several decades to develop. Thus, even if many hundreds or even a thousand people have been exposed at a site such as Love Canal, the latent period required for the development of cancer may make it very difficult to measure any pathological effects unless those effects are overwhelming. If there were a tripling in the incidence of leukemia from 6 to 18 per 100,000 per year, one can imagine how long it would take to show an effect in a population of 5,000, the number exposed at Love Canal. For the most part, exposures have been minor and of relatively small populations, and their effects have apparently not been large enough to be discerned with any confidence.

Occupational Exposures

If environmental pollution is a factor in causing cancer in Western industrial society, and if most of the polluting substances result from industrial processes, the individuals who work in the industries that use these processes should be at substantially increased cancer risk. There is evidence of carcinogenicity in a number of industrial substances. Exposure to the organic aromatic hydrocarbons—petroleum, coal, and their by-products—has been shown to increase the risk of cancer of the lung, skin, and bladder. Exposure to benzene can induce leukemia. Mustard gas workers have been found to have elevated levels of lung cancer. Vinyl chloride exposure induces liver cancer. Arsenic exposure increases the risk of cancer of the lung and skin; chromium, the risk of cancer of the lung. Asbestos has been convincingly demonstrated to increase the risk of cancer of the pleura, mediastinum, and peritoneum (Cole and Merletti 1984).

A number of other substances are suspected to be carcinogens, although it has been impossible to generate firm evidence that the risks imposed are appreciable. The already noted long latency period between exposure and the appearance of cancer is one of the chief difficulties in the establishment of an associaton between occupational exposure and cancer. During this latency period, which may extend twenty years, workers may have

changed jobs many times; with each switch, they may be exposed to a number of different compounds. Thus, among individuals diagnosed with a given cancer, such a melange of individual exposures may have occurred that it would be nearly impossible to assess which of these exposures were responsible.

Even if a substance has been identified as a carcinogen, it is difficult to assess the amount of exposure that is "safe." A laudable goal would be to eliminate exposure to any dangerous substance, but eliminating some such exposures would be impossible or at least extremely costly if industry were to continue widely using some industrial processes. Arriving at decisions regarding strategies for the elimination of dangerous exposures will require careful thinking about the costs and benefits of various policies.

The complexity of considerations in assessing solutions to these problems is immense. For example, we can recognize that asbestos in the workplace, in a building where it is used as a heat insulator and a fireproof substance, very definitely increases the risk of the cancers noted above. These cancers are rare. In addition, asbestos is probably responsible for a very small proportion of cancers of the lung. One solution may be to substitute another substance for asbestos (rockwool or glasswool), which also may insulate or serve as a fireproof material. The difficulty is that we have had long experience with asbestos; we know its risks and how to reduce those risks. But in the case of newer substitute substances, we have no idea of their special pathogenic qualities, and, if they are responsible for only a small amount of pathology over several decades, we are not likely to find out soon.

Moreover, asbestos is an especially good fire retardant and insulator. It probably saves many lives each year through its fireproofing qualities, and it greatly reduces energy expenditures through its insulating properties. Many more lives may be lost each year through fire than through asbestos-related cancers. Thus, the decision to remove asbestos from the work and living space has to involve consideration of these varying factors, and the decision is not as easy as may first appear.

Irradiation

Heavy exposure to ionizing radiation clearly induces cancer. This holds for leukemia, cancer of the thyroid, female breast, lung, stomach, colon, and liver cancer, and for a nontrivial number of other cancers (Jablon and Bailar 1980). We found that medical irradiation not only increases the risk of leukemia in individuals but that irradiation of the fetus, or of the mother and father prior to conception, increases risk of leukemia in the child. However, the major source of exposure to ionizing radiation in the United States today is the natural cosmic background. This includes cosmic ray bombardment and exposure to radionuclides in natural biologic and physical materials. Such exposures account for over half of the typical individual's total environmental exposure to ionizing radiation (Jablon and Bailar 1980).

Medical irradiation accounts for some 40 percent of total exposure, mostly for diagnostic purposes. Nuclear weapons fallout may account for some 2.5 to 4 percent of total exposure, and a similar amount may result from exposure to the processing of radioactive materials (e.g., mining and milling of uranium). Jablon and Bailar estimated that some 5,000 cancers per year are induced by total natural background radiation exposure. Another 4,250 are induced by the use of medical irradiation. Two hundred fifty to 500 per year result from nuclear weapons testing fallout, and about 250 per year result from the processing of radiation-emitting materials. Ten cases per year may result from radiation emitted by nuclear energy facilities, and about 2 result from exposure to consumer products that emit ionizing radiation. Another 60 per year are induced among occupations in which there is exposure to substantial amounts of radiation or radioactive materials. These occupatons are located in medical nuclear energy facilities, research activities, naval reactors, and nuclear weapons research and development. These deaths total some 10,000 or approximately 2 to 2.5 percent of total cancer mortality in the United States in a given year.

While it is certainly desirable to limit exposure to ionizing radiation where possible, these figures imply that limiting exposures will have little impact on the total incidence of cancer in the United States. Some limitation of medical irradiation is already taking place. For example, enthusiasm about the use of mammography for early identification of breast cancers among women less than forty-five years of age has declined markedly in recent years. It has been reasoned that breast cancer is rare enough among young women that the number of cases discovered will only approximate the number induced. In contrast, for certain categories of women known to be at high risk for breast cancer, for example, those whose mothers have had cancer of the breast, who had no children, or had them late in life, annual mammograms after age forty are a good idea. Such weighing of costs and benefits in consideration of needs of various people at different risks must be undertaken before intelligent decisions can be made about exposures to irradiation. It must also be recognized that a substantial portion of diagnostic radiation is used with individuals who are seriously ill. The likelihood that many of these individuals will survive long enough to develop cancer, even if it were induced by such irradiation, may be small.

It is clearly desirable to limit irradiation exposure resulting from nuclear weapons testing fallout. It is also desirable to limit exposures generated by nuclear energy facilities, mining, and other industrial facilities. Energy decisions, however, cannot be taken lightly. A number of factors must be considered. For example, the levels of industrial exposures of workers today are small, and no evidence shows that such exposures are pathogenic in any major way. Many traditional occupations also engender substantial risks. The deaths attributed to coal mining amount to some 150 annually in the United States. These deaths are accepted as part of the cost of obtaining this form of energy. The number of deaths associated with mining uranium and operating nuclear energy facilities is only a tiny fraction of that number.

Diet

Three types of evidence suggest that components of diet may be important determinants of the risk of certain cancers. The first involves international variation in cancer mortality. It is clear that, in the Westernized countries, cancers of the colon, rectum, breast, and prostate are elevated. The diet in these countries tends to contain relatively high amounts of meat and fat, and relatively low amounts of fruits, vegetables, and whole grain. The bread in these countries tends to have most of its fiber removed during processing. In certain other countries, stomach cancer rates are consistently elevated. Japan, China, and many other Asian countries have high rates of cancer of the stomach and esophagus. The diet in these countries tends to contain relatively large amounts of starch, small amounts of meats and fats, and includes frequent use of pickled, salted, smoked, or otherwise preserved foods. One could hypothesize that the lowered incidence of cancer of the stomach and esophagus in industrialized countries may be related to their use of meats and fats, which could figure in their higher incidence of cancer of the colon. Cancer of the stomach or esophagus, on the other hand, may result from starchy food, or from pickled or preserved food consumption.

It is tempting to suspect that the significant differences in the diets of people of these countries have something to do with the very substantial differences observed in patterns of cancer risk, but the perils of deriving explanations from ecological data have been well documented (Robinson 1950). It is particularly pertinent to cancer epidemiology that the countries mentioned differ in far more than diet: their social patterns, stress, exercise, and environmental pollution also vary substantially.

Another source of evidence on the relevance of diet to cancer is derived from migrant studies. Certain cancer rates of migrants tend within their lifetime to assume a level approximately between those of the countries of their origin and destination. It is reasonable to suspect that dietary change is responsible for these shifts. Generally, studies of migrants have tended to support findings derived from ecological studies.

Finally, evidence has come from individual-based studies, both retrospective and prospective. The retrospective, or case-control method, by far the most widely used in studies of diet and cancer, involves the assessment of the diets of newly diagnosed cases and those of controls. The rationale for this approach is that, if a certain diet increases cancer risk, cases will have consumed that diet to a greater degree than controls. Use of the prospective method, on the other hand, requires assessment of study participant diets at the beginning of the study period. Those participants are then watched and the rate at which they become cancer patients noted. The period of observation may

extend several years. It is reasoned that, if a specific substance in the diet increases cancer risk, the cancer rate of those whose diets contain more of that food will be elevated. The most consistently observed result of both retrospective and prospective studies has been that a diet high in fruits and vegetables confers some protection against cancer and that dietary fats may increase cancer risk.

For example, the consumption of green and yellow vegetables appears to reduce risk of lung cancer by as much as 50 percent, even with adjustment for smoking practices. This result appears to come from the carotene in such foods (Mettlin and Graham 1979); Hinds et al. 1984; Byers et al. 1984).

Similar patterns of protection resulting from the use of vitamin A–containing foods have been observed for cancer of the bladder (Mettlin, Graham, and Swanson 1979), esophagus (Mettlin et al. 1981), larynx (Graham et al. 1981), cervix (Marshall et al. 1983), and mouth (Marshall et al. 1982). The consumption of some vegetables appears to protect against cancer of the colon and rectum, although the findings of studies of these sites are not consistent (Graham et al. 1978; Miller et al. 1978). Finally, although vegetable consumption has been shown to protect a number of cancer sites, some evidence shows that it may increase the risk of cancer of the prostate (Graham et al. 1983; Kolonel 1983; Hirayama 1979).

Although, as noted, little is known about how diet influences individual risk, the massive differences between countries in cancer risk and the suspicion that the diet may be an important factor in these differences have generated interest among researchers and policymakers. The National Cancer Institute is currently sponsoring a number of epidemiologic studies of diet and cancer. These include retrospective studies and intervention trials to determine whether cancer risk can be reduced. The interventions involve increasing vitamins or lowering fat ingestion by individuals who are, by several criteria, high in cancer risk.

Sexual Practices

One of the earliest observations relating sexuality to cancer risk was that women who married early and bore large numbers of children experienced an elevated risk of cervical cancer, while nuns had almost no such risk. Subsequent studies have consistently shown that women who commence sexual activity at a young age and have contact with large numbers of sexual partners are at an increased risk (Graham et al. 1979). Substantial evidence shows that cervical cancer may in fact be a venereal disease. Thus, we and others (Martinez 1969) have found that women whose husbands had cancer of the penis had a higher risk of developing cervical cancer (Graham et al. 1979). A large number of studies suggest that cervical cancer patients are more likely than control women to have antibodies to Herpes Simplex Virus Type 2, a virus that can be transmitted through sexual activity. There is evidence, also, that another virus transmitted through sexual contact, human papilloma virus, could be involved (zur Hausen 1977) in the genesis of cervical cancer.

Homosexuality among men has recently been shown to be associated with an increase in risk of a cancer, Kaposi's sarcoma, this risk resulting from acquired immunodeficiency syndrome (AIDS). The ultimate cause of AIDS is likely to be communicable via microorganisms carried by blood, feces, and semen. This disease is spreading at a very fast rate; the case fatality rate (the proportion of cases that die of the disease) is very high. The skyrocketing increase in incidence is probably related to the fact that some male homosexuals have extremely large numbers of sexual contacts and that individuals can have AIDS for some time before experiencing symptoms that might reduce their sexual activity.

In addition, AIDS is apparently transmitted by other exposures to infected blood; these may occur while injecting drugs or transfusing blood. As with smoking and lung cancer, we have a key to reducing the incidence of AIDS, even before understanding completely the mechanism of its occurrence. The greatest proportion of AIDS occurs among male homosexuals, and many of these victims had engaged in sex with large numbers of partners. The potential for exposure to pathogenic microorganisms is greatly enhanced among individuals who have large numbers of intimate contacts. Clearly, one measure for the reduction of risk is to reduce the number of sexual contacts an individual has. This probably is already occurring, as evidenced by the recent reduction in the incidence of gonorrhea within the homosexual community. Similarly, stocks of blood for transfusion are carefully screened now that a microorganism linked to AIDS has been identified.

Social and Psychological Stress

Social scientists are sometimes tempted to hypothesize that risk of cancer may be increased among individuals suffering social or psychological stress of one sort or another. However, there is little evidence for any site (Funch and Marshall 1983). The few sites that have been studied show only weak relationships. Perhaps the episodes of relevant stress occurred at the time of the initiation of the cancer, some twenty or thirty years prior to its expression as a symptomatic tumor. Nevertheless, stress is a ubiquitous part of human existence; whether it would be possible to discern differences in stress experience between cases and controls is extremely problematic.

Smoking

As noted earlier, smoking is the most important pathogen in Western industrialized society. Not only is it responsible for hundreds of thousands of deaths from cancer of the lung but it is also an important cause of cancer of the mouth, larynx, and bladder and of many thousands more deaths from coronary heart diseases and emphysema.

Smoking is a factor that by itself greatly increases risk; in synergy with other factors, such as exposures to irradiation, metal or coal dust, asbestos, or other substances, it helps magnify risk many times. Despite the fact that tobacco has been a known carcinogen for several decades, relatively little has been done to control this scourge. The policy implication is clear; everything possible should be done to eradicate smoking. But many people in the United States, France, England, and other countries benefit economically from tobacco. In each country, the government either obtains significant revenues from taxes on tobacco, or, as in France and Denmark, administers a tobacco monopoly. American tobacco farmers are engaged in an intensive type of agriculture involving very small acerage. It would be difficult for them to shift from growing tobacco to another crop that would be equally remunerative. Retail outlets, ranging from "Mom-and-Pop" to large chain stores, and the communication and advertising industries all profit from tobacco. They constitute strong political forces.

It is anomalous that, in the United States, we have a tobacco-growing industry subsidized in part by federal monies, that the federal government obtains excise taxes through the sale of cigarettes, and that the National Cancer Institute and the National Heart, Lung, and Blood Institute spend large sums of money to combat the use of tobacco. In the best of all possible worlds, knowing what we do, we would erase tobacco from our society in a trice. But tobacco has been built into the fabric of society since the sixteenth century; it will take a long time and much effort and consideration of some powerful potential economic options to rid ourselves of it. Nevertheless, no more important public health problem exists, and those interested in the public health should make every effort to accomplish this end.

Conclusion

We have seen that the large group of different diseases known as cancer exacts a tremendous toll on the population of the United States and of other countries in the Western world. Not only is therapy frequently ineffective, it is often disfiguring, maiming, and incapacitating. It is preferable in many circumstances only to death.

At the same time, it is possible to avoid the necessity for therapy by preventing the disease from developing in the first place. We have ready some solutions to the problem of prevention. These solutions derive from research on the relationship between exposures of various sorts to subsequent risk of cancer at various sites. Industrial exposures such as asbestos, benzene, and irradiation are responsible for a small number of cancers. Other human behavioral characteristics, such as sex behavior, diet, and most important, smoking, have been implicated as risk factors for cancers at various sites. The most important of these is smoking, which, if eliminated, could save hundreds of thousands of deaths per year from cancer and other diseases. Currently, research is in progress to find ways of applying what we have learned through our epidemiological studies. Studies of behavioral change are now examining ways to help people stop smoking and stop other damaging behaviors. As research continues and identifies dietary or other means of avoiding cancer, principles of behavioral change may also provide new strategies for future preventive efforts.

References

Ackerman, L., and J. del Regato. 1970. *Cancer: Diagnosis, treatment, and prognosis.* 4th ed. St. Louis: C. V. Mosby.

American Cancer Society. 1984. *Cancer facts and figures.* New York: American Cancer Society.

Byers, T., J. Vena, C. Mettlin, M. Swanson, and S. Graham. 1984. Dietary vitamin A and lung cancer risk: An analysis by histologic subtypes. *American Journal of Epidemiology* 120:769–776.

Cole, P., and F. Merletti. 1984. Personal communication.

Funch, D., and J. Marshall. 1983. The role of stress, social support, and age in survival from breast cancer. *Journal of Psychosomatic Research* 27:77–83.

Graham, S., H. Dayal, M. Swanson, A. Mittelman, and G. Wilkinson. 1978. Diet in the epidemiology of cancer of the colon and rectum. *Journal of the National Cancer Institute* 61:709–714.

Graham, S., B. Haughey, J. Marshall, R. Priore, T. Byers, T. Rzepka, C. Mettlin, and J. Pontes. 1983. Diet in the epidemiology of carcinoma of the prostate gland. *Journal of the National Cancer Institute* 70:687–692.

Graham, S., C. Mettlin, J. Marshall, R. Priore, T. Rzepka, and D. Shedd. 1981. Dietary factors in the epidemiology of cancer of the larynx. *American Journal of Epidemiology* 113:675–680.

Graham, S., R. Priore, M. Graham, R. Browne, W. Burnett, and D. West. 1979. Genital cancer in wives of penile cancer patients. *Cancer* 44:1870–1874.

Graham, S., and L. Reeder. 1972. Social factors in the chronic diseases. In *Handbook of medical sociology*, ed. H. Freeman, S. Levine, and L. Reeder, pp. 63–107. New York: Academic Press.

Hinds, M., L. Kolonel, J. Hankin, and J. Lee. 1984. Dietary vitamin A, carotene, vitamin C, and risk of lung cancer in Hawaii. *American Journal of Epidemiology* 119:227–236.

Hirayama, T. 1979. Epidemiology of prostate with special reference to the role of diet. *National Cancer Institute Monograph* 53:149–155.

Jablon, S., and J. Bailar. 1980. The contribution of ionizing radiation to cancer mortality in the United States. *Preventive Medicine* 9:219–226.

Jacques, P., S. Hartz, R. Tuthill, and C. Hollingsworth. 1981. Elimination of "lead time" bias in assessing the effect of early breast cancer diagnosis. *American Journal of Epidemiology* 113:93–97.

Kolonel, L. 1983. Vitamin A in the epidemiology of prostate cancer. Paper presented at the Meeting of the Society for Epidemiologic Research, Winnipeg, Manitoba, Canada.

Marshall, J., W. Burnett, and J. Brasure. 1983. On precipitating factors: Cancer as a cause of suicide. *Suicide and Life-Threatening Behavior* 13:15–27.

Marshall, J., S. Graham, T. Byers, M. Swanson, and J. Brasure. 1983. Diet and smoking in the epidemiology of cancer of the cervix. *Journal of the National Cancer Institute* 70:847–851.

Marshall, J., S. Graham, C. Mettlin, D. Shedd, and M. Swanson. 1982. Diet in the epidemiology of oral cancer. *Nutrition and Cancer* 3:145–149.

Martinez, I. 1969. Relationship of squamous cell carcinoma of the cervix uteri to squamous cell carcinoma of the penis. *Cancer* 24:777–780.

Mettlin, C. 1984. Personal communication.

Mettlin, C., and S. Graham. 1979. Dietary risk factors in human bladder cancer. *American Journal of Epidemiology* 110:255–263.

Mettlin, C., S. Graham, R. Priore, J. Marshall, and M. Swanson. 1981. Diet and cancer of the esophagus. *Nutrition and Cancer* 2:143–147.

Mettlin, C., S. Graham, and M. Swanson. 1979. Vitamin A and lung cancer. *Journal of the National Cancer Institute* 62:1435–1438.

Miller, A., A. Kelley, N. Choi, V. Matthews, R. Morgan, L. Munan, J. Burch, J. Feather, G. Howe, and M. Jain. 1978. A study of diet and breast cancer. *American Journal of Epidemiology* 107:499–509.

Moss, R. 1980. *The cancer syndrome*. New York: Grove Press.

Pike, M., R. Gordon, B. Henderson, et al. 1975. Air pollution. In *Persons at high risk of cancer: An approach to cancer etiology and control*, ed. J. Fraumeni, pp. 225–240. New York: Academic Press.

Robinson, W. 1950. Ecological correlations and the behavior of individuals. *American Sociological Review* 15:351–357.

Rosenman, R., R. Brand, C. Jenkins, M. Friedman, R. Straus, and M. Wurm. 1975. Coronary heart disease in the Western Collaborative Group Study: Final follow-up experience of eight and one-half years. *Journal of the American Medical Association* 233:827–877.

Sontag, S. 1978. *Illness as metaphor.* New York: Farrar,Straus and Giroux.

U.S. Department of Health and Human Services. 1983. *NCI Fact Book.* Bethesda, Md.:NIH.

Vena, J. 1982. Air pollution as a risk factor in lung cancer. *American Journal of Epidemiology* 116:42–56.

zur Hausen, H. 1977. Human Papilloma viruses and their possible role in squamous cell carcinomas. *Current Topics Microbiology and Immunology* 78:1.

Chapter 10

Mental Illness

George W. Brown

The much debated third edition of the *American Psychiatric Association Diagnostic and Statistical Manual of Mental Disorders* (DSM-3) lists some three hundred diagnoses (Spitzer, Endicott, and Robins 1978; Klerman et al. 1984). The relevance of psychosocial factors is made clear throughout its commentary. By contrast, the discussion in this chapter focuses only on two conditions— schizophrenia and depression. Because even with this narrowing of focus the span of topics is still too broad for a single chapter, I will disproportionately discuss work of research groups with which I have been associated. While this approach overemphasizes my own work, the advantage is that I know it in depth.

In the field of psychiatry, social science has been concerned with case finding and demographic description in the hope of gaining insights about etiology; for some social scientists there has also been the hope that some insight about society could be achieved as well. Carol Gilligan (1984) notes how Sigmund Freud and John Bowlby relied on the "magnification of pathology to reveal what is otherwise invisible." In a similar sense it is possible to consider the workings of social institutions by using the lens of mental illness. Emile Durkheim's *Suicide*, published in 1897, is an early and illustrious example. The study of depression is particularly critical for such an approach because it is common as well as linked to broad social experiences and the person's own milieu. It becomes clear, for instance, that self-esteem is involved in depression's genesis, and its genesis in turn is influenced by success in the social roles to which a person is committed. Much social science input in the 1960s and 1970s, particularly that associated with the so-called antipsychiatry movement, chose schizophrenia as such a magnifier. Unfortunately, while there is little doubt that the course of a schizophrenic disorder is related to the patient's immediate social setting, it has not been easy to connect the development of this particular disorder, the milieu of the individual (particularly the family), and wider societal structures.

Rates of Disorder

Several studies begun about the same time in North America pointed to a surprisingly high prevalence of psychiatric disorder (e.g., Leighton et al. 1963, Leighton 1965, Srole et al. 1962). These studies were met with a good deal of skepticism especially as they used global mental status measures based on questionnaires to estimate rates of general psychological impairment. The extremely high proportion of individuals (81 percent) said to suffer from some symptoms in the midtown Manhattan study has often been used to illustrate the absurdity of such claims. None the less, this early survey in fact concluded that 23 percent of a sample of 1,660 inhabitants were psychiatrically impaired (Langner and Michael 1963), and this figure has proved to be reasonably close to estimates of subsequent studies using more sophisticated and clinically based measures. There is some hope that such work will in time inform decisions concerning allocation of resources and treatment options (Boyd and Weissman 1981). The key advance has been that the use of semistructured interviews has made it possible to identify persons in the general population with conditions comparable to those treated by psychiatrists. In the United Kingdom, work with general population samples using the Present State Examination (PSE) began in 1970 (Brown, N. Bhrolchain, and Harris 1975; Brown and Harris 1978; Wing et al. 1977). In the United States this step was first taken in 1975–1976 in New Haven (Weissman and Myers 1980) and based on diagnostic techniques (SADS-RDC) developed by Spitzer, Endicott, and Robins (1978). Of particular interest are recent studies carried out in Edinburgh (Dean, Surtees, and Sashidharan 1983) and in Islington, London (Brown, Craig, and Harris 1985) since they have combined the most popular U.K. and U.S. approaches to case finding.

This context is not appropriate for a general review of epidemiological surveys. (For details, the reader should consult Boyd and Weissman 1981; Dean, Surtees, and Sashidharan 1983; Dohrenwend and Dohrenwend 1974; Dohrenwend et al. 1980). The one-month prevalence of psychiatric morbidity using newer case-finding methods, has usually been found to range from 8 percent to 15 percent, with depression and anxiety much the most common conditions. Rates for depression, as for psychiatric disorder in general, have consistently been found to be higher for women (Bebbington et al. 1981; Kessler and McRae 1981; Weissman and Klerman 1977). Women are between two and three times more likely than men to report a history of affective disorder (Al-Issa 1982). Other forms of psychopathology appear to be unrelated to sex or to occur more commonly in men (Dohrenwend and Dohrenwend 1976). There has been a good deal of imaginative discussion of the reasons for sex differences in depression, although for convincing conclusions the research itself has been too distant from detailed study of the lives of men and women who have developed disorders (e.g., Gove 1972; Kessler 1979; Kessler and McRae 1984).

In a recent Edinburgh survey a one-year period prevalence for psychiatric disorder for women (based on SADS-RDC) was 25 percent (Dean, Surtees, and Sashidharan 1983). In early work in Camberwell, using what is probably a somewhat stricter criterion of disorder or "caseness," the rate was 17 percent (Brown and Harris 1978); this rate was doubled if conditions of lesser severity were included. The most common disorder in both surveys was depression. Both studies concluded that about half the women with conditions at a caseness level had had them for over one year, and that the severity of the conditions was such that it "would be both inappropriate and misleading to classify them as either 'minor' or as a transitory form of 'demoralisation'" (Surtees, Sashidharan, and Dean 1984).

There is also general agreement that a considerable social class difference exists in rates of mental illness (Schwab and Schwab 1978). This difference is reflected in treatment statistics (Rosen 1977) and in rates in the general population (Dohrenwend et al. 1980; Kessler and Cleary 1980). In the first Camberwell survey, which included 458 women between the ages of eighteen and sixty-five, disorder (most of a depressive nature) was far more common among working-class than middle-class women— 23 percent versus 6 percent in the three months before interview. And

differences were greatest for women with at least one child at home (Brown and Harris 1978). These results have been confirmed in the recent Edinburgh survey of 576 women (Dean, Surtees, and Sashidharan 1983; Surtees 1984; Surtees et al. 1983), and a second and later survey in Camberwell is not inconsistent (Bebbington et al. 1981, 1984). In the New Haven survey social class differences were found only among those suffering minor depression (Weissman and Myers 1978). Unfortunately only 54 percent of the original cohort on which the study was based was followed up, which may have resulted in relatively more lower-class individuals with affective disorder dropping out. In sum, it appears that a higher rate of affective disorder exists among working-class groups, but this result may hold only for urban areas. (For studies of rural populations, see Brown and Prudo 1981, Leighton et al. 1971).

In comparison, rates of schizophrenia in Britain are extremely low, with a prevalence rate of about 3.3 per 1,000 (Cooper 1978) and an inception rate based on first-ever contact with psychiatric services of between 11 and 14 per 100,000 (Wing and Fryers 1976). (More "lenient" diagnostic practices in the United States inflate these figures somewhat.)

Schizophrenia and Its Course

A program of research, begun in the MRC Social Psychiatry Research Unit in 1956 and currently being pursued in a number of other countries, has established that psychosocial factors play a part in the course of a schizophrenic illness. The emphasis has been on the course of the illness, although by implication any factor found to be of importance may also turn out to play some part in original onset. The research has proceeded by refining crude risk factors in a series of inquiries.

The first study was a simple one dealing with male patients who, against all the odds, had managed to leave hospital after staying continuously for at least two years. The follow-up study showed that, if the subjects had been diagnosed as schizophrenic, they were more likely to relapse if they returned to live with parents or wives than if they went to live in lodgings or with brothers and sisters. This finding did not hold for other diagnoses such as depression. Other findings from the same study suggested that the social environment might play an important part in the return of florid symptomatology and, because of this, return to hospital (Brown, Carstairs, and Topping 1958; Brown 1959a). It seemed possible that the schizophrenic patients were often reacting adversely to close ties *and* that patients with this diagnosis, because of some underlying predisposition, were particularly sensitive to such influences—that is, to too much emotional arousal.

The next project was longitudinal and confirmed, by direct measures of family interaction at the time of discharge, the relevance of this insight (Brown et al. 1962). Still more specific and sensitive measures of feelings expressed in a family were developed for a second longitudinal study. In this study it was found that a measure of "expressed emotion" of family members, made when they were talking about the patient, based on the number of critical comments and amount of emotional overconcern, was highly predictive of the return of florid symptoms once the patient had been discharged (Brown, Birley, and Wing 1972).

This finding applied to patients returning to any family setting and involved the kind of feelings that might occur in ordinary families. The finding differed from the emphasis on the overriding importance of deeply disturbed relationships with parents found in most other research on schizophrenia and the family (Hirsch and Leff 1975). Such disturbed relationships certainly occur, but it seemed unlikely that they could provide a general explanation of exacerbations of symptoms and rehospitalization. The expressed emotion (EE) measure reflected phenomena that are a good deal more commonplace; trained interviewers took into account by means of rating scales a range of feelings and emotions found in ordinary families—criticism, dissatisfaction, hostility, and the like. The final index used to predict relapse was based on critical comments made about the patient and on the amount of emotional overconcern expressed by key household members. Hostility proved to be redundant, and the other measures were unrelated to relapse once the index was taken into account (Brown, Birley, and Wing 1972). The results were replicated in an independent study two years later. Combining both studies, 51 percent of patients returning to high and 13 percent to low EE homes relapsed with florid symptoms (Vaughn and Leff 1976).

Research in hospital settings confirmed the importance of emotional arousal; and with this finding a full theory dealing with secondary disabilities, such as lack of confidence in one's ability to hold down a job, was developed. A schizophrenic patient can have florid symptoms (e.g., delusions, hallucinations, incoherence of thought and speech, overactivity) and negative symptoms (e.g., social withdrawal, flatness of effect, poverty of speech, slowness); the latter was particularly common among long-stay hospital patients and relates to understimulating rather than overstimulating social conditions (Wing 1966; Wing and Brown 1970). Many schizophrenic patients appear to be biologically vulnerable to environments in which very little occurs and are liable to respond by a marked increase in social withdrawal. A study of 233 female long-stay patients over an eight-year period showed that negative symptoms improved when the environment changed in a way consistent with the theory. (Research dealing with rehabilitation of schizophrenic patients has confirmed this—e.g., Wing 1978; Watts and Bennett 1983). However, if such changes are too extensive and too sudden, florid symptoms emerge. Therefore, for schizophrenic patients things can go wrong in two quite distinct ways. In correcting overstimulation, psychiatrists and families can easily go too far in creating an environment leading to social withdrawal and negative symptoms.

Part of the theory concerning overstimulating conditions can be linked with research on life events. Patients had a three times greater chance of experiencing a significant life event in the three weeks immediately prior to a florid attack, and this held for first and subsequent episodes (Birley and Brown 1970; Brown and Birley 1968). The events can be quite minor—being called on by a policeman with news of a distant relative's hospital admission or moving with parents to the other side of the same town could be enough to trigger a florid episode. The result has been replicated in a series of studies (e.g., Day 1986; Jacobs, Prusoff, and Paykel 1974; Leff and Vaughn 1980; Paykel 1978).

Schizophrenia and Social Intervention with Families

Schizophrenia is today no longer seen in terms of progressive deterioration; it is recognised that the illness can follow a fluctuating or chronic course (Bleuler 1974). Analyses based on the expressed emotion research also showed that for those in high EE homes, decreased contact with relatives or neuroleptic medication reduced chances of relapse and that the two effects were additive. Particularly intriguing is evidence that life events can serve to provoke relapse in patients protected by medication. Indeed, together with exposure to EE relatives, such life events may explain most instances of florid relapse even of those patients still on maintenance doses of neuroleptic drugs (Leff and Vaughn 1981; Leff et al. 1973).

Until recently the direction of causality could not be established beyond doubt (Hirsch 1983). As in science as a whole, it is desirable to follow correlational findings for possible confounding factors, however subtle their control, with an experimental approach where changes made in relation to causal factors in the theory can be shown to be followed by changes in the dependent variable. Several intervention studies have now been carried out in the United Kingdom and United States. (Barrowclough and Tarrier 1984 give a recent review.)

The first study dealing with expressed emotion was conducted by members of the MRC Social Psychiatry Research Unit. The investigators suggested that if a high level of contact with high EE families leads to relapse, then the 50 percent relapse rate over a nine-month period among patients taking medication who live with high EE relatives should fall if either the patients reduced contact with their relatives or the relatives reduced their expressed emotion. In a randomized trial, twenty-four patients were either treated in an ordinary outpatient clinic or placed in an intensive family treatment program. All were given maintenance doses of neuroleptic drugs. The family treatment condition included two talks about the nature of schizophrenia; also, a relatives' group helped those with high expressed emotion deal with everyday contact with the patient. And meetings were held with the patient and relative to try to reduce expressed emotion and with the patient to reduce face-to-face contact. There was a significant reduction in critical comments or contact between patient and relative in eight of the eleven experimental families and no reduction in the control families; as predicted, the relapse rate fell in the experimental group to below 15 percent (Leff et al. 1982). (In terms of previous experience the expected rate, and that found in the control group, was 50 percent.) The results go a considerable way to support the original theory and raise hopes about effective intervention. Similar work has been done in the United States, and these studies on the whole support the effectiveness of intervention. The recent research of Gerry Hogarty and his colleagues in Pittsburgh is of considerable interest, but on balance clear-cut evidence for the importance of social intervention has not emerged (Barrowclough and Tarrier 1984; Hogarty et al. 1974a, 1974b, 1979). Research in California by Michael Goldstein and Ian Falloon and their colleagues concerned "family therapy" and produced findings consistent with that in the London study (Goldstein and Kopeikin 1981; Falloon et al. 1982). In the Falloon study, for example, only one patient (6 percent) relapsed in the family therapy group compared with eight relapses (44 percent) in an individual therapy group during a nine-month follow-up. After two years, only 17 percent of the latter had remained stable throughout compared with 83 percent of the family-treated patients (Falloon, Boyd, and McGill 1984). A recent analysis has used new measures of "affective style" to gain further insights into the favorable impact of the family treatment on relapse and on social functioning.

Particularly interesting are the insights on the time needed to reduce the amount of affect-laden comments within a family (Doane et al. 1985).

Schizophrenic patients form a large part of the pool of the chronically mentally ill who have significant impairments. Although they are estimated at no more than 1 percent of the total population, they constitute a major burden on the community (Goldman, Gattozzi, and Taube 1981). David Mechanic has outlined the variety of forces that have dramatically reshaped the mental health services system and location of care in the United States in the past thirty years; much of the same argument holds for the United Kingdom (Mechanic 1985). A dramatic reduction has occurred in the public mental hospital population, and in this context excellent research has documented that hospital stay is not essential for the great majority of patients. However, effective alternatives are extremely demanding of effort and organization and may well be as expensive as inpatient care. One significant experiment in Wisconsin, reported by Leonard Stein and Mary Ann Test, involved comparing a training program in community living with a progressive hospital care unit (Stein and Test 1978, 1980; Test and Stein 1980; Weisbrod, Test, and Stein 1980). The experimental group was assisted in developing an independent living situation in the community, given social support, and taught simple living skills such as budgeting, job hunting, and using public transportation. The encouragement of such skills is undoubtedly an important complement to the family intervention already described, and such skills are often essential for patients living outside a family setting. The experimental group did better on a variety of measures, including having fewer symptoms and expressing more satisfaction with their lives. Sadly, and not unexpectedly in light of previous research, when the support was withdrawn after thirteen months and patients were returned to the more traditional (but nonetheless still substantial) services, the experimental group by and large quickly reverted to the level of functioning of the control series. Stein and Test conclude that for a large number of chronically disabled psychiatric patients, treatment must be an ongoing rather than a time-limited endeavor. One particularly impressive aspect of this program was the way the staff went out of their way to include patients: "the program must be assertive, involve patients in their treatment, and be prepared to 'go to' the patient to prevent dropout. It must also actively insure continuity of care among treatment agencies rather than assume that a patient will successfully negotiate the often difficult pathways from one agency to another on his own" (Stein and Test 1980, 393). This assertive attitude was probably critical for the program's success because the most handicapped schizophrenic patients are the ones most likely to be out of touch with community services, even when these are considerably developed (Brown et al. 1966).

There are three major and related issues concerning such services. The first is to establish the methods and the principles on which effective intervention is based. Clearly, considerable progress has been made here. The second need is to bring this knowledge to bear on the provision of care in a national population as a whole, not merely in terms of special inquiries. Mechanic has discussed the extraordinary difficulties, not least in funding, faced by any attempt at widespread introduction of a progressive program such as that in Wisconsin outlined earlier (Mechanic 1985). He concludes that the "single most important contribution to patient care we could make in coming years is to consolidate funding sources at the local level, allowing rational calculations and decision-making among alternatives." But there is a third, perhaps equally difficult issue: innovations tend to deteriorate.

Alexander Leighton's account of the history of a Community Health Centre in Nova Scotia is only one of a number of eloquent case descriptions of the tendency of such organizations to decline in efficacy and morale (Leighton 1983). Particularly persuasive is a description of the creation (and decline) of treatment programs based on the personal experience of one clinical psychologist (Sarason 1972.

The actual process of reform and decline within the hospital setting itself was documented in an eight-year study of long-stay schizophrenic patients. Before the study began in 1960, two of the three hospitals had carried out major reforms in the care of long-stay patients; these hospitals continued to improve. But after 1962 both declined for the next six years until restrictiveness of ward regime and quality of life of the patients had regressed to the 1960 level. The third hospital had begun its reform, with the appointment of a new medical superintendent, just at the time of the research workers' first contact with it. Here reform largely petered out by 1966, and by this time some of the least handicapped of the patients had been allowed to become less active. At all hospitals the patients' mental state worsened with the decline in quality of care (Wing and Brown 1970).

A number of fascinating historical accounts have been written of such processes (e.g., Grob 1966; Bockhoven 1956). The reasons for such decline are complex and have been of sociological concern since Max Weber's classic discussion of charisma and routinization (Weber 1948). Factors at many levels are undoubtedly involved—from decisions at the highest level about the way resources are allocated to factors influencing the morale of those immediately in contact with patients (Brown 1973). One of the major challenges for social science is to learn more about such processes.

As far as the family studies of expressed emotion are concerned, important matters of interpretation must still be sorted out—measurement, type of intervention, impact on other outcome criteria and theory—but the program of research appears to have come successfully full circle. A psychosocial theory based on evidence provided by a crude cross-sectional study has guided work of increasing sophistication, resulting in research involving direct and apparently effective intervention.

One interesting conclusion that

can be drawn is the importance of taking into account the social context in which drugs are given. In the early research, neuroleptic drugs appeared to be far more effective in high expressed emotion homes, and it was concluded that perhaps they were effective only in such settings. However, Julian Leff and Christine Vaughn have added an interesting and important caveat. When patients in low EE homes were followed up for a period longer than nine months, there was a definite indication that drugs reduced relapse for this group as well. Leff and Vaughn's (1981) interpretation is interesting—that a maintenance dose had a prophylactic effect because it helped protect schizophrenics from the impact of critical life events that inevitably occurred in the course of time. While this interpretation is speculative, it is clear that viewing drug treatment in the social context in which it is given is important.

The Etiology of Depression

There is evidence that certain stressors play a major etiological role in a wide range of depressive conditions; but only life events with severe long-term threats or ongoing difficulties, which are both markedly unpleasant and have gone on for some time, can act as such "provoking agents" (Brown and Harris 1978, 1986). Moreover, such events work because of their meaning rather than through any change in a person's customary habits and routines. The words *loss,* *failure, abandonment, rejection,* and *disappointment* sum up well the meaning that is critical for depression. About 80 percent of all depressive conditions that develop in the general population appear to be brought about by a loss—loss not so much of a person but of an idea or an aspiration (Finlay-Jones and Brown 1981). The comparable proportion among persons who are already psychiatric patients is less clear; although if the small group of bipolar depressive conditions are excluded, the proportion is unlikely to be much less than two-thirds (Brown and Harris 1978, 1986).

Only a minority develop depression, even following the severest of life's crises. Therefore, we must seek sources of vulnerability to such crises. One way of doing this is to identify factors that relate to risk of depression only when there is also a stressor. In the early research in Camberwell in London, lack of an intimate tie with a husband acted as a vulnerability factor. (Others included early loss of mother by death or separation, and three or more children less than fifteen years old at home.) In conjunction with this two-factor model the following speculative theory was developed, emphasizing the critical importance of the generalization of hopelessness in response to a particular stressor. Given a major loss or disappointment the average person would feel some hopelessness, and this feeling would tend to be specific to the crisis. The more vulnerable, in contrast, go on to generalize these feelings, applying them to life as a whole. Such generalization in turn is more likely to occur in the context of ongoing feelings of low self-esteem. And it is more difficult to imagine oneself emerging from the privation when self-esteem is low. Finally, we speculated that vulnerability factors, such as lack of intimacy with husband, play an etiological role because they relate to ongoing feelings of low self-esteem (Brown and Harris 1978).

This early research therefore pinpointed the issue of vulnerability —why only one in five women experiencing a major loss or disappointment goes on to develop a depressive disorder. In planning new research it was essential to recognize the danger that attempts to answer this question can become self-fulfilling if the depression starts to color the subject's accounts of herself and her contacts; that she will perhaps look back and describe herself quite misleadingly as just as lonely and worthless before onset as she feels now she is ill. To avoid this reporting bias, information was collected about self-esteem and social support at a time prior to the onset of any depression. And only onsets in the year following the first interview were used in the analysis. (These were established at the interview carried out a year later.)

The site of the research, Islington, is an inner-city area in North London. A random sample of some four hundred women, all of whom had a child living at home, were seen. A fifth were single parents—a proportion far in excess of the national average and an indicator of the kind of adversity to be found in the population. In keeping with previous estimates, 22 percent of these working-class women experienced a psychiatric disorder at a case level in the year before interview. As in previous surveys half of these disorders were "chronic" in the sense of lasting continuously for a year or more (Brown, Craig, and Harris 1985).

There has been growing interest in the possibility that social support might provide protection from the impact of major stressors, even when vulnerability factors such as low self-esteem are present (Cassel 1974, 1976; Caplan 1974; Cobb 1976). Unfortunately much of the work on social support is methodologically weak and conceptually confused. A useful recent review based on the best studies concludes that particular and limited types of support, especially having a confidant and perceiving that one has access to broad-based crisis support, have a stress-buffering effect. Evidence for the importance of more extensive networks of ties is far less impressive (Kessler and McLeod 1984). One important recent prospective study in Canberra, concentrating on general social support, found no evidence that social support as traditionally conceived, that is as external to the person, plays any part in protecting against a depressive disorder (Henderson, Byrne, and Duncan-Jones 1981).

By contrast, the importance of the quality of relationship with a husband as a vulnerability factor in depression has now been confirmed in a series of studies (e.g., Brown and Prudo 1981; Campbell, Cope and Teasdale 1983; Costello 1982; Finlay-Jones 1986; Murphy 1982; Paykel et al. 1980; Parry and Shapiro 1986). Only one study has failed to replicate the finding (Bebbington et al. 1984). The prospective study in Islington produced unequivocal evidence in support of the earlier speculative theory. Low self-esteem was measured by negative comments the woman made about herself during the first interview. Those with low self-esteem were only at increased risk when exposed to a stressor. Depression was more than twice as likely to occur following a stressor among those with low self-esteem—33 percent (18/54) versus 13 percent (12/96). Unlike the Canberra study, the role of lack of social support was also clear, probably because the measures concentrated on particular core relationships and not on more extensive networks as in the Australian study. For married women the quality of marriage (taking account of reports about arguing, strain, violence, indifference, and coldness), as in earlier research, was critical.

Another measure of support concerned persons the woman named as "very close," excluding a child at home, husband, or boyfriend. All but a fifth of the women named at least one person, with an average of two, as being very close. However, there was a considerable range in the quality of the contact. Women were therefore characterized as having a "true" very close relationship only when there was both confiding about intimate matters and regular contact at least every two to three weeks (O'Connor and Brown 1984).

Quality of marriage was highly related to risk of depression among the married women with a stressor. And, as might be expected, negative inter-action in marriage and negative evaluation of self were highly associated. In this sense both can be seen as vulnerability factors, and much evidence suggested that the poor quality of marriage had often served to lower self-esteem. However, leaving the relationship with husband aside, a very close tie was only associated with a reduced risk for single parents. And here those with a "true" very close relationship were at a particularly low risk—4 percent with a true, 29 percent with a nontrue, and 44 percent with no very close relationship developed depression once a stressor had occurred. A wide range of other measures of the social network were examined to try to take account of every potentially supportive relationship, but none were associated with risk of depression.

However, these analyses took account only of social support before the first interview. This is not the same as support actually mobilized in any crisis in the follow-up year (Gore 1985). When such crisis support was considered, it became clear that women were particularly likely to develop depression in the setting of a major loss or disappointment if support they had every reason to expect was not forthcoming. Furthermore, for married women the measure of true very close relationship did not predict very well who outside their immediate families would give support in a crisis. The upshot is that it was possible to show that actual support mobilized in a crisis was highly related to risk of depression and that such support from a person named as very close at first interview was related to reduced risk of depression for married women as well as single parents (Brown, Craig, and Harris 1985). The difference between married women and single parents was that it was impossible to predict for married women whom among those named as very close at first interview would turn out to give support in a crisis.

Various minor riders must be added to these findings, but enough has been said to make clear my conclusion that psychosocial factors explain to a considerable degree high rates of depression among working-class women in urban settings. Low self-esteem (or negative evaluation) in Islington seemed in considerable part an understandable reaction to a current climate of adversity, disappointment, and failure, and support mobilized in a crisis was critical in the development of depression. In addition, certain other results have dealt with chronic difficulties. First, that events linked to an ongoing difficulty were much more likely to bring about depression (Brown, Harris, and Bifulco 1986). Second it has also been established that chronic depression appears to be, in part at least, sustained by a climate of current difficulty and failure. Indeed, over half of those experiencing chronic depressive conditions who recovered in the two-year follow-up period did so after a "positive" event helped clear up or neutralize a long-term difficulty — often the direct consequence of the original stressor. The results as a whole underline the argument of several workers who have urged greater attention to chronic role-related stresses, maintaining that too much

emphasis has been given to life events by themselves (Kanner et al. 1981; Pearlin and Schooler 1978).

Mental Illness and Pathways to Care

An important program of research initiated by the General Practice Unit at the Institute of Psychiatry in London has succeeded in throwing light on how general practitioners deal with psychiatric disorder in the population. David Goldberg and Peter Huxley (1980) offer an illuminating discussion of pathways to psychiatric care, particularly of the extent to which milder conditions tend to be "filtered out" by referring agencies. The main task of detection and management of psychiatric disorder, both in the United States and the United Kingdom, falls on the shoulders of physicians in primary care. Goldberg and Huxley deal with five levels of care and the filters through which one must pass to move from one level to another. Level 1 represents the group of people shown by studies of psychiatric morbidity to be distributed in the population as a whole. Level 2 represents those who are disturbed among those consulting primary care physicians. The first filter, linking these two levels, often involves "illness behavior," reflecting the fact that patients have chosen to seek advice about their symptoms. However, some patients may visit the doctor for an unrelated ailment and happen at the same time to be suffering from a psychiatric disorder.

Almost all those with an affective disorder appear to contact their general practitioner for some reason during the course of their disorder. But many will make either no reference or only a tangential one to their psychological symptoms. And, as already noted, perhaps only half will pass through the next filter to have their disorder recognized by their general practitioners. Level 3 consists of those patients, consulting primary care physicians, who are identified as "psychiatrically sick" by their doctor. Goldberg and Huxley estimate that on average no more than half of those visiting a doctor, who are suffering from a psychiatric disorder, are recognized by their doctor as disturbed. Doctors differ considerably in the proportion of disturbed whom they recognize as requiring help (Goldberg and Huxley 1980, 94–114). Level 4 represents patients attending psychiatric outpatient clinics or private offices; as already noted, the primary care physician is usually critically placed to determine who will be referred. (This is less true in the United States.) Level 5 represents patients admitted to psychiatric hospitals. It is now recognized that only a small minority at levels 1, 2, and 3 enter levels 4 and 5. The final filters are particularly difficult to cross. Goldberg and Huxley estimate that in the United Kingdom only some one in fourteen of those suffering from a psychiatric disorder pass these final filters, and evidence shows that much the same order of probabilities holds in the United States. The exact probabilities, of course, depend on the definition of a "case" that is utilized (Regier, Goldberg, and Taube 1978).

One important finding is that general practitioners typically do little more than prescribe drugs for those they recognize as suffering from a psychiatric disorder. The evaluation of the effectiveness of such drugs is still controversial, although there can be no doubt that at times they do have a beneficial effect. However, in the context of everyday general practice the present situation is not a happy one. In an intensive study of forty-five women suffering from a definite depressive disorder, three things became clear (Ginsberg and Brown 1982). Although, as previous research had suggested, almost all the women saw their doctor during their depression, only about half had their depression acknowledged. Furthermore, this acknowledgment usually consisted of no more than a minimal recognition that the patient might be suffering from a psychiatric disorder; no exploration was undertaken of the range of symptoms or the nature of any difficulties that might have led to the depression. In almost every instance where the doctor acknowledged the depression, a prescription for psychotropic drugs was given. But at the same time, on the woman's part there was a low level of satisfaction with the care received. Most of the women made clear when interviewed in the course of the research that they would prefer to talk rather than receive drugs. Finally, the study revealed how difficult it was for a woman to get her family or friends to recognize that she needed help; it was extremely difficult to have the depression unequivocally acknowledged, in spite of the widely held belief that depressive symptoms are common among women. A recurrent theme was the way in which family and friends explained away and "normalized" the patient's depression.

Fortunately sufficient research has now been carried out to suggest that effective intervention is possible in a general practice setting. For example, Johnstone and Goldberg (1976) showed that the recognition of "hidden psychiatric disorder" by general practitioners apparently led to a quicker recovery and fewer symptoms at follow up one year later. However, much remains to be done to establish just what is possible, particularly in terms of the severity and duration of disorders (e.g., Corney 1981). In particular, what role drug treatment should play is unclear. Many patients with depressive illness will improve without drug treatment. As David Goldberg (1982) notes, a significant proportion of depressed patients receiving placebos will get better. In some studies this effect is so marked that those taking antidepressants are not at an advantage (Porter 1970; Raskin 1974).

The possible practical relevance of the research on depression is clear. However, unlike the research on schizophrenia reviewed earlier, none of the many interesting intervention programs for depressives have been properly evaluated. In any case, much remains to be done to integrate these findings with the kind of research and theory that I have outlined (for reviews see Iscoe and Harris 1984; Kessler, Price, and Wortman 1984).

The Study of Bereavement

So far I have reviewed research employing systematic methods of measurement in which what was to be collected and how it was to be collected was settled before the main inquiry. This method particularly holds for the life-event research, based on population samples, that attempts to deal with the full range of crises and difficulties that can afflict us. However, another type of life-event research typically is based on small samples of people who have been victimized by a particular crisis such as widowhood or rape. Much of the research is probably best seen as exploratory and not designed to test particular ideas or theories (Silver and Wortman 1980). There are exceptions. Bolton and Oatley (1983), for instance, in a prospective matched control study have documented the link between unemployment due to redundancy and the development of depression in men. And some areas such as bereavement have received a great deal of research attention.

Epidemiological studies of the health consequences of bereavement contain many inconsistencies, even when hard variables such as mortality are considered. Indeed, the recent report by the Committee for the Study of the Health Consequences of the Stress of Bereavement concludes that there is convincing evidence that bereavement only increases risk of death for men. It does not appear to do so for the first year for women, and evidence thereafter is equivocal (Osterweis, Solomon, and Green

1984). However, such inconsistency is just what would be expected if death of a husband differs in meaning from that of a wife, and if persons vary in their vulnerability and resources. It is perhaps no accident that death of a child shows particularly powerful effects since it is an event for which there is probably far less variation in meaning. Given the research on life events already reviewed, it is difficult to believe that death of a spouse is not a potential stressor of considerable importance. But, as with severe loss in general, it may have health consequences for only a minority.

Qualitative studies have dealt far more convincingly with meaning. The particular strengths in this research have been the insights provided on the processes of coping and support as ongoing activities. The approach typically relies on intensive interviews, only part of which are couched in the form of standard questions. Robert Weiss, working over a twenty-year period, illustrates particularly well the strengths of qualitative studies as an approach when researching in the general area of marriage and health. He has developed seminal ideas about the nature of social support (e.g., 1973, 1976a, 1976b) and, with Murray Parkes, has provided insights into the process of bereavement and its impact on health (Parkes and Weiss 1983). This longitudinal effort studied fifty-nine recently bereaved widows and widowers and a comparison series from the same population who had not lost a partner. Those experiencing loss but reporting high conflict in their marriage had particularly poor outcomes

when judged two to four years later. When seen a few weeks after the loss, however, this group showed far less grief and emotional upset than others. In a fascinating use of case material, three alternative explanations are suggested, all running against the popular explanation provided by Freud in *Mourning and Melancholia* and based on the idea that the lost figure has somehow been incorporated within the mourner. First, Parkes and Weiss suggest that the poor outcome (often with depressive features) stems from awareness that the relationship for which the remaining partner is grieving has never been as wanted—that is the "survivor mourns not only for the marriage that was, but also for the marriage that could have been, and was not" (Parkes and Weiss 1983, 122). A second interpretation is even more subtle—that pervasive problems in relationships with others can underlie an adverse response to loss and that these problems stem from earlier experiences in people's lives. Parkes and Weiss cite the influential work of John Bowlby (1969, 1973, 1980) and the possibility that particular kinds of early experience lead to certain long-term styles of attachment. One widow, with a very troubled marriage to a man who drank heavily and was often not home, noted how her hurried early commitment to her future husband when both were still very young had been driven by insecurity: "In a desperate need for affection she had chosen a partner who seems to have been incapable of giving her the security she craved."

But such examples illustrate a more profound point than that "personality" plays a role. They suggest that decisions made at key points in life can have fateful long-term consequences; that, in this example, perhaps the chief function of the "weakness" in personality was to lead the woman to make a "wrong" decision early in her life; furthermore, that the impact of her personality has to be taken in conjunction with the response of her husband. Parkes and Weiss note, as a third interpretation, that the marriage itself is best seen as a long-term learning situation. "Just as a well-functioning marriage can foster growth through the adult years, an unsatisfactory marriage can confirm and reinforce lack of trust in oneself and others."

In fact, more systematic inquiries have begun to produce reasonably convincing evidence about such effects. And surprisingly, these have emerged from research in an area that has been plagued by the inconsistency of its findings—the long-term impact of loss of a parent in childhood on functioning in adult life (Harris and Brown 1985; Harris, Brown, and Bifulco 1986a; Rutter 1981).

Studies of Childhood and Adolescence

Michael Rutter, in 1966, reviewed clinical evidence for a link between psychiatric disorders in parents receiving treatment and their children, something that had also been noted in large-scale studies of general practice records (Buck and Laughton 1959). Population studies not relying on clinic or hospital referrals have since made it clear that such a link exists (e.g., Richman, Stevenson, and Graham 1982; Rutter and Quinton 1984).

The quality of family life plays a critical role in linking parental and childhood disorder (Rutter and Quinton 1984). In a prospective study of children with a parent receiving psychiatric care matched with a comparison group from the general population, children with a mentally ill parent did not show a greater risk of emotional or behavioral disturbance when families were matched for marital discord and family disruption. In both groups psychiatric disorder in the children was most frequent when there was a combination of different family adversities. Rutter and Quinton conclude that, for the most part, parental mental disorder does not give rise to an increased risk for the children, which is independent of the family's psychosocial circumstances as a whole; and that it is family disorder and parental aggression toward the children that are the most powerful risk factors. They note that this picture is general and that more specific risk factors may involve a genetic component. In this context Myrna Weissman's group in New Haven, in a detailed family study, have shown higher risk of depression in children of depressed parents, although the interpretation of this interesting observation is by no means clear (Weissman et al. 1984).

Such work can be linked with the study of long-range effects of family disruption and the insight it throws on the impact of early loss of a parent.

Here there has been a growing realization that nothing short of the study of the life course or biography of the person will suffice (Rutter 1982). The study of various life stages in a series of separate studies is of limited use. For many problems it is necessary to follow an individual from childhood through adult life to determine how various experiences interrelate. Ideally this requires long-term prospective inquiries, although intensive interviews at one point in time do provide a reasonably accurate picture of many aspects of the past, which can serve as an invaluable introduction to time-consuming and costly longitudinal inquiries.

The links between early adaptations and later disorder are complex, and a number of possible pathways have been identified (Sroufe and Rutter 1984). The simplest link would be that experiences in childhood bring about disorder which then persists into adult life; alternatively, the experiences could lead to other changes in the child (but not psychological disturbance), which in turn influence later functioning and increase risk of psychiatric disorder. Or perhaps early experience actually brings about important environmental changes (say in family or school life) which in turn influence opportunities and behavior in adult life. And, of course, these possibilities may combine. With these in mind, there begins to converge the opinion that the launching period between childhood and adult life is of the greatest importance in "transmitting" early adverse experiences.

Quinton and Rutter, in a longitudinal study of forty-seven girls in local authority care, and a comparison group of forty-seven girls from the same London borough with no history of local authority care, have shown large differences in subsequent parenting, marital relationships, and psychiatric health (Quinton and Rutter 1984a, 1984b, 1984c). At the follow-up interview, fifteen years after first contact, it was found that far more of the ex-care young women had become pregnant by the age of nineteen (42 percent versus 5 percent) and fewer were in stable cohabiting relationships at time of interview (78 percent versus 100 percent). In addition there were serious problems in their motherhood roles; a fifth of their children had been taken into care by the time of the follow-up interview and an additional 18 percent had young children they were no longer looking after. This was true of none of the comparison women. Ex-care mothers also had greater difficulty relating to their children, and they displayed poorer control, lower sensitivity, lower warmth, and higher hostility. However, the quality of child care was highly associated with marital support and psychosocial problems in the spouse. The rate of good parenting among ex-care women with a supportive spouse was the same as for the comparison women. Of particular interest is the finding that the presence of a "deviant" spouse (one with either psychiatric disorder, criminality, an alcohol or drug problem, or longstanding difficulties in relationships) related to the amount of planning before marriage or cohabitation and not to the woman's own "deviance" in childhood. (Evidence of planning involved knowing the man for over six months before cohabiting and having positive reasons for living together without the external pressures of a pregnancy or being driven out of an unhappy home.) The lack of planning in marriage or cohabitation was higher amongst women with local authority care backgrounds and was linked to unsupportive marriages and to poor parenting.

Another aspect of the study involved a retrospective analysis of the reports of mothers with children in local authority care (Quinton and Rutter 1984b). Experiences similar to those of their own children had occurred to these mothers in their early life. More of the mothers with children in care than comparison mothers had been in care themselves in childhood or separated from parents in childhood as a result of family discord. They were more likely to have suffered difficulties during teenage years; twice as many had left home by age nineteen or were pregnant at this age, or had left home for negative reasons such as rejection by parent. At time of interview the mothers of children in care were in worse housing conditions and were more likely to be single parents. They had much higher rates of psychiatric disorder and exhibited poorer parenting. Thus an identical cycle was uncovered across the two generations through both retrospective and prospective research design. Both studies indicate that while there is a good deal of continuity, discontinuity is also common and there is nothing inevitable about the transmission of psychiatric disorder via these mechanisms.

The life course approach has also been adopted in the study of lifetime risk for depression; a biographical etiological model was developed by focusing in a similar way on the "launching" stage of early adulthood and the circumstances surrounding motherhood in this period. In the initial Camberwell study of depression, vulnerability or risk factors for depression included loss of a mother before age eleven. Research in Walthamstow, northeast London, has now studied 170 women especially selected because of a parental loss in childhood or adolescence (defined by death or separation from either parent, for over a year, before the child reaches the age of seventeen), together with a comparison group of women with no such parental loss (Brown, Harris, and Bifulco 1986; Harris, Brown, and Bifulco 1986a, 1986b, 1986c). Detailed questioning in the women's homes covered experiences, both before and after the loss, dealing with quality of parental care, relations with parent figures, discord in the home, and level of disruption in childhood as a result of the loss. Information was also collected on the "launching" period between childhood and adult life, with particular attention to circumstances surrounding relations with boyfriends, marriage, and first pregnancy.

Results confirmed that loss of mother in childhood was associated with an increased risk of depression, both at time of interview and in terms of a lifetime prevalence. Among women with such a loss of mother, 22 percent were depressed in the year before interview compared with 7 percent with no parental loss or loss of father only. The most important feature of childhood experience associated with depression in adulthood was lack of adequate care by parents or parental substitutes; this feature was also highly associated with the loss of a mother. "Lack of care" was based on ratings of high indifference and low control by parents or parent substitutes; concrete and detailed examples of neglect, disinterest, or lack of discipline were required for "lack of care" ratings to be made.

Premarital pregnancy was highly related to loss of mother before age seventeen and was also related to depression in the year of interview—42 percent compared with 15 percent of the rest of the women. In addition, premarital pregnancy related to lack of care in childhood. There was also a greatly increased risk of working-class status in adulthood among women who had experienced such a pregnancy, and a reduced chance of women having an intimate and confiding relationship with a husband, particularly among the working class.

The resulting biographical model of depression emphasizes the effect of two distinct strands (one "environmental" and the other "psychological") in leading to later depression, both of which emanate from lack of parental care in childhood rather than from early loss as such. The environmental strand involves premarital pregnancy, teenage marriage, low social class, lack of a supportive husband, and psychological factors such as childhood and adult helplessness and atypical attachment styles (Bowlby 1980).

The finding that premarital pregnancy increased the risk of later depression was of particular interest since it is linked to both strands in the model. The way women coped at this point was important, with those undergoing terminations or consciously delaying marriage until sure of their decision faring much better in terms of subsequent social class position and later depression. Effective coping involved avoiding entrapment in an undesirable relationship, either with a man or with a child; less effective coping involved marrying solely because of the pregnancy, or trying to bring up the child by oneself. Effective coping related to middle-class status at time of interview and to a reduced rate of depression. Here childhood social class based on father's occupation and adult social class based on husband's occupation must be distinguished. Premarital pregnancy was unrelated to childhood social class but was highly related to adult social class. Therefore, although not deriving from lower-class status, premarital pregnancy was related to subsequent working-class status. And here, effectiveness of coping at time of the pregnancy was vital—twice the number of those with middle-class status in adulthood had coped effectively.

Biographical approaches to the study of adult disorder have therefore begun to identify certain key points in an individual's life, crossroads when a downward path toward depression can be embarked upon and after which the risk of becoming depressed at some point is greatly increased. One such crossroads occurs in women before age twenty-five or so, when an unplanned pregnancy occurs outside marriage. The decisions and choices made at this point can entail stepping onto an "escalator" of adverse circumstances, involving marital difficulties, lower social class and attendant material difficulties, and a negative cognitive set of helplessness. These in turn affect the likelihood of the woman experiencing provoking agents in years to come and weaken her resistance to them, thus leading to depression. However, both of the studies reviewed suggest that such risks are reversible—although doubtless with time this becomes more difficult.

Conclusion

I have used research in the area of depression and schizophrenia to illustrate the kind of development and testing of theoretical ideas about etiology and course that has dominated social science interest in psychiatry in recent years and the way these interests in time link with work on experimental intervention. I am conscious that I have neglected the concern of many social scientists studying other issues—the organization of services, their evolution in a broad political and cultural context, and the need to evaluate the vast financial expenditures involved and the effectiveness of the services in alleviating suffering and disabilities that characterize mental illness. I have also said nothing about the way these problems extend well beyond the mentally ill themselves, affecting families, work relationships, and community life as a whole (e.g., Clausen and Huffine 1979; Mechanic 1985; Yarrow, Clausen, and Robbins 1955). Nor have I dwelt on the impact

of the recent revolutionary changes in the organization of care for the most disabled, particularly those who have been chronic inmates in mental hospitals in the past, or those who would have been (e.g., Lamb 1979; Mollica 1983). It will, of course, be essential to integrate the results of the kind of research I have outlined with broader issues of social policy and the multifactorial impact of mental illness on society. However, I have not hidden the difficulty of any translation of knowledge about etiology and course into effective intervention. There is no easy road from knowledge about mechanisms to effective intervention. That we may understand the risk certain kinds of marriages hold for the development of complicated bereavement reaction tells little about how we might change matters for the better before or after such a loss. However, clearly we are already learning some important lessons. The implications of the studies highlighting the crucial role of decisions about life plans such as marriage, motherhood, and employment in late teenage or early adulthood must obviously vary in terms of different cultures and subcultures. There can be no universal prescription outlining advice to a young woman who has become pregnant out of wedlock. However, discussion with a counselor, who can emphasize the importance of, say, a future, long-term supportive relationship with a partner, may help such a young woman decide with more insight whether to marry the father or not, and this may in turn afford her some protection in the future. But in any case, such practical implications are not everything. Indeed, the "application" of any such knowledge often may be through pressure to rethink established ideas as much as through recommendations or pressure for particular changes.

References

Al-Issa, I. 1982. Gender and adult psychopathology. In *Gender and psychopathology*, ed. I. Al-Issa. New York: Academic Press.

Barrowclough, C., and N. Tarrier. 1984. "Psychosocial" interventions with families and their effects on the course of schizophrenia: A review. *Psychological Medicine* 14:629–642.

Bebbington, P., J. Hurry, C. Tennant, E. Sturt, and J. K. Wing. 1981. Epidemiology of mental disorders in Camberwell. *Psychological Medicine* 11: 561–579.

Bebbington, P., E. Sturt, C. Tennant, and J. Hurry. 1984. Misfortune and resilience: A community study of women. *Psychological Medicine* 14: 347–363.

Birley, J. L. T., and G. W. Brown. 1970. Crises and life changes preceding the onset and relapse of schizophrenia: Clinical aspects. *British Journal of Psychiatry* 116:327–333.

Bleuler, M. 1974. The long-term course of the schizophrenic psychoses. *Psychological Medicine* 4:244-254.

Bockhoven, J. S. 1956. Moral treatment. *American Psychiatry Journal of Nervous and Mental Disease* 74:167–194, 292–321.

Bolton, W., and K. Oatley. 1983. A prospective study of unemployment and a theory of depression. *Bulletin of the British Psychological Society* 36:A46 (abstract).

Bowlby, J. 1969. *Attachment and loss*, vol. 1: *Attachment*. New York: Basic Books.

————. 1973. *Attachment and loss*, vol. 2: *Separation: Anxiety and anger*. New York: Basic Books.

————. 1980. *Attachment and loss*, vol. 3: *Loss: Sadness and Depression*. New York: Basic Books.

Boyd, J. H., and M. Weissman. 1981. Epidemiology of affective disorders: A reexamination and future directions. *Archives of General Psychiatry* 38: 1039–1046.

Brown, G. W. 1959a. Experience of discharged chronic schizophrenic patients in various types of living group. *Millbank Memorial Fund Quarterly* 37:105.

————. 1959b. Social factors influencing length of hospital stay of schizophrenic patients. *British Medical Journal* 2:1300.

————. 1960. Length of hospital stay and schizophrenia: A review of statistical studies. *Acta Psychiatrica Neurologiza Scandinavica* 35:414.

_____. 1981. Life events and psychiatric illness: Some thoughts on methodology and causality. *Journal of Psychosomatic Research* 16:311–320.

_____. 1973. The mental hospital as an institution. *Social Science and Medicine* 7:407–424.

Brown, G. W., B. Andrews, T. Harris, Z. Adler, and L. Bridge. 1986. Social support, self-esteem, and depression. *Psychological Medicine* (in press).

Brown, G. W., and J. L. T. Birley. 1968. Crises and life changes and the onset of schizophrenia. *Journal of Health and Social Behaviour* 9:203.

Brown, G. W., J. L. T. Birley, and J. K. Wing. 1972. Influence of family life on the course of schizophrenic disorders: A replication. *British Journal of Psychiatry* 121: 241–258.

Brown, G. W., M. Bone, B. Dalison, and J. K. Wing. 1966. *Schizophrenia and social care*. London: Oxford University Press.

Brown, G. W., G. M. Carstairs, and G. Topping. 1958. Post-hospital adjustment of chronic mental patients. *Lancet* 2:685.

Brown, G. W., T. K. J. Craig, and T. O. Harris. 1985. Depression: Distress or disease? Some epidemiological considerations. *British Journal of Psychiatry* 147:612–622.

Brown, G. W., and T. O. Harris. 1978. *Social origins of depression: A study of psychiatric disorder in women*. London: Tavistock Publications; New York: Free Press.

_____. 1982. Disease, distress, and depression: A comment. *Journal of Affective Disorders* 4:1–8.

_____. 1986. Establishing causal links: The Bedford College studies of depression. In *Life events and psychiatric disorders*, ed. H. Katschnig. Cambridge: Cambridge University Press.

Brown, G. W., T. O. Harris, and A. Bifulco. 1986. Long-term effect of early loss of parent. In *Depression in children: Developmental perspectives*, ed. M. Rutter, C. E. Izard, and P. B. Read, pp. 251–290. New York: Guildford Press.

Brown, G. W., E. M. Monck, G. M. Carstairs, and J. K. Wing. 1962. Influence of family life on the course of schizophrenic illness. *British Journal of Preventative Social Medicine* 16:55.

Brown, G. W., M. Ni Bhrolchain, and T. O. Harris. 1975. Social class and psychiatric disturbance among women in an urban population. *Sociology* 9:225–254.

Brown, G. W., and R. Prudo. 1981. Psychiatric disorder in a rural and an urban population, 1: Aetiology of depression. *Psychological Medicine* 11: 581–599.

Buck, C., and K. Laughton. 1959. Family patterns of illness: The effect of psychoneurosis in the parent upon illness in the child. *Acta Psychiatrica Neurologiza Scandinavica* B4:165–175.

Campbell, E. A., S. J. Cope, and J. D. Teasdale. 1983. Social factors and affective disorder: An investigation of Brown and Harris's Model. *British Journal of Psychiatry* 143:548–553.

Cannon, W. B. 1939. *The wisdom of the body.* New York: Norton.

Caplan, G. 1974. *Support systems and community mental health.* New York: Behavioral Publications.

Cassel, J. 1974. Psychosocial processes and "stress": Theoretical formulations. *International Journal of Health Services* 4:471–482.

———. 1976. The contribution of the social environment to host resistance. *American Journal of Epidemiology* 104:107–123.

Clausen, J. A., and C. L. Huffine. 1979. The impact of parental mental illness on children. In *Research in community and mental health,* ed. R. Simmons, pp. 183–214. Greenwich, Conn.: JAI Press.

Cobb, S. 1976. Social support as a moderator of life stress. *Psychosomatic Medicine* 38:300–314.

Cooper, B. 1978. Epidemiology. In *Schizophrenia: Towards a new synthesis,* ed. J. K. Wing. London: Academic Press.

Corney, R. H. 1981. Social work effectiveness in the management of depressed women: A clinical trial. *Psychological Medicine* 11:417–423.

Costello, C. G. 1982. Social factors associated with depression: A retrospective study. *Psychological Medicine* 12:329–339.

Craig, T. K. J., G. W. Brown, and Z. Alder. 1984. Psychiatric disorder in an urban population: Three diagnostic systems compared. Typescript.

Day, R. 1981. Life events and schizophrenia: The "triggering" hypothesis. *Acta Psychiatrica Neurologiza Scandinavica* 64:97–122.

Day, R. 1986. Stressful Life events preceding the acute onset of schizophrenia: a cross-national study from the World Health Organization. *Culture, Medicine, and Psychiatry* (in press).

Dean, C., P. G. Surtees, and S. P. Sashidharan. 1983. Comparison of research diagnostic systems in an Edinburgh community sample. *British Journal of Psychiatry* 142: 247–256.

Doane, J. A., I. R. H. Falloon, M. J. Goldstein, and J. Mintz. 1985. Parental affective style and the treatment of schizophrenia. *Archives of General Psychiatry* 42:34–42.

Dohrenwend, B. P., and B. S. Dohrenwend. 1974. Psychiatric disorders in urban settings. In *American handbook of psychiatry,* vol. 11: *Child and adolescent psychiatry, sociocultural and community psychiatry,* ed. G. Caplan. New York: Basic Books.

———. 1976. Sex differences and psychiatric disorders. *American Journal of Sociology* 81(1):1447–1454.

Dohrenwend, B. P., B. S. Dohrenwend, M. S. Gould, B. Link, R. Neugebauer, and R. Wunsch-Hitzig. 1980. *Mental illness in the United States.* New York: Praeger.

Durkheim, E. 1952. *Suicide: A study in sociology.* London: Routledge and Kegan Paul.

Falloon, I. R. H., J. L. Boyd, and C. W. McGill. 1984. *Family care of schizophrenia: A problem-solving approach to the treatment of mental illness.* New York: Guildford Press.

Falloon, I. R. H., J. L. Boyd, C. W. McGill, J. Razani, H. B. Moss, and A. M. Gilderman. 1982. Family management in the prevention of exacerbations of schizophrenia. *New England Journal of Medicine* 306 (24):1437–1440.

Finlay-Jones, R. 1986. Anxiety. In *Life events and illness*, ed. G. W. Brown and T. Harris. New York: Guildford Press.

Finlay-Jones, R., and G. W. Brown. 1981. Types of stressful life event and the onset of anxiety and depressive disorders. *Psychological Medicine* 11:803–815.

Freud, S. 1971. *Mourning and melancholia*. In *Collected Papers*, vol. 4. London: Hogarth.

Gilligan, C. 1984. Remapping the moral domain: New images of self in relationship. Paper presented at the conference Reconstructing Individualism, Stanford Humanities Center.

Ginsberg, S., and G. W. Brown. 1982. No time for depression: A study of help-seeking among mothers of pre-school children. In *Monographs in psychosocial epidemiology, 3: Symptoms, illness behaviour, and help-seeking*, ed. D. Mechanic. New York: Neale Watson Academic Publications.

Goldberg, D. 1982. The concept of a psychiatric "case" in general practice. *Social Psychiatry* 17:61–65.

Goldberg, D., and P. Huxley. 1980. *Mental illness in the community: The pathway to psychiatric care*. London and New York: Tavistock Publications.

Goldman, H. H., A. A. Gattozzi, and C. A. Taube. 1981. Defining and counting the chronically mentally ill. *Hospital and Community Psychiatry* 32:21–27.

Goldstein, M. J., and H. S. Kopeikin. 1981. Short and long term effects of combining drug and family therapy. In *New developments in intervention with families of schizophrenics*, ed. M. J. Goldstein, pp. 5–26. San Francisco: Jossey-Bass.

Goldstein, M. J., E. H. Rodnick, J. R. Evans, P. R. A. May, and M. R. Steinberg. 1978. Drug and family therapy in the aftercare of acute schizophrenics. *Archives of General Psychiatry* 35:1169–1177.

Gore, S. 1985. Social support and styles of coping with stress. In *Social support and health*, ed. S. Cohen and L. Syme. New York: Academic Press.

Gove, W. R. 1972. The relationship between sex roles, marital status, and mental illness. *Social Forces* 51:34–44.

Grob, G. N. 1966. *The state and the mentally ill*. Chapel Hill: University of North Carolina Press.

Gunderson, E. K., and R. H. Rahe, eds. 1974. *Life stress and illness*. Springfield, Ill.: Charles C. Thomas.

Harris, T. O., and G. W. Brown. 1985. Interpreting data in aetiological studies of affective disorder: Some pitfalls and ambiguities. *British Journal of Psychiatry* 147:5–15.

Harris, T. O., G. W. Brown and A. Bifulco. 1986a. The impact of loss of parent in childhood upon adult psychiatric health: The Walthamstow Study, 1. The Role of Lack of Adequate Parental Care. *Psychological Medicine* (in press).

———. 1986b. The impact of loss of parent in childhood upon adult psychiatric health: The Walthamstow Study, 2. The Role of Social Class Position and Premarital Pregnancy. Typescript.

———. 1986c. The impact of loss of parent in childhood upon adult psychiatric health: The Walthamstow Study, 3. The role of cognitive sets with special reference to situational helplessness. Typescript.

Heath, C. W. 1945. *What people are.* Cambridge: Harvard University Press.

Henderson, A. S., D. G. Byrne, and P. Duncan-Jones. 1981. *Neurosis and the social environment.* Sidney, Australia: Academic Press.

Hirsch, S. R. 1983. Psychosocial factors in the cause and prevention of relapse in schizophrenia. *British Medical Journal* 286:1600–1601.

Hirsch, S. R., and J. P. Leff. 1975. *Abnormalities in the parents of schizophrenics.* Maudsley Monograph No. 22. London: Oxford University Press.

Hogarty, G., S. Goldberg, N. R. Schooler, R. F. Ulrich, and Collaborative Study Group. 1974a. Drug and sociotherapy in the aftercare of schizophrenic patients, 2: Two-year Relapse Rates. *Archives of General Psychiatry* 31:603–608.

———. 1974b. Drug and sociotherapy in the aftercare of schizophrenic patients, 3: Adjustment of non-relapsed patients. *Archives of General Psychiatry* 31:609–618.

Hogarty, G., N. R. Schooler, R. Ulrich, F. Mussare, P. Ferro, and E. Herron. 1979. Fluphenazine and social therapy in the aftercare of schizophrenic patients. *Archives of General Psychiatry* 36:1283–1294.

Iscoe, I., and L. C. Harris. 1984. Social and community interventions. *Annual Review Psychology* 35:333–360.

Jacobs, S. C., B. A. Prusoff, and E. S. Paykel. 1974. Recent life events in schizophrenia and depression. *Psychological Medicine* 4:444–453.

Johnstone, A., and D. Goldberg. 1975. Psychiatric screening in general practice. *Lancet* 1:605–608.

Kanner, A. D., J. C. Coyne, C. Schaefer, and R. S. Lazarus. 1981. Comparison of two modes of stress measurement: Daily hassles and uplift versus major life events. *Journal of Behavioral Medicine* 14:1–39.

Kessler, R. C. 1979. Stress, social status, and psychological distress. *Journal of Health and Social Behavior* 20:259–272.

Kessler, R. C., and P. D. Cleary. 1980. Social class and psychological distress. *American Sociological Review* 45:63–78.

Kessler, R. C., and J. D. McLeod. 1984. Sex differences in vulnerability to undesirable life events. Typescript.

Kessler, R. C., and J. A. McRae, Jr. 1981. Trends in the relationship between sex and psychological distress, 1957–1976. *American Sociological Review* 46:443–452.

———. 1984. A note on the relationships of sex and marital status to psychological distress. *Research in community and mental health* 4: 109–130.

Kessler, R. C., R. H. Price, and C. B. Wortman. 1984. Psychopathology: Social approaches. *Annual Review of Psychology* 36 (in press).

Klerman, G. L., G. E. Vaillant, R. L. Spitzer, and R. Michels. 1984. Commentary: A debate on DSM-3. *American Journal of Psychiatry* 141(4):539–553.

Lamb, H. R. 1979. The new asylums in the community. *Archives of General Psychiatry* 36:129–134.

Langner, T. S., and S. T. Michael. 1963. *Life stress and mental health.* London: Collier-Macmillan.

Leff, J. P., S. R. Hirsch, R. Gaird, P. D. Rhodes, and B. C. Stevens. 1973. Life events and maintenance therapy in schizophrenic relapse. *British Journal of Psychiatry* 123:659–660.

Leff, J., L. Kuipers, R. Berkowitz, R. Eberlein-Vries, and D. Sturgeon. 1982. A controlled trial of social intervention in the families of schizophrenic patients. *British Journal of Psychiatry* 141:121–134.

Leff, J. P., and C. Vaughn. 1980. The interaction of life events and relatives' expressed emotion in schizophrenia and depressive neurosis. *British Journal of Psychiatry* 136:146–153.

———. 1981. The role of maintenance therapy and relatives' expressed emotion in relapse of schizophrenia: A two-year follow-up. *British Journal of Psychiatry* 139:102–104.

Leighton, A. H. 1965. Poverty and social change. *Scientific American* 212:21–27.

———. 1983. *Caring for the mentally ill: Psychological and social barriers in historical context.* Cambridge: Cambridge University Press.

Leighton, D. C., O. Hagnell, A. H. Leighton, J. S. Harding, S. R. Kellert, and R. A. Danley. 1971. Psychiatric disorder in a Swedish and a Canadian Community: An exploratory study. *Social Science and Medicine* 5:189–209.

Leighton, D. C., J. S. Harding, D. B. Macklin, A. M. MacMillan, and A. H. Leighton. 1963. *The character of danger.* New York: Basic Books.

Mechanic, D. 1980. *Mental health and social policy.* 2nd ed. Englewood Cliffs, N.J.: Prentice-Hall.

———. 1985. Mental health and social policy: Some needed initiatives for the 1980s. *Health Affairs* (in press).

Mollica, R. F. 1983. From asylum to community: The threatened disintegration of public psychiatry. *New England Journal of Medicine* 308:367–373.

Murphy, E. 1982. Social origins of depression in old age. *British Journal of Psychiatry* 141:135–142.

O'Connor, P., and G. W. Brown. 1984. Supportive relationships: Fact or fancy? *Journal of Social and Personal Relationships* 1:159–175.

Osterweis, M., F. Solomon, and M. Green, eds. 1984. *Bereavement reactions, consequences, and care.* Washington, D.C.: National Academy Press.

Parkes, Murray C., and R. S. Weiss. 1983. *Recovery from bereavement.* New York: Basic Books.

Parry, G., and D. A. Shapiro. 1986. Social support and life events in working-class women: Stress buffering or independent effects? *Archives of General Psychiatry* (in press).

Paykel, E. S. 1978. Contribution of life events to the causation of psychiatric illness. *Psychological Medicine* 8:245–253.

Paykel, E. S., E. M. Emms, J. Fletcher, and E. S. Eassaby. 1980. Life events and social support in puerperal depression. *British Journal of Psychiatry* 136:339–346.

Pearlin, L. I., and C. Schooler. 1978. The structure of coping. *Journal of Health and Social Behavior* 19:2–21.

Porter, A. M. 1970. Depressive illness in general practice: A demographic study and a controlled trial of imipramine. *British Medical Journal* 1:773–778.

Quinton, D., and M. Rutter. 1984a. Family pathology and child psychiatric disorder: A four-year prospective study. In *Longitudinal studies in child psychology and psychiatry: Practical lessons from research experience,* ed. R. Nicol. Chichester: Wiley.

———. 1984b. Parents with children in care, 1: Current circumstances and parenting. *Journal of Child Psychology Psychiatry* 25:211–229.

———. 1984c. Parents with children in care, 2: Intergenerational continuities. *Journal of Child Psychology Psychiatry* 25:231–250.

Rahe, R. H. 1969. Life crisis and health change. In *Psychotropic drug response: Advances in prediction,* ed. P. R. A. May and J. R. Winterborn. Springfield, Ill.: C. C. Thomas.

Raskin, A. 1974. A guide for drug use in depressive disorders. *American Journal of Psychiatry* 131:181–185.

Regier, D., I. D. Goldberg, and C. Taube. 1978. The de facto US mental health services system: A public health perspective. *Archives of General Psychiatry* 35:685–693.

Richman, N., J. Stevenson, and P. J. Graham. 1982. *Pre-school to school: A behavioural study.* London: Academic Press.

Rosen, B. M. 1977. Mental health and the poor: Have the gaps between the poor and the "nonpoor" narrowed in the last decade? *Medical Care* 15:647–661.

Rutter, M. 1981. *Maternal deprivation reassessed.* 2d ed. Harmondsworth: Penguin Books.

———. 1982. Epidemiological-longitudinal approaches to the study of development. In *The concept of development: The Minnesota symposia on child psychology* 15, ed. W. Andrew Collins. Hillsdale, N.J.: Lawrence Erlbaum.

Rutter, M., and D. Quinton. 1984. Parental psychiatric disorder: Effects on children. *Psychological Medicine* 14:853–880.

Sarason, S. B. 1972. *The creation of settings and the future societies.* San Francisco: Jossey-Bass.

Schwab, J. J., and M. E. Schwab. 1978. *Sociocultural roots of mental illness: An epidemiologic survey.* New York: Plenum Publishing.

Selye, H. 1956. *The stress of life.* New York: McGraw-Hill.

Silver, R., and C. B. Wortman, 1980. Coping with undesirable life events. In *Human helplessness: Theory and applications,* ed. J. Gerber and M. E. P. Seligman. New York: Academic Press.

Spitzer, R., J. Endicott, and E. Robins. 1978. Research diagnostic criteria. *Archives of General Psychiatry* 34:773–782.

Srole, L., T. S. Langer, S. T. Michael, M. K. Opler, and T. A. C. Rennie. 1962. *Mental health in the metropolis.* New York: McGraw-Hill.

Sroufe, L. A., and M. Rutter. 1984. The domain of developmental psychopathology. *Child Development* 55:17–29.

Stein, L. I., and M. A. Test. 1980. Alternatives to mental hospital treatment, 1: Conceptual model, treatment program, and clinical evaluation. *Archives of General Psychiatry* 37:392–397, 412.

—————, eds. 1978. *Alternatives to mental hospital treatment.* New York: Plenum Publishing.

Stokes, P. E., P. M. Stoll, S. H. Koslow, J. W. Maas, J. M. Davis, A. C. Swann, and E. Robins. 1984. Pretreatment DST and hypothalmic-pituitary-adrenocortical function in depressed patients and comparison groups. *Archives of General Psychiatry* 41:257–267.

Surtees, P. 1984. Kith, kin, and psychiatric health: A Scottish survey. *Social Psychiatry* 19:63–67.

Surtees, P. G., C. Dean, J. G. Ingham, N. B. Kreitman, P. McC. Miller, and S. P. Sashidharan. 1983. Psychiatric disorder in women from an Edinburgh community: Associations with demographic factors. *British Journal of Psychiatry* 142:238–246.

Surtees, P. G., Sashidharan, S. P., and Dean, C. 1986. Affective disorder amongst women in the general population: A longitudinal study. *British Journal of Psychiatry* 148:176–186.

Test, M. A., and L. I. Stein. 1980. Alternatives to mental hospital treatment 3: Social cost. *Archives of General Psychiatry* 37: 409–412.

Vaughn, C. E., and J. P. Leff. 1976. The influence of family and social factors on the course of psychiatric illness: A comparison of schizophrenic and depressed neurotic patients. *British Journal of Psychiatry* 129:125–137.

Watts, F. N., and D. H. Bennett, eds. 1983. *Theory and practice of psychiatric rehabilitation.* Chichester: John Wiley and Sons.

Weber, M. 1948. *From Max Weber: Essays in sociology,* ed. H. H. Gerth and C. Wright Mills. London: Routledge and Kegan Paul.

Weisbrod, B. A., M. A. Test, and L. I. Stein. 1980. Alternatives to mental hospital treatment 2: Economic benefit-cost analysis. *Archives of General Psychiatry* 37:400–405.

Weiss, R. S. 1973. *Loneliness: The experience of emotional and social isolation.* Cambridge: M.I.T. Press.

———. 1976a. The emotional impact of marital separation. *Journal of Social Issues* 32:135–145.

———. 1976b. Transition states and other stressful situations: Their nature and programs for their management. In *Support systems and mutual help: Multidisciplinary explorations,* ed. Gerald Caplan and Marie Killilea. New York: Grune and Stratton.

Weissman, M. M., and G. L. Klerman. 1977. Sex differences and the epidemiology of depression. *Archives of General Psychiatry* 34:98–111.

Weissman, M. M., and J. K. Myers. 1978. Affective disorders in a United States urban community: The epidemiological survey. *Archives of General Psychiatry* 35:1304–1311.

———. 1980. Use of a self-report symptom scale to detect depression in a community sample. *American Journal of Psychiatry* 137:1081–1084.

Weissman, M. M., B. A. Prusoff, G. D. Gammon, K. R. Merikangas, J. F. Leckman, and K. F. Kidd. 1984. Psychopathology in children (ages 6–18) of depressed and normal women. *Journal American Academy of Child Psychiatry* 23:74–84.

Wing, J. K. 1966. Social and psychological changes in a rehabilitation unit. *Social Psychiatry* 1:21–30.

———, ed. 1978. *Schizophrenia: Towards a new synthesis.* London: Academic Press.

Wing, J. K., and G. W. Brown. 1970. *Institutionalism and schizophrenia.* Cambridge: Cambridge University Press.

Wing, J. K., and T. Fryers. 1976. Psychiatric services in Camberwell and Salford. MRC Social Psychiatry Research Unit, Institute of Psychiatry, London.

Wing, J. K., J. Nixon, S. A. Mann, and J. P. Leff. 1977. Reliability of the PSE (ninth edition) used in a population study (1977). *Psychological Medicine* 7:505–516.

Yarrow, M. R., J. A. Clausen, and P. R. Robbins. 1955. The social meaning of mental illness. *Journal of Social Issues* 11:33–48.

Chapter 11

The Assessment of Health Status

John E. Ware, Jr.

At least three developments present a formidable challenge to health status assessment. First, issues of cost containment continue to dominate the policy debate regarding the relative merits of strategies for organizing and financing health care services. Can health assessment become a useful tool in evaluating these strategies and in addressing other policy issues? Second, with increasing frequency, the definitions of outcomes in clinical trials are beginning to consider more than survival and the biomedical parameters that have traditionally been measured. What role can health assessment play in evaluating patient outcomes in these trials? Third, the focus of one-on-one clinical practice is broadening to include physical, mental, and social functioning and general health perceptions. Can measures of these concepts become the new "laboratory tests" in clinical practice?

This chapter examines whether the evolving field of health assessment is sufficiently well developed to meet these challenges. Two distinct issues must be addressed in answering this important question. The first issue is conceptual: What is health? What is known about health? The second is methodological: What is the state of the art of health status assessment? What dimensions of health are reflected in different health status measures?

This chapter presents a conceptual framework for assessing health status and an overview of major health concepts. It also discusses specific health measures. The discussion is directed to those who are interested in the use of health status measures in policy analysis, clinical trials, and clinical practice and thus avoids detailed discussion of technical issues.

Conceptualizing Health Status

Health problems are many and varied, but they all usually affect quality of life, functioning, and longevity. Length of life can be expressed in terms of average life expectancy, mortality rates, deaths due to specific causes, and other such indicators (National Center for Health Statistics 1981). In developed countries, however, mortality rates are of little value in estimating the health of the general population (Elinson 1979). Quality of life, as traditionally defined, is a much broader concept than personal health status. In addition to health, quality of life encompasses such life factors as family circumstances, finances, housing, and job satisfaction (Andrews and Withey 1976). It is becoming fashionable in the clinical literature to equate all concepts beyond survival and biological functioning with quality of life. This practice has some value because it provides a unifying theme for discussing concepts other than disease and infirmity in the literature on clinical trials and clinical practice (Wenger 1984; Wenger et al. 1984). Quality of life in this context is likely to be a source of some confusion, however, because it encompasses many factors outside the purview of the health care system (Ware 1984). The health component of quality of life, namely personal health status, should be emphasized.

Conceptually and practically, an important feature of health is its dimensionality. Health is composed of distinct components that must be measured and interpreted separately. Health connotes "completeness"—nothing is missing from the person; it connotes "proper function"—all is working efficiently; it also suggests "well-being"—health is more than just freedom from disease but includes "soundness" and "vitality." Dictionary definitions emphasize both physical and mental dimensions of health.

In addition to conceptual arguments, empirical evidence supports the distinction between physical and mental health. For example, the correlation between an aggregate measure of physical functioning (limitations in performance of self-care, mobility, and physical activities due to poor health) and an aggregate measure of mental health (anxiety, depression, and psychological well-being) is significant but weak ($r = 0.206$, $p < .001$, $N = 4,681$) in the general population of adults enrolled in the Rand Health Insurance Experiment. For those with one or more chronic medical problems (e.g., chronic obstructive pulmonary disease, diabetes), a correlation of similar magnitude was observed ($r = 0.261$, $p < .001$, $N = 1,115$). Factor analytic studies (e.g., Ware, Davies-Avery, and Brook 1980; Allen and Ware, in press) and studies of health effects on subsequent medical expenditures also strongly support a multidimensional model of health status (Manning, Newhouse, and Ware 1982). In both kinds of multivariate analysis, a multidimensional specification of health explained the data better than the best unidimensional model.

While dictionary definitions emphasize physical and mental well-being, the World Health Organization (1948) defines health as a "state of complete physical, mental, and *social* well-being and not merely the absence of disease or infirmity" (emphasis added). Is social well-being a dimension of personal health status? Physiologic, physical, and mental dimensions of health are similar in that they "end at the skin." They do not consider other people or factors outside the individual. By contrast, the concept of social well-being extends beyond the individual to encompass the quantity and quality of social contacts and resources across distinct domains of life, including community, family, and work (Kaplan 1975; Donald et al. 1978; Donald and Ware 1984). Hence, social well-being is an attribute of an individual in a particular set of social circumstances.

Another conceptual distinction should be made between social circumstances and the physical and mental dimensions of health. Individual differences in preferences for social circumstances seem to be greater than those for physical and mental health dimensions. Without doubt, virtually everyone would rather be able to walk than not. Whether all people prefer more social interaction (e.g., more visits with friends, more memberships in organizations) to less is not as clear. Thus, determining what constitutes "good" social health is problematic. Whatever one's viewpoint, there are good reasons to include measures of social functioning in any battery of outcome measures

(Levine and Croog 1984). The community places a high value on social functioning and particularly on the performance of usual role activities. Thus, from this perspective, social functioning is the "bottom line." In other words, when everything is added up, is an individual a productive member of society?

While multidimensional, health is more than just the sum of its parts and it is not enough to just measure its parts. Health means different things to different people. Physical, mental, and social dimensions of health are not valued equally by everyone (Ware and Young 1979). Well-being is a state of mind. For these and other reasons, a very personalized and integrative concept—the perception of health in general—should be considered as well (Davies and Ware 1981).

Review of Concepts and Measures

I now examine in greater detail varying definitions, elaborate on important conceptual issues, assess the content of selected standardized instruments, and comment on the interpretation of some of the more widely used measures. Much of this discussion is based on my experience with empirical studies of these or very similar measures and on the literature. Content analyses of widely used measures of physical, mental, and social health and general health perceptions are available elsewhere (Stewart et al. 1978; Ware et al. 1979; Donald et al. 1978; Davies and Ware 1981). Empirical evidence that supports the conclusions summarized here includes multivariate analyses of health measures (Ware, Davies-Avery, and Brook 1980; Davies and Ware 1981; Allen and Ware, in press). Readers interested in reviewing the background information should consult these and other references cited.

Table 11.1 presents specific operational definitions that might be adopted when measuring six health concepts: physical functioning, mental health, social well-being, role functioning, general health perceptions, and symptoms. The concepts defined would be appropriate to test hypotheses about health outcomes in analyses of health care policy options and to describe individual differences in patients' health in clinical trials and practice. The choice among specific operational definitions should depend on which concepts are most relevant to the intervention and population of interest. Table 11.1 also includes a few examples of the content of standardized measures. While the examples selected reflect the health concepts in question, they do not necessarily represent the complete content of the instruments that contain them. Readers should personally examine the content of referenced instruments before deciding what is most appropriate for a particular study.

Table 11.2 presents information about the dimensions of health assessed by some of the more widely used standardized measures. Table 11.2 is useful in determining an appropriate interpretation of results for each kind of measure. The six health concepts defined in table 11.1 are included. The categories of measures

within each concept were selected by examining the content of the measures. The entries in each row of table 11.2 are based on empirical results. The examples presented in table 11.2 were selected to distinguish measures having a straightforward interpretation from those that do not. Four different patterns are illustrated:

1. Measures that relate substantially to only one dimension of health (indicated by one solid circle and no other entries in the same row of table 11.2). The interpretation of these measures is straightforward because they reflect differences in only one major health dimension; they are not comprehensive measures of health.

2. Measures that relate substantially to more than one health concept (indicated by two solid circles in the same row). These are good general measures, but they do not distinguish different health dimensions.

3. Measures that relate substantially to one health concept and show noteworthy relationships with other health concepts (indicated by one solid and one open circle in the same row). These are good measures of their primary concept (solid circle) but they are subject to an alternative interpretation (open circle).

4. Measures that do not relate substantially to any of the three major health concepts (open circles only in the same row). Such measures are least useful in detecting differences in the three major health concepts.

Physical Functioning

As defined in table 11.1, physical functioning includes the performance

TABLE 11.1
Definitions of Selected Health Concepts

Concepts	Definition	Abbreviated Items	References
Physical			
Physical limitations	Performance of self-care, mobility, and physical activities.	Independence in bathing, dressing. In bed, chair, couch, for most of day. Do not walk at all.	Katz et al. 1963 Kaplan, Bush, and Berry 1976 Bergner et al. 1976
Physical abilities	Ability to perform everyday activities.	Able to walk uphill, upstairs. Able to participate in sports, strenuous activities. Unable to walk without assistance.	Stewart, Ware, and Brook 1981 Stewart, Ware, and Brook 1981 Hulka and Cassel 1973
Days in bed	Number of days health keeps one in bed all or most of the day.	During past 30 days, number of days health keeps one in bed all day or most of day. Staying in bed most of time.	NCHS 1981 Bergner et al. 1976
Mental			
Anxiety/ depression	Feelings of anxiety, nervousness, tenseness, depression, moodiness, downheartedness during specified period.	Depressed or very unhappy. Bothered by nervousness or nerves.	Bradburn 1969 Dupuy 1972, 1984
Psychological well-being	Frequency and intensity of general positive affect (happy, cheerful, full and satisfying life) during specified period.	Happy, pleased, satisfied with life. Wake up expecting an interesting day. Feel cheerful, lighthearted.	Dupuy 1972, 1984 Costello and Comrey 1967 Dupuy 1972, 1984

Behavioral/ emotional control	Control of behavior, thoughts, and feelings during specified period.	Felt emotionally stable. Lose control of behavior, thoughts, feelings. Laugh or cry suddenly. Life is not worth living.	Dupuy 1984 Veit and Ware 1983 Bergner et al. 1976 Hunt 1984
Social			
Visits with friends and relatives	Frequency of visits with friends and relatives, during a specified period of time.	Number of friends visited. Going out less often to visit people.	Donald and Ware 1984 Bergner et al. 1976 Bergner 1984
Telephone contacts	Frequency of telephone contacts with close friends or relatives during specified period of time.	How often on telephone with close friends/relatives, past month.	Donald and Ware 1984
Close friends	Number of close friends, relatives, neighborhood acquaintances.	Number of close friends, people to talk with.	Donald and Ware 1984
Role			
Role func- tioning	Freedom from limitations in performance of usual role activities (e.g., work, housework, school) due to poor health.	Limited in kind or amount of major role activity. Working shorter hours. Health causes problem at work. Unable to work because of health.	NCHS 1981 Bergner et al. 1976 Hunt 1981 Stewart et al. 1981
General Perceptions			
EGFP rating	Rating of health in general in terms of excellent, good, fair, or poor.	In general, is health excellent, good, fair, or poor?	NCHS 1981

TABLE 11.1 (*continued*)

Concepts	Definition	Abbreviated Items	References
Current health	Self-assessment of health in general at present.	Health is excellent. Energy, pep, vitality. Been feeling bad lately.	Davies and Ware 1981 Dupuy 1984 Davies and Ware 1981
Pain	Ratings of the intensity, duration, and frequency of pain as well as limitations in usual activities due to pain.	During the past three months, how much pain have you had? How much pain interfered with things?	NCHS 1981 Daut, Cleeland, and Randall 1985
Symptoms Physical	Reports of physical symptoms during specified period of time. Symptoms (e.g., shortness of breath with light exercise or light work) and minor symptoms (e.g., cough without fever for less than one week).	Did you have any of the following symptoms during the past month?	Aday, Andersen, and Fleming 1980 Shapiro, Sherbourne, and Ware 1985
Psycho-physiologic	Reports of symptoms likely to have a psychological component (including upset stomach, headaches, trembling) during specified period of time.	Did you have any of the following symptoms during the past month?	Shapiro, Ware, and Sherbourne 1986

of or capacity to perform self-care activities (e.g., eating, bathing, dressing), mobility, and physical activities. Health-related limitations in these activities are frequently measured because they are socially relevant, directly interpretable (see table 11.2), and easily verified. For example, a person either can or cannot walk up a flight of stairs, and this behavior can be observed. Physical functioning is socially relevant because an individual's performance of everyday physical activities is prerequisite to being a productive member of society, determines the level of dependence on others, and at the extreme indicates whether institutionalization is required.

Measures of physical functioning differ greatly in their focus, including both the specific concept and the range of severity measured (see table 11.2). For example, self-care limitations are rare in a general population; less than 0.5 percent report limitations in eating, dressing, bathing, or using the toilet due to poor health (Stewart, Ware, and Brook 1981). Thus, in studies of general populations, items that focus on these limitations should be selected sparingly; this principle also applies to studies of many patient populations. In studies of the severely ill, however, an entire battery of measures focused on self-care activities may be appropriate (Katz et al. 1963; Kane and Kane 1981).

Physical health represents more than the performance of physical activities. Two individuals may each walk up a flight of stairs; one may require markedly more effort or assistance because of weakness or poor

motor control, for example, and may suffer greater pain. Many widely used measures of physical functioning fail to capture these differences. Exceptions include functional capacity scales that go beyond performance by assessing pain and difficulty (Jette 1980; Fries et al. 1980). Measures of physical capacity (as opposed to performance) have been criticized as overstating functional status because capacity (ability) is an ambiguous concept (Bush 1984). As summarized in table 11.2, it is well documented that both performance and capacity measures are directly interpretable as measures of physical functioning (Stewart et al. 1978; Stewart, Ware, and Brook 1981; Ware, Davies-Avery, and Brook 1980; Allen and Ware, in press). For many purposes, the extra information about pain and difficulty will prove useful.

The distinction between more general as compared with disease- or problem-specific measures of physical functioning is often important in clinical applications of functional status instruments. Measures of the concepts defined in table 11.1 are general and would be expected to capture gross differences in physical limitations among those in a general population as well as among most clinic patients (Nelson et al. 1983). Such broad measures are likely to miss relatively specific effects of disease or treatment. To guard against this problem, generic measures should be supplemented with highly focused measures of disease impact. Consider, for example, the assessment of functional status using the Physical Functioning Index (PFI). The PFI, a general measure, distinguishes between adults

TABLE 11.2
Dimensions of Health Assessed by Widely Used Standardized Measures

Measures	Physical	Mental	Social
Physical			
Limitations in physical performance	●		
Physical capacities	●		
Days in bed due to poor health	●		
Mental			
Anxiety/depression		●	
Behavioral/emotional control		●	
General positive affect		●	○
Social			
Visits with friends/relatives			●
Telephone contacts			●
Close friends		○	●
Role			
Unable to work due to poor health	●		
Working shorter hours	●		
General Perceptions			
EGFP rating	●	●	
Current health	●	●	
Pain	●	○	
Symptoms			
Physical	○	○	
Psychophysiologic	○	●	

with and without arthritis (Brook et al. 1983, table 1). The PFI does not assess many arthritis-specific limitations (e.g., difficulties with grip, reach); other instruments do (Fries et al. 1980). Generic and arthritis-specific measures of functioning have been compared by Spiegel and her colleagues (1985) with clinical measures of disease activity. Similar studies of patients with other chronic conditions would greatly facilitate the selection of the most appropriate measures for those groups (see, for example, Bergner 1984).

Mental Health

Whereas physical functioning is manifested in behavioral performance, mental health encompasses feelings that cannot be observed. Thus, the assessment of general mental health requires measures of psychological states (e.g., self-reports of the frequency and intensity of psychological distress and psychological well-being). To determine how happy or sad someone is you will have to ask him (Irwin, Kamman, and Dixon 1979).

The content of some general mental health measures based on self-reports of behavioral dysfunction (e.g., certain Sickness Impact Profile scales; Bergner 1984) show similarities to the content of some self-reports of psychological distress (e.g., the Mental Health Inventory described by Ware, Veit, and Sherbourne 1986). Therefore, empirical studies should confirm that they have similar interpretations in relation to general mental health.

Contrary to Dohrenwend and his colleagues (1980, 1981), mental health as defined in table 11.1 is a multidimensional concept. In other words, there are distinct mental health dimensions that should be measured and interpreted separately before reliance on a summary score. The distinction between two of these concepts—psychological distress and psychological well-being—is an important development in the conceptualization of mental health. Strong empirical evidence supports the distinction between these two concepts (Bradburn 1969; Veit and Ware 1983). The addition of psychological well-being to general mental health measures is a relatively recent event (Bradburn 1969; Dupuy 1972; Goldberg 1978; Veit and Ware 1983).

Measures of mental health like those defined in table 11.1 do not overlap much with the physical dimension of health. This pattern of results contrasts with that observed for measures of general health and symptoms (see table 11.2). It is for this reason that general health ratings and reports of physical and psychophysiologic symptoms should be scored and interpreted separately in testing hypotheses about mental health as defined in table 11.1.

Interestingly, measures of psychological well-being correlate highly with mental health, and also correlate significantly with the social health dimension (see table 11.2). This overlap with social health does not hold for measures of other mental health concepts, such as depression and anxiety.

Clinically and socially relevant changes in mental health are not always captured by measures of psychological distress (see, for example, anxiety and depression in table 11.1). The impact of disease, infirmity, stressful life events, and treatment are sometimes captured only by measures of psychological well-being. In other words, the psychological impact of these events amounts to "taking the top off" of a person's life. Life becomes less enjoyable or less interesting—there is less to be happy and cheerful about. Capturing this effect requires measures of psychological well-being, in addition to psychological distress, in studies of mental health outcomes (Bradburn 1969; Dupuy 1972, 1984; Goldberg 1978; Veit and Ware 1983).

Spiegel and her colleagues (1985) describe an interesting example of this phenomenon in clinical practice. In a study of patients with rheumatoid arthritis, they estimated the strength of associations between five physical health measures—disease severity (e.g., manual dexterity), activities of daily living, mobility, household activities, and physical activities—and three measures of mental health (anxiety, depression, and psychological well-being). Controlling statistically for sociodemographic variables and measures of arthritis and general health, the psychological well-being measure correlated significantly and positively with all five physical health measures; the measures of psychological distress (anxiety and depression) did not relate significantly to any of the physical health measures.

Are differences in psychological well-being socially relevant? While critics might argue that measures of psychological well-being assess nothing more than karma, results from Rand's Health Insurance Experiment argue to the contrary. People who enjoyed greater psychological well-being at the beginning of the experiment were significantly less likely to receive mental health care in subsequent years (Ware et al. 1984). This analysis controlled statistically for other initial health variables, study site, insurance coverage, sociodemographic characteristics, and other variables (Ware et al. 1984).

Measures of psychological distress, psychological well-being, and other general mental health concepts described above are not appropriate for diagnosing specific mental disorders. Noteworthy advances have been made in the development of interview schedules designed to standardize the diagnosis of selected mental disorders. These contributions include the Diagnostic Interview Schedule (DIS), which allows both lay interviewers and clinicians to be used in psychiatric epidemiologic studies of specific mental disorders (Robins et al. 1981). In contrast to earlier mental health surveys that sampled symptoms associated with a limited set of disorders, the DIS provides a comprehensive assessment of criteria necessary to diagnose a large number of conditions. The Schedule for Affective Disorders and Schizophrenia (SADS) is another example of a methodology for standardizing the diagnosis of mental disorders (Endicott and Spitzer 1978). The SADS also provides information regarding the severity of the condition.

Although cognitive functioning does not appear in table 11.1, it is an important mental health concept, particularly in some clinical applications of mental health measures. This concept includes orientation with respect to time and place and such mental processes as memory, comprehension, abstract reasoning, and problem solving. Kane and Kane (1981) present an excellent overview of cognitive functioning and available measures.

Social Well-being

As defined in table 11.1, social well-being includes two distinct categories of concepts (Donald and Ware 1984): (1) social contacts and other activities (e.g., visits with friends and relatives), and (2) social ties or resources (e.g., close friends and relatives who can be relied upon for tangible and intangible support). Social contacts can be observed and, thus, represent the more objective of the two categories.

However, one criticism of social contact measures is their focus on events and activities without respect to how the events are personally experienced. Merely counting social activities is analogous to counting the number of feelings while ignoring whether they were good or bad.

Unlike social contacts, social resources cannot be directly observed. For the most part they exist in the mind of the individual and are best measured by asking the individual or significant others about them directly. Social resources represent personal evaluations of the adequacy of interpersonal relationships, including linkages with people who will listen to personal problems and provide tangible support and needed companionship. People who are satisfied with their social resources feel "plugged in" or "connected" with others; they feel cared for, loved, and wanted (Cobb 1976). Not surprisingly, given the personal evaluation of well-being inherent in an assessment of social resources, measures of these resources seem to overlap empirically with the mental dimension of health (see table 11.2). This overlap has been observed for measures of close friends and for other measures of social resources not included in table 11.2 (e.g., neighborhood acquaintances). Measures of feeling cared for, loved, and wanted assess mental health (e.g., depression and anxiety) much more than they measure social well-being, as defined in table 11.1.

Social well-being is more heterogeneous than the physical and mental dimensions of health. In other words, one kind of social circumstance does not predict well another kind of social circumstance. This observation has been confirmed empirically in studies of the social health measures fielded in the Rand Health Insurance Experiment (Donald and Ware 1982, 1984) and in studies of social interaction measures included in the Sickness Impact Profile (Bergner et al. 1976). There is a real danger of reaching inappropriate conclusions when aggregate measures of social well-being are interpreted before examining the consistency of results across specific social concepts. For example, social contacts decrease and social resources increase, respectively, with age. Not surprisingly, a summary index that aggregates these two concepts shows no association with age (Donald and Ware 1982).

Individual differences in social well-being generate considerable interest because they have been linked to medical complications in specific patient populations (Nuckolls, Cassel, and Kaplan 1972) and to survival in a general population (Berkman and Syme 1979). A popular research topic is whether social supports serve as "buffers" of the effects of illness and other stressful life events on mental health (Lin et al. 1979; Williams, Ware, and Donald 1981). Recently reviewed by Wortman (1984), this literature offers evidence that links social circumstances to both physical and mental health outcomes. Thus, measures of social well-being have considerable potential value in clinical practice. For example, they could be used to identify patients at risk of poor outcomes or patients likely to be high users of medical care services because of social isolation.

Although studies linking social factors to survival (e.g., Berkman and Syme 1979; Berkman and Breslow 1983) have been widely quoted, they should be interpreted cautiously because of relatively weak control for individual differences in initial health status. Do individuals who are more socially active live longer because they have better social networks or because they enjoyed better health to begin with?

To choose between these alternative interpretations would require a comprehensive battery of initial health measures. Further, each health concept must be measured with precision, and a multivariate specification of initial health variables (as opposed to an arbitrary aggregation) is required. Differences in predictions across models differing in health status specification have been well documented in studies of medical expenditures (Manning, Newhouse, and Ware 1982). The same principles should be applied to studies of social factors and survival.

Role Functioning

Historically, role functioning has had a special meaning in the health literature. It refers to health-related limitations in the performance of or capacity to perform usual role activities, including formal employment, school work, and housework (see table 11.1). Although discussions of health outcomes often interchange the concept of role functioning and social functioning, the two concepts are distinct. This distinction, as defined in table 11.1, is illustrated in table 11.2.

Measures of role functioning have a completely different interpretation than measures of social functioning in relation to the physical, mental, and social dimensions of health. In most populations, measures of health-related limitations in role performance reflect physical health. At the extreme, severe psychological impairment also disrupts role performance; however, this is rare relative to the incidence of role limitations due to poor physical health. Further, severe psychological impairment is less likely to be detected by typical measures of role limitations (e.g., those in table 11.1) because personal and emotional problems are often not equated with "health problems."

Measures of role functioning are sometimes aggregated with measures of physical functioning (Patrick, Bush, and Chen 1973; Reynolds, Rushing, and Miles 1974). There are good reasons to keep them separate in studies of health in both general and patient populations. Role performance reflects physical health status and the physical demands of usual role activity. Thus, one would expect considerable discrepancy between disease state, physical functioning, and role performance, and such discrepancies are typically observed. For example, role limitations are often observed in the presence and in the absence of physical limitations (Stewart, Ware, and Brook 1981). Pending further research, it is best to measure and interpret measures of physical and role limitations separately before aggregating them. Standardized measures that distinguish the two concepts are available for this purpose (e.g., Bergner et al. 1976; Bergner 1984; Stewart et al. 1978; Stewart, Ware, and Brook 1981).

General Health Perceptions

There is much to be said for the notion that your health is what you think it is. Certainly, self-ratings of health in general are among the most commonly used measures of health and well-being (Davies and Ware 1981). Almost everyone has been asked to provide a rating of their health as "excellent," "good," "fair," or "poor" (National Center for Health Statistics 1981). These ratings are considered measures of general health for two reasons. They do not focus on a specific dimension of health (see table 11.1). Further, they have been linked empirically to a wide range of health concepts (Davies and Ware 1981) and to both physical and mental health dimensions (see table 11.2). They are considered ratings rather than reports because they reflect individual differences in the evaluation of information people have about their health; they are self-assessments.

Measures of general health perceptions are often criticized as subjective and unreliable. Their subjectivity is their strength because they reflect personal evaluations of health not captured by the other measures defined in table 11.1. Who is more qualified to apply a person's values in a health formulation than the person in question (McCullough 1984)? There should be no doubt that general health perceptions can be measured reliably. Even with very brief instruments, these perceptions can be reliably measured in both general and patient populations (Davies and Ware 1981; Lurie et al. 1984; Ware et al., in press).

Measures of general health perceptions could be very useful in clinical practice because they are among the best predictors of patient-initiated physician visits, including both general medical and mental health visits (Manning, Newhouse, and Ware 1982; Wells et al. 1982). However, physicians in practice rarely attempt to understand the reasons behind these perceptions in any systematic way. An interesting question is whether standardized measures of these perceptions would prove valuable in the management of patients. What does it mean when doctor and patient hold disparate views regarding the patient's health? Are the "worried well" really well? Studies addressing these issues are underway (Nelson et al. 1983; Rubenstein et al. 1985; Smith, Monson, and Ray, in press).

An interesting example of results from a systematic comparison between doctor and patient ratings of health was recently reported for patients with somatization disorder (Smith and Monson 1983). This psychiatric disorder is characterized by frequent medical complaints in the absence of demonstrated medical problems. Measures of physical and mental health and general health perceptions were administered to patients with this disorder and to their primary care physicians. Patient and physician ratings of the patient's health in general showed good agreement, but for very different reasons. Patients saw themselves in poorer physical health (82 percent of the time) and doctors rated them lower in mental health (75 percent of the time). Interventions that might correct these misperceptions and reduce unnecessary demand for care are currently being evaluated.

Finally, an example of the potential value of a short-form measure of general health perceptions is found in a recent controlled study of medically indigent adults (MIAs) forced to leave their usual source of care because of loss of benefits (Lurie et al. 1984). MIAs with hypertension and diabetes were followed for six months after benefits were lost. A control group that maintained their benefits was also followed. The baseline and follow-up health assessments for both groups (N = 278) included measures of diastolic blood pressure, blood sugar control, and a four-item general health perceptions scale (Davies and Ware 1981). While the control group showed no changes in health status, the MIAs were significantly worse off in blood pressure, blood sugar control, and showed significantly less favorable perceptions of health (− 8 on a 100-point scale). These results suggest that short-form measures of general health perceptions may be able to detect differences in health outcomes when they are relatively large.

Symptoms

Measures of symptoms reflect acute and chronic problems involving one or more of the body's functional systems. As illustrated in table 11.1, items in symptom inventories can be classified in terms of their content into two major categories: physical symptoms (e.g., toothache, sore throat with fever, swollen ankles when you wake up) and psychophysiologic symptoms (e.g., low energy, headaches, upset stomach). Psychological symptoms (e.g., feeling nervous, depressed, anxious) were discussed above in relation to mental health. The major distinction between physical and psychophysiologic symptoms is that the latter are more likely to reflect an underlying psychological problem.

Consistent with the observations offered above, the kinds of symptoms most often included in mental health instruments has shifted over the past few decades. Early mental health instruments (e.g., Macmillan 1957; Gurin, Veroff, and Field 1960; Langner 1962) included measures of physical, psychophysiologic, and psychological symptoms. More recent instruments focus almost exclusively on psychological symptoms (see table 11.1). Some measures that include both psychological and psychophysiologic symptoms contain scales for each that can be interpreted separately (e.g., Derogatis et al. 1974).

Physical symptoms are very heterogeneous. They correlate only weakly with each other, and, as indicated in table 11.2, batteries of physical symptoms are only weakly associated with the physical dimension of health (as defined in table 11.1). Further, measures of physical symptoms do not discriminate well between physical and mental health problems, even when purged of all psychophysiologic items.

When using symptom inventories to assess health outcomes, it is useful to distinguish between physical symptoms that are serious (e.g., shortness of breath with light exercise, chest pain when exercising) and physical symptoms that are minor (e.g., cough without fever for less than one week, cold with nose stopped up). Analyses of serious and minor symptoms in the Rand Health Insurance Experiment produced very different patterns of results (Shapiro, Ware, and Sherbourne 1986). The prevalence of serious symptoms was substantially correlated with other health measures, was relatively stable over time, increased with age, decreased with income, and was affected by health insurance plan. By contrast, the prevalence of minor symptoms was correlated only weakly with other health measures, was relatively unstable over time, decreased with age, increased with income, and was not affected by health insurance plan.

Physiologic Status and Other Risk Factors

Physiologic status is a core health status concept. From a traditional medical perspective, which emphasizes measurable physiologic parameters of disease, it represents "real health." Physiologic measures do not detect changes in physical, mental, or social functioning, as defined above; thus,

they are not included in table 11.1 or 11.2.

The physiologic dimension of health is very heterogeneous. The distinct parameters are only weakly, if at all, related. Measures of physiologic status are disease or problem specific. A measure that is valid for monitoring the course of one disease is usually or not valid for another. Interventions that target a specific physiologic parameter should be evaluated in terms of highly focused measures.

The technology for measuring the biology and chemistry of disease and the modalities for treatment of these abnormalities have advanced markedly during the past thirty years. This technology is important because longitudinal epidemiologic studies have linked biomedical parameters to the length and quality of life. Measures of other risk factors that reflect lifestyle (e.g., smoking, exercise, alcohol consumption) should be considered for the same reason. Both kinds of risk factors serve a useful role in assessing health outcomes—they introduce prognosis into the health status equation.

Some interventions may affect more than one physiologic parameter or risk factor. If these effects are slight, they are likely to be missed by highly focused measures. An example of an intervention that might produce diffuse but slight effects is a change in overall access to medical care. How could such effects be detected? An interesting strategy is to use an index that combines more than one physiologic parameter or risk factor. One way to combine these variables is in terms of their impact on survival estimated from longitudinal epidemiologic studies. An example is the Risk of Dying Index developed for use in comparing different health care financing arrangements in the Rand Health Insurance Experiment (Brook et al. 1983, 1984; Ware et al., in press). This index combined measures of physiologic status (serum cholesterol and systolic blood pressure) and behavior (smoking) to estimate an overall change in risk of dying.

Although measures of physiologic status are often interpreted as outcomes in clinical trials and in clinical practice from the broader perspective of health status assessment, they actually represent "proximate" outcomes. A cancerous tumor is of concern because some cancers set upper limits on the length and quality of life (Kaplan 1984). Cancer would be of little concern if it did not. Because of preoccupation with length of survival in most longitudinal epidemiologic studies, little is known about the effect of differences in physiologic parameters on physical, mental, and social functioning in subsequent years. This is unfortunate because the impact of differences in physiologic health and other risk factors on subsequent physical, mental, and social functioning may be as great, in the aggregate, as their impact on survival.

Conclusion

The challenge to health status assessment from policymakers, clinical investigators, and health care providers is great. Fortunately, many interesting developments have occurred in the past few decades, including greater breadth of measurement and refinements in standardized instruments. The need and the potential for further progress are also great.

The state of the art of measurement does not pose the only constraint to applying health assessment to clinical medicine and health policy analysis. Progress is also hampered by a limited understanding of health as a concept, including its normal life course, its meaning across subgroups of the population (Mechanic 1983), the nature of its response to specific medical care interventions and outside factors, and the difference between statistically significant and clinically and socially relevant effects of treatment on health. Methodologists working in this field need to be guided. On what concepts should measurement be focused? Are the expected effects of interventions large, medium, or small?

It has become increasingly common to survey patients directly about their health; people are an obvious source of information. A by-product of this development is the recognition of concepts that have been included in general population health surveys for decades but are only rarely considered in assessing outcomes in clinical trials or in clinical practice. Included are physical and role functioning, psychological distress and psychological well-being, and general health perceptions. With increasing frequency, practical considerations have encouraged reliance on self-administered instruments. Given the volume of information required for a comprehensive assessment of health, reliance on less expensive data collection methods is desirable whenever possible. Self-administered surveys can achieve a high level of data quality with considerable cost savings in research applications and in clinical practice.

Adoption of health status instruments would be greatly facilitated by the development of short-form measures. In their absence, clinicians and researchers with limited time or resources are often faced with the choice between measuring one health concept well or measuring multiple health concepts using single-item measures or ad hoc instruments that are not likely to produce valid scores. Good short-form measures are best developed following careful analyses of longer instruments. In fact, it is experience with longer instruments that make good short-forms possible. One example is a seventeen-item survey instrument constructed from scales used in Rand's Health Insurance Experiment. Despite its brevity, this instrument yields scores for physical functioning, general mental health, role functioning, and general health perceptions (Ware, Sherbourne, Davies et al., in press). In a recent telephone survey of adults representing U.S. households, the instrument required about four minutes to administer and achieved a high level of reliability.

Given that health is a multidimensional concept, an appropriate standard for judging a health status measure is its comprehensiveness in terms of major health dimensions. Another important feature of health is the range of functioning and well-being represented. Again, health is more than just the absence of disease or infirmity. Health encompasses well-being and vitality. Thus, health measures should be judged in terms of whether they assess the full range of functioning within each health dimension. The range of measurement is an important consideration in adapting measures of general health concepts across community and patient populations. However, most patients score in the "well" range.

Psychometric standards (e.g., reliability, validity) are also important because adherence to them can greatly increase the likelihood of success in measuring health status (American Psychological Association 1974). The standards have served the behavioral and social sciences well for a century, and they have much to offer those interested in health assessment. Issues of practicality (e.g., acceptability of methods to patients and providers, respondent burden, data collection costs) should be considered along with method of scale construction (topics included, range of differences measured, and coarseness of the scale), distribution of scores in the population of interest, and appropriate occasions for totaling measures.

Trends toward an expanded focus in health assessment are not universal. Information about the level of general mental health in the U.S. population is limited, in part, because of the narrow focus of health surveys fielded by the National Center for Health Statistics (NCHS). In contrast to the 1975 National Health and Nutrition Examination Survey, which assessed general mental health (Dupuy 1972, 1984), more recent NCHS surveys have excluded mental health altogether (e.g., National Center for Health Statistics 1981).

This discussion would be incomplete without comment on the assessment of health status in the Rand Health Insurance Experiment (HIE). The HIE represents the most ambitious attempt yet to evaluate a comprehensive set of health outcomes in a randomized groups experiment. It has taught many lessons about health and its measurement. Much of this experience is summarized in journal articles and in technical reports, including those referenced in this chapter. However, analyses of these data completed to date only scratch the surface. Public use files, which are now becoming available, will be a valuable resource for decades to come.

Methodological lessons from the HIE are beyond the scope of this chapter; some of them are discussed elsewhere (Ware 1984). Information about other methodological developments is available in bulletins published by the National Clearinghouse on Health Status Indexes (National Center for Health Statistics, 3700 East-West Highway, Hyattsville, Md. 20782). Other noteworthy sources of information about methodological issues include books by Berg (1973), Elinson and Siegmann (1979), Mushkin and Dunlop (1979), and Kane and Kane (1981), and the Winter 1976 issue of *Health Services Research.* Interest in improving health outcome assessment prompted the National Heart, Lung, and Blood Institute to host a 1984 workshop on clinical applications of health measures. An excellent reference document entitled *Assessment of Quality of Life in Clinical Trials of Cardiovascular Therapies* was produced (Wenger et al. 1984). It reviews conceptual and methodological issues, and specific health status instruments, and discusses health assessment for patients with specific medical conditions.

Much can be learned about health and health outcomes over the next ten years if there is a concerted effort to apply health assessment methods in clinical trials and in clinical practice. The methods required have not been perfected, but good measures are available. One of the most important discoveries thus far is that people, regardless of their disease status, vary greatly in physical, mental, and social functioning. The explanation of these differences and the mastery of functional outcomes are the challenges of the future.

Acknowledgments

Preparation of this chapter was supported by grants for the National Study of Medical Care Outcomes from the Robert Wood Johnson Foundation and from the Henry J. Kaiser Family Foundation and by the Health Insurance Experiment grant from the U.S. Department of Health and Human Services. The views expressed are those of the author and do not necessarily reflect the views of the sponsors or the Rand Corporation. The author gratefully acknowledges the helpful comments received from Allyson Ross Davies and David Mechanic in response to an earlier draft.

References

Aday, L. A., R. Anderson, and C. V. Fleming. 1980. *Health care in the U.S.: Equitable for whom?* Beverly Hills: Sage Publications.

Allen, H., and J. E. Ware. In press. *Defining physical, mental, and social health in general populations: A multivariate model.* Santa Monica, Calif.: Rand Corporation. (in Press)

American Psychological Association. 1974. *Standards for educational and psychological tests.* Washington, D.C.: American Psychological Association.

Andrews, F. M., and S. B. Withey. 1976. *Social indicators of well-being.* New York: Plenum Press.

Berg, R. L., ed. 1973. *Conference on a health status index.* Chicago: Hospital Research and Educational Trust.

Bergner, M. 1984. The sickness impact profile. In *Assessment of quality of life in clinical trials of cardiovascular therapies,* ed. N. K. Wenger et al. New York: LeJacq Publishing.

Bergner, M., R. A. Bobbitt, W. E. Pollard, D. P. Martin, and B. S. Gilson. 1976. The sickness impact profile: Validation of a health status measure. *Medical Care* 14(1):57–67.

Berkman, L. F., and L. Breslow. 1983. *Health and ways of living.* New York: Oxford University Press.

Berkman, L. F., and S. L. Syme. 1979. Social networks, host resistance, and mortality: A nine-year follow-up study of Alameda County residents. *American Journal of Epidemiology* 109(2):186–204.

Bradburn, N. M. 1969. *The structure of psychological well-being.* Chicago: Aldine Publishing.

Brook, R. H., J. E. Ware, W. H. Rogers et al. 1984. *The effect of coinsurance on the health of adults.* Rand R-3055-HHS. Santa Monica, Calif.: Rand Corporation.

Brook, R. H., J. E. Ware, W. H. Rogers, E. G. Keeler et al. 1983. Does free care improve adults' health? Results from a randomized control trial. *New England Journal of Medicine* 309(23):1426–1434.

Bush, J. W. 1984. General health policy model/quality of well-being (QWB) scale. In *Assessment of quality of life in clinical trials of cardiovascular therapies,* ed. N. K. Wenger et al. New York: LeJacq Publishing.

Cobb, S. 1976. Social support as a moderator of life stress. *Psychosomatic Medicine* 38:300–314.

Costello, C. G., and A. L. Comrey. 1967. Scales for measuring depression and anxiety. *Journal of Psychology* 66:303–313.

Daut, R. L., C. S. Cleeland, and C. F. Randall. 1985. Development of the Wisconsin brief pain questionnaire to assess pain in cancer and other diseases. Department of Neurology, University of Wisconsin, Madison. Typescript.

Davies, A. R., and J. E. Ware. 1981. *Measuring health perceptions in the health insurance program.* Rand R-2711-HHS. Santa Monica, Calif.: Rand Corporation.

Derogatis, L. R., R. S. Lipman, K. Rickels, E. H. Uhlenhuth, and L. Covi. 1974. The Hopkins symptom checklist (HSCL): A self-report inventory. *Behavioral Science* 19:1–5.

Dohrenwend, P. B., L. Oskenberg, P. E. Shrout et al. 1981. What brief psychiatric screening scales measure. In *Health Survey Research Methods* (DHHS Publication No. PHS 81-3268). Washington, D.C.: Government Printing Office.

Dohrenwend, B. P., P. E. Shrout, G. Egri, and F. S. Mendelsohn. 1980. Nonspecific psychological distress and other dimensions of psychopathology. Measures for use in the general population. *Archives of General Psychiatry* 37(11)1229–1236.

Donald, C. A., and J. E. Ware. 1982. *The quantification of social contacts and resources.* Rand R-2937-HHS. Santa Monica, Calif.: Rand Corporation.

———. 1984. The measurement of social support. In *Research in community and mental health,* ed. J. R. Greenley, 4:325–370. Greenwich, Conn.: JAI Press.

Donald, C. A., J. E. Ware, R. H. Brook, and A. Davies-Avery. 1978. *Conceptualization and measurement of health for adults in the health insurance study,* vol. 4: *Social Health.* Rand R-1987/4-HEW. Santa Monica, Calif.: Rand Corporation.

Dupuy, H. J. 1972. The psychological section of the current health and nutrition examination survey. In *Proceedings of the public health conference on records and statistics meeting jointly with the national conference on health statistics.* Washington, D.C.: National Conference on Health Statistics.

———. 1984. The psychological general well-being (PGWB) index. In *Assessment of quality of life in clinical trials of cardiovascular therapies,* ed. N. K. Wenger et al. New York: LeJacq Publishing.

Elinson, J. 1979. Introduction to the theme: Sociomedical health indicators. In *Socio-medical health indicators,* ed. J. Elinson and A. E. Siegmann. Bloomingtondale, N.Y.: Baywood Publishing.

Elinson, J., and A. E. Siegmann, 1979. *Socio-medical health indicators.* Bloomingdale, N.Y.: Baywood Publishing.

Endicott, J. and R. L. Spitzer. 1978. A diagnostic interview: The schedule for affective disorders and schizophrenia. *Archives of General Psychiatry* 35:837–844.

Fries, J. F., P. Spitz, R. G. Kraines, and H. R. Holman. 1980. Measurement of patient outcome in arthritis. *Arthritis and Rheumatism* 23(2):137–145.

Goldberg, D. 1978. *Manual of the general health questionnaire.* Windsor, England: NFER Publishing.

Gurin, G., J. Veroff, and S. Field. 1960. *Americans view their mental health: A nationwide interview survey.* New York: Basic Books.

Hulka, B. S., and J. C. Cassel. 1973. The AAFP-UNC study of the organization, utilization, and assessment of primary medical care. *American Journal of Public Health* 63:494–501.

Hunt, H. J. 1984. Nottingham health profile. In *Assessment of quality of life in clinical trials of cardiovascular therapies*, ed. N. K. Wenger et al. LeJacq Publishing.

Irwin, R., R. Kammann, and G. Dixon. 1979. If you want to know how happy I am you'll have to ask me. *New Zealand Psychologist* 8:10–12.

Jette, A. M. 1980. Functional capacity evaluation: An empirical approach. *Archives of Physical Medicine and Rehabilitation* 61:85–89.

Kane, R. A., and R. L. Kane. 1981. *Assessing the elderly*. Lexington, Mass.: Lexington Books.

Kaplan, B. H. 1975. An epilogue: Toward further research on family health. In *Family and health: An epidemiological approach*, ed. B. H. Kaplan and J. C. Cassel, pp. 89–100. Chapel Hill: Institute for Research and Social Science, University of North Carolina.

Kaplan, R. M. 1984. The connection between clinical health promotion and health status. *American Psychologist* 39(7):755–765.

Kaplan, R. M., J. W. Bush, and C. C. Berry. 1976. Health status: Types of validity and the index of well-being. *Health Services Research* 11(4): 478–507.

———. 1979. Health status index: Category rating versus magnitude estimation for measuring levels of well-being. *Medical Care* 17:501–525.

Katz, S., A. B. Ford, R. W. Moskowitz et al. 1963. Studies of illness in the aged. *Journal of the American Medical Association* 185(12):94–99.

Langner, T. S. 1962. A twenty-two item screening score of psychiatric symptoms indicating impairment. *Journal of Health and Human Behavior* 3:269–276.

Levine, S., and S. H. Croog. 1984. What constitutes quality of life? A conceptualization of the dimensions of life quality in healthy populations and patients with cardiovascular disease. In *Assessment of quality of life in clinical trials of cardiovascular therapies*, ed. N. K. Wenger et al. New York: LeJacq Publishing.

Lin, N., R. S. Simeone, W. M. Ensel, and W. Kuo. 1979. Social support, stressful life events, and illness: A model and an empirical test. *Journal of Health and Social Behavior* 20:108–119.

Lurie, N., N. B. Ward, M. F. Shapiro, and R. H. Brook. 1984. Termination from Medi-Cal: Does it affect health? *New England Journal of Medicine* 311:480–484.

McCullough, L. B. 1984. Philosophical and ethical dimensions of the quality of life: Relationship to cardiovascular care. *Quality of Life and Cardiovascular Care* 1(1):18–28.

Macmillan, A. M. 1957. The health opinion survey: Technique for estimating prevalence of psychoneurotic and related types of disorder in communities. *Psychological Reports* 3:325–339.

Manning, W. G., Jr., J. P. Newhouse, and J. E. Ware. 1982. The status of health in demand estimation; or beyond excellent, good, fair, poor. In *Economic aspects of health*, ed. V. R. Fuchs, pp. 143–184. Chicago: University of Chicago Press.

Mechanic, D. 1983. The experience and expression of distress: The study of illness behavior and medical utilization. In *Handbook of health, health care, and the health professionals*, ed. D. Mechanic. New York: Free Press.

Medical Outcomes Study. 1985. Overview of the national study of medical care outcomes. Santa Monica, Calif.: Rand Corporation.

Mushkin, S. J., and D. W. Dunlop. 1979. *Health: What is it worth?* New York: Pergamon Press.

National Center for Health Statistics. 1981. *Health: United States* U.S. Department of Health and Human Services. Washington, D.C.: Government Printing Office.

Nelson, E., B. Conger, R. Douglass, D. Gephart, J. Kirk, R. Page, A. Clark, K. Johnson, K. Stone, J. Wasson, and M. Zubkoff. 1983. Functional health status levels of primary care patients. *Journal of the American Medical Association* 249(24):3331–3337.

Nuckolls, K. B., J. Cassel, and B. H. Kaplan. 1972. Psychosocial assets, life crisis, and the prognosis of pregnancy. *American Journal of Epidemiology* 95:431–441.

Patrick, D. L., J. W. Bush, and M. M. Chen. 1973. Methods for measuring levels of well-being for a health status index. *Health Services Research* 8: 228–245.

Reynolds, W. J., W. A. Rushing, and D. L. Miles. 1974. The validation of a functional status index. *Journal of Health and Social Behavior* 15:271–288.

Robins, L., J. Helzer, J. Croughan, and K. Ratcliff. 1981. The National Institute of Mental Health Diagnostic Interview Schedule: Its history, characteristics, and validity. *Archives of General Psychiatry* 38:381–389.

Rubenstein, L. V., D. R. Calkins, A. Fink, R. T. Young, P. D. Cleary, A. M. Jette, J. Kosecoff, A. R. Davies, T. L. Delbanco, and R. H. Brook. 1985. How to help your patients function better. *Western Journal of Medicine* 143(1)114–117.

Shapiro, M. F., J. E. Ware, and C. D. Sherbourne 1986. Effects of cost-sharing on seeking care for serious and minor symptoms. Annals of Internal Medicine, 1986.

Smith, R. G., and R. A. Monson. 1983. Assessment of health status. *Journal of the American Medical Association* 250(23):3163–3164.

Smith, R. G., R. A. Monson, and D. C. Ray. In press. *Patients with multiple unexplained symptoms: Their characteristics, functional health, and health care utilization.* Little Rock: University of Arkansas Press.

Spiegel, J. S., N. C. Ward, R. L. Kane, H. E. Paulus, B. Leake, T. M. Spiegel, and J. E. Ware. 1985. What are we measuring: An examination of disease activity and functional measures for arthritis patients. Los Angeles: UCLA School of Medicine.

Stewart, A. L., J. E. Ware, and R. H. Brook. 1981. Advances in the measurement of functional status: Construction of aggregate indexes. *Medical Care* 19(5):473–488.

Stewart, A. L., J. E. Ware, R. H. Brook, and A. Davies-Avery. 1978. *Conceptualization and measurement of physical health for adults in the health insurance study,* vol. 2: *Physical health in terms of functioning.* Rand R-1987/2-HEW. Santa Monica, Calif.: Rand Corporation.

Valdez, R. B., R. H. Brook, W. H. Rogers, J. E. Ware, E. B. Keeler, C. A. Sherbourne, K. N. Lohr, G. A. Goldberg, P. Camp, and J. P. Newhouse. 1985. The consequences of cost sharing for children's health. *Pediatrics* (in press).

Veit, C. T., and J. E. Ware. 1983. The structure of psychological distress and well-being in general populations. *Journal of Consulting and Clinical Psychology* 51(5):730–742.

Ware, J. E. 1984. Methodological considerations in the selection of health status assessment procedures. In *Assessment of quality of life in clinical trials of cardiovascular disease,* ed. N. K. Wenger et al., pp. 87–111. New York: LeJacq Publishing.

Ware, J. E., R. H. Brook, W. H. Rogers, E. B. Keeler, A. R. Davies, C. D. Sherbourne, G. A. Goldberg, P. Camp, and J. P. Newhouse. In press. *How do health outcomes at an HMO compare with those of the fee-for-service systems of care: Rresults from a randomized controlled trial among non-aged adults.* Santa Monica, Calif.: Rand Corporation.

Ware, J. E., A. Davies-Avery, and R. H. Brook. 1980. *Conceptualization and measurement of health for adults in the health insurance study,* vol. 6: *Analysis of relationships among health status measures.* Rand R-1987/6-HEW. Santa Monica, Calif.: Rand Corporation.

Ware, J. E., S. A. Johnston, A. Davies-Avery, and R. H. Brook. 1979. *Conceptualization and measurement of health for adults in the health insurance study,* vol. 3: *Mental health.* Rand R-1987/3-HEW. Santa Monica, Calif.: Rand Corporation.

Ware, J. E., W. G. Manning, N. Duan, K. B. Wells, and J. P. Newhouse. 1984. Health status and the use of outpatient mental health services. *American Psychologist* 39(10):1090–1100.

Ware, J. E., C. D. Sherbourne, A. R. Davies, and A. L. Stewart. In press. *General health* A Short Form Survey. Santa Monica, Calif.: Rand Corporation.

Ware, J. E., C. T. Veit, and C. A. Sherbourne. 1986. *Refinements in the measurement of mental health for adults in the health insurance experiment.* Santa Monica, Calif.: Rand Corporation.

Ware, J. E., and J. Young. 1979. Issues in the conceptualization and measurement of value placed on health. In *Health: What is it worth?* ed. S. J. Mushkin and D. W. Dunlop, pp. 141–166. New York: Pergamon Press.

Wells, K. B., W. G. Manning, N. Duan, J. E. Ware, and J. P. Newhouse. 1982. *Cost sharing and the demand for ambulatory mental health services.* Rand R-2960-HHS. Santa Monica, Calif.: Rand Corporation.

Wenger, Nanette K. 1984. The concept of quality of life. *Quality of Life and Cardiovascular Care* 1(1):8–14.

Wenger, N. K., M. E. Mattson, Curt D. Furberg, and J. Elinson. 1984. *Assessment of quality of life in clinical trials of cardiovascular therapies.* New York: LeJacq Publishing.

Williams, A. W., J. E. Ware, and C. A. Donald. 1981. A model of mental health, life events, and social supports applicable to general populations. *Journal of Health and Social Behavior* 22:324–336.

World Health Organization. 1948. Constitution of the World Health Organization. In *Basic Documents.* Geneva: World Health Organization.

Wortman, C. B. 1984. Social support and the cancer patient: Conceptual and methodologic issues. *Cancer* 53(10):2339–2359.

Chapter 12

Social Experiments in Health

Joseph P. Newhouse

Experimentation has long been accepted in clinical research, and over the years it has become ever more widespread. Indeed, the words *randomized controlled trial* (RCT) have become the gold standard for determining the efficacy of a new clinical procedure and are required in the case of a new drug. Experiments or RCTs —I shall use the words interchangeably—are less well accepted in the world of health policy. Nonetheless, their use has greatly expanded in the last decade.

In this chapter I wish to demonstrate (1) that randomized controlled trials (RCTs) in the area of health policy are feasible for many problems, and (2) that when feasible, the RCT is generally desirable. Although more expensive than an observational study, the difference in cost is often surprisingly little. Finally, I offer some guidelines or hints for those contemplating or designing an experiment in the health policy area.

Feasibility and Desirability

A description of several RCTs that have been conducted in health policy supports both their feasibility and their desirability. The following list is by no means exhaustive; for example, almost all the examples discussed are from the United States, although any number of important and well-designed trials have been conducted in other countries.

Health Insurance Study

Field work for the Health Insurance Study, a controlled trial of health care

229

financing and organization, was conducted between 1974 and 1982. Participants (6,970) were randomized to one of fourteen different insurance plans or to a health maintenance organization. Additionally, a random sample of 733 individuals already enrolled at the health maintenance organization was included. The insurance plans varied the cost of care to the families. Some families paid nothing for their medical care; others paid 25, 50, or 95 percent of their medical bills up to a $1,000 maximum out-of-pocket expense per year per family. The out-of-pocket maximum was scaled down for poor families. One plan approximated a $150 per person per year deductible, but the cost sharing applied only to outpatient services; inpatient services were free.

The objectives were to ascertain the effect of variation in cost sharing (or the effect of using a health maintenance organization) on the use and cost of services, health status, quality of care, and patient satisfaction. Additionally, the study sought to determine whether these effects differed among subgroups of the population —for example, individuals, in poor families, who began the experiment sick.

Initial Results

Analysis is still not complete, but the following results are known (Newhouse et al. 1981; Brook et al. 1983; Manning, Leibowitz et al. 1984):

1. Use in the fee-for-service system responds importantly to cost sharing. Expenditures per person per year were about 50 percent higher in the free plan than in the plan with 95 percent coinsurance. Visits rose from about 3.5 per person per year to 5.5 per person per year, while the percentage of individuals admitted to a hospital in a year rose from around 8 percent to around 10 percent. The responsiveness of hospital admissions, however, was entirely among adults; admission rates for children were unaffected by plan.

2. Except for hospital admissions for children, all groups changed their use by roughly similar amounts as the plan changed. This included individuals in small towns and large cities, in high-income and low-income groups, and in large and small families. More precisely, there were no detectable interactions between insurance plan and other covariates.

3. Once admitted to the hospital, expenditure seemed unaffected by plan. This was not surprising, given that 70 percent of those hospitalized exceeded their out-of-pocket maximum and received all additional services free. But it implies that cost sharing does little to affect hospital cost per stay (or cost per day), the most rapidly rising component of hospital cost.

4. The health maintenance organization also reduced the use of services. Because of randomization, the families assigned to the health maintenance organization were similar to those in the free care plan; in particular, both faced no cost sharing. The rate of expenditure was some 28 percent less than in the free plan; the pattern of reduction, however, was quite different from the pattern caused by cost sharing. Virtually all

the reduction occurred from reduced hospital admissions, which were some 40 percent less than in the free fee-for-service plan. Outpatient visit rates were similar to those in the free fee-for-service plan. The reduced use of hospital services was found in both the group randomized into the health maintenance organization and the group that was already enrolled there, implying no selection of risks for or against the health maintenance organization in this case.

5. Within the fee-for-service system the change in use caused by free care (relative to cost sharing) produced very modest changes in health among the average adult participant. Those whose uncorrected vision was worse than 20/20 had a gain in corrected vision from 20/22.5 to 20/22. Diastolic blood pressure improved by about 0.8 mmHg.

6. The improvement in health appeared concentrated in poor individuals who began the experiment in poor health. Their diastolic blood pressure on average improved by about 2 mmHg, with a corresponding decrease in the risk of death from 2.1 times the average risk of death at any age to 1.9 times the average risk of death.

Kansas Trial of More Generous Outpatient Coverage

The Kansas study was conducted in 1968 in Wichita. The Kansas Blue Cross–Blue Shield Association agreed to provide $200,000 of outpatient benefits for a randomly chosen sample of their subscribers. The hypothesis examined was that lack of outpatient coverage artificially inflated hospital admission rates and hospital expenditure. The principal comparison, then, was hospitalization among families with the experimental benefit and families with no such benefit. The experimental benefit provided payment for physician services in the home, office, and emergency room, as well as laboratory and X-ray services wherever done; no well care benefits were provided. Approximately 5,000 families were given these benefits; 10,000 other families were studied as a control group.

The primary result of the study was that outpatient coverage did not serve to reduce hospital admissions; if anything, it increased them (Hill and Veney 1970; Lewis and Keairnes 1970). Although free outpatient care may have caused physicians to move the location of some procedures to an outpatient setting, these instances appear to be outweighed by a countervailing phenomenon. The outpatient coverage increased the rate at which patients sought office care from the physician. (For example, 39 percent of the experimental group saw a physician during a ten-week period, whereas only 34 percent of the control group did. It seems that the more frequently a patient seeks care, the more likely the physician will observe some pathology that in his or her opinion merits hospitalization. The experiment terminated when the $200,000 fund was spent; no offsetting savings had appeared. Effects of the experimental insurance coverage appeared somewhat muted because over half the experimental participants disclaimed knowledge of their additional experimental coverage.

The finding of the Kansas study—that more generous coverage of outpatient services does not reduce impatient use of services—is reaffirmed by the results from the Health Insurance Study. In that study one group of participants had free inpatient care and costly outpatient care, whereas another group received both services free of charge. Hospitalization rates and expenditure were higher in the group that received all services free.

These results of the two randomized studies, however, stand in contrast to a noncontrolled "experiment" with the California Medicaid population conducted in 1972. In this experiment certain Medicaid beneficiaries were charged $1 for the first two office visits and 50 cents for the first two drug prescriptions in each month. Utilization experience was followed for six months before the copayments took effect and for twelve months following the copayments.

The results of the experiment appeared to show that the copayments decreased office visits but dramatically increased hospitalization (Roemer et al. 1975; Helms, Newhouse, and Phelps 1978). The net effect on expenditure was positive, though insignificantly different from zero.

The differences between the California Medicaid "experiment" results and the two randomized experiment results are highly suggestive of the advantages of controlled experiments. In particular, in the California Medicaid experiment the poorer of the Medicaid population was exempted from copayment, which was only imposed on those with higher income levels. If hospitalization in the prior year depressed income levels, those who were hospitalized in the before period would have been more likely to have been assigned to the no-copayment group. In such a case this group would have exhibited a decline in hospital use (i.e., regression to the mean) that would not have been mirrored in the experimental population; the decline in use would have been attributable solely to the nonrandom assignment. An alternative explanation is that a Medicaid population may behave differently with respect to cost sharing than does a non-Medicaid population, but no evidence in the Health Insurance Study results suggests that the utilization response among the poor is different from the average response. In light of two randomized trials that come to the opposite conclusion, it is a reasonable inference that the nonrandomized study yielded a false result.

Colorado Clinical Psychologist/ Expanded Mental Health Benefits Experiment

The Colorado experiment was conducted between 1976 and 1978 using all Medicare beneficiaries in the state of Colorado, about one hundred forty thousand people (Health Care Financing Administration 1981). The Medicare beneficiaries were randomly assigned to one of four treatment groups, which varied along two dimensions. Two groups retained the previous Medicare coverage for mental health services, a 50 percent coinsurance rate together with a maximum payment of $250 per year, while two other groups received a more generous benefit of 20 percent coinsurance and a maximum payment of $400 per year. Each of these two groups was in turn split into two groups, one that could contact a clinical psychologist as an independent practitioner and one that could only receive Medicare benefits for clinical psychologists if a physician supervised the psychologist.

The experiment was evaluated only with respect to the effects of the changes on use and cost; effects on mental health were not measured. For the most part the changes in financing seemed to have little or no effect; there were no statistically significant differences in use among the four groups, although both a lower coinsurance rate and direct access to clinical psychologists appeared to raise expenditures.

The lack of a statistically significant effect of the change in coinsurance stands in contrast to a result from the Health Insurance Study. In that experiment, more complete coverage of mental health services nearly doubled the proportion seeking care, from around 4.5 to around 9 percent (Manning, Wells et al. 1984). Although age differences in the samples studied might account for the differences in outcome, more likely they are attributable to the Colorado beneficiaries' lack of understanding of the new benefits; in a separate questionnaire only around 1 percent of the participants exhibited any accurate knowledge of the experiment (Health Care Financing Administration 1981). Perhaps for the same reason,

the ability to seek care from a clinical psychologist practicing independently did not appear to affect behavior. Fewer than 2 percent of the mental health services were delivered by clinical psychologists who were practicing and billing independently.

Burlington Randomized Trial of the Nurse-Practitioner

The Burlington Randomized Trial was conducted in Burlington, Ontario, for twelve months in 1971 and 1972. Two family physicians agreed to introduce nurse-practitioners into their practice by randomizing primary care patients to them. The study groups consisted of 1,058 families divided equally between each physician as the primary care giver and 540 families divided equally between the two nurse-practitioners as the primary care giver.

The success of the trial was judged by utilization, health status, and quality-of-care outcomes (Spitzer et al. 1974; Sackett et al. 1974). On all these dimensions, care delivered by the nurse-practitioner appeared to be an improvement over conventional care. The services provided by each nurse-practitioner were valued at $16,000, and almost half of those services were delivered without supervision. The authors do not tell us how much the nurses were paid, but the average hourly wage of nurses in the United States in 1969 was $3.53 (Fuchs 1976), suggesting that the value of services the nurses provided may have been as much as double their salary. (In light of the potential economic gain, one might ask why physicians had not added nurse-practitioners previously. The answer is that payment for nurse-practitioners as independent practitioners was not possible under the Ontario health insurance scheme. As a result, during the twelve months of the trial practice, revenue declined 5 percent despite the increase in services.) Indexes of physical, mental, and social functioning appeared unaffected by the primary care giver's identity. Quality of care also appeared unaffected: in 392 episodes of care, management of the condition was rated as adequate in an insignificantly greater number of cases among those treated by the nurse-practitioners.

Wadsworth VA Trial of Hospice Care

The Wadsworth trial was held in the early 1980s (Kane et al. 1984). Terminally ill cancer patients being cared for at a Veterans Administration facility were randomly assigned to receive hospice or conventional care. The hospice in this case was an eleven-bed unit staffed by two physicians, nineteen nurses, a social worker, a chaplain, and about thirty volunteers. Additionally, a home care program serving about twenty-five patients at any one time was in place.

The objectives of the trial were to determine the effect of the hospice on the cost of care and on such patient outcomes as pain control and satisfaction with care. Prior studies of hospice care were largely anecdotal but appeared to indicate that the hospice dominated conventional care on all dimensions. Such studies, however,

were based on patients who had been assigned on a nonrandom basis to hospice care; they may have been less costly to care for than those who received conventional care. Moreover, those who expected to like hospice care better may have been those who used it.

The trial found little difference in cost between hospice care and conventional care. If anything, hospice costs were higher. Outcome measures used included scales for measuring pain, depression, anxiety, functional status, and patient satisfaction. In general, the outcomes were not very different. Survival curves for the two groups were coterminous. Satisfaction was greater in the hospice group, but other outcome measures did not differ between the two groups.

A large evaluation of hospice care was conducted at approximately the same time, but in this project patients were not randomized to hospice care. The project involved fourteen hospital-based hospices and eleven home-care-based hospices. Fifteen months into the project preliminary findings were published that drew on the experience of 1,143 hospital-based hospice patients, 2,746 home-care-based hospice patients, and 334 conventional care patients with terminal cancer (Greer and Mor 1984).

Because of the lack of randomization, the evaluators must attempt to control for differences in the types of patients using hospices and conventional care—a quite difficult task. For example, patients in hospital-based hospices received on average eighteen days of inpatient care, while patients in home-care hospices received only five days. It seems possible that this large difference was in part due to differences in characteristics of patients rather than solely in the care given by the two types of hospices. When making comparisons among the three treatments (two hospice treatments and conventional care), the evaluators controlled for such factors as the patient's age, sex, cancer, length of time since diagnosis, and health care cost per week in the period prior to entering the hospice. The degree to which controlling for such variables can serve to standardize the groups is judgmental.

A smaller sample was chosen for final evaluation (Greer et al., in press). The results indicated that hospital-based hospices were approximately as expensive as conventional care, but home care hospices, by contrast, were 30 percent cheaper than both hospital-based hospices and conventional care when adjusted (as described earlier) for patient characteristics. Hospital-based hospice patients reported less pain than conventional care patients in the last three weeks of life, but the amount of pain reported by home-care hospice patients did not differ from that reported by those in conventional care. No significant differences were found in reported satisfaction by patients, although a close relative was more satisfied with care in hospital-based hospices. The investigators concluded that with small exceptions, quality of life was similar among patients in the three systems.

Comparison of these results with those of the randomized trial is difficult because the hospice used in the randomized trial was hospital based but had a home care component. The randomized trial reports no saving in money, but the observational study suggests that home-care-based hospices may produce savings. The savings, however, appear in part because family members provide direct care, and no cost is imputed for this care. The randomized trial found greater satisfaction among the hospice patients but no difference in pain; the observational study of hospital-based hospices reports no difference in satisfaction (when reported by patients) but reduced pain. Whether these differences between the findings are due to differences in design (i.e., randomization versus nonrandomization with lack of complete standardization) or to a difference in the sample of hospices studied (i.e., one hospice versus fourteen hospices) is speculative. Although the conclusion from both studies marginally favors hospice care, the expectation in many quarters that hospice care is less expensive than conventional care has no support in the case of hospital-based hospices. Home care hospices, by contrast, do appear to save third parties money by substituting the time of family members for the time of health professionals; but a skeptic can still wonder whether the statistical controls are adequate to justify even this conclusion.

National Preventive Dentistry Demonstration Program

The Preventive Dentistry Program began in the fall of 1977 in ten cities (Bell et al. 1984; Foch et al. 1984; Robert Wood Johnson Foundation 1983). It involved about thirty thousand children in first, second, and fifth grades and ran for four years in nine sites and three years in a tenth. Children were sampled by school; each school at a site was assigned to one of five treatment programs or to a control group. The five treatment programs consisted of a preventive dentistry program in a clinic setting, two programs of varying comprehensiveness in a classroom setting, and two programs of varying comprehensiveness that used both clinic and classroom settings. The assumptions behind the program were that preventive dentistry was efficacious and that the classroom was a relatively low-cost delivery site.

In one sense the program was effective. The two clinic programs prevented about half the decay that might otherwise have occurred. However, the incidence of decay among the control group was so low that the gains from the various treatment alternatives amounted to only one to two carious surfaces after a four-year period. Moreover, this effect was almost entirely due to relatively expensive sealants, which in 1981 dollars cost over $90 per child per year. By comparison, roughly similar effects are available from water fluoridation, which costs less than $1 per person per year.

The findings ran counter to the prevailing views at the outset of the program. The chairman of the advisory committee to the project concluded that "Providing routine, standardized, individually applied preventive dental procedures to all children can no longer be justified"; one of the investigators concluded that "the cost of such a program for all children is prohibitive" (Robert Wood Johnson Foundation 1983).

The program did find, however, that 20 percent of the children account for around 60 percent of the caries. The investigators who carried out the program strongly suggested targeting preventive services at this high-risk group.

The major reason the preventive program proved less beneficial than expected was that the control group had fewer caries than had been anticipated on the basis of previous studies. In retrospect, the earlier studies, which suggested a rather large effect of treatment, were flawed. Some of these studies were performed in a "laboratory" setting rather than as true field programs; in such a setting the investigator maintains better control of the treatment program, and thus the program might be expected to show a larger effect. Other studies performed under field conditions were not randomized studies and had no true control group. Often the "control" group was the amount of decay in the community prior to introduction of the program. In an era when decay rates were falling generally, this led to an overestimate of the effect on decay of the preventive programs.

Hypertension Detection and Follow-up Program

The Hypertension Detection Program was a community-based experiment involving just under eleven thousand men and women between the ages of thirty and sixty-nine (Hypertension Detection and Follow-up Program Cooperative Group 1976, 1977, 1979a, 1979b, 1982). These participants all had a diastolic blood pressure equal to or greater than 90 mmHg upon entry into the program. They were randomized to two groups; one received a cost-free standardized program of pharmacologic therapy at one of fourteen participating clinical centers. The "control" group was referred to their usual source of care, and a notification of the individual's blood pressure was sent to that source. The program lasted for five years, from 1974 to 1978.

The intervention appeared to be successful. Among white men, for example, diastolic blood pressure fell by 10 mmHg in the conventional care group and by 15 mmHg in the "treatment" group. (The decline in the conventional care group and part of the decline in the treatment group is attributable to regression toward the mean.) The additional reduction in blood pressure in the treatment group had important payoffs. Mortality from all causes after a five-year period was 17 percent lower in the treatment group; the incidence of stroke was reduced by a third, and death rates from strokes were reduced 45 percent. The mortality rate from stroke among this hypertensive population approached the rate in a general population. The decline in diastolic blood pressure in this trial was greater than that achieved by free care in the Health Insurance Study, perhaps because the treatment was focused on hypertension.

Multiple Risk Factor Intervention Trial

The Multiple Risk Factor Intervention Trial (MRFIT) involved 12,866 men aged thirty-five to fifty-seven who were at high risk of cardiovascu-

lar disease but had no clinical evidence of such disease (Multiple Risk Factor Intervention Trial Research Group 1976, 1982). The high-risk group was defined as those in the upper 10 to 15 percent of risk for disease based on their blood pressure, smoking habits, and serum cholesterol. (Men with serum cholesterol of 350 mg/dl or more and men with diastolic blood pressure of 115 mmHg or higher were, however, excluded, as were men with weight exceeding 150 percent of their ideal weight, men with angina pectoris, and men with treated symptomatic diabetes.) Entry into the trial occurred between December 1973 and February 1976; all the men were followed for at least six years, with the average time in the trial about seven years.

The men were randomized into two groups. The "control" group continued to see their usual source of care; additionally, their physicians were notified of the initial screening results, and the men were asked to take an annual examination. The "treatment" received by the other group depended upon their condition. If they were hypertensive, they received a stepped-care drug treatment very much like that in the Hypertension Detection and Follow-up Program; if they were smokers, they received counseling by a physician and were treated with behavioral modification techniques. The latter were administered in ten-week group sessions or five-day quit clinics. If they had elevated cholesterol levels, they received a dietary treatment that focused on lowering the consumption of saturated fat and cholesterol. (Specifically, after 1976 the recommendation was that saturated fat be less than 8 percent of total calories and dietary cholesterol be less than 250 mg/day.) In general, participants in the treatment group were seen at least every four months by a team of physicians, nurses, nutritionists, and health counselors; usually a behavioral scientist headed this team.

The trial focused on mortality from coronary heart disease, from cardiovascular disease, and from any cause, as well as actual levels of the risk factors. The mean levels of risk factors notably improved in the treatment group: after six years diastolic blood pressure was 3 mmHg less in the treatment group (about the same reduction as occurred in the Hypertension Detection and Follow-up Program), the reported number of cigarette smokers was 13 percentage points less, and serum cholesterol was 5 mg/dl less. An analysis using these values to predict mortality indicates that mortality from cardiovascular disease should have been lowered 22 percent in the treatment group.

In fact, the actual death rate was 2 percent higher in the treatment group. This highly unexpected finding has not yet been well explained. Some individuals at high risk of cardiovascular disease had been excluded from the trial; this may have reduced the likelihood of observing reductions in mortality from the intervention. Still, it seems unlikely that this fact by itself can explain the findings.

Another possibility is that the unanticipated decline in cardiovascular disease in the population at large during this period (its causes still poorly understood) led to relatively few deaths in both groups; thus, any effects of the program were hard to detect. For example, although deaths from coronary heart disease were 7 percent less in the treatment group, the 90 percent confidence interval on the change in coronary heart disease that the intervention may have caused is quite wide, ranging from −25 percent to +15 percent.

The pattern of decline in mortality was not uniform among subgroups. For example, in contrast to the average 7 percent decline, there was a 49 percent lower death rate from coronary heart disease among those men who began the study as smokers and with elevated cholesterol levels. Interestingly, this result is consistent with the results of a similar intervention among men in Olso, Norway, who were smokers with elevated cholesterol levels. The Olso trial showed a significant decline in the incidence of myocardial infarction and sudden death (Hjermann et al. 1981).

Those who designed the MRFIT considered three explanations for the failure to find the expected mortality reduction.

1. The intervention program was without benefit relative to the control group, either because no true benefit existed or because the control group also benefited. For example, the control group and their physicians may have been sensitized to cardiovascular disease and to their high level of risk and therefore altered their behavior (Lundberg 1982). This argument, however, seems inconsistent with the greater reduction in risk factors in the treatment group.

2. There was a favorable effect on mortality, but for statistical reasons

it was not detected. Given the large confidence intervals mentioned above, this explanation seems plausible, although it was not the explanation favored by the designers of the trial.

3. The designers argue that a favorable effect occurred in certain subgroups but that it was offset by unfavorable effects in other subgroups. In particular, they point to the unfavorable effects in men who were hypertensive and exhibited abnormal electrocardiograms at entry. The designers mention the possibility that the drugs used to treat the hypertension of these men raised cardiovascular mortality; no theoretical reason is presented, however, as to why this might have happened. In light of the Hypertension Detection and Follow-up Program result and the relatively large confidence intervals associated with the MRFIT results (the unfavorable effects are not significant at the 5 percent level even without adjusting for the multiple comparisons being made), it seems plausible that the adverse effects occurred by chance.

The investigators in the Oslo study mentioned earlier subsequently commented on the MRFIT (Olso Study Research Group 1983). They focused on the differences in the two studies rather than on the similarities. They believe one reason the Olso trial experienced different results was that one person directed it, whereas the MRFIT involved twenty-eight institutions with 250 investigators. Also, they imply that the effect of the MRFIT treatment may have been weakened by a lack of standardization. This argument does not seem consistent with the similar reduction in risk factors in the two trials among those who smoked and had elevated cholesterol levels.

Stanford Three-Community Study

The Stanford experiment was conducted in the early 1970s in three California communities of fifteen thousand each. In two of the communities, experimental efforts were mounted to decrease the levels of cardiovascular risk factors; the third community served as a control. In both experimental communities, health education campaigns involved direct mailings, newspaper columns, billboards, and public service announcements on radio and television. Additionally, in one of the communities a program of small-group instruction on risk-factor reduction was implemented among two-thirds of those in the upper quartile of cardiovascular risk (Maccoby et al. 1977; Stern et al. 1976; Farquhar et al. 1977; Fortmann et al. 1982). The campaign continued for about two-and-one-half years. The study sample included men and women between the ages of thirty-five and fifty-nine; about four hundred subjects completed the study in each site.

The effort appeared effective. Both the mass media campaign and personal counseling led to lower dietary cholesterol and daily consumption of saturated fat (a 20 to 40 percent reduction) among the men and women studied. Knowledge of risk factors also increased. Among those with small-group counseling, a decrease in the number of cigarettes smoked was evident. The favorable effects found for smoking and cholesterol are consistent with those found in the MRFIT; the Stanford study is novel in its effective mounting of a public education campaign.

Generalizations Based on Prior Social Experiments in Health

What conclusions about social experiments in health can be drawn from these studies?

1. A randomized study sometimes produces a different conclusion than a nonrandomized study. Examples include the effects of more complete insurance coverage of outpatient medical services as well as the school-based preventive dental programs described above. When the findings of randomized and nonrandomized studies conflict, the randomized study tends to be believed. Hence, a randomized study is preferable, provided it is feasible.

One objection to a randomized study is its cost, but the cost of randomization per se is often not very great; rather, large costs tend to be associated with primary data collection efforts whether they are observational studies or randomized trials.

2. Interventions in health should be evaluated using health outcome measures. A number of early studies simply measure cost or utilization (e.g., the Kansas study or the Colorado mental health study), but most of the studies reviewed above mea-

sured outcomes. Ten years ago it might have been possible to argue that measurement of health outcomes was too difficult and expensive. Relatively inexpensive, reliable measures of health outcomes have now been developed, however. At this time there is little excuse for not measuring both the cost and health status consequences of interventions in medical care delivery or health policy.

One aspect of health that is still relatively expensive to measure is physiologic outcomes such as blood pressure. Nonetheless, many such measures can be gathered at a screening examination center, and their collection does not require a physician. Such physiologic measures showed effects of variation in medical care use in the Health Insurance Experiment, whereas more general measures did not (Brook et al. 1983). Because much medical intervention is directed at altering such measures, their collection as part of an outcome evaluation is highly desirable.

3. If a behavioral intervention is being evaluated, care must be taken to inform the consumers about the intervention. In both the Kansas and the Colorado experiments, surveys of participant knowledge of the intervention showed a surprisingly high level of ignorance. As noted earlier, in the Kansas experiment fewer than half the participants showed an awareness of their experimental benefits; in the Colorado experiment fewer than 1 percent were aware of their benefits. Thus, in both of these trials the results might have been different if participant knowledge had been greater, as might have been the

case in a program of indefinite length. Indeed, the results from the Health Insurance Study, where knowledge was much greater, suggest that the quantitative effects observed in both the Kansas and Colorado studies would have been much greater with greater knowledge.

4. The experimenter must maintain close control over the treatment administered. Clearly any variation in treatment across subjects will obscure the results; some argue that this occurred in the MRFIT study (Oslo Study Research Group 1983). Brown (1984) and Archibald and Newhouse (1980) discuss management of social experiments in some detail.

5. The number of observed events may fall short of the number expected when sample size is determined. In the MRFIT a society-wide decline in mortality from coronary heart disease occurred; in the Preventive Dentistry Project a society-wide decline in tooth decay occurred during the lifetime of the projects. Such declines appear to have adversely affected the precision of inferences drawn at the conclusion of the MRFIT study. One should not only routinely calculate power (i.e., expected precision) when determining sample size for an experiment, one should also consider a safety factor when determining sample size.

6. A randomized controlled trial is no guarantor of truth. By definition, some percentage of the time (e.g., 5 percent) one will draw an inference of an association when there is none. Depending on power, there may be a considerably greater chance of drawing an inference of no association when there is an association (or even an inference of a negative effect when there is a positive one). On the basis of their results, the designers of the MRFIT suggested that antihypertensive drugs may be harmful to certain individuals (especially those with a cardiac abnormality). The drugs may indeed be harmful. But the outcome of the MRFIT that hints at such an effect may simply be attributable to chance.

When Not To Conduct an Experiment

Experiments conducted using households or individuals as units of observation are almost always feasible technically. The experiments described above were of this type, although in some of them the generalizations one seeks to draw are hazardous. For example, the Stanford Three-Communities Study showed that a mass media campaign was effective in two towns of fifteen thousand. Would it be effective in towns of a million or more? The Health Insurance Study showed that one HMO reduced expenditure 28 percent. Would other HMOs behave similarly?

Two straightforward issues that militate against an experiment using households or individuals may arise: (1) the value of the knowledge to be gained may not be worth the costs of generating it; (2) ethical considerations may preclude an experiment.

If the unit of observation is not an individual or household but a large collection of individuals, both experiments and nonrandomized studies tend to become less conclusive. Consider, for example, a hypothetical experiment to determine the competitive effects of health maintenance organizations. In this case, the unit of observation would be a local health care market; one wants to know if communities with a high market penetration of HMOs have lower costs or lower rates of increase in costs than communities with little or no HMO market penetration. An observational study faces the problem that communities with a high natural penetration of HMOs may be different in other, unmeasured respects from communities with low natural penetration. An experiment, however, would have to start HMOs. The resulting difficulty would seem to preclude a genuine experiment of this type.

Advice for Those Contemplating an Experiment

Several principles useful in designing and operating a successful experiment can be enumerated. More advice of this nature and more detail can be found in Archibald and Newhouse (1980) and Brown (1984).

1. A major concern of most individuals who appraise an experiment will be whether refusals to participate or attrition from the experiment have biased the results. Refusals to participate can be random, in which case there is no problem. If they are nonrandom, but similarly nonrandom between experimental and control groups (or among experimental groups), one cannot generalize to the entire population without adjusting for the nonrandom nature of the refusal; that may be difficult to do with any confidence. If the refusal rate is relatively small, however, failure to adjust for refusal is unlikely to cause a problem. The most serious problem is nonrandom refusal that affects different groups differently. For example, if sick individuals elect not to participate in the experimental group but are happy to participate in the control group, the groups will not be comparable. Similar comments apply to attrition from the experiment.

In many clinical experiments, the participant is blind to treatment. In that case, the alternative treatments (including control group status) can be explained to the participant, and his or her consent can be obtained to be randomized to one treatment. If the participant is blind to treatment, any further refusal should be both small and random. Hence, the treatment and control groups will be comparable. In most social experiments it will be difficult or impossible to keep the participant blind to treatment. (For example, if one is changing the individual's insurance plan, not only must the individual know the plan, but the experimenter wants the individual to know the plan.) Hence, if one follows the clinical method of randomizing after obtaining consent, one runs the risk that a participant states that he will participate in order to see the results of the randomization; then if he is randomized to a treatment he does not like, he withdraws, and conversely. Because withdrawal must always be an option for ethical reasons, nothing can be gained by following the clinical model of enrollment prior to randomization. Indeed, there is a reason not to do so —explaining all the alternative treatments may confuse the individual and will certainly take the individual's time and the experimenter's effort.

The major control of refusal and attrition must be in the design of the treatment; that is, individuals must want to enroll and to continue to participate in the experiment. An obvious incentive is money, though one need not always use money; for example, the Colorado experiment offered an improved insurance benefit. If money is used, minimization of attrition may require that at least part of the money be paid for completing the experiment. Thus, never during the life of the experiment is there a financial inducement to withdraw.

2. Adequate time must be allowed in the design of the experiment to produce an acceptable design. At the beginning of the experiment there is likely to be a great deal of pressure to get the experiment underway. The sooner it is underway, the sooner there will be results, and the designer of an experiment may consequently feel pressure to commit to a quite optimistic schedule. These pressures should be resisted. Failure in the design stage will guarantee failure in the analytical stage. The need for careful design of the experiment to minimize refusal and attrition was just noted, but numerous other features of the design must be fleshed out at the beginning of the project. Moreover, any new instrumentation

(e.g., questionnaires) must be developed at this time. There is a heavy penalty to changing instrumentation midway through the project. Suppose, for example, that because of haste in fielding the experiment a very sketchy measure of mental health is used. Later the mistake is realized. The designer now faces an unappetizing choice of either keeping the flawed instrument or redesigning it. If the designer opts for the latter course, the end-of-the-experiment measures of mental health will differ from the initial measures. This is a minor analytical problem as well as a data management problem. In a large-scale experiment the data management problem can become critical if measures are redesigned more than once or if many measures are redesigned.

The early stages should allow time for a pretest or pilot sample. Usually an experiment is trying to do something not done before; it is unlikely that a designer will anticipate all the problems that will arise. If an unanticipated problem does arise, the designer faces an even worse choice than in the case of a flawed interview instrument—a choice between going forward with a flawed experiment or throwing out all that has happened and beginning again.

3. One should consider splitting the sample if a measurement technique is thought to affect behavior. One issue raised about many experiments is whether participants (and sometimes those who implement the treatment) behaved as they would if the program were of indefinite length. (Sometimes this is referred to as a Hawthorne effect.) Creation of subsamples that do not receive certain

instrumentation can lay the ground-work for assessing the magnitude of such effects.

One design that can sometimes be implemented is the following: There is a series of treatment groups, a control group, and a control-on-control group. The control group receives all the instrumentation that the treatment group does, and a comparison of the treatment group with the control group thus reveals the effects of the treatment. The control-on-control group receives as little instrumentation as possible; thus, a comparison of the control group with the control-on-control group reveals the effect of the instrumentation. Administrative records or medical charts that show behavior of individuals who are not enrolled are an ideal source of data for a control-on-control group, provided such records exist.

4. Contrary to the impression one might receive from textbooks, the designer should probably not attempt to eliminate bias. Eliminating bias has costs. With a constrained budget for the experiment, the last few dollars spent eliminating bias may be better spent in other ways, such as procuring additional respondents.

An example arises in sampling. Suppose that households living in a random sample of dwelling units are selected for a baseline interview and that some of them are subsequently chosen for participation in the experiment. But after the baseline interview some households selected for enrollment move to another city. Maintenance of an unbiased sampling frame would require following those households. An alternative rule is to substitute the household now residing at the dwelling unit. In practice, this method may introduce some bias; nonetheless, it is probably better to accept the bias and not incur the costs of pursuing the households that moved.

5. Making the distribution of characteristics of households or persons on one treatment similar to that of another is usually a good idea. A device for doing this is now available, the Finite Selection Model (Morris 1979).

6. Do not strongly oversample a group whose membership is not well defined. Many experiments may be differentially interested in certain groups, such as sick individuals who are poor. The textbook advice in such instances is to oversample cases. If the members of the favored group do not change status over time (e.g., individuals who have lost a limb), the textbook advice is correct. If they do change status (e.g., individuals with low incomes at one point in time may not have low incomes later), the experimenter can actually lose by trying to oversample the group he or she is most interested in (Morris, Newhouse, and Archibald 1979). That is, the precision with which the response of even the favored group can be determined may be reduced by oversampling. Departures from proportional sampling should thus be undertaken cautiously.

Concluding Comment

Both the technology of social experimentation and the scope with which it is being applied in health made large strides during the 1970s. The past five years, however, have seen something of a retrenchment; in particular, the very large scale experiments of the 1970s are less numerous.

Nonetheless, the experimental technique has certainly demonstrated its value, and its basic principles, especially randomization or a variant of it, seem likely to become ever more widespread.

References

Archibald, R., and J. P. Newhouse. 1980. *Social experimentation: Some whys and hows.* Publication No. R-2479-HEW. Santa Monica, Calif.: Rand Corporation.

Bell, R. M., S. P. Klein, H. M. Bohannan, J. A. Disney, R. C. Graves, and R. Madison. 1984. *Treatment effects in the National Preventive Dentistry Demonstration Program.* Publication No. R-3072-RWJ. Santa Monica, Calif.: Rand Corporation.

Brook, R. B., J. E. Ware, Jr., W. H. Rogers, E. B. Keeler, A. R. Davies, C. A. Donald, G. A. Goldberg, K. N. Lohr, P. C. Masthay, and J. P. Newhouse. 1983. Does free care improve adults' health? Results from a randomized controlled trial. *New England Journal of Medicine* 309: 1426–1434.

Brown, M. 1984. *Lessons learned from the administration of the Rand Health Insurance Experiment.* Publication No. R-3095-HHS. Santa Monica, Calif.: Rand Corporation.

Farquhar, J. W., N. Maccoby, P. D. Wood, J. K. Alexander, H. Breitrose, B. W. Brown, Jr., W. L. Haskell, A. L. McAlister, A. J. Meyer, J. D. Nash, M. P. Stern. 1977. Community education for cardiovascular health. *Lancet* 1:1192–1195.

Foch, C. B., S. P. Klein, H. M. Bohannan, P. E. Anderson, F. H. Leone, J. A. Disney, and M. Oshiro. 1984. *Cost of treatment procedures in the national preventive dentistry demonstration program.* Publication No. R-3034-RWJ. Santa Monica, Calif.: Rand Corporation.

Fortmann, S. P., P. T. Williams, S. B. Hulley, N. Maccoby, and J. W. Farquhar. 1982. Does dietary health education reach only the privileged? The Stanford three community study. *Circulation* 66: 77–82.

Fuchs, V. R. 1976. The earnings of allied health personnel: Are health workers underpaid? *Explorations in Economic Research* 3:414.

Greer, D. S., and V. Mor. 1984. *A preliminary report of the national hospice study.* U. S. Department of Health and Human Services, Health Care Financing Administration, Office of Research and Demonstrations. Working Paper Series No. 84–5. Washington, D.C.: Government Printing Office.

Greer, D. S., V. Mor, J. N. Morris, S. Sherwood, D. Kidder, and H. Birnbaum. In press. An alternative in terminal care: Results of the National Hospice Study. *Journal of Chronic Diseases.*

Health Care Financing Administration. 1981. *Evaluation of the Colorado clinical psychology/expanded mental health benefits experiment: Executive summary.* HCFA Publication No. 03130. Baltimore, Md.

Helms, L. J., J. P. Newhouse, and C. E. Phelps. 1978. Copayments and demand for medical care: The California Medicaid experience. *Bell Journal of Economics* 9:192–208.

Hill, D. B., and J. E. Veney. 1970. Kansas Blue Cross/Blue Shield outpatient benefits experiment. *Medical Care* 8:143–158.

Hjermann, I., K. Velve Byre, I. Holme, and P. Leren. 1981. Effect of diet and smoking intervention on the incidence of coronary heart disease. *Lancet* 2:1303–1310.

Hustead, E. C., and S. S. Sharfstein. 1978. Utilization and cost of mental illness coverage in the Federal Employees Health Benefits Program, 1973. *American Journal of Psychiatry* 135:315–319.

Hypertension Detection and Follow-up Program Cooperative Group. 1976. The hypertension and follow-up program. *Preventive Medicine* 5: 207–215.

———. 1977. Blood pressure studies in 14 communities. *Journal of the American Medical Association* 237:2385–2391.

———. 1979a. Five year findings of the Hypertension Detection and Follow-up Program, 1: Reduction in mortality of persons with high blood pressure, including mild hypertension. *Journal of the American Medical Association* 242:2562–2571.

———. 1979b. Five year findings of the hypertension detection and follow-up program, 2: Mortality by race-sex and age. *Journal of the American Medical Association* 242:2572–2577.

———. 1982. Five year findings of the Hypertension Detection and Follow-up Program, 3: Reduction in stroke incidence among persons with high blood pressure. *Journal of the American Medical Association* 247:633–638.

Kane, R. L., J. Wales, L. Bernstein, A. Leibowitz, and S. Kaplan. 1984. A randomized controlled trial of hospice care. *Lancet* 1:890–894.

Lewis, C. E., and H. W. Keairnes. 1970. Controlling costs of medical care by expanding insurance coverage: Study of a paradox. *New England Journal of Medicine* 282:1405–1412.

Lundberg, G. D. 1982. MRFIT and the goals of the journal. *Journal of the American Medical Association* 248:1501.

Maccoby, N., J. W. Farquhar, P. W. Wood, and J. Alexander. 1977. Reducing the risk of cardiovascular disease: Effects of a community-based campaign on knowledge and behavior. *Journal of Community Health* 5:100–114.

McGuire, T. G. 1981. *Financing psychotherapy: Costs, effects, and public policy.* Cambridge, Mass.: Ballinger.

Manning, W. G., A. Leibowitz, G. A. Goldberg, and J. P. Newhouse. 1984. A controlled trial of the effect of a prepaid group practice on use of services. *New England Journal of Medicine* 310:1505–1510.

Manning, W. G., K. B. Wells, N. Duan, J. P. Newhouse, and J. E. Ware, Jr. 1984. Cost sharing and the use of ambulatory mental health services. *American Psychologist* 39:1077–1089.

Morris, C. 1979. A finite selection model for experimental design of the Health Insurance Study. *Journal of Econometrics* 11:43–61.

Morris, C., J. P. Newhouse, and R. Archibald. 1979. On the theory and practice of obtaining unbiased and efficient samples in social surveys and experiments. In *Experimental Economics*, ed. V. Smith, vol. 1. Westport, Conn.: JAI Press.

Multiple Risk Factor Intervention Trial Research Group. 1976. Multiple Risk Factor Intervention Trial: A national study of primary prevention of coronary heart disease. *Journal of the American Medical Association* 235: 825–827.

———. 1982. Multiple Risk Factor Intervention Trial: Risk factor changes and mortality results. *Journal of the American Medical Association* 248:1465–1477.

Newhouse, J. P., W. G. Manning, C. N. Morris, L. L. Orr, N. Duan, E. B. Keeler, A. Leibowitz, K. H. Marquis, M. S. Marquis, C. E. Phelps, and R. H. Brook. 1981. Some interim results from a controlled trial of cost sharing in health insurance. *New England Journal of Medicine* 305:1501–1507.

Olso Study Research Group. 1983. MRFIT and the Olso study. *Journal of the American Medical Association* 249:893–894.

Reed, L. S. 1975. *Coverage and utilization of care for mental health conditions under health insurance: Various studies.* Washington, D.C.: American Psychiatric Association.

Reed, L. S., E. Myers, and P. Scheidemandel. 1972. *Health insurance and psychiatric care: Utilization and cost.* Washington, D.C.: American Psychiatric Association.

Robert Wood Johnson Foundation. 1983. *Special report: National preventive dentistry demonstration program.* Princeton: Robert Wood Johnson Foundation.

Roemer, M. I., C. E. Hopkins, L. Carr, and F. Gartside. 1975. Copayments for ambulatory care: Penny-wise and pound-foolish. *Medical Care* 13:457–476.

Sackett, D. L., W. O. Spitzer, M. Gent, and R. S. Roberts. 1974. The Burlington randomized trial of the nurse practitioner: Health outcomes of patients. *Annals of Internal Medicine* 80:137–142.

Spitzer, W. O., D. L. Sackett, J. C. Sibley, R. S. Roberts, M. Gent, D. J. Kergin, B. C. Hackett, and A. Olynich. 1974. The Burlington randomized trial of the nurse practitioner. *The New England Journal of Medicine* 290:251–256.

Stern, M. P., J. W. Farquhar, N. Maccoby, and S. H. Russell. 1976. Results of a two-year health education campaign on dietary behavior: The Stanford three community study. *Circulation* 54:826–833.

Part III

Health and Illness over the Life Cycle

Chapter 13

The Management of Reproduction
Social Construction of Risk and Responsibility

Catherine Kohler Riessman and Constance A. Nathanson

I n years past in our society, and still in many parts of the world today, the conscious "management" of reproduction would have been perceived as a contradiction in terms. All societies, of course, have social norms that specify the timing of reproductive events in the life cycle, the circumstances under which these events are to occur, and the rituals that will surround them. Nevertheless, for much of history the conceiving and bearing of children have been culturally defined as "acts of God," or the inevitable consequences of sexual intercourse, with which humans interfered at their peril. The incentives for childbearing and the social structural arrangements within which birth and child rearing occur have been "built in" to each society; rarely were they questioned.

Today, in the United States, almost every aspect of these arrangements is being subjected to intense scrutiny; this change in orientation had its beginnings in the nineteenth century and has recently escalated to almost a fever pitch. What accounts for the emergence of reproduction as a "social problem" and for the remarkable societal concern with how this problem is, or should be, managed?

Reproductive processes have lost their "taken-for-granted" status as part of a complex and interrelated set of demographic and social changes occurring over the past 150 years. Although we cannot specify precise causal relationships, a brief review of these changes will place the issue of reproductive management in its proper historical context.

The first set of factors is demographic. With the exception of the 1950s baby boom the birthrate in the United States has been declining steadily for the past 150 to 200 years (Ryder 1980). Although the point is controversial (see, e.g., Easterlin 1980), the consensus of scholarly opinion holds that the "baby boom" was a historically unique phenomenon; the long-term trend in U.S. fertility is downward (Westoff 1978; Cherlin 1981). This conclusion is supported by data on women's expectations for their future family size; if women born in the 1950s have the number of children they expect, average family size will decline to about two children (U.S. Department of Commerce, Bureau of the Census 1983).

Within this overall context of decreasing birth rates, two recent changes in fertility patterns are particularly important to our argument: first, the delay of childbearing *within* marriage and, second, adolescents' increased fertility *outside* of marriage. The recent rise in age at marriage and decline in first birth rates within marriage represent a return to the family formation patterns of earlier cohorts rather than a new demographic phenomenon (Thornton and Freedman 1983). Nevertheless, changes in the social context of childbearing (to be more fully described later) have led to

predictions that as many as 30 percent of U.S. women now of childbearing age will remain childless (Westoff 1978; Bloom 1982) and that the remainder will have very small families. At the same time that married women are delaying reproduction or foregoing it altogether, increasing rates of sexual activity, pregnancy, and birth have been documented among unmarried teenage women (Zelnik and Kantner 1980). These latter changes, together with marked increases in single parenthood (the outcome of high divorce rates as well as of births outside of marriage) and in "living together" without marriage have contributed heavily to public perception of reproductive processes as "problematic."

Social structural changes provide a second, and closely related, set of conditions behind the increasing concern with the management of reproduction. These include both the actual changes that have occurred in women's roles (principally, increased participation in explicitly "nonreproductive" work outside the home) and the social movements that have been fueled by these changes and have drawn public attention to their implications for the future of the family. The facts of married women's employment are familiar: in 1982 over half of all married women, including 49 percent of mothers of preschool children, held paid jobs outside the home. Even more impressive are recent marked changes in sex role attitudes (Cherlin 1981; Thornton, Alwin, and Camburn 1983). Women are increasingly prepared not only to engage in paid work but to assert the legitimacy of their extrafamilial roles. The rise of the women's movement in the 1960s and subsequent controversies over abortion and the Equal Rights Amendment have meant that these changes at the statistical level have become the subject of intense debate at the public-policy level, thereby adding further to public consciousness of reproduction as a "problematic" issue.

Finally, technological developments yield a third set of factors. Reproduction is problematic because of the widespread availability and employment of effective means for the control of reproductive processes. The term *control* is used advisedly to refer not only to the prevention of births through contraception, abortion, or sterilization but also to birth selection by amniocentesis and abortion, to manipulation of conception using a variety of artificial fertilization techniques, and to the potential that exists for intervention in almost all aspects of childbirth itself. The technological revolution in reproductive management has created both the possibility and the pressure for a vast expansion in the scope of reproductive choice.

The changes that have been described create a set of conditions in which the "naturalness" and "inevitability" of reproductive processes— conception, pregnancy, and birth— are no longer taken for granted. Most obviously, women's commitment to the traditional feminine role— motherhood and sex in the service of motherhood—has been called into question. But even when motherhood is accepted, movements to change the conditions of childbirth, as well as widespread experimentation (not all

of it voluntary, of course) with unconventional family forms, raise doubts about the strength of social commitment to the structural arrangements within which reproductive processes have traditionally occurred. Finally, at the very same time that the survival of the family is being questioned, declining numbers of births to each couple, together with an enormous expansion in both the ability and the will to control all aspects of conception, pregnancy, and birth, have led to a vast increase in the personal and social significance of individual reproductive events.

Against this background of increasing individual and social concern with reproduction, certain issues in reproductive management have emerged as distinctively "public" problems, in Gusfield's (1981) sense of problems that become matters for "conflict and controversy in the arena of public action." Our purpose in this chapter is to demonstrate how the ways in which these problems are socially constructed influence and constrain the public policy options offered for their "solution." We will do this through the detailed examination of two specific issues: the management of teenage pregnancy and the management of childbirth.

We selected these two issues for closer examination for several reasons. Most obvious, there is considerable controversy around both teenage pregnancy and childbirth, in contrast to other areas of women's health that are not considered "problematic" at the present time (such as married women's contraceptive use). The examples also illuminate the contrasting ways in which social control operates in the daily practice of medicine. The first example—teenage pregnancy—illustrates how moral values influence the general approach taken to the problem as well as the specific response of nurses to it. The second example—childbirth— highlights how medical technology and physicians' professional power combine to limit the options available for managing birth. Both examples reveal how social and value choices are embedded in the practice of medicine and nursing.

We approach teenage pregnancy and childbirth within the framework proposed by Gusfield (1981). As he observes, neither "problems" nor their "solutions" are inherent in particular objective conditions. There are multiple ways of defining the "reality" of a problem and, consequently, multiple possibilities of resolution; however, how a problem is perceived largely determines what strategies for resolution are adopted. Furthermore, and perhaps of most importance, adoption of a particular "way of seeing" may foreclose alternative perspectives and alternative managerial options. This "homogenous consciousness" is, as Gusfield notes, a powerful form of social control; unlike more overt conflicts of power, "it goes unrecognized. What we cannot imagine, we cannot desire" (1981,7).

less by the practice itself than by the visibility of its consequences in the form of pregnancy and (particularly out-of-wedlock) birth. It is these consequences that are problematic, given the well-established relationship between poverty and single-headed households. More to the point of this chapter, however, teenage pregnancy and birth call public attention to widespread normative violations and raise questions about the effectiveness of traditional means of social control of sexuality.

In this section, we will show how successive redefinitions of the problem of teenage pregnancy have taken place since the 1960s, and further, how these redefinitions reflect deep ambivalence about adolescent sexuality. Instead of focusing on the social consequences of teenage childbearing, as many other investigators have done (see Furstenberg and Brooks-Gunn in this volume), our focus will be on the ways in which moral issues are embedded in health policies in general and in provider practices in particular. It will be argued that American social values about sex find expression in the medical strategies that have been selected to control the problem of adolescent fertility. We will pay special attention to how public health nurses attempt to reconcile the moral and the medical in their work.

Teenage Women and Birth Control

Historically, societal concern with adolescent sexuality has been aroused

Defining the Problem

In the United States, "adolescent sexuality and its consequences burst upon the consciousness of federal administrators in the 1970's" (Steiner

1981). Specifically, in 1972 Congress amended the Social Security Act to single out "sexually active minors" as a category of clients for whom federally funded agencies were specifically required to provide birth control services. This occurred despite the fact that during the decade from 1960 to 1970, the rate of adolescent childbearing actually declined (Vinovskis 1981). The upsurge of concern can best be understood in the light of changes in the demographic and social patterns of fertility among teenagers.

Among changes noted by Furstenberg, Lincoln, and Menken (1981) are the following: (1) a near doubling in the birthrate to unmarried teenagers (from 12.6 to 22.4 per 1,000) between 1950 and 1970, resulting primarily from sharp increases in out-of-wedlock births to white girls; (2) a decrease in the number of conceptions legitimized by marriage; (3) an increase in the proportion of pregnant young women who remained in school. Prior to the 1970s "illegitimacy" was seen as largely a problem of low-income blacks (Ryan 1976); out-of-wedlock pregnancy among white teenagers was "managed" by adoption, abortion, or marriage. Once these mechanisms went out of fashion or, as in the case of abortion, became all-too-publicly fashionable, the universality of adolescent sexuality could no longer be concealed. Adding to their impact, these changes in adolescent fertility behavior took place in the context of, first, a sharp rise in the sheer number of adolescents at risk of pregnancy as baby boom babies reached the teen years and, second, a marked decline in the fertility of older, married women. As a proportion of total births, births to adolescents peaked in 1975 (approximately eighteen years after the crest of the baby boom) and have now begun to decline toward their 1960 level. In sum, the greater visibility of the deviant behavior and its changing social distribution, rather than an increase in frequency, led to the designation of teenage pregnancy as a social problem.

In Gusfield's (1981) sense, the allocation of federal funds to solve the problem marked the "coming of age" of adolescent out-of-wedlock pregnancy as a public problem, with agencies—such as federally funded family planning clinics, the federal Office of Adolescent Pregnancy Programs—officially dedicated to working for its solution. In the initial stages of its development as a public problem, the "solution" to adolescent pregnancy adopted by the federal government was to increase adolescent women's access to birth control methods, as reflected in the 1971 legislation. In adopting this approach, the government was, at least by implication, throwing its weight behind a conception of adolescent pregnancy as a "medical" problem and fixing responsibility upon the medical profession to find a solution to it. However, it is also important to note that the government's initial response to adolescent pregnancy—to medicalize it—did not remain uncontested for long. By "making manifest" the politics of this issue (cf. Gusfield 1981,13) and the terms of the debate that have ensued, we can see some of the major dilemmas inherent in the medical management of a social problem.

In an address to the National Association of Evangelicals on March 8, 1983, President Ronald Reagan made the following comments in reference to the federal government's recent unsuccessful attempt to require federal notification when contraceptives were prescribed to teenagers seventeen and under:

Girls termed "sexually active"— that has replaced the word "promiscuous"—are given [birth control drugs and devices by federally subsidized clinics] in order to prevent illegitimate birth or abortion. [In discussions of this issue] no one seems to mention morality as playing a part in the subject of sex. Is all of Judeo-Christian tradition wrong? Are we to believe that something so sacred can be looked upon as a purely physical thing with no potential for emotional and psychological harm? And isn't it the parents' right to give counsel and advice to keep their children from making mistakes that may affect their entire lives? (*New York Times*, March 9, 1983)

In these remarks, the lines of battle are clearly drawn. Reagan explicitly attempts to invoke an earlier definition of adolescent pregnancy as a moral rather than as a medical issue. Girls who have sexual intercourse outside of marriage are described in moral ("promiscuous") as opposed to clinical ("sexually active") terms; responsibility for control of their behavior is assigned to parents rather than to "federally subsidized clinics"; and the means of control suggested are "counsel and advice," not "birth control drugs and devices." One could hardly find a more telling illustration of Gusfield's thesis that "modes of conceiving of the reality of a phenomenon are closely related to the activities of resolution" (1981,6). However, in ironic testimony to the continuing power of the medical model, a major argument employed by the U.S. Department of Health and Human Services in defending its proposed parental notification rule was that it was necessary to protect the "health" of adolescents (U.S. Department of Health and Human Services 1983).

The Medical Solution

From the perspective of the helping professions, the central figure in the drama of adolescent fertility is the unwed teenage mother. "More to be pitied than censored," she is portrayed as the tragic victim not of a scheming man but of an insufficiently concerned and caring society (Alan Guttmacher Institute 1976, 1981). In recent years a substantial body of scholarly literature has been generated documenting adverse consequences of early childbearing for both mother and infant (Furstenberg, Lincoln, and Menken 1981). To policymakers, the plight of the teenager mother has been described in harrowing, and often highly personalized, terms (Bogue 1977; U.S. Congress, House of Representatives 1978).

However justified this portrait may be, it has clear, and often intended, implications for the management strategies that are proposed. Importantly, by selecting certain strategies, others are foreclosed. For example, by focusing our attention on the individual adolescent girl (not only verbally, but also pictorially, as in the well-illustrated publications of the Alan Guttmacher Institute), we are led to think that the problem is soluble by intervention at the individual level. Furthermore, it is the representation of adolescent childbearing as a "serious threat to the life and health of a young woman" (Bogue 1977, 2) that provides the principal rationale for specifically medical intervention: threats to life and health fall clearly within the medical domain. However, other approaches to adolescent out-of-wedlock fertility become possible if we broaden our perceptions and examine the full process from sex to motherhood.

Applying a scheme originally proposed by Davis and Blake (1956), Cutright (1971) defines four stages of unwed motherhood: the unmarried woman must have sexual relations; she must use ineffective or no contraception; failing to have either a spontaneous or induced abortion, she must carry a pregnancy to term; and she must not get married before the birth occurs. If the aim of social policy is to prevent unwed motherhood, then intervention at any one of these four stages would be equally effective. In other words, the alternative that is advocated at a particular time and place reflects prevailing institutional and value climates. For example, as a consequence of legal and social constraints, prevention at the level of stages two and three—contraception and abortion—did not become publicly discussed options in the United States until the 1970s. Although unwed motherhood gained recognition as a "social problem" during the 1960s, the problem was labeled by the deviant status of the child (illegitimacy) rather than by that of the mother (adolescent pregnancy) (Roberts 1966). Ameliorative efforts were directed by social workers, not physicians, and took the form of treatment as opposed to prevention: aiding the mother to care for her "illegitimate" child through programs such as AFDC or arranging for the child's placement with foster or adoptive parents.

In the early 1970s, the problem was redefined as one of pregnancy prevention through the correct application of medical technology (see, e.g., "Medical Services for Sexually Active Teenagers," an editorial in the *American Journal of Public Health*, April 1973). More recently, continued high rates of adolescent out-of-wedlock pregnancy, combined with an increasingly conservative value climate, have led some observers to question the effectiveness of the medical model and to advocate intervention at the very first stage, before sexual relations are initiated (U.S. Congress, House of Representatives 1984; Schwartz and Ford 1982). Proposals in this vein would take responsibility for control of adolescent fertility out of the hands of professionals altogether and assign this responsibility to the young woman's family.

The recent career of the medical model of adolescent pregnancy provides an almost classic example of a process described by Schneider and Conrad in which the failure of medical control of deviance to produce immediate and demonstrable results creates "currents toward demedicalization and either recriminalization or social disapproval" (1980, 42). To understand this development we must briefly review the history of the provision of "medical services for sexually active teenagers," so enthusiastically heralded by the *American Journal of Public Health.*

In the early 1970s, when "adolescent sexuality and its consequences" first entered the public arena, two major obstacles to a medical resolution of the problem were perceived: legal requirements for parental consent to the medical treatment of a minor under age eighteen and insufficient availability of "sex-related medical services" (Pilpel and Wechsler 1969; Cutright 1971; House 1973). Optimism was expressed in these early writings both that the characteristics of effective programs were known and that, once in place, they would be used, particularly with the aura of legitimacy provided by federal funding. Medical contraceptive methods backed up by legal abortion in case of contraceptive failure would substantially reduce unwed motherhood.

Over the suceeding decade (1970–1980) the major legal restrictions on "mature" minors' access to contraceptive and abortion services without parental consent virtually disappeared. Writing in 1980, Furstenberg, Lincoln, and Menken were able to state that "long a source of resistance to change, the legal system during the past decade has been a principal agent of it. . . . The rights of a mature minor . . . have been firmly established" (1981, 385). During the same time period, the federal government's constant dollar investment in family planning services increased by over tenfold, from $13.5 million in 1968 to an estimated $142 million in 1979 (Torres, Forrest, and Eisman 1981). The impact of this investment on the use of services by teenage women was considerable. Between 1970 and 1975, the number of fifteen- to nineteen-year-olds served annually by organized family planning programs was estimated to have increased from 300,000 to 1,175 million; the largest percentage increase occurred between 1970 and 1972 (Dryfoos and Heisler 1978). Recently, program participation has increased more slowly; the estimated number of teenagers served in 1979 was 1,478 million (Torres, Forrest, and Eisman 1981). An alternative way of evaluating program impact is in terms of the percentage of teenagers "at risk" of unwanted pregnancy who are receiving contraceptive services. Torres, Forrest, and Eisman (1981) estimate that, in 1979, 56 percent of young women at risk were "served," slightly more than half by organized clinics and the remainder by private physicians.

Thus, it is incontestable that the availability of medical contraceptive methods to teenage women increased over the decade of the 1970s; evidence from service statistics is supported by survey data showing increases in contraceptive use (Zelnick and Kantner 1980). Yet, during this same time period, contrary to the optimistic expectations with which the decade opened, the birthrate for unmarried women under twenty rose by 21 percent (Ventura 1984). In part, this increase is explained by the declining propensity to legitimize out-of-wedlock pregnancies by marriage; however, had it not been for the simultaneous increase in use of abortion (reaching 41 percent of teenage pregnancies in 1980), the birthrate would have been much higher. Thus, not only did increased contraceptive availability fail to reduce adolescent out-of-wedlock pregnancy, the pregnancy-coping strategies employed by adolescents had the effect of markedly increasing the visibility of their sexual behavior.

The reluctance of adolescent birth and pregnancy rates to behave as predicted by the medical model resulted in a shift in research priorities: from the effects of adolescent parenthood to the description and interpretation of adolescent sexual behavior and patterns of contraceptive use. The focus is still on the individual adolescent, but the question has become why does she not use contraception or why does she not use it effectively. The volume of literature generated by these questions is both large and inconclusive. (Work published through 1980 is reviewed in Chilman 1978, 1980; and in Nathanson and Becker 1983; examples of more recent studies are Zabin and Clark 1981, 1983; Furstenberg et al. 1983, 1984; Shea, Herceg-Baron, and Furstenberg 1984.) A wide range of sociodemographic, situational, and psychological predictors have been explored, and over time a considerable increase has occurred in methodological sophistication. Nevertheless, the amount of explained variation in adolescent contraceptive use remains disappointingly small. To cite one of the most recently published, and among the most careful, studies, "only 14 percent of the variance is explained by all 13 variables" examined; only four variables reached even the customary .05 level of significance (Furstenberg et al. 1983). The unpredictable quality of adolescent contraceptive behavior has made substantial inroads in the optimism of an earlier era: "Given the available techniques of contraception, we do not hold out any hope of perfect compliance, even with far more effective sex education and family planning programs than we currently have" (p. 217).

Although the argument for medical intervention to control adolescent fertility is couched almost entirely in terms of the hazards of adolescent child*bearing*, programs have concentrated on the far more difficult task of preventing pregnancy itself, thereby accommodating to normative and regulatory constraints on abortion. Adolescent women, confronted with the reality of an unplanned child, have increasingly chosen the easier route of abortion. They have resisted control by "approved" medical methods and have increasingly resorted to highly visible, "disapproved" medical methods. This shift has provided the entering wedge for groups and individuals wishing to challenge the medical model of adolescent fertility: "amply warned of the disastrous consequences of giving birth out of wedlock, and *accustomed to seeking medical solutions to their 'reproductive health' needs*, young people dutifully trooped off to the abortion clinics in ever-increasing numbers as the promise of contraceptive protection proved false for them, and they found themselves unintentionally pregnant" (Schwartz and Ford 1982, 155; emphasis ours).

These authors attribute increased adolescent sexual activity and the associated rise in "unintentional" pregnancy to the "approval of premarital intercourse," which they believe to be implicit in the very existence of birth control clinics. An equally critical, if more moderately worded, appraisal of the medical model was expressed by Rep. Thomas J. Bliley in opening hearings of the House Select Committee on Children, Youth, and Families, held in 1983: "we have been working under the assumption that increased use of medical methods of contraception must necessarily bring down the teen pregnancy rate.... Apparently, we were missing something ... it seems to be time to examine our assumptions, to examine the conventional mechanistic approach to pregnancy prevention" (U.S. Congress, House of Representatives 1984, 3). In these remarks, continued high rates of teenage pregnancy and birth are attributed to the failure of preventive strategies. We believe that the problem does not lie with these strategies themselves, but with how they are applied in a society that remains fundamentally ambivalent toward the sexual behavior of adolescents.

Provider Perspectives:
The Dilemma of
Social Control

Adolescent sexuality and out-of-wedlock fertility violate deeply held social norms concerning when and for whom these behaviors are appropriate. The apparent failure of the medical "solution" to decrease the visibility of adolescents' deviant behavior has created the conditions for these norms to resurface in a new and vigorous form. Yet as Schneider and Conrad point out, "deviance is a *social* construction. The nature of medical care, however, is *individual*-centered. If one sets out to 'cure' deviance—which is a social attribution—by individual-centered technologies, how can one expect success?" (1980, 43).

The dilemma of social control presented by adolescent out-of-wedlock pregnancy is reflected not only in pregnancy, birth, and abortion rates but also in the immediate experiences of service providers: physicians, nurses, and counselors with direct responsibility for carrying out the medical mandate. A small body of literature exists on the moral conflicts of abortion service workers, suggesting that complicity in normatively disapproved behavior can be a source of considerable strain, even when that behavior is ideologically or intellectually supported by providers as individuals (Such-Baer 1974; Joffe 1978, 1979; Nathanson and Becker 1977). No comparable work on family planning workers has as yet been published (but see Nathanson and Becker 1985). However, results from a recently completed study of county health department family planning clinics suggest that responsibility for teenage pregnancy and, in particular, the elusive quality of "success" in this endeavor, create profound dilemmas for physicians and nurses who provide contraceptive services for teenage women.

As background, health department

clinics provide about 25 percent of medical contraceptive services received by U.S. teenagers. From the present perspective the most important distinguishing features of the health department setting are its goals—teenagers are provided with preventive medical care at little or no cost—and its staffing patterns—the dominant professionals in this setting are nurses. Health departments, like hospitals and private physicians' offices, but unlike Planned Parenthood clinics, are fundamentally health care institutions. Expectations for behavior in these medical settings tend to be structured in terms of the traditional doctor-patient relationship: the client is exempted from responsibility for her condition and is, in turn, expected to trust the provider and to comply with his or her advice (Parsons 1951).

Interviews with health department family planning nurses reflect the problems they confront in applying this model in interaction with teenage contraceptive clients. Although it has been suggested by some advocates of birth control that, once initiated, sexual intercourse is addictive (see, e.g., Brozan 1982), thereby qualifying as behavior for which young women are not responsible, this classic justification for medical intervention is not widely accepted by the nurses studied. By background and orientation, these are women with highly traditional moral values; from their perspective, sexual intercourse is quintessentially behavior for which the individual is personally responsible. Thus, they find themselves in the uncomfortable position of being socially mandated to provide an essen-

tially medical, that is nonpunitive, service directed toward preventing young women from experiencing the consequences of what many nurses regard as irresponsible, if not immoral, behavior. Compounding nurses' dilemma is their limited ability to obtain compliance with their contraceptive instructions. As has been noted in other contexts (Zola 1972; Schneider and Conrad 1980), the further that medical behavioral control is extended outside the consulting room into the most intimate arenas of daily life, the more problematic effective control becomes. Thus, the role of the family planning nurse requires that she assist her client to avoid the consequences of "irresponsible" behavior under conditions where her real authority to influence that behavior is severely restricted.

Nurses' response to the dilemmas they confront is to structure their encounters with teenage clients to maximize the client's responsibility for the "outcome" of treatment and to minimize that of the provider. In the clinic setting, "virtue" has been redefined from chastity to contraceptive responsibility, that is, autonomous adherence to a set of detailed procedures for birth control use. Education and counseling sessions are the vehicles through which responsibility is taught; nurses frequently evaluate their own behavior on the basis of whether or not it fosters client "responsibility." By structuring contraceptive compliance in essentially moral terms, nurses attempt to extend their control of client behavior into the private settings where conception actually occurs. Furthermore, they do so in such a way that the burden of failure falls squarely on the client. The teenager who uses her method incorrectly and becomes pregnant as a result demonstrates a defect of character, not the imperfection of contraceptive methods or the inflexibility of clinic procedures.

The deflection of responsibility for failure away from the provider onto the client is supported by clinic ideology. *Responsibility* is defined not only as conformity to clinic procedures but also as autonomy. The ideal client is one who makes her decision to attend the clinic free of any external influence, makes an independent choice of contraceptive method, and does not blame the clinic when things go wrong. An ideology that defines client responsibility as an end in itself also absolves the provider of responsibility if the outcome is untoward.

The foregoing observations are, of course, based on data from only one among several types of settings where birth control services to teenagers are provided. Nevertheless, we would argue that issues surrounding the allocation of responsibility are generic not only to provider-client interaction in these settings but to interaction in other "reproductive management" settings as well (on abortion clinics, see, for example, Joffe 1978, 1979; on genetic counseling, Lippman-Hand and Fraser 1979a, 1979b; Kessler 1979). Medical providers of reproductive health care share the common problem of affecting behavior that takes place outside of their organizational domain and beyond the range of their surveillance. This same problem is present, although to a lesser extent, when providers try to change other "life-style" behaviors.

Both our own work and that of others suggest that this problem is resolved in two ways: first, by elevating the concept of "personal responsibility" into a moral imperative and, second, by structuring interaction with clients to inculcate a notion of responsibility that is consonant with provider values. The subsequent failure of clients to conform with those values may be imputed to defects of moral character or possibly to imperfect counseling procedures (Kessler 1979; Grobstein 1979), but seldom to the underlying premises on which interaction is based. Although moral judgments implicit in the notion of "noncompliance" with a medical regimen have been noted in the literature on medicalization (cf. Zola 1972), less well recognized is the extent to which attributions of client responsibility protect the provider under circumstances where "compliance" is, indeed, highly problematic.

Consequences of Medicalization for Control of Teenage Pregnancy

The most important consequence of medicalization is to locate both the origin and the treatment of the "teenage pregnancy problem" in the individual unmarried teenager—principally, the individual teenage woman. Thus, the contribution of larger social forces to the production of the problem tend to be overlooked. For example, recent research (Rothenberg and

Varga 1981; Zuckerman et al. 1983) indicates that the physical hazards of teenage childbearing are socially rather than biologically induced. In other words, age alone does not have an independent effect on fetal and maternal health. Rather, it is the environment in which teenage childbearing occurs that appears to cause adverse outcomes. Further, the problem itself may be misspecified with a focus on the unmarried status of the individual teenager. After a detailed literature review, Chilman (1980) concludes that the consequences of teenage motherhood "may be less severe if the young woman does *not* marry" (p. 75). Perhaps of most importance, an exclusive focus on the "willful" ("immature," "irresponsible") teenager as the obstacle to effective intervention acts to deflect attention from other possible loci of responsibility for continued high rates of teenage pregnancy and birth: the organizational structure of contraceptive services; the inadequacies of available contraceptive methods; the ambivalence of adult society (including the families of sexually active adolescents) toward teenage sex, contraception, and abortion; the circumstances under which teenagers have sex and use contraception; and the complex agendas of teenagers themselves.

In concluding this section, it may be useful to reemphasize that the "problem" of teenage pregnancy is itself a socially constructed category. We do not deny that having a child may have severe social and economic consequences for individual teenage women, in large part because of the paucity of social supports for mothering outside of traditional marital arrangements. Nevertheless, in this society, teenage pregnancy has been defined in such a way as to mitigate against either a wholehearted commitment to prevention or a wholehearted commitment to the economic and social support of the teenage unwed mother herself: social policies and practices directly reflect the deep ambivalence about adolescent sexuality that exists within the dominant culture. However, as the sheer numbers of teenage women "at risk" of pregnancy continue to decline, as sex prior to marriage is increasingly taken for granted (facilitating open discussion of contraception), as single parenthood becomes an increasingly "acceptable" option, and as abortion remains an available option, teenage pregnancy as a public problem may simply disappear, not because a "solution" has been found but because social change has caused this construction of the problem to become obsolete.

The next section of this chapter focuses on another facet of women's reproductive health: the management of childbirth. Like teenage pregnancy, it has been socially constructed in ways that dictate particular modes of management and foreclose others.

Childbirth: A Risky Business

A paradox exists in the management of childbirth in the United States today. In this century an unprecedented decline in deaths associated with birth has occurred. For example, in 1915 maternal mortality claimed sixty women out of every ten thousand live births; in 1980 the figure was less than one. In 1915 neonatal mortality occurred in forty-four out of every one thousand live births; in 1980 the figure was eight (Institute of Medicine 1982). In a word, maternal and infant death rates are at an all time low. With respect to the risk of death, birth is safer than it has ever been; paradoxically, however, the concept of risk in childbirth is expanding. (Let us not underestimate the problems in U.S. mortality levels: rates for blacks exceed rates for whites by a considerable margin, and the United States lags behind many other industrialized countries.)

A second and closely related trend in childbirth practice is greater use of medical technology, including the almost routine use of ultrasound, fetal monitoring, and surgical procedures. Although cesarean sections are not routine, they comprise 20 percent of all births nationally; rates in many hospitals are considerably higher (Taffel, Placek, and Moien 1985). Simply stated, American childbirth has become a technologically managed medical event. Birth technologies are used in the belief that they will improve further the health of mothers and infants. Paradoxically, however, history tells us that changes in the social environment, rather than specific medical measures, have been responsible in large part for declines in morbidity and mortality (Dubos 1959). To be sure, particular scientific discoveries—such as the adoption of sulfonamides and then the antibiotics—

were responsible in part for the decline in maternal deaths that occurred after 1935. Similarly, in the contemporary period, infant survival has improved as a result of neonatal intensive care. But for most of human history, "upstream" rather than "downstream" efforts—such as nutrition, housing, and general economic well-being—have led to dramatic improvements in the nation's health (McKinlay 1981). Why, then, is there such a strong emphasis on medical measures and the risk of childbirth? This section of the chapter will explore the reasons for this paradox.

Defining the Problem

In the medical literature on obstetrics, a new disease vocabulary is emerging. In this literature, there is no such thing as a "normal" birth, only a "low-risk" one. While medical science no longer defines pregnancy and birth as pathological events, as it did at the turn of the century (Kobrin 1966), the contemporary "solutions" to these problems still assume a disease orientation. Martin Stone (1979), a past president of the American College of Obstetrics and Gynecology (ACOG), has stated that "the trip through the birth canal is the most dangerous trip we will ever take with the greatest chance of our dying of any one day in our lives." The ACOG has made explicit its ambivalence about the normalcy of birth, stating that "labor and delivery, while a physiologic process, clearly presents potential hazards to both mother and fetus before and after birth" (ACOG 1975). Because of these hazards,

ACOG has taken a position against home births as well as against midwife-attended births unless supervised by physicians. According to this view, birth is a medical event that requires the attendance of physicians, the setting of a hospital, and the availability of the latest technology in order to be safe.

A few facts about adverse outcomes may be helpful in placing the issue of risk, and the use of medical technology to combat it, in its proper context. First, most infant deaths result from low birth weight (McCormick 1985), not from unanticipated emergencies in women delivering full term. In the event of signs of premature labor, referral to a hospital equipped with neonatal intensive care could be made by either obstetrician or midwife. Second, the risk of unexpected adverse outcomes is small for women giving birth at full term. Research suggests that out-of-hospital birth for these women is quite safe. In spite of this fact, however, beliefs about how birth should be handled have severely constrained good evaluation research on alternative birth settings and on different providers. Thus, research on safety and efficacy has been limited to descriptive studies and medical record reviews—research designs that do not take into account the characteristics of women seen in different birth settings. Although this method limits the generalizability of results, the findings suggest that out-of-hospital birth may, in fact, be less risky. For example, a descriptive study of a stratified sample of 1,938 women who began labor in eleven freestanding birth centers staffed by certified nurse-midwives found excellent maternal and fetal outcomes. In addition, 89 percent of the deliveries were spontaneous, only 4 percent were assisted by forceps, and only 5 percent ended in cesarean section at a back-up hospital (Bennetts and Lubic 1982). In another study of a center in Texas serving migrant Mexican American women, the prematurity rate was almost half the rate for the state as a whole (Murdaugh 1976). A medical record study comparing matched pairs of home births and hospital births found no significant differences in neonatal and fetal mortality. On a series of other indicators, hospital births were found to be more dangerous; these women had significantly higher rates of forceps deliveries, cesarean sections, and lacerations. Their infants were more likely to have birth injuries and respiratory distress syndrome (Mehl and Peterson 1976; Mehl et al. 1977). The Institute of Medicine of the National Academy of Sciences has called for rigorous research to promote informed debate and policy development on the safety and efficacy of various birth settings (Institute of Medicine 1982).

Yet in spite of these facts about safety, the problem of "risk" has emerged as the centerpiece in the debate about appropriate childbirth practice. We believe that this is because the concept of risk is essential to the maintance of an orientation to birth as a medical problem. Although concern about the relationship between safety and the qualifications of various birth attendants is not a new issue (see Williams 1912; Leavitt 1983; Drachman 1979), as sociologists we must account for the upsurge of concern rather than accept the notion that risk is in the nature of pregnancy and birth. From this standpoint, let us analyze the structure of the "risk problem," the reasons for this orientation, and the consequences of this "way of seeing" for health policy.

The Medical Solution

All would agree that a certain percentage of women are in genuine need of medical measures to assure a healthy mother and infant, although there is considerable disagreement about the size of this pool. According to conservative estimates, morbidity can be expected in mother or neonate in approximately 5 to 10 percent of cases (Apgar 1953; Wertz and Wertz 1979). Situations that, by their very nature, "cause" a risk include a pelvis too small to deliver through, an Rh factor, a premature labor, an excessively long labor, and so forth. The emergency nature of these atypical conditions generally emerges well in advance of the moment of birth, thus allowing for the orderly use of a hospital. What is significant, however, is the expanding nature of risk in both pregnancy and childbirth. As Rothman (1982) suggests, conditions that would have been considered normal or marginal in the past are now labeled "high risk."

Why is the average woman treated as if she had one of these unfortunate conditions? After all, there is a risk of death or maiming when we cross the street, a risk of choking when we swallow a piece of food, a risk of crib death in the first year of life. (In fact, sudden infant death syndrome is the leading cause of death for infants between one week and one year old.) Yet for none of these risks does public policy mandate hospitalization for the entire population who can potentially experience these calamities.

As in the case of teenage pregnancy, government played a role in structuring the problems in certain ways. The targeting of funds for "high-risk" populations forced upon the consciousness of physicians the notion of risk; they had to think about the complicating conditions of pregnancy in these terms. In the late 1960s and early 1970s, federal funds assisted the development and diffusion of a variety of risk-detecting technologies (such as fetal monitors and sonography) which were then recommended routinely for all pregnant women. Considerable effort went into the development of indexes to identify "high-risk" pregnancies through social area analysis of census tracts as well as through the analysis of individual characteristics of pregnant women themselves. (It is noteworthy that working-class women tend to score high on these various indexes; yet as Hurst and Summey (1984) point out, middle-class women actually receive more of the procedures, such as cesarean delivery, developed for "high-risk" pregnancies. This finding suggests that the use of medical technology hinges on a set of social, as opposed to scientific, factors—a point we will return to later. (See Guillemin 1981.)

In spite of the effort to develop a "science" of risk assessment, the prediction of complicating conditions of pregnancy for individual women remains remarkably poor. After reviewing the various measures for obstetrical risk assessment, a study committee of the Institute of Medicine noted a number of serious methodological problems. They concluded that although several of the research instruments may be of some use in large-scale evaluation studies of alternative birth settings, they are not appropriate for predicting risk for individuals. Instead, the committee recommended that "clinical judgment is appropriate in determining treatment for an individual woman," with objective assessment of risk only a "useful adjunct" (Institute of Medicine 1982, 52). Thus, subjective criteria ("clinical judgment") rather than reliance on objective scientific knowledge must guide physicians' assessments of their individual patients' chances for successfully completing a given pregnancy.

At the same time that physicians' training as medical scientists encourages them to rely on "objective facts," their orientation as clinicians leads them to use their subjective judgments and clinical experience in defining and interpreting risk for individual patients. Subjective judgments in medical decision-making give the practitioner a great deal of freedom in the interpretation of physical signs as indicators of risk, especially in situations that are ambiguous. The average patient, who has limited knowledge, cannot contest medical evaluations of her progress in labor (DeVries 1981). Too often, the language of science obscures these processes at work in medicine to both patient and practitioner. In the words

of Gusfield (1981, 20), the "facts" of childbirth risk "are picked out of a pile, scrubbed, polished, highlighted here and there, and offered as discoveries in the context of the particular and practical considerations of their finders."

Although not the focus of this chapter, alternative conceptions of the "reality" of the problem of childbirth risk do exist. Competing definitions have been put forward by governmental groups (U.S. Congress, House of Representatives 1980; U.S. Federal Trade Commission 1981), by professional associations (American Public Health Association 1983), and by individual physicians themselves ("Whose Baby Is It Anyway?" 1980; Duff 1980; Hamburg 1983). Certified nurse-midwives and lay midwives have different conceptions of the "reality" of childbirth risk—different both from each other and from the dominant medical perspective—and therefore have alternative "solutions" to the problem (Peterson 1983; Diers 1981; Rothman 1983). These practitioners emphasize the risks associated with the typical hospital birth: greater probability of induction of labor, overmedication, routine use of instruments and technologies, cesarean section, and separation of the family unit. Finally, pregnant women of different social classes have their own distinct perspectives on the "reality" of the risk problem (Graham and Oakley 1981; Nelson 1983; McClain 1983). The competing definitions have led to considerable ferment, particularly with the increasing number of freestanding birth centers established by nurse-midwives (see Riessman 1984). As competing "solutions" have become institutionalized, organized medicine has been united in defending its jurisdiction over birth against the encroachment of these alternative perspectives.

Determinants of the Dominant Perspective of the Problem

Despite the existence of competing "realities," and attendant differences in the definition of what constitutes risk, why has the problem of risk been constructed in the terms that it has —emphasizing the risk of non-physician-attended, nonhospital births? We shall suggest a set of interrelated factors that are shaping current discussions of risk. At the most basic level are economic and political considerations of physicians. Less obvious are cognitive and organizational factors embedded in the very culture of medicine itself. Finally, the medical industries and clients themselves have also played a role in constructing the risk problem.

While not necessarily a conscious motive, it is clear that the expansion of nurse-midwifery threatens obstetrician/gynecologists' economic control over the market, especially in light of a rising supply and a declining demand. The federal government estimates that the supply of obstetrician/gynecologists will increase from the 1970 figure of 9.3 per 100,000 population to 13.6 per 100,000 population in 1990 (U. S. Department of Health, Education, and Welfare 1974). At the same time, the population trends reviewed earlier suggest that the long-term trend in U.S. fertility is downward. Under these conditions, it makes sense to create demand with a rhetoric that emphasizes the hazards of childbearing.

Professional dominance (Freidson 1970) is also undermined by the expansion of nurse-midwifery, particularly when practiced outside of hospital settings. Physicians have gained autonomy over their work and thus freedom from control by others. As an effectively organized occupational group, they have established a strong labor market shelter (Freidson 1982). This shelter assures the profession an effective monopoly of opportunity over the performance of a particular set of tasks—performed under desirable conditions and on favorable terms. In order to maintain shelter in the labor market of healing, physicians need to control the supply of labor entering the market to perform this particular set of tasks as well as to control the substance of demand for what they supply. Such control presupposes "either a binding agreement by all potential consumers to use only members of the occupation for supplying a defined kind of labor" (Freidson 1982, 47) or legal sanctions that will make it difficult for consumers to use others to supply the service. Social claims about risk serve to remind consumers that they should rely only on bona fide members of the profession of medicine to manage their births.

Until recently, obstetricians' occupational success was evidenced by the state-sponsored, quasi monopoly they held over childbirth practice, except in medically underserved areas where nurse-midwives were allowed to practice. With the expansion of nurse-midwifery, especially in middle-class areas, this monopoly is breaking down. Under these conditions, efforts to move birth out of the organizational settings where physicians have their greatest authority will be resisted. Stated differently, professional dominance can be more easily assured in the hospital, where the physician is dominant in the division of labor, than in the home or freestanding birth center. In these latter settings, the balance of power will shift, and defining birth as a medical affair run by medical professionals will be less possible.

In addition to political/economic reasons, physicians want to preserve traditional practice structures for other reasons as well. Innovations that incorporate "nontraditional" approaches to women's health tend to be resisted by physicians, particularly in hospitals with strong obstetrical departments (Nathanson and Morlock 1980). Social innovations (such as having fathers involved in delivery) disrupt the organization of physicians' work. Customary work patterns would be altered even more extensively if physicians provided emotional support to the laboring woman in lieu of painkilling medications or if they taught the mother to give birth rather than "delivering" her. In contrast, seeing birth in terms of "risk" assures the preservation of work structures that maintain the traditional practice of medicine.

Finally, the construction of the risk problem can be understood in light of the cognitive orientations of physicians themselves. Doctors are trained to look for disease. Because they are overtrained for normal childbirth

cases, thinking in risk terms may be a way of making an interesting case out of one that is routine and perhaps boring. In addition, as Scheff (1966) has noted, physicians are more likely to err on the side of hypothesizing that disease is present when, in fact, it is absent (Type II error). As a consequence of this orientation, there is a bias toward action—intervention in the disease process. In obstetrics, this approach is best illustrated by the advice of Walter Channing, professor of obstetrics at Harvard in the midnineteenth century. An axiom of practice ever since, he stated that when called to attend laboring women, the doctor "must do something. He cannot remain a spectator merely" (as quoted in Leavitt 1983).

Professional socialization influences physicians' orientation to birth in other ways. Socialization occurs in hospitals—not in the home or the freestanding birth center—where physicians are trained in particular modes of thinking about human problems as well as in particular work structures. As Rosengren and De Vault (1963) found, the maintenance of a "correct tempo" is necessary for the smooth hospital management of birth. Thus, physicians are taught to rationalize, control, and make predictable what are inherently uncertain and unpredictable natural events, such as birth. They are taught to think about disease as a state within the individual body, for which there is a specific etiology and hence a specific cure (Mishler 1981). They are taught to think about the body as a machine—a set of parts subject to breakdown but also amenable to repair (Osherson and AmaraSingham

1981). They are taught a particular view of medical technology and are socialized to seek technical solutions to problems they encounter in patients. They are taught to think about physiological processes according to particular medical timetables (Roth 1963). These timetables, in turn, construct medical birth by dividing it into stages, each of which is supposed to last a specified period of time. When deviations from these statistical norms occur in individual cases, the situation is often defined as "high risk," necessitating medical intervention (Rothman 1983). Stated somewhat differently, physicians are taught to adopt "treatment stereotypes" as the functional units in which the business of curing gets done. As Scheff (1973) notes, physicians tend to accept these stereotypic descriptions of cases with only a very minimal attempt to see if they fit the particular case at hand. These "normal cases" (Scheff 1973) standardize diagnosis, prognosis, and treatment, making it possible for the physician to manage work in a routinized fashion. Categories of risk are among the conceptual packages that obstetrical physicians use to standardize medical work.

In addition, the fear of malpractice suits may foster Type II thinking (seeing disease when, in fact, it is absent). In such a climate, physicians prefer erring on the side of active intervention rather than using a "wait and see" approach. Obstetricians persist in this activist approach to childbirth, despite the evidence that greater damages are awarded in malpractice suits for overmanagement than for the opposite (Lubic 1981).

In addition to the role that physicians have played in constructing a "risk problem," some childbearing women and their families may have participated unwittingly in the process. Their collaborative roles can be best understood in light of demographic trends cited earlier, for a transformation in the meaning of birth has occurred in this low-birth-rate society. Of course, the meaning of pregnancy is different for different women: for some it is unwanted, for others it is routine, for still others it is a longed-for event—occurring after an intentional delay or, perhaps, after years of effort. Especially for middle-class professionals, a particular pregnancy may be highly salient if the woman has had to postpone motherhood until late in her reprductive career and, in some cases, has had to struggle with the decision to bear children. On the one hand, these new meanings lead to greater scrutiny of the various options for giving birth, as these women seek birth experiences that are psychologically satisfying as well as safe. On the other hand, the greater salience of pregnancy may lead some middle-class women to participate with physicians in viewing birth within a risk framework. Obviously, women do not create the framework. But they may be responsive to it because of their own interests, thereby fueling its development. This process has been observed in the medicalization of other health problems in women (Riessman 1983).

Lastly, the emergence of technology has played a part in the construction of the "risk problem" in childbirth. Medical technology is implicated in at least four ways. First, certain birth technologies themselves may lead to iatrogenic effects when they are used routinely rather than selectively. For example, electronic fetal monitoring does not permit laboring women to be ambulatory, which, in turn, may lead to longer labors and increase the subjective experience of pain. To deal with these effects, further procedures and medications that carry added risks may be used. In this example, the problem is the technology itself and what it sets in motion. Second, the technology may be misused. The most obvious example is cesarean sections. In a study of a sample of sixteen communities in Massachusetts, rates ranged from 22 to 48 percent—a rate most obstetricians would consider excessively high (Health Planning Council for Greater Boston 1984). National data show that rates of cesarean section are highest for women with private health insurance (Taffel, Placek, and Moien 1985), although, as a group, these women should be at lower risk due to their advantaged socioeconomic status. In this case, the problem appears to be the inappropriate use of the technology by individual physicians practicing within a particular reimbursement system.

Third, reliance on technology may be substituted for direct observation, inference, and clinical judgment, which in turn may lead to increased risk for the patient. To return to the example of electronic fetal monitors, there is evidence that abnormal tracings occur in up to 40 percent of all monitored labors and that this sign does not, in itself, signify the need to terminate the labor (National Institute of Child Health and Human De-

velopment 1979). Yet experimental research has shown that decision making is strongly affected by physicians' prior attitudes toward the technology. In one study, those who relied on monitors in their practices were significantly more likely to recommend a cesarean section when presented with an equivocal and slightly ominous tracing, especially if the hypothetical patient was identified as "high risk" than were physicians who relied less on this technology (Helfand, Marton, and Ueland in press). Other studies have found that routine use of electronic fetal monitoring increases the incidence of cesarean section (Banta and Thacker 1979). In this case, the problem is the substitution of technology for subjective judgment and clinical acumen, resulting in the greater probability of unnecessary and expensive surgical births.

Finally, and perhaps most important, medical technology is problematic because it transforms the ways medical scientists think about human problems. Mishler (1984) has called this tendency the "triumph of the technocratic consciousness." This mentality has a limited view of the causes of problems that patients bring to physicians at the same time that it reifies technical solutions to these problems. It encourages interventionist approaches to human problems like birth and death, for the body is viewed as a machine in need of repair. In a reciprocal fashion, birth technologies shape physicians' solutions to the management of labor and delivery at the same time that the development of technology itself is fueled by the technocratic consciousness.

Reproductive technologies have developed in a particular economic context. Over the last several decades, the electronics industry has diversified into health care, leading to a burgeoning industry in medical technology and equipment. As old markets have become saturated, new ones are developed to keep profits up (Waitzkin 1979). Yet explaining the growth of the medical industry solely on the basis of the profit motive is far too simple. As Bell (in press) has shown in the case of the drug Diethylstilbestrol (DES), new technologies are developed and are brought into medical practice out of particular ways of seeing and solving human problems; in addition, they are spurred on by the conflictual interests of a variety of communities —professional, business, and governmental—with each dependent on the others for the realization of their particular interest.

In sum, despite the prevailing view that reproductive technologies are examples of "medical progress" which give women more "choice," a deeper analysis suggests that the reality is more complicated (see Arditti, Klein, and Minden 1984; Young 1982). On the one hand, there are clear instances where the timely use of specific technologies has assured the survival of individual patients. Neonatal intensive care, for example, has been responsible for saving many low-birth-weight babies (McCormick 1985). On the other hand, the routine use of other birth technologies—such as fetal monitors, sonography, and surgical interventions—has created new medical problems, as noted earlier. In addition to the ways these

technologies have transformed the meaning and experience of birth, the long-term effects of some of these technologies—ultrasound, for example—are far from certain (Bolsen 1982). Even neonatal intensive care is not without its dark side: surviving low-birth-weight babies have more chronic disease morbidity, such as neurodevelopmental problems, congenital anomalies, and respiratory conditions, than do babies born full term (McCormick 1985). Research has yet to determine the effects of exposure to the substances, machines, and environmental conditions of neonatal intensive care units.

Perhaps most important, medical technologies do not always expand and contract according to acceptable rules of scientific evidence. As one physician stated to a congressional committee, there has been less scrutiny of medications, monitors, and other "scientific procedures than the scrutiny to which midwives' services currently are being subjected" (Arden Miller, M.D., as quoted in U.S. Congress, House of Representatives 1981). As scholars have pointed out with other medical technologies, diffusion often occurs before anyone establishes efficacy or decides whether diffusion is a wise public action (Banta 1980).

This analysis suggests there are multiple reasons for the "risk problem." The reasons the problem has been constructed the way it has are structural and interactive, involve a number of actors, and are not a result of the sinister motivations of individual doctors. Yet it is important to state that while seeing childbirth as inherently dangerous may be sociologically understandable, it may not be desirable. This way of thinking about childbirth has far-reaching consequences for health policy.

Consequences of the Dominant Perspective of the Problem

The adoption of a risk framework for managing birth will increase costs because the thrust will be for more and better hospital-based obstetrical units. Rather than traditional labor and delivery room arrangements, the growth may be in birthing rooms—innovations that have been called "concessions without conviction" (U.S. Congress, House of Representatives 981, 117). Yet, the evidence suggests that many women will be "risked out" of these facilities (Rothman 1982), experiencing birth instead in technology-intensive, physician-controlled environments where the iatrogenic risks will continue to be high.

For third-party payers, managing normal births in high-technology obstetrical units of general hospitals and reimbursing specialist physicians for attendance will be far more costly. A recent survey found the average cost for a birth in a freestanding birth center was $801, with a range from $200 to $1,700. The average comparable hospital care was $1,713, with a range from $550 to $3,750. Thus birth center charges are roughly 48 percent of hospital charges (Cooperative Birth Center Network 1983). In other words, maternity center births, managed by nurse-midwives in consultation with obstetrical specialists, are more cost-effective than traditional hospital and physician-attended births. This is because birth centers have lower overhead, rely less on expensive technologies, have lower induction and cesarean section rates, and, to provide care, use professionals who earn considerably less than physicians. (Nurse-midwives' incomes, on the average, are one-fifth the incomes of obstetrician-gynecologists; Cooperative Birth Center Network 1983.)

Finally, the social causes of complicating conditions of pregnancy and delivery will not be addressed by a health care policy that emphasizes only high-technology care of the individual patient. For example, it is well known that low-income women are more likely than middle-class women to experience complications in childbirth and to deliver low-birth-weight babies due to a combination of factors: their younger age, poorer nutrition, and prepregnancy health status, as well as lack of prenatal care. Black women are particularly vulnerable: their infants are more than twice as likely to weigh 2,500 grams or less than are infants born to white women (McCormick 1985). If we are serious about prevention, we need to look beyond individual characteristics and focus on conditions in the home, the school, the workplace, as well as the clinic.

Up to now, the thrust in American health policy has been primarily on intensive services for the mother at the time of birth and for the infant during the neonatal period. Few have addressed why so many babies are in neonatal intensive care in the first place. Although there is little doubt that these units have resulted in greater survival for low-birth-weight babies born to poor women, officials are now warning that this approach to the problem may have reached its limits in pushing down infant mortality for this group because infant deaths are now leveling off (American Public Health Association 1985). To improve the picture, the Institute of Medicine is now calling for a major shift toward prevention in the care of expectant and even potential mothers, including the provision of a broad range of "nontraditional" services (Institute of Medicine 1985).

To return to McKinlay's (1981) metaphor, if we are to improve further the health of mothers and infants, we need to look "upstream" rather than concentrating resources solely on "downstream" efforts. An "upstream" approach to risk would stress changing the environment that gives rise to the conditions promoting infant mortality and disease. By contrast, a more narrow technological approach would stress the establishment of more high-risk obstetrical services, more neonatal intensive care units, the diffusion of technology into low-income areas, and the like. Both approaches involve large costs. However, the social approach attacks the causes of the problem, in addition to benefiting communities as a whole. (More research is needed to further specify the particular components that should be included in social programs aimed at combating the high infant mortality and disease morbidity evident in low-income communities.)

In sum, by expanding our "ways of seeing" the risk problem in childbirth, we are led to a variety of possible "solutions." A health care policy that supported various options for the management of childbirth—such as the home, freestanding birth center, or birthing room, with hospital backup as necessary—becomes possible when, in Gusfield's (1981) terms, we do not allow alternative definitions of the problem to be rendered "unthinkable."

Conclusion

This chapter has examined, against a backdrop of changes in fertility both inside and outside of marriage, the ways in which the management of reproduction has become "problematic" in the contemporary period. Our focus has been on two issues that have become matters of considerable conflict and controversy—teenage pregnancy and the management of childbirth. We have explored how the ways that these problems are socially constructed influence and constrain public policy options that are offered for their solution. Practitioners evoke notions of "responsibility," in the case of teenage contraception, and "risk," in the case of childbirth, to legitimize particular modes of management. Yet these "solutions" create additional problems for individual practitioners and for health policy more generally. In the case of teenage contraceptive use, the attribution of responsibility to the teenager creates dilemmas for nurses, while simultaneously freeing them from responsibility when contraceptive failures occur. In the case of childbirth, emphasis on potential hazards creates new risks while more successfully managing old ones.

In a more general sense, our analysis has pointed to the ways that social control operates in the daily practice of medicine and nursing. When situations become "public problems," health professionals often are charged with eliminating or containing them. This "medicalization" of human problems is a powerful force in American society and has evoked a large body of social science analysis and commentary (Kittrie 1971; Zola 1972; Janowitz 1979; Conrad and Schneider 1980; Riessman 1983).

Comparing the two examples of reproductive medicalization is instructive; their differences illuminate the underlying politics at work. In the case of childbirth, the concept of *risk* and its elaboration in clinical practice represent an active effort to extend and consolidate the medical mandate; the invocation of risk legitimizes physician control and undermines the legitimacy of nonphysician intruders into the medical domain. By contrast, *responsibility* is employed to limit the medical mandate under conditions where its reach exceeds its grasp. The effectiveness of the "risk" strategy owes much to the fact that childbirth, unlike conception, is normatively "public" and, consequently, directly available to surveillance and control by outside observers. When surveillance is limited, it is failure of control—not its extension —that requires rationalization.

In both teenage pregnancy and the management of childbirth, medicalization is a vehicle for dealing with essentially social dilemmas. Medical "solutions" for these problems bring in their stead a series of different yet far-reaching consequences for women, practitioners, and policymakers.

References

Alan Guttmacher Institute. 1976. *11 million teenagers.* New York: Planned Parenthood Federation of America.

————. 1981. *Teenage pregnancy: The problem that hasn't gone away.* New York: Alan Guttmacher Institute.

American College of Obstetrics and Gynecology. 1975. Statement of policy on safety in childbirth.

American Public Health Association. 1983. Guidelines for licensing and regulating birth centers. Policy Statement 8209. *American Journal of Public Health* 73:331–334.

————. 1985. A slowdown in decline reported: US looks at infant deaths issue as report on health published. *Nation's Health* 15(4):1,4.

Apgar, V. A. 1953. A proposal for a new method of evaluation of the newborn infant. *Current Research in Anesthesia and Analgesia* 32:260–267.

Arditti, R., R. D. Klein, and S. Minden eds. 1984. *Test-tube women: What future for motherhood?* Boston: Routledge and Kegan Paul.

Banta, H. D. 1980. The diffusion of the computed tomography (CT) scanner in the United States. *International Journal of Health Services* 10:251–269.

Banta, H. D., and S. B. Thacker, 1979. *Costs and benefits of electronic fetal monitoring: A review of the literature.* DHEW Publication No. (PHS) 79-3245. Washington, D.C.: Government Printing Office.

Bell, S. E. In press. A new model of medical technology development: A case study of DES. In *Research in the sociology of health care*, vol. 4, ed J. Roth and S. Ruzek. Greenwich, Conn.: JAI Press.

Bennetts, A. B., and R. W. Lubic. 1982. The free-standing birth center. *Lancet,* pp. 378–380.

Bloom, D. E. 1982. What's happening to the age at first birth in the United States? A study of recent cohorts. *Demography* 19:351–370.

Rogue, D. J., ed. 1977. *Adolescent fertility.* Chicago: University of Chicago, Community and Family Study Center.

Bolsen, B. 1982. Question of risk still hovers over routine prenatal use of ultrasound. *Journal of American Medical Association* 247:2195–2197.

Brozan N. 1982. Adolescents, parents, and birth control. *New York Times* 131:20.

Cherlin, A. J. 1981. *Marriage, divorce, remarriage.* Cambridge: Harvard University Press.

Chilman, C. S. 1978. *Adolescent sexuality in a changing American society: Social and psychological perspectives.* NIH Publication No. 79-1426. U.S. Department of Health, Education, and Welfare. Washington, D.C.: Government Printing Office.

———. 1980. Social and psychological research concerning adolescent childbearing, 1970–1980. *Journal of Marriage and the Family* 42:67–79.

Conrad, P., and J. W. Schneider. 1980. *Deviance and medicalization: From badness to sickness.* St. Louis: C.V. Mosby.

Cooperative Birth Center Network. 1983. *CBCN News* (Perkiomenville, Pa.) 1:4.

Cutright, P. 1971. Illegitimacy: Myths, causes, and cures. *Family Planning Perspectives* 3:26–48.

Davis, K., and J. Blake. 1956. Social structure and fertility: An analytic framework. *Economic Development and Cultural Change* 4:211–214.

DeVries, R. G. 1981. Birth and death: Social construction at the poles of existence. *Social Forces* 59:1047–1093.

Diers, D. K. 1981. Nurse-midwifery as a system of care: Provider process and patient outcome. In *Health policy and nursing practice*, ed. L. Aiken, pp. 73–89. New York: McGraw-Hill.

Drachman, V. G. 1979. The Loomis trial: Social mores and obstetrics in the mid-nineteenth century. In *Health care in America: Essays in social history*, ed. S. Reverby and D. Rosner, pp. 67–83. Philadelphia, Pa.: Temple University Press.

Dryfoos, J. G., and T. Heisler. 1978. Contraceptive services for adolescents: An overview. *Family Planning Perspectives* 10:223–233.

Dubos, R. 1959. *Mirage of health.* Garden City, N.Y.: Anchor.

Duff, R. S. 1980. Care in childbirth and beyond (editorial). *New England Journal of Medicine* 302:685–686.

Easterlin, A. 1980. *Birth and fortune: The impact of numbers on personal welfare.* New York: Basic Books.

Freidson, E. 1970. *Profession of medicine.* New York: Dodd, Mead.

———. 1982. Occupational autonomy and labor market shelters. In *Varieties of work,* ed. P. L. Steward and M. G. Cantor, pp. 39–54. Beverly Hills: Sage.

Furstenberg, F. F., Jr., R. Herceg-Baron, J. Shea, and D. Webb. 1984. Family communication and teenagers' contraceptive use. *Family Planning Perspectives* 16:163–170.

Furstenberg, F. F., Jr., R. Lincoln, and J. Menken, eds. 1981. *Teenage sexuality, pregnancy, and childbearing.* Philadelphia, Pa.: University of Pennsylvania Press.

Furstenberg, F. F., Jr., J. Shea, P. Allison, R. Herceg-Baron, and D. Webb. 1983. Contraceptive continuation among adolescents attending family planning clinics. *Family Planning Perspectives* 1615:211–217.

Graham, H., and A. Oakley. 1981. Competing ideologies of reproduction: Medical and maternal perspectives on pregnancy. In *Women, health, and reproduction,* ed. H. Roberts, pp. 50–74. Boston: Routledge and Kegan Paul.

Grobstein, R. 1979. Amniocentesis counseling. In *Genetic counseling: Psychological dimensions,* ed. S. Kessler, pp. 107–113. New York: Academic Press.

Guillemin, J. 1981. Babies by cesarean: Who chooses, who controls? *Hastings Center Report* 11:15–18.

Gusfield, J. R. 1981. *The culture of public problems.* Chicago: University of Chicago Press.

Hamburg, P. 1983. Humanization of birthing practices. Letter in *Journal of Pediatrics* 102:486.

Health Planning Council for Greater Boston. 1984. Surgical utilization in Massachusetts communities. Typescript.

Helfand, M., K. Marton, and K. Ueland. In press. Factors involved in the interpretation of fetal monitor tracings. *American Journal of Obstetrics and Gynecology.*

House, E. 1973. Medical services for sexually active teenagers. *American Journal of Public Health* 63:285–287.

Hurst, M., and P. S. Summey. 1984 Childbirth and social class: The case of cesarean delivery. *Social Science and Medicine* 18:621–663.

Institute of Medicine. 1982. *Research issues in the assessment of birth settings.* Publication No. IOM-82-04. Washington, DC: National Academy Press.

———. 1985. *Preventing low birth weight.* Washington, D.C.: National Academy Press.

Janowitz. M. 1979. *The last half century: Societal change and politics in America.* Chicago: University of Chicago Press.

Joffe, C. 1978. What abortion counselors want from their clients. *Social Problems* 26:112–121.

———. 1979. Abortion work: Strains, coping strategies, policy implications. *Social Work* 24: 485–490.

Kessler, S. 1979. The counselor-counselee relationship. In *Genetic counseling: Psychological dimensions,* ed. S. Kessler, pp. 53–63. New York: Academic Press.

Kittrie, N. N. 1971. *The right to be different: Deviance and enforced therapy.* Baltimore: Johns Hopkins University Press.

Kobrin, F. E. 1966. The American midwife controversary: A crisis of professionalization. *Bulletin of the History of Medicine* 40:350–363.

Leavitt, J. W. 1983. "Science" enters the birthing room: Obstetrics in America since the eighteenth century. *Journal of American History* 70:281–304.

Lippman-Hand, A., and F. C. Fraser. 1979a. Genetic counseling: Provision and reception of information. *American Journal of Medical Genetics* 3:113–127.

———. 1979b. Genetic counseling: The post-counseling period, II. Making reproductive choices. *American Journal of Medical Genetics* 4:73–87.

Lubic, R. W. 1981. Evaluation of an out-of-hospital maternity center for low risk patients. In *Health policy and nursing practice,* ed. L. Aiken, pp. 90–116. New York: McGraw-Hill.

McClain, C. S. 1983. Perceived risk and choice of childbirth service. *Social Science and Medicine* 17:1857–1865.

McCormick, M. C. 1985. The contribution of low birth weight to infant mortality and childhood morbidity. *New England Journal of Medicine* 312: 82–90.

McKinlay, J. B. 1981. A case for refocussing upstream: The political economy of illness. In *The sociology of health and illness: Critical perspectives,* ed. P. Conrad and S. Kern, pp. 613–663. New York: St. Martin's Press.

Mehl, L. and G. H. Peterson. 1976. Home birth versus hospital birth. Paper presented at annual meeting. American Public Health Association, Miami, Fla.

Mehl, L., G. H. Peterson, M. Whitt, and W. F. Hawes. 1977. Outcomes of elective home births: A series of 1,146 cases. *Journal of Reproductive Medicine* 19:281–290.

Mishler, E. G. 1981. Viewpoint: Critical perspectives on the biomedical model. In *Social contexts of health, illness, and patient care,* ed. E. G. Mishler et al., pp. 1–23. New York: Cambridge University Press.

———. 1984. *The discourse of medicine: Dialectics of medical interviews.* Norwood, N.J.: Ablex.

Murdaugh, A. 1976. Experience of a new migrant health clinic. *Women and Health* 1:25–29.

Nathanson, C. A. In press. Family planning and contraceptive responsibility.

In *Towards a contraceptive ethos: Reproductive rights and responsibilities*, ed. W. Bondeson, H. T. Engelhardt, Jr., and S. Spicker. Boston: Reidel.

Nathanson, C. A., and M. H. Becker. 1977. The influence of physicians' attitudes on abortion performance, patient management, and professional fees. *Family Planning Perspectives* 9:158–163.

————. 1983. Contraceptive behavior among unmarried young women: A theoretical framework for research. *Population and Environment* 6:39–59.

————. 1985. The influence of client-provider relationships on teenage women's subsequent use of contraception. *American Journal of Public Health* 75:33–38.

Nathanson, C. A., and L. Morlock. 1980. Control structure, values, and innovations: A comparative study of hospitals. *Journal of Health and Social Behavior* 21:315–333.

National Institute of Child Health and Human Development. 1979. *Antenatal diagnosis: Report of a consensus development conference.* Washington, D.C.: Government Printing Office.

Nelson, M. K. 1983. Working class women, middle class women, and modes of childbirth. *Social Problems* 30:284–297.

Osherson, S., and L. AmaraSingham. 1981. The machine metaphor in medicine. In *Social contexts of health, illness, and patient care*, ed. E. G. Mishler, et al., pp. 218–249. New York: Cambridge University Press.

Parsons, T. 1951. *The social system.* New York: Free Press.

Peterson, K. J. 1983. Technology as a last resort in home birth: The work of lay midwives. *Social Problems* 30:273–283.

Pilpel, H. F., and N. H. Wechsler. 1969. Birth control, teenagers, and the law. *Family Planning Perspectives* 1:29–36.

Riessman, C. K. 1983. Women and medicalization: A new perspective. *Social Policy* 14:14–23.

————. 1984. The use of health services by the poor: Are there any promising models? *Social Policy* 14:30–40.

Roberts, R. W., ed. 1966. *The unwed mother.* New York: Harper and Row.

Rosengren, W. R., and S. DeVault. 1963. The sociology of time and space in an obstetric hospital. In *The hospital in modern society*, ed. E. Friedson, pp. 284–285. New York: Free Press.

Roth, J. 1963. *Timetables: Structuring the passage of time in hospital treatment and other careers.* Indianapolis, Mo.: Bobbs Merrill.

Rothenberg, P. B., and P. E. Varga. 1981. The relationship between age of mother and child health and development. *American Journal of Public Health* 71:810–817.

Rothman, B. K. 1982. *In labor.* New York: Norton.

————. 1983. Midwives in transition: The structure of a clinical revolution. *Social Problems* 30:262–271.

Ryan, W. 1976. *Blaming the victim.* Rev. ed. New York: Vintage.

Ryder, N. B. 1980. Components of temporal variations in American fertility. In

Demographic patterns in developed societies, ed. Robert W. Hines, pp. 15–54. London: Taylor and Francis.

Scheff, T. J. 1966. Decisions in medicine. In *Being mentally ill: A sociology theory*, pp. 105–127. Chicago: Aldine.

———. 1973. Typification in rehabilitation agencies. In *Deviance: The interactionist perspective*, ed. E. Rubington and M. Weinberg, pp. 128–131. New York: Macmillan.

Schneider, J. W., and P. Conrad. 1980. The medical control of deviance: Causes and consequences. In *Research in the sociology of health care*, ed. J. Roth, pp. 1–53. Greenwich, Conn.: JAI Press.

Schwartz, M., and J. H. Ford. 1982. Family planning clinics: Cure or cause of teenage pregnancy? *Linacre Quarterly* 49:143–164.

Shea, J. A., R. Hercog-Baron, and F. F. Furstenberg, Jr. 1984. Factors associated with adolescent use of family planning clinics. *American Journal of Public Health* 74:1227–1230.

Steiner, G. Y. 1981. *The futility of family policy*. Washington, D.C.: Brookings Institution.

Stone, M. L. 1979. Presidential address. *ACOG Newsletter* 25:4–6.

Such-Baer, M. 1974. Professional staff reaction to abortion work. *Social Casework* 55:435–441.

Thornton, A., D. F. Alwin, and D. Camburn. 1983. Causes and consequences of sex-role attitudes and attitude change. *American Sociological Review* 48:211–227.

Thornton, A., and D. Freedman. 1983. The changing American family. *Population Bulletin* 38 (October).

Torres, A., J. D. Forrest, and S. Eisman. 1981. Family planning services in the United States, 1978–1979. *Family Planning Perspectives* 13:132–141.

U.S. Congress. House of Representatives. 1981. *Nurse midwifery: Consumers' freedom of choice*. Hearing before Subcommittee on Oversight and Investigations, Committee on Interstate and Foreign Commerce. Series No. 96-236. Washington, D.C.: Government Printing Office.

———. Select Committee on Children, Youth, and Families. 1984. *Teen parents and their children: Issues and programs*. Washington, D.C.: Government Printing Office.

———. Select Committee on Population, 1978. *Fertility and contraception in America: Adolescent and pre-adolescent pregnancy*. Washington, D.C.: Government Printing Office.

U. S. Department of Commerce. Bureau of the Census. 1983. Fertility of American women, 1981. In *Current population reports*, series P-20, no. 378. Washington, D.C.: Government Printing Office.

U.S. Department of Health and Human Services. 1983. Parental notification requirements applicable to projects for family planning services. *Federal Register* 48:3600–3614.

U.S. Department of Health, Education, and Welfare. 1974. *The supply of health manpower: 1970 profiles and projections to 1990.* DHEW Publication No. (HRA) 75-38. Washington, D.C.: Government Printing Office.

U.S. Federal Trade Commission. 1981. *Competition among health practitioners: The influence of the medical profession on the health manpower — case study: The childbearing center.* Typescript.

Ventura, S. J. 1984. Trends in teenage childbearing: United States, 1970–81. In *Vital and health statistics,* series 21, no. 41. U.S. Department of Health and Human Services, Public Health Service, National Center for Health Statistics. DHHS Publication No. (PHS) 84-1919. Washington, D.C.: Government Printing Office.

Vinovskis, M. A. 1981. An "epidemic" of adolescent pregnancy? Some historical considerations. *Journal of Family History* 6:205–230.

Waitzkin, H. 1979. A Marxian interpretation of the growth and development of coronary care technology. *American Journal of Public Health* 69:1260–1268.

Wertz, R. W., and D. C. Wertz. 1979. *Lying in: A history of childbirth in America.* New York: Schocken.

Westoff, C. F. 1978. Marriage and fertility in the developed countries. *Scientific American* 239:51–57.

Whose baby is it anyway? 1980. *Lancet,* pp. 1284–1285.

Williams, J. W. 1912. Medical education and midwife problem in the United States. *Journal of the American Medical Association* 58:1–7.

Young, D., ed. 1982. Obstetrical intervention and technology in the 1980's. *Women and Health* 7:(3&4).

Zabin, L.S., and S. D. Clark, Jr. 1981. Why they delay: A study of family planning clinic patients. *Family Planning Perspectives* 13:205–217.

———. 1983. Institutional factors affecting teenagers' choice and reasons for delay in attending a family planning clinic. *Family Planning Perspectives* 15:25–29.

Zelnik, M., and J. F. Kantner. 1972. Sexuality, contraception, and pregnancy among young unwed females in the United States. In *Commission on population growth and the American future, research reports,* vol. 1: *Demographic and social aspects of population growth,* ed., Charles Westoff and Robert Parke, Jr., pp. 355–374. Washington, D.C.: Government Printing Office.

———. 1980. Sexual activity, contraceptive use, and pregnancy among metropolitan area teenagers, 1971–1979. *Family Planning Perspectives* 12:230–237.

Zola, I. K. 1972. Medicine as an institution of social control. *Sociological Review* 20:487–504.

Zuckerman, B., J. J. Alpert, E. Dooling, R. Hingson, H. Kayne, S. Morelock, and E. Oppenheimer. 1983. Neonatal outcome: Is adolescent pregnancy a risk factor? *Pediatrics* 61:489–493.

Chapter 14

Implications of Recent Changes in Infant Mortality

Marie C. McCormick

Ⓘn the past two decades, the infant mortality rate in the United States has declined sharply. This now-well-established trend has elicited great interest, in part, because it follows a period of almost equal duration when the infant mortality rate remained relatively constant despite intense efforts to decrease it. More important, however, the nature of the current changes in infant mortality raises serious questions about the efficacy of preventive services in the antenatal period, the role of perinatal intensive care services, and the implications of changes in infant mortality for the burden of morbidity experienced in childhood. In view of the recent dramatic changes in infant mortality, an overview of what is currently known about the major causes of infant mortality and morbidity is helpful in understanding these changes and identifying areas for future policy concern.

The changes in infant mortality and its causes over the course of this century have been dramatic. In 1900 the infant mortality rate was over 100 infant deaths per 1,000 live births. Over the first half of the century, infant mortality rates declined to levels about half those seen in 1900 or to about 50 per 1,000 live births. When these changes were examined according to the age at which the infant died, most of the decline could be attributed to sharp decreases in mortality among infants older than one month, decreases in post-neonatal mortality. Deaths in this age range are frequently due to infectious conditions such as gastroenteritis (vomiting and diarrhea) and respiratory infections (e.g., pneumonia). Thus, these decreases in post-neonatal mortality are believed to reflect improvements in environmental conditions and nutrition, which reduced the impact of infectious disease (Shapiro, Schlesinger, and Nesbit 1968; Pharoah and Morris 1978).

With the reduction in post-neonatal mortality, a shift occurred in the timing of infant death: by 1950 two-thirds of all infant deaths occurred in the neonatal period—the first month of life. The major causes of neonatal deaths reflected antenatal and intrapartum events such as birth injury, asphyxia, congenital malformations, and "immaturity." One indicator of the latter was low birth weight ($\leq$ 2,500 grams or 5.5 pounds). In 1950 the proportion of newborns weighing 2,500 grams or less was less than 10 percent, but these infants accounted for two-thirds of the neonatal deaths (Shapiro, Schlesinger, and Nesbit 1968).

These changes established the context in which modern perinatal care emerged. Further reductions in infant mortality would require addressing the problems of the neonatal period. In this chapter, I will discuss two major contributors to neonatal mortality: low birth weight and congenital anomalies. The former is both proportionately and numerically the most important determinant of neonatal mortality. Addressing the prevention of low birth weight illustrates the complexity of child health problems partially related to socioeconomic disadvantage. Approaches to the prevention of congenital anomalies encounter other issues surrounding pregnancy and childbirth. Both problems illustrate some of the dilemmas emanating from the current capabilities of modern intensive care to sustain the lives of very tiny or very sick newborns. This chapter will address what we know about the contribution of these conditions to infant mortality and childhood morbidity and the risk factors for each. It will conclude with an overview of implications for the future.

Contribution of Low Birth Weight to Mortality

Recent figures for the United States indicate that 7.0 percent of all newborns weigh 2,500 grams or less. This figure represents a 13.5 percent decline from the rates in 1968–1970. Almost no change in the proportion of infants born at very low birth weight (1,500 grams or less, or 3.3 pounds) has occurred, and these infants constitute 1.15 percent of all births. Thus, of the 3,494,398 live births in 1979, 252,511 weighed 2,500 grams or less, and 40,186, 1,500 grams or less (U.S. Department of Health and Human Services 1982).

Assessing the contribution of low-birth-weight infants to mortality and morbidity requires birth-weight-specific mortality rates derived from files containing infant death certificates matched to the corresponding birth certificate, as well as morbidity information on surviving children. Unfortunately, such data are not available for the United States as a whole. However, some indirect evidence of an association between low birth weight and mortality on a national level can be gleaned from differences in neonatal mortality by race.

Black newborns are twice as likely to weigh 2,500 grams or less than white ones (12.7 percent versus 5.9 percent); this increased risk also pertains to the proportion in the lowest birth weight group of 1,500 grams or less (2.4 percent versus 0.9 percent). Parallel to this difference in birth weight distribution is a difference in infant mortality. For 1977–1979 the infant mortality rate was 13.6 per 1,000 live births, 11.9 for white births, and 22.8 for black births. In this period blacks accounted for 16.5 percent of all live births, but 30 percent of all low-birth-weight newborns, 34 percent of very-low-birth-weight newborns, and 28 percent of infant deaths (U.S. Department of Health and Human Services 1982).

More direct estimates of the effect of birth weight on mortality can be derived from several recent large-scale analyses relying on the type of matched infant death and birth files noted above. While these analyses do not deal with the United States as a whole, the results are likely to be generalizable.

The relationship between birth weight and infant mortality had been repeatedly documented in a variety of settings. The lowest mortality rates are experienced by infants weighing 3,500 grams (or 7.7 pounds). For infants born weighing 2,500 grams or less, the mortality rate rapidly increases with decreasing birth weight such that most of the infants weighing 1,000 grams (1.5 pounds) or less die. Compared to normal-birth-

weight infants, low-birth-weight infants are almost forty times more likely to die in the neonatal period; for very-low-birth-weight infants the relative risk of a neonatal death is almost two hundred times greater (Shapiro et al. 1980).

Not only are low-birth-weight infants at increased relative risk of neonatal mortality, but the attributable risk or proportion of all neonatal deaths occurring among low-birth-weight infants is also high. Infants born weighing 2,500 grams or less still account for two-thirds of neonatal deaths; those 1,500 grams or less, half of neonatal deaths (Shapiro et al. 1980). As mortality among normal-birth-weight infants decreases, this attributable risk is likely to increase. Thus, in industrialized populations, the proportion of very-low-birth-weight infants is a major predictor of neonatal mortality. Even controlling for other factors known to affect the risk of neonatal mortality, low birth weight remains the major determinant of neonatal mortality.

In the postneonatal period, low-birth-weight infants remain at increased risk of death. The relationship between post-neonatal mortality and birth weight is not as large as that for neonatal mortality, however. Low-birth-weight infants are five times more likely than normal-birth-weight infants to die later in the first year; they account for 20 percent of all post-neonatal deaths. For very-low-birth-weight infants, the relative risk of post-neonatal death is twenty times that of normal-birth-weight infants, and these infants account for up to 25 to 30 percent of post-neonatal deaths. As suggested by previous reports, the effect of birth weight on post-neonatal mortality is modified by socioeconomic factors (Shapiro et al. 1980).

Within birth-weight groups, the risk of mortality is not uniform and varies with gestational age. For a given birth weight, the longer the duration of gestation up to forty-two weeks, the lower the mortality. Alternatively, for a given gestational age, again up to forty-two weeks, the heavier infants experience lower mortality rates (Williams et al. 1982).

While variation in birth-weight-specific mortality with gestational age is well recognized, in the clinical setting the more usual distinction is between those infants whose birth weight falls within the normal range given the duration of gestation (the appropriate-for-gestational-age infant) and those whose birth weight is much lower than expected in view of the duration of gestation (the small-for-gestational-age infant). This distinction is clinically useful because for a given birth weight, appropriate- and small-for-gestational-age infants differ in the health problems present in the neonatal period and in prognosis for mortality. Small-for-gestational-age infants have lower neonatal and post-neonatal mortality rates than appropriate-for-gestational-age infants of comparable birth weights, with the exception of the full-term infant weighing 2,500 grams or less (Starfield et al. 1982). For populations in which the proportion of infants of low birth weight exceeds 10 percent, small-for-gestational-age infants represent the majority of low-birth-weight infants. At lower rates, 5 to 7 percent, truly premature, appropriate-for-gestational-age infants are in the majority (Essel, Villar, and Berendes 1984).

The relative contribution of appropriate- and small-for-gestational-age infants to neonatal mortality in the United States is not well established. Despite the difference in mortality rates between these two groups of infants at a given birth weight, the shift toward a higher proportion of appropriate-for-gestational-age infants is unlikely to affect by much the estimate of the proportion of perinatal deaths accounted for by low-birth-weight infants. Where the relative effects of birth weight and gestational age on mortality have been examined, birth weight appears to be the dominant factor.

Besides gestational age, other factors are also associated with an increased risk of neonatal mortality. Race is a major factor; others include maternal age at the extremes of the childbearing age range (younger than eighteen or older than thirty-four years of age), low maternal educational attainment, and a history of prior adverse obstetric outcome such as fetal death. These risk factors also increase the risk of low birth weight. Controlling for birth weight distribution sharply reduces or eliminates the differentials in neonatal mortality associated with a number of these factors, namely nonwhite race, adolescent motherhood, and low maternal educational attainment. This finding indicates that the proportion of low-birth-weight infants largely accounts for the adverse neonatal mortality experiences of these subgroups (Shapiro et al. 1980).

Differences in birth weight do not

eliminate the increased risk of neonatal death associated with advanced maternal age and prior history of fetal loss. These factors are associated with both an increased risk of low birth weight and an increased obstetric vulnerability leading to poor neonatal outcome (Shapiro et al. 1980).

The situation is different for post-neonatal mortality. Even after controlling for birth weight, post-neonatal mortality rates remain higher for nonwhite infants, and infants of adolescent mothers and of mothers of low educational attainment. Thus, factors indicative of socioeconomic disadvantage are linked to increased infant mortality through both an association with higher low-birth-weight rates and an increased risk of post-neonatal death, regardless of birth weight (Shapiro et al. 1980; McCormick, Shapiro, and Starfield 1984).

Factors Affecting Changes in Low Birth Weight and Changes in Mortality

After relative stagnation in the 1960s, the infant mortality rate began a rapid decline. In 1980 the infant mortality rate was 13.1 per 1,000 live births, a 47 percent decrease from the rate in 1965 (U.S. Department of Health and Human Services 1982). In contrast to the first half of the century, however, this recent change is primarily the result of a decrease in neonatal mortality.

While mortality rates of normal-birth-weight infants have been declining, the accumulating evidence indicates that a major factor in this rapid decline has been the increased survival of low-birth-weight infants, in part as the result of more intensive, hospital-based management.

The results of several different types of studies provide support for this conclusion (McCormick 1985).

1. The decrease in neonatal mortality has occurred in the context of only modest decreases in the proportion of low-birth-weight infants.

2. A progressive decline in neonatal mortality has occurred among very-low-birth-weight infants who receive intensive care.

3. Decreases in neonatal mortality for geographically defined areas have followed the introduction of perinatal intensive care units.

4. Low-birth-weight infants born in hospitals with intensive care facilities have a higher survival rate than infants born in hospitals without such units, even after controlling for other risk factors known to affect survival. This enhanced survival rate persists even when infants born in hospitals with intensive care facilities are compared to those transported to such hospitals shortly after birth.

5. Decreases in neonatal mortality in geographically defined regions have been shown to accompany an increase in the proportion of low-birth-weight and very-low-birth-weight infants born in tertiary centers.

The net result is that in many areas of the country, birth-weight-specific mortality rates are now similar for both high- and low-risk groups, which suggests that sustaining the decline in neonatal mortality will require prevention of low-weight births and increased attention to the efficacy of services in the prenatal period. The concern about the potential for prevention has been reinforced by the observation that the relatively modest decline in the proportion of low-birth-weight deliveries has occurred in the context of substantial increases in the proportion of women beginning their preganacy care in the first trimester, such that the majority of women now begin their care in the first trimester. In some areas, this number includes the majority of those giving birth to low-birth-weight infants. In addition, studies of prenatal care do not provide as clear agreement about effectiveness as those of hospital-based services. The implications of these changes will be discussed at the end of the paper.

Contribution of Low Birth Weight to Morbidity

The contribution of low birth weight to morbidity in childhood is less well established than its contribution to infant mortality. In part, this results from the relative lack of population-based morbidity data sufficient to ascertain the morbidity attributable to low birth weight, as noted earlier. In addition, the types of morbidity that occur in low birth weight, especially among the smallest survivors, are still being defined. Finally, perinatal events are only one determinant of

child health, and disentangling the effect of low birth weight alone or in interaction with other factors has proven difficult. Despite these reservations, the existing literature indicates that low-birth weight infants appear at increased risk for a number of health problems, and that this increased risk has implications for health and educational services as well as for family functioning.

The prevalence of neurodevelopmental handicap has been a primary focus in the follow-up of low-birth-weight infants since the increased risk of these infants for cerebral palsy, seizure disorders, and other neurodevelopmental problems was documented in the 1950s. At that time, the risk for all low-birth-weight infants was three times that of normal-birth-weight infants; the risk for very-low-birth-weight infants was ten times that of normal-birth-weight infants (Hardy, Drage, and Jackson 1979).

In view of the very high mortality rates and high risk of neurodevelopmental handicap, much of the recent literature has focused on the very-low-birth-weight infants. Recent reviews of this literature have concluded that the prevalence of neurodevelopmental handicap among very-low-birth-weight survivors appears to be decreasing, although variations in data suggest the need for cautious interpretation. Despite the evident of a decrease, low-birth-weight infants remain three times as likely as normal-birth-weight infants to experience adverse neurologic sequelae; the risk increases with decreasing birth weight such that 8 to

19 percent of very-low birth-weight infants may be severely affected (Budetti et al. 1980; Stewart 1981).

Less well established is the risk for other developmental problems, especially those related to success in school. It appears, however, that low birth weight is a significant predictor of school failure, and this may be particularly characteristic of those who are small for gestational age. Even in this latter group, however, the proportion handicapped may be dependent on the presence of birth asphyxia rather than on birth weight per se (Klein et al. 1985).

The risk of developmental delay is not independent of factors that act to increase the risk of low birth weight. Thus, low-birth-weight infants of disadvantaged mothers are more likely to experience school failure or to have lower intelligence quotients than infants of similar birth weights in more advantaged families (Escalona 1982; Ramey et al. 1978).

Although less intensively studied, the increased risk of congenital anomalies among low-birth-weight survivors is well documented. As compared to normal-birth-weight infants, low-birth-weight infants are twice as likely to have a nontrivial anomaly; very-low-birth-weight infants are three times as likely. Among low-birth-weight infants, the risk of an anomaly is higher among those small for gestational age rather than those whose birth weight is more consistent with the duration of gestation (Starfield et al 1982; Christianson et al. 1981).

Congenital anomalies and neuro-developmental handicap are not mutually exclusive occurrences. The percentage of infants affected with one or both ranges from 19 percent of normal-birth-weight infants to 42 percent of very-low-birth-weight infants; those severely affected range from 2 percent of normal-birth-weight to 14 percent of very-low-birth-weight infants (Shapiro et al. 1980).

Intensive care technology required for the survival of these infants is not without hazard and may result in complications. The most well known is retinopathy of prematurity (formerly referred to as retrolental fibroplasia), which is associated with oxygen administration to immature infants. Other early diagnostic and therapeutic techniques have also been shown to be hazardous (Silverman 1980). Current special care units provide exposure to many substances, machines, and environmental conditions. The potential side effects are still being defined.

Early studies suggested that low-birth-weight infants might be at greater risk for illness in general. Relatively few studies have examined this issue, however, and early studies vary in their findings. More recent data indicate that very-low-birth-weight infants may be at increased risk of relatively serious or protracted illness. By one year of age, about 40 percent of these infants will have an illness requiring hospitalization or prolonged care, as compared to 20 percent of all low-birth-weight infants and 8.7 percent of normal-birth-weight infants. This percentage may vary with age because the proportion of very-low-birth-weight infants with selected chronic conditions varies from 23 percent at forty weeks of age (corrected for duration of gestation) to 3 percent at twenty months. The susceptibility of high-risk survivors to acute or less serious illness remains to be established (McCormick, Shapiro, and Starfield 1980; Hack et al. 1981).

Finally, the risk of low-birth-weight infants for accidental injury remains relatively unexplored. Up to one year of age, little difference in the risk of injury by birth weight occurs. Beyond that, few population-based data have been published. The relatively extensive literature identifying low birth weight as a risk factor for intentional injury (abuse) has recently been reviewed; the conclusion reached was that the evidence for such an association is not strong (McCormick, Shapiro, and Starfield 1981b; Leventhal 1981).

Morbidity among low-birth-weight infants also has implications for health services use and the family. Most of the attention on medical care use by low-birth-weight infants has focused on the intensive care required, in the neonatal period, to increase the survival of very-low-birth-weight infants. During this period the average length of stay for infants who survive to the first year of life averages 3.5 days for normal-birth-weight infants but is much longer for smaller infants: 24 days for those 1,501 to 2,000 grams, 57 days for those ≤ 1,500 grams at birth, and 89 days for those ≤ 1,000 grams. The length of stay for nonsurviving infants tends to be much less, although not proportionately less expensive. Wide variations in both length of stay and direct medical costs per day occur within birth weight groups, depending on the need for ventilation, the presence of congenital anomalies, and the need for surgery, among other things (*Preventing Low Birthweight* 1985).

The cost-effectiveness of neonatal intensive care has been reviewed and the conclusion reached that neonatal intensive care is generally cost-effective, although doubts remain whether this conclusion will hold for the very smallest infants, depending on the adjustments made for future costs incurred by handicapped survivors (Budetti et al. 1981).

Besides the prolonged hospitalization at birth, a substantial proportion of very-low-birth-weight infants are rehospitalized during the first year. Up to 40 percent of these infants will be hospitalized twice for an average of 16 days total, all hospitalization combined. This compares with 19 percent of all low-birth-weight infants, who average 12.5 days, and 8.7 percent of normal-birth-weight infants, who average 8 days. A major determinant of rehospitalization for all birth weight groups is the presence of a chronic condition, congenital anomaly, or poor developmental outcome. After infancy, hospital use diminishes sharply (McCormick, Shapiro, and Starfield 1980; Hack et al. 1981).

The average number of physician visits is also higher for low-birth-weight infants than for normal-birth-weight infants, but the relationship to birth weight is not as large as with hospitalization. Average visits in the first year ranged from fourteen to sixteen for those ≤ 1,500 grams at birth to ten for normal-birth-weight infants. As with hospitalization, a major determinant of physician utilization is the presence of a congenital anomaly or developmental delay (McCormick, Shapiro, and Starfield 1981a).

Worth emphasizing, on a population basis, are the conditions for which use of medical services are similar for infants of all birth weights. These conditions include congenital anomalies, respiratory infections such as pneumonia, bronchiolitis and otitis media, and gastrointestinal problems. The increased use of services among low-birth-weight infants reflects the increased prevalence of these conditions. The etiologic basis for this increased morbidity and increased use of services is only partially known. Contributing factors may include biologic vulnerability due to immaturity or therapeutic maneuvers required to support the infant, the socioeconomic disadvantage characteristic of many low-birth-weight infants, and increased surveillance by health care providers and parents (Green and Solnit 1964; Leventhal 1981; Lozoff et al. 1977).

Finally, the birth of a high-risk infant may have major implications for family functioning. In early attempts at managing low-birth-weight infants, an apparent decrease in the attachment of mother and surviving infant was noted. Much recent work suggests that the bond between mother and critically ill infant may be disrupted such that inappropriate parenting results. In the extreme this may result in overprotectiveness or physical abuse, although the data on the latter may be questioned on methodological grounds. More subtle indications of this disruption include altered perceptions and attitudes toward the infant which might have adverse consequences on the child's future development (Green and Sonit 1964; Lozoff et al. 1977).

The etiology of this maladaptive parenting remains unclear. Early investigators linked these changes to separation of the mother and infant in the course of intensive management of the high-risk infant. Other work has suggested that the physical appearance of the child, parental anxiety generated by the critical status of the infant at birth, continued illness after discharge from the nursery, and temperamental differences in the infant may also contribute to altered parent-child interactions. Most likely many of these factors operate together.

Beyond the parent and infant interaction literature, the effect of high-risk infants on other aspects of family functioning has received little attention. Evidence from studies of children with other chronic or catastrophic illness suggests, however, that the usual patterns of family functioning may be substantially disrupted. Serious or chronic illness in children has been associated with marital instability, altered parental employment opportunities and family income, decreased social contacts and vacations as a result of the burden of care for the child and the lack of alternate care-givers, problems in other children in the family, and an increased workload for mothers. While the longer-term assessments of functioning in the families of low-birth-weight infants are just beginning to be addressed, at least one study supports these concerns. In this study, high levels of behavior problems were found among preschool very-low-birth-weight infants; these problems were associated with decreased performance on standardized IQ tests (Escalona 1982).

Finally, the degree of financial stress experienced by the families of high-risk infants is unknown. In the neonatal period, a substantial proportion of direct medical charges may be borne by the parents, up to 5 percent of the total for those with insurance and up to a third for those without insurance. The amount of postdischarge care, both inpatient and ambulatory, absorbed by the family is not known but likely to be high. In general 15 to 20 percent of the costs of hospital care and 70 percent of the costs of outpatient care and medical supplies for children are paid out of pocket by the family. Insurance coverage affects use of inpatient services regardless of health problems for low-birth-weight infants, and, in addition to insurance, family income affects the use of ambulatory services. Almost no information is available on indirect costs that are due to alterations in opportunities for maternal participation in the work force, time lost from work to obtain medical care, and other such factors, although the costs of visiting the child in the neonatal period have recently been estimated. Whatever the amount of the expenditures, the stress in some families is likely to be high because many are young parents just beginning their working lives.

The literature cited above indicates that low-birth-weight infants are at increased risk for a relatively lengthy list of health problems. In the terms introduced earlier in this report, the relative risk of morbidity increases for low-birth-weight infants compared to normal-birth-weight infants. In contrast to mortality, however, the magnitude of the increased relative risk is modest. By the end of the first year of life, low-birth-weight infants are only 1.6 times, and very-low-birth-weight infants 3.3 times, more likely to have a congenital anomaly or developmental delay than normal-birth-weight infants. Low-birth-weight infants account for 6 percent of all children with these conditions —about their representation in the population (Shapiro et al. 1980). Since the proportion of very-low-birth-weight survivors with serious illnesses diminishes rapidly after the first year, the effect of low-birth-weight infants on morbidity later in the preschool period is likely to be small. The potential of such infants later to experience school failure or behavioral problems cannot be estimated, but again the figure is unlikely to be as overwhelming as the effect of low birth weight on mortality.

At first this result seems inconsistent with data on increased relative risk of morbidity. However, birth weight confers a different relative risk for mortality than for morbidity; compared to a normal-birth-weight infant, an infant born weighing 1,500 grams or less is two hundred times more likely to die but only ten times more likely to experience developmental delay. In addition, because of their higher mortality rates, low-birth-weight infants constitute a lower proportion of survivors than other infants. This assessment must be tempered, however, by the realization that the full range of morbidity experienced by these infants is still being defined, that the full range may well be affected by changes in perinatal care, and that outcomes among the most recent group of very small babies, those ≤ 1,000 grams, are unclear. Moreover, although they represent a relatively small proportion of surviving children, these high-risk infants represent a relatively new population whose health problems require special services. This notion suggests that more research is required into the morbidity experiences of these infants and into effective management strategies.

Contribution of Changes in Mortality to Changes in Morbidity

Recent reviews of the outcomes among survivors of intensive care have documented decreases in the proportion of infants who experience adverse outcomes over time. The interpretation of such reviews must be cautious, however, since different studies show wide variation in the proportion who experience adverse outcome, and selection factors affecting referral to intensive care units might affect the results (Budetti et al. 1980; Stewart 1981).

More recent data based on clinical series and population-based morbidity surveys indicate that the increased survival of low-birth-weight infants has not been associated with an increase in the number with handicapping conditions. The proportion with severe congenital anomalies or developmental delay has remained the same; whereas, the proportion with less severe morbidity associated with antenatal and intrapartum events has declined. However, as noted earlier, concerns remain about the effect of increased survival of the very smallest infants, those less than 1,000 grams (Hack, Fanaroff, and Merkatz 1979; Shapiro et al. 1983).

Contribution of Congenital Malformation to Infant Mortality and Morbidity

Since many of the issues surrounding low birth weight also pertain to congenital malformations, this discussion will be brief and aimed at contrasting the two. The infant mortality rate due to malformations is about 2 per 1,000 live births. Malformations, however, are a major cause of mortality among normal-birth-weight infants, infants who would otherwise be at very low risk of adverse outcome.

In contrast, the neonatal mortality rate due to congenital malformations has remained relatively stable despite significant advances in techniques for the diagnosis and management of these conditions (Manniello and Farrell 1974). To understand this lack of change, consideration of the epidemiology of congenital anomalies is required.

There are four broad classes of causes for congenital malformations, and these account for varying percentages of major malformations. Many conditions are caused by single major mutant genes, for example, phenylketonuria (PKU), sickle-cell anemia, and hemophilia; collectively, monogenic conditions account for 7.5 percent of malformations. Another 6 percent can be attributed to chromosomal abnormalities like those causing Down syndrome. Conditions that appear to be due to interactions between hereditary susceptibility and some-as-yet-undefined nongenetic factor such as neural tube defects may account for another 20 percent. The etiology of the remainder can be attributed either to maternal illness or exposure to unidentified factors. Among maternal conditions, maternal illness (i.e., infection and diabetes) accounts for 3.5 percent of malformations, but the total contribution of maternal exposure to teratogenic or malformation-causing agents such as environmental chemicals, drugs, alcohol, and nutritional factors is unknown. Thus, less than half of major malformations have identifiable or predictable causes (Kalter and Warkany 1983).

Several problems emerge which affect the potential for reduction in mortality due to congenital anomalies:

1. The most successful prevention techniques apply only to the most infrequent conditions. The techniques thought most successful, for example, screening of high-risk populations and immunization against conditions that may cause intrauterine infections, all require that a specific cause or characteristic of the defect be detectable before an affected child is born or becomes symptomatic. As noted above, the majority of congenital anomalies do not have identifiable or predictable causes.

2. The multiplicity of types of congenital anomalies and the relatively low frequency of single anomalies is such that reduction in any single anomaly does not markedly affect mortality from these conditions as a whole.

3. Many preventive techniques are aimed less at altering mortality than long-term handicap. For example, among the most cost-effective programs are those that screen neonates for the presence of PKU and congenital hypothyroidism (or cretinism) in order to institute early treatment. Such programs, however, do not prevent the birth of children with these disorders.

4. Many potential techniques also involve parental awareness of risk to initiate behavioral changes before conception that will reduce risk prior to conception. Such changes include adequate nutrition, assessment of obstetric risk (e.g., immunization status for rubella, preexisting conditions such as high blood pressure), and changing adverse health habits such as smoking and drinking. Such approaches require a more deliberate approach to conception than is indicated by the current literature. In general, only a slight majority of women plan or intend their pregnancies, and those at highest risk for adverse pregnancy outcome are least likely to have a planned or intended pregnancy (Klerman and Jekel 1984). The very individual who could most benefit from prepregnancy interven-

tions may be least likely to receive them.

Estimates of the proportion of surviving children with congenital malformations depends to some extent on the data source used. Birth certificate data are the most comprehensive source but produce a substantial underestimate because many malformations are not recognized until after the infant goes home from the hospital. Establishing a more exact estimate of the prevalence of malformations depends on special studies of children systematically followed over time. These studies reveal that 1 percent of children will be recognized as having a severe malformation at birth; 2 percent will be recognized at one year of age; and 4 percent by age five. For total malformations, the figures are 3 percent, 9 percent, and 15 percent respectively (Christianson et al. 1981).

The overall contribution of congenital malformations to morbidity is difficult to assess because few data address this issue. Congenital malformations represent a major predictor of the use of hospital and ambulatory services in infancy. In addition, the increase in survival of infants with malformations may be contributing to the increase in the proportion of children reporting limits in activities of daily living due to health (Newacheck, Budetti, and McManus 1984). The reasons for this latter change remain to be determined, however.

The morbidity associated with specific conditions is better documented; for conditions like spina bifida, the morbidity and its attendant health care use is substantial. In fact, for some infants with malformations

the prognosis for future function is so limited that the use of intensive medical interventions to achieve survival may be questioned.

Risk Factors for Morbidity and Mortality

Not all infants are equally at risk for morbidity and mortality. Factors that alter the risk of illness include characteristics of the family and environment.

Socio-Demographic Characteristics

Characteristics of the family which affect the risk of illness in infancy are more well defined. The exact mechanism by which the risk is increased or decreased is not always clear.

Race. In the United States, black children are twice as likely as white children to be born at low birth weight and, as a result, experience twice the neonatal mortality rate. Black infants also experience higher rates of post-neonatal mortality, but this finding is not explained by lower birth weight (*Preventing Low Birthweight* 1985; Shapiro et al. 1980).

While many of the adverse health outcomes experienced by black infants are attributed to socioeconomic disadvantage, the exact mechanism is often unclear. This is particularly true regarding birth weight. Birth weight differentials between white and black infants persist even after controlling for socioeconomic factors such as maternal education. Moreover, other groups such as Hispanics who also experience socioeconomic disadvantage do not have the same level of adverse preganacy outcome. Interpretation of the data for the latter group is complicated because Hispanics represent an immigrant group that is known to be relatively healthier (*Preventing Low Birthweight* 1985).

In contrast to low birth weight, blacks are not at increased risk for congenital malformation on a population basis. Clearly, however, they are at increased risk for some specific conditions such as sickle-cell anemia.

Maternal Age. Maternal age at both extremes of the childbearing age-range increases the risk of infant mortality and morbidity. The reasons are different for younger as contrasted with older mothers.

The infants of young mothers are at increased risk of low birth weight, which accounts for their higher neonatal mortality rates. These infants also experience higher post-neonatal mortality and morbidity. The high risk of adverse infant outcome associated with adolescent preganacy may persist even when the mother grows older; the subsequent children of women who initiated their childbearing before age seventeen are also at high risk for neonatal and post-neonatal problems. Programs directed toward the problems of the adolescent mother are able to reduce the risk of adverse outcome but not able to achieve the low levels characteris-

tic of older, more advantaged mothers. In contrast to older mothers, young mothers are not at increased risk of congenital malformations (McCormick, Shapiro, and Starfield 1984).

Older maternal age (≥35) also increases the risk both of low birth weight and neonatal mortality. Even controlling for birth weight, however, neonatal mortality rates are still higher for infants of mothers thirty-five years or older. In part, this finding is explained by the increased risk of congenital anomalies which comes with advanced maternal age; the finding is paralled by increased risk of congenital anomalies and developmental delay among survivors. The infants of older mothers are not at increased risk for health problems in the post-neonatal period (Shapiro et al. 1980).

Maternal Education and Other Indicators of Socioeconomic Status. Maternal educational attainment is the most often used indicator of socioeconomic status and a strong correlate with many child health problems. Low maternal educational attainment is associated with higher neonatal morality as a result of an increased risk of low birth weight. The infants of mothers with low educational attainment also experience higher rates of post-neonatal mortality and illness due to environmentally related problems.

Prior Maternal Reproductive History

Previous adverse pregnancy outcome such as habitual spontaneous abortion, prior premature infants, difficulty in conceiving a child, short intervals between births, and previous stillbirth are all associated with increased risk of low birth weight and with neonatal mortality independent of birth weight factors. In addition, the proportion of children with congenital anomalies is also increased for women with prior adverse outcomes. Post-neonatal mortality and morbidity are not affected, however (Shapiro et al. 1980). Prior first trimester therapeutic abortions appear to confer little increased risk for adverse outcome in subsequent pregnancies in most situations (*Preventing Low Birthweight* 1985).

Parental Health Habits

Parental health habits also affect the risk of illness in their infants. For example, late or no prenatal care is associated with an increased risk of low birth weight. Both maternal cigarette and alcohol use increase the risk of low birth weight, although cigarette use is the greater contributer, and heavy maternal alcohol use increases the risk of the constellation of malformations labeled fetal alcohol syndrome. Finally, maternal exposure to radiation, certain drugs, and possibly some chemicals early in pregnancy may explain some malformations (*Preventing Low Birthweight* 1985).

As a general summary, risk factors associated socioeconomic disadvantage (young maternal age) confer a double hazard. With such factors the risk of low birth weight (and, therefore, death in the neonatal period) is increased, as is the risk of infection and deprivation, thus increasing the risk of ill health in the post-neonatal period. The risk of congenital malformations, however, is unaffected. In contrast, risk factors that reflect reproductive hazards (advanced maternal age) increase the risk of adverse neonatal outcome by increasing the risk of low birth weight and the risk of malformations.

Implications for Further Reductions in Infant Mortality and Morbidity

The extent to which some degree of morbidity and even mortality in infancy is unavoidable remains to be established. However, comparison with other developed countries suggests that using currently available techniques, the United States could lower its infant mortality substantially. Countries such as Sweden and Japan, and even Ireland and Spain, experience mortality rates lower than that of the United States (Wegman 1984). When rates for U.S. black and white births are compared separately, white mortality rates are comparable to those in other developed countries but black mortality rates are disproportionately high.

Three main approaches to reducing infant mortality appear possible. The first would rely on reducing the number of infants conceived or born to women at high risk of adverse outcome. This strategy, in turn, relies on risk identification and effective provision of family planning services or therapeutic abortion. With regard to low birth weight, this strategy has focused primarily on encouraging birth control among sexually active adolescents and among women with a previous low-birth-weight infant to achieve adequate spacing of subsequent pregnancies. The former group is of particular concern because, although women younger than twenty years of age account for 15 percent of the births in the country, they may account for about 25 percent of the low-birth-weight births. Moreover, their children remain vulnerable to a variety of health problems that partly reflect the limited social, emotional, and financial resources available to young mothers (Wegman 1984; McCormick, Shapiro, and Starfield 1984). The difficulties in providing services to adolescents are well known and include lack of education regarding sexuality and contraception, lack of access to contraceptive services due to financial barriers, geographic inaccessibility of family planning services, and attitudinal and legal restrictions on providing reproductive health services to young people.

Older women with many or frequent pregnancies contribute less to the overall low-birth-weight rate than do younger mothers. But targeting family planning services to older women offers the potential for reducing congenital malformations. However, the number of older mothers whose infants experience both problems is relatively small, so reduction of high-risk deliveries in this group is unlikely to affect by much the total number of infants born with problems.

Identifying other high-risk women involves screening procedures in groups known to carry genetic disorders (e.g., Tay-Sacks disease in Ashkenazi Jews; sickle-cell disease in blacks) or in families in which one or more affected children have already been born. Since relatively few such conditions occur, the use of this strategy is limited.

Alternatively, identification of women at risk due to adverse health and reduction of risk prior to conception appears to have greater potential. In particular, discouraging cigarette and alcohol use prior to conception offers opportunities for reducing adverse outcome. But because many women do not visit an obstetric health provider until after conception, the methods to encourage other types of health providers to initiate preventive strategies need to be developed.

For both low birth weight and malformation, access to therapeutic abortion is an additional strategy for preventing the birth of an affected infant. With regard to low birth weight, access to abortion is most important for adolescent women. With regard to malformation, this strategy must be coupled with screening procedures to identify affected fetuses; such procedures include amniocentesis to recover fetal cells for culture, which predicts chromosomal and chemical abnormalities, or maternal serum alpha-fetal protein screening, which predicts open spina bifida.

Indirect evidence suggests that the prevention of conception or birth among high-risk women has contributed to recent declines in infant mortality. For example, the birth rate has declined, and these declines have occurred disproportionately among older women with large numbers of children. In addition, neonatal mortality rates have declined in areas with access to family planning and abortion services. Finally, the age of mothers delivering children with chromosomal anomalies (e.g., Down's syndrome) has shifted downward as older women (>35 years of age) avail themselves of amniocentesis and abortion. Nonetheless, the magnitude of the effect is small, accounting for less than 20 percent of the decline in neonatal mortality (Morris, Idry, and Chase 1975; Hadley 1982).

The extent to which more aggressive policies with regard to family planning services and therapeutic abortion might affect infant mortality and morbidity is difficult to estimate. Moreover, implementation of such strategies may be difficult for the following reasons:

1. As noted earlier, groups at greatest risk for adverse outcome may be least able to implement preventive approaches. I have indicated some of the barriers confronting adolescent women, but these problems are not unique to young women. Further work is required to identify and reduce the financial and cultural barriers to family planning services.

2. Many high-risk women are among those least likely to plan their pregnancies. Currently, about 50 percent of pregnancies are planned or intended, but among disadvantaged women less than 25 percent are planned.

3. Both of the above concerns suggest that strategies that rely on immediate preconceptional care may be limited. More generalized approaches that might involve aggressive provision of prepregnancy care in school or work settings by screening for risk factors run the risk of reinforcing the stereotype that all women are always at risk of being pregnant. Depending on the circumstances, such strategies may appear inappropriate (e.g., for adolescents whose psychological immaturity limits any sexual activity) or offensive. Such approaches are also relatively new, and their efficacy needs to be established.

4. Strategies of early detection and termination of affected fetuses involve technical concerns about the timing, availability, precision, and adverse effects of screening procedures. In addition, current techniques require precise gestational age information (i.e., duration of pregnancy) because the standards for many tests and ability to perform amniocentesis and abortion pertain to a relatively limited interval in pregnancy. Therefore, access to and early initiation of prenatal care is required.

5. Ethical beliefs may affect decisions regarding abortion, even when the procedure is technically feasible. Thus, programs aimed at reducing the birth of affected infants, especially those with malformations, may never achieve expected goals.

6. Although the etiology of most malformations, and the exact precipitating factors for preterm labor leading to low birth weight, are unknown, characteristics of women's work environments have been suspect. With malformations, concerns include exposure to potentially teratogenic chemicals; with low birth weight, ex-

posure to physical fatigue and psychological distress. In either case, policies directed toward reduction of workplace risks raise questions concerning legal liability and equal workforce participation by women.

7. Finally, the risk of adverse outcome is still relatively low. Only about 7 percent of infants have low birth weight; 2 percent have serious malformations. Preconceptional strategies to prevent adverse outcomes may involve substantial changes in personal habits (e.g., smoking cessation, change in work activities, etc.), which may be perceived as disproportionate to risk. More needs to be known about how women make decisions about such trade-offs.

The second major approach involves improving pregnancy outcomes among fetuses recognized as having a malformation or at high risk of low birth weight. For malformations, techniques for detecting malformation or altering outcome are limited. Only a few conditions can be treated with fetal surgery or transfusion. Such approaches and other potential fetal therapies are very preliminary, and their effectiveness remains to be established.

In contrast, prenatal intervention with current techniques holds more promise for the prevention of low birth weight. To address this issue, however, the distinction between low birth weight due to preterm delivery and that due to intrauterine growth retardation assumes importance. Also, the efficacy of specific interventions compared to the package of services called "antenatal care" require discussion.

Low-weight births appear to have declined primarily among the segment characterized by intrauterine growth retardation; in proportion, little change has occurred among low-weight births considered preterm. This finding suggests that intervention aimed at preventing intrauterine growth retardation has been more successful than that aimed at preterm delivery, but the identification of which strategies have produced the change is difficult. First, a large number of conditions, each contributing only a small percentage of cases, may result in intrauterine growth retardation. Conditions range from intrauterine infections such as congenital rubella (German measles) to maternal conditions such as hypertension (high blood pressure) and diabetes. The range of preventive interventions is also broad, from immunization programs in infancy to screening and treatment for chronic maternal illnesses. In addition, some conditions may not become apparent until pregnancy or may be worsened by pregnancy and may not be modifiable by prepregnancy strategies. Much of the routine screening and monitoring in the course of antenatal care is aimed at the detection and management of such conditions, particularly in the last third of pregnancy. The decline in births with insufficient growth for any gestation duration provides some support for such activities as a whole but does not make clear the most effective activities or future directions for improving services (*Preventing Low Birthweight* 1985).

In contrast, interventions to prevent preterm deliveries are now being developed. To some extent, the development of such strategies is dependent on research into the basic mechanisms that result in the initiation of labor and delivery before term. At least two approaches are currently being assessed. One emerges from the observation that the placental tissues in preterm deliveries exhibit more evidence of inflammation and that women with preterm deliveries have higher rates of a variety of vaginal infections. These findings have led to a trial of earlier, more aggressive screening and treatment of vaginal infections to prevent preterm delivery. Another approach reflects the observation that preterm labor may be heralded by specific symptoms experienced by the mother or changes in the appearance of the cervix. Potentially, these signs and symptoms could lead to treatment (such as bed rest and labor-inhibiting drugs) at a stage when progress to delivery could be halted. Currently being tested is a program for women at high risk for preterm delivery; the program combines education in the symptoms and responses to uterine contractions that might result in labor, a more intensive schedule of antenatal visits, and earlier intervention with labor-inhibiting regimens (*Preventing Low Birthweight* 1985).

Other specific strategies have been directed toward low birth weight in general. These include smoking cessation programs, nutritional supplements, and efforts to provide psychosocial support and reduce physical and psychological stress, especially among high-risk women. Among these strategies, smoking cessation may offer the most potential of any single intervention for increasing birth weight (*Preventing Low Birthweight* 1985).

While increasing nutritional intake makes intuitive sense when trying to increase growth, the results of specific nutritional intervention studies have been disappointing. Although increase in birth weight has been reported, the amount of weight gained on average has been very small (one to two ounces). Larger increases in birth weight have been reported for women receiving nutritional supplements through a special program (Supplemental Food Program for Women, Infants, and Children— [WIC]), but various interpretations of these findings are possible. The characteristics of women who receive WIC and those who do not are very different; the complex character of the program itself, which is designed to assure access to services as well as food, makes a specific interpretation difficult.

Least well supported by evidence of effectiveness are interventions designed to enhance participation in antenatal care and to alleviate environmental stress. Again such programs make intuitive sense based on the vast literature documenting financial and cultural barriers to health services, the levels of environmental stress in the lives of disadvantaged women, and the potential for strenuous physical activities to precipitate preterm labor. While interventions such as outreach, advocacy, counseling, and rest may be helpful, documentation of their efficacy is fraught with methodological pitfalls, including definition of the risk factors (e.g., psychosocial stress) and determination of the appropriateness and power of currently available interventions to relieve the effects of these risk factors (*Preventing Low Birthweight* 1985).

The foregoing shows that the problem of low birth weight may involve several causes; its prevention may require an equal number of interventions that must be tailored to needs of individual women. The services may also vary from site to site, depending on the expertise of the staff, and over time, as new knowledge evolves concerning risks and treatments. With this heterogeneity, documenting the effect of the package of services called "prenatal care" proves difficult. Nonetheless, with certain caveats, the evidence supports the conclusion that antenatal care reduces low birth weight. The evidence is of two types:

1. From data on the birth certificate, many studies have shown a clear association between the start of antenatal care (or number of visits) and birth weight. Those who start care early (or have an appropriate number of visits) have better outcomes. Even controlling for factors known to affect outcome (e.g., maternal age) or probability of receiving adequate care (i.e., adjusting the number of visits for the duration of gestation) does not eliminate this effect.

2. Specific programs aimed at providing prenatal care (or enhancing it) to high-risk populations have shown increases in birth weight among women enrolled in the programs.

While the evidence generally supports a positive effect of prenatal care in reducing the rate of low-birth-weight infants, estimating the potential effect of increased access to prenatal services proves difficult. In part this difficulty reflects the fact noted earlier that "prenatal care" is not a single, well-defined set of services but varies in content from site to site and over time. In addition, in the absence of true experimental designs that are ethically impossible, factors that encourage women to enroll for prenatal care at different times and in different programs may substantially affect the outcome of pregnancy independent of the type of services provided. Moreover, particularly with birth certificate data, the quality of the information that characterizes prenatal care may be inadequate. Information on other factors affecting pregnancy outcome may be unavailable. For special programs, information not only on the content of the program but also on the effect of the novelty of any new effort on both providers and patients may not be specified. The effect of regionalized services in reducing neonatal mortality by increasing the proportion of infants delivered in and receiving intensive care has been already noted. Whether such organized services contribute to decreases in low-birth-weight rates remains to be established.

The third major approach is to increase the survival of high-risk infants, in part through the increased use of intensive care. Besides the cost and risk of adverse sequelae associated with this approach, concerns have emerged about the limits of current technology. Over the past few years, the survival rates among infants admitted to intensive care units appear to have stabilized. Continued declines reflect increases in the proportion of high-risk infants born in or transported to these tertiary centers.

In many areas, however, the majority of such infants are already being born in tertiary centers; thus we may be reaching the potential limits of current technology to reduce further neonatal mortality.

Three generic issues underlay all three major approaches: availability of providers, access to services and payment for services. Any discussion of the availability of providers involves the type and number, their education, and their geographic distribution. The major providers of prenatal and neonatal services are obstetricians-gynecologists, family practitioners, nurse-midwives, and neonatologists. Despite increases in the number of family practitioners and nurse-midwives, obstetrician-gynecologists still deliver most of reproductive care to women, including family planning, and prenatal and delivery services. However, many obstetrician-gynecologists are focusing more on gynecologic (e.g., gynecologic surgery, preventive care, etc.) than on obstetric services due to the rapid increase in malpractice insurance for obstetric practice and the inadequacy of payment, especially public payment, for obstetric services. The alternative of replacing obstetricians with family practitioners and nurse-midwives applies only to low-risk pregnancies. Even for a low-risk practice, malpractice and payment issues may affect family practitioners as well. The use of nurse-midwives has been advocated to provide services for low-risk pregnancies, and to provide additional supportive and educational services to disadvantaged women in conjunction with routine obstetric care. Only limited data are available to assess the poential effect of the deployment of such providers in improving obstetric outcome, and the issues concerning the training and independence of nurse-midwives remain to be resolved. While these pressures move to reduce or at least maintain the status quo of obstetric providers, the alternative pressure of an excess number of physicians may increase physician obstetrical services and availability, but at the potential of increasing costs.

In contrast to obstetricians, neonatologists are sufficiently available and may actually exceed the number required to provide services. An excessive number of such subspecialists also presents problems. It encourages the development of intensive care units in smaller community hospitals where the number of high-risk neonates may not be large enough to maintain intensive care skills among providers. Pressures to maintain high occupancy rates in order to pay for these expensive services will discourage referrals to centers better able to manage the infants. Thus, the development of such units in community hospitals may lead to disruption of referral patterns and regional organization of services, which have contributed to the current decline in neonatal mortality. Reduction in the number of new neonatologists requires altering staffing patterns in university neonatal intensive care units, which depend heavily on trainees for services.

Access to services is dependent on physical availability, knowledge, cultural acceptability, and adequate financing. Indirect evidence suggests that in some areas, adequate family planning, and prenatal, and perinatal services may not be available. The constraints on provider participation have been noted. Anecdotal evidence suggests that the current rearrangement and reduction of federal funding has reduced availability for some subgroups. Finally, attitudes and inadequate knowledge about appropriate use of services may hamper receipt of services for some subgroups in the population. The extent to which these factors account for adverse neonatal outcome is unknown. Equally uncertain are the potential gains from a variety of strategies aimed at increasing use of reproductive services. This is not to argue that other substantial benefits may not result from providing outreach workers, and transport and child care services, to facilitate use of health care, but little data exists to allow estimates of potential effects.

More substantial evidence underlies the assertion that the financing of care, especially for diadvantaged groups, is inadequate. Disadvantaged groups have to rely on a nonsystematic patchwork of services, each with different eligibility requirements and benefits, funded by a variety of federal agencies: WIC through the Department of Agriculture; special maternal and child health programs funded by the Department of Health and Human Services; public health departments (state, county, and city); and joint federal/state programs such as Medicaid, Crippled Children's, and family planning services. Even those with private insurance may find that pregnancy care or hospital care for neonates born with congenital malformations or at low birth weight is not covered, resulting in high out-of-pocket costs or debt for young families with few resources. Thus, the efficacy of prenatal and neonatal services may not be realized because of lack of access. Barriers may result from lack of financial resources or inability to negotiate the complex system of public support for these services.

Moreover, current approaches to cost containment may exacerbate the difficulty of obtaining care for certain subgroups in the population. Such strategies as "case management" in which the primary care provider coordinates services for patients and is at financial risk for referral services, and "preferred provider options" in which the full cost of care is insured only if the patient uses specified providers and hospitals, may limit access to special services required by the relatively few women with problems and may disrupt existing referral networks designed to deal with such problems.

In summary, changes in infant mortality early in the century shifted the major causes of infant loss to events during pregnancy and delivery. We have examined two broad categories of such events: low birth weight and congenital malformations. For both groups, current decreases in mortality have resulted from the application of hospital-based technology in the perinatal period. Further reduction in infant mortality will require the prevention of these high-risk births, but preventive strategies raise a host of questions concerning individual and social attitudes toward childbearing and the efficacy of current preventive techniques.

Acknowledgment

Part of this chapter appeared in a modified version of a report prepared for the Committee for the Study of Strategies for the prevention of Low Birthweight, Institute of Medicine, National Academy of Sciences, Washington, D.C., and subsequently published in the *New England Journal of Medicine* 312 (1985): 82–90.

References

Budetti, P., P. McManus, H. Banand, and L. Heinen. 1980. *The implications of cost-effectiveness analysis of medical technology.* Background paper no. 2: *Case studies of medical technologies (neonatal intensive care).* Office of Technology Assessment, OTA-BO-H-9(10). Washington, D.C.: Government Printing Office.

Christianson, R. E., B. J. Van den Berg, L. Milkovich, and F. W. Oeschli. 1981. Incidence of congenital anomalies among white and black births with long-term follow-up. *American Journal of Public Health* 71:1333–1341.

Escalona, S. K. 1982. Babies at double hazard: Early development of infants at biologic and social risk. *Pediatrics* 71:376–382.

Green, M., and A. J. Solnit. 1964. Reactions to the threatened loss of a child: A vulnerable child syndrome: Pediatric management of the dying child. *Pediatrics* 34:58–66.

Hack, M., D. DeMonterice, I. R. Merkatz, and A. M. Fanaroff. 1981. Rehospitalization of the very low birthweight infant: A continuation of perinatal and environmental morbidity. *American Journal of the Disease of Children* 135:263–266.

Hack, M., A. A. Fanaroff, and I. R. Merkatz. 1979: The low-birthweight infant: Evolution of a changing outlook. *New England Journal of Medicine* 301: 1162–1165.

Hadley, J. 1982. *More medical care, better health?* Washington D. C.: Urban Institute.

Hardy, J. B., J. S. Drage, and E. C. Jackson. 1979. *The first year of life: the collaborative perinatal study of the National Institute of Neurologic and Communicative Disorders and Stroke.* Baltimore: Johns Hopkins University Press.

Kalter, H. and J. Warkany. 1983. Congenital malformations: Etiologic factors and the role in prevention. *New England Journal of Medicine* 308:424–431, 491–497.

Kessel, S. S., J. Villar, and H. W. Berendes. 1984. The changing pattern of low birthweight in the United States, 1970–80. *Journal of the American Medical Association* 251:1978–1982.

Klein, N., M. Hack, J. Gallagher, and A. M. Fanaroff. 1985. Preschool performance of children with normal intelligence who were very low-birth-weight interests. *Pediatrics* 75:531:537.

Klerman, L. V., and J. F. Jekel. 1984. Unwanted pregnancy. In *Perinatal epidemiology*, ed. M. B. Bracken. New York: Oxford University Press.

Leventhal, J. M. 1981. Risk factors for child abuse: Methodologic standards in case-control studies. *Pediatrics* 68:684–690.

Lozoff, B., G. M. Brittenham, M. A. Trause, J. H. Kennell, and M. H. Klaus. 1977. The mother-newborn relationship: Limits of adaptability. *Journal of Pediatrics* 91 (1977):1–12.

McCormick, M. C. 1985. Contribution of low birthweight to infant mortality and childhood morbidity. *New England Journal of Medicine* 312:82–90.

McCormick, M. C., S. Shapiro, and B. H. Starfield, 1980. Rehospitalization in the first year of life for high-risk survivors. *Pediatrics* 66:991–999.

――――. 1981a. Factors associated with the use of hospital ambulatory and preventive services among infants using different sources of ambulatory care. Paper presented at the Ambulatory Pediatric Association meeting, San Francisco, Calif.

――――. 1981b. Injury and its correlates among 1-year-old children. *American Journal of the Disease of Children* 135:159–163.

――――. 1984. High-risk mothers: Infant mortality and morbidity in four areas of the United States, 1973–1978. *American Journal of Public Health* 74:18–23.

Maniello, R. L., and P. M. Farrell, 1977. Analysis of United States neonatal mortality statistics from 1968 to 1974, with specific reference to changing trends in major casualties. *American Journal of Obstetrics and Gynecology* 129:667–674.

Morris, N. M., J. R. Idry, and C. L. Chase. 1975. Shifting age-parity distribution of births and the decrease in infant mortality. *American Journal of Public Health* 65:359–362.

Newacheck, P. W., P. P. Budetti, and P. McManus. 1984. Trends in childhood disability. *American Journal of Public Health* 74:232–236.

Pharoah, P. O. D., and J. N. Morris. 1978. Post-neonatal mortality. *Epidemiological Reviews* 1:170–183.

Preventing low birthweight. 1985. Washington D.C.: National Academy of Sciences/Institute of Medicine.

Ramey, C. T., D. J. Stedman, A. Borders-Patterson, and W. Mengel. 1978. Predicting school failure from information available at birth. *American Journal of Mental Deficiency* 82:525–534.

Shapiro, S., M. C. McCormick, B. H. Starfield, and B. Crawley. 1983. Changes in morbidity associated with decreases in neonatal mortality. *Pediatrics* 72:408–415.

Shapiro, S., M. C. McCormick, B. H. Starfield, J. P. Krischer, and D. Bross. 1980. Relevance of correlates of infant deaths for significant morbidity at 1 year of age. *American Journal of Obstetrics and Gynecology* 136:363–373.

Shapiro, S., E. R. Schlesinger, and R. E. L. Nesbitt. 1968. *Infant, perinatal, ma-*

ternal, and childhood mortality in the United States. Cambridge: Harvard University Press.

Silverman, W. A. 1980. *Retrolental fibroplasia: A modern parable.* New York: Grune and Stratton

Starfield, B., S. Shapiro, M. C. McCormick, and D. Bross. 1982. Mortality and morbidity in infants with intrauterine growth retardation. *Journal of Pediatrics* 101:978–983.

Stewart, A. L. 1981. Outcomes of infants of very low birthweight: Survey of world literature. *Lancet* 1:1038–1041.

U.S. Department of Health and Human Services. 1982. *Health United States.* Publication No. (PHS)83-1232. Hyattsville, Md.: Government Printing Office.

Wegman, M. E. 1984. Annual summary of vital statistics, 1983. *Pediatrics* 74 (1984):981–990.

Williams, R. L., R. K. Creasy, G. C. Cunningham, W. E. Hawes, F. D. Norris, and M. Tashiro. 1982. Fetal growth and perinatal viability in California. *Obstetrics and Gynecology* 59:624–632.

Chapter 15

Teenage Childbearing
Causes, Consequences, and Remedies

*Frank F. Furstenberg, Jr., and
Jeanne Brooks-Gunn*

ll societies devise means of managing sexuality in order to regulate reproduction. The task is rarely accomplished without some strain. Control of youthful sexuality was considered a problem in American society long before the 1960s, when the so-called sexual revolution occurred. Nonvirginity at marriage was common at the beginning of the century; by the 1950s, it is estimated that a quarter of all marriages involved pregnant teenage brides (Kinsey et al. 1953; Degler 1980). Since the 1960s, however, adolescent pregnancy has increasingly aroused public concern. This chapter reviews recent evidence on the causes and consequences of childbearing among adolescents, especially those under eighteen, and assesses what is presently known about preventive and ameliorative strategies. Our summary draws upon our own research and also makes use of several excellent sourcebooks. Since we cannot give full treatment to many important topics, readers may wish to consult the following references for more detailed information: Alan Guttmacher Institute 1981; Chilman 1983; Furstenberg, Lincoln, and Menken 1981; McAnarney and Schreider 1984; Moore and Burt 1982. Our aim is to identify and discuss key research issues of interest to practitioners and policy analysts.

Changing Patterns of Adolescent Sexual Activity, Pregnancy, and Childbearing

Adolescent fertility has decreased in recent decades, but authorities today probably view the issue with greater concern than they did two decades ago when the incidence of early childbearing was much higher. The following section addresses this apparent contradiction.

Table 15.1 displays different indicators of trends in adolescent fertility. The data are shown by race because a substantial and disproportionate share of early childbearing occurs among blacks. In absolute numbers, fewer teenage females among both whites and nonwhites are becoming mothers today than a decade ago. Since 1960, just after the peak of the baby boom, rates of early childbearing have been declining. Even among teens under eighteen the rates have decreased, although the decline is much less dramatic among whites than blacks.

In contrast with earlier periods, the majority (51 percent) of teens who bear children today do so out of wedlock. Most teens who became mothers in the 1950s and 1960s were married before or soon after they became pregnant. Indeed the incidence of nonmarital childbearing among the young has increased over the past several decades as is shown in table 15.2. Twenty-seven percent of black and 4 percent of white unmarried adolescents born in the late 1950s be-

came mothers by the end of their eighteenth year (U.S. Dept. of Commerce, Bureau of Census 1984).

Were it not for the legalization of abortion, the incidence of early childbearing would be much higher (Dryfoos 1982). About half of all pregnancies among teenagers under the age of eighteen are terminated voluntarily. The incidence of abortion has not increased in the past few years, but the overall number of abortions among teenagers is an area of major political concern (Petchesky 1982).

Two conspicuous demographic changes largely account for the growth of abortion and the rising proportion of out-of-wedlock births. Starting in the 1960s and accelerating in the 1970s, a sharp increase took place in the incidence of sexual activity among adolescents. It was accompanied by other changes in the lifestyle of youth—increased drug and alcohol use and probably greater tolerance for nonconforming behavior in general. Some of these changes can be traced to the emergence of "youth culture" in the Vietnam era, the cultivation of a huge youth market by commercial interests, and the gradual decline of restrictive sexual standards in the adult population. The availability of oral contraceptives, and eventually, legalized abortions, probably also contributed to the changing sexual climate, though these factors are probably best seen as both causes and consequences of the sexual transformation.

The proportion of teenage women who had experienced intercourse rose by two-thirds during the 1970s. The increase was especially large for whites and younger teens because

TABLE 15.1

Adolescent Fertility by Race, 1955–1983

Age/Race	1955	1960	1970	1980	1983
	Number of Births (in thousands)				
15–19					
Total**	484	587	645	552	489
White	373	459	464	388	338
Black	111*	129*	172	150	137
18–19					
Total	334	405	421	354	317
White	269	329	320	260	229
Black	65*	76*	95	84	79
15–17					
Total	150	180	224	198	173
White	104	130	144	128	110
Black	46*	53*	77	66	58
<15					
Total	6	7	12	10	10
White	2	3	4	4	4
Black	4*	4*	7	6	5
	Birthrates (per 1,000 women)				
15–19					
Total	90.3	89.1*	68.3	53.0	51.7
White	79.1	79.4	57.4	44.7	43.6
Black	167.2*	156.1*	147.7	100.0	95.5
18–19					
Total	—	—	114.7	82.1	78.1
White	—	—	101.5	72.1	68.3
Black	—	—	204.9	138.8	130.4
15–17					
Total	—	—	38.8	32.5	32.0
White	—	—	29.2	25.2	24.8
Black	—	—	101.4	73.6	70.1
10–14					
Total	0.9	0.8	1.2	1.1	1.1
White	0.3	0.4	0.5	0.6	0.6
Black	4.8*	4.3*	5.2	4.3	4.1

(continued on next page)

TABLE 15.1 (continued)
Adolescent Fertility by Race, 1955–1983

Age/Race	1955	1960	1970	1980	1983
Out-of-Wedlock Birthrates (per 1,000 unmarried women)					
15–19					
Total	15.1	15.3	22.4	27.6	29.7
White	6.0	6.6	10.9	16.2	18.5
Black	77.6*	76.5*	96.9	89.2	86.4
Out-of-Wedlock Births (per 1,000 births)					
15–19					
Total	143	148	295	476	534
White	64	72	171	330	391
Black	407*	421*	628	851	883
18–19					
Total	102	107	224	398	457
White	49	54	135	270	323
Black	324*	337*	521	792	835
15–17					
Total	232	240	430	615	676
White	102	116	252	452	527
Black	524*	543*	760	928	948
<15					
Total	663	679	808	887	904
White	421	475	579	754	799
Black	801*	822*	935	985	984

Sources: Moore, Simms, and Betsey 1984; Collaborative Perinatal Study 1984; U.S. Department of Commerce, Bureau of the Census 1984; National Center for Health Statistics 1985.

* Includes all nonwhites, not only blacks.

**All totals include all nonwhites, which is somewhat more than the sum of whites plus blacks.

they started from a lower baseline. By 1979 close to half of all teen females were sexually active; about a third of those between ages fifteen and seventeen were nonvirgins (Zelnik and Kantner 1980).

Marital timing also contributed in important ways to the growth of out-of-wedlock pregnancies and child-bearing among the young. During the baby boom period, marriage age had declined significantly; in the 1960s it reversed direction, and throughout the 1970s to the present has continued to rise. In 1970, 31.2 percent of all females were married by the age of

TABLE 15.2

Women Aged 18 or Younger Having a First Birth, by Race, Birth Cohort, and Marital Status (percentage)

Birth Cohort of Women	1935–1939	1945–1949	1955–1959
All Races			
Married	12.9	9.3	8.5
Unmarried	4.5	5.0	7.1
Whites			
Married	13.1	9.5	9.1
Unmarried	2.7	2.7	3.9
Blacks*			
Married	12.1	9.0	5.2
Unmarried	18.8	23.6	26.9

*Nonwhite
Source: National Center for Health Statistics 1985.

nineteen. By 1983 this proportion had dropped to 16.6 percent (U.S. Dept. of Commerce, Bureau of the Census 1983b). There are probably many reasons for this change: the extension of education; the poor job prospects for young adults; the entrance of women into the labor force in greater numbers; the acceptability of cohabitation and nonmarital sex; and, perhaps, the declining social value placed on marriage (Thornton and Freedman 1983). In the 1950s most teenagers were able to delay intercourse until they were of marriageable age, even if they often did not wait until they were actually married. Today, if teenagers employed a similar strategy, they would need to wait until they were in their early or middle twenties. Thus, the once-secure connection between the onset of sexual activity and marriage has been severed, providing no anchor point for the sexual debut.

All studies of the antecedents of sexual activity in early adolescents show that the major contributing factors to the sexual transition may greatly differ for blacks and whites and certainly vary for males and females (McAnarney and Schneider 1984; Zelnik, Kantner and Ford 1981). Existing research indicates that most teens do not consciously plan to become sexually active, and they often do not foresee the first sexual experience. As such, it frequently is not experienced as a decision but rather as something that happens to them (Frank 1983; Rains 1971; Chilman 1983).

A larger proportion of younger than older teens are initiated into sexual activity by friends or acquaintances than by steady dating partners (Zelnik, Kantner, and Ford 1981; Zelnik and Shah 1983). Younger females are often pressured or coerced into having sex by males who are ill prepared to assume responsibility should a pregnancy occur. The timing of sexual activity is also clearly affected by the immediate social world of the teenager (Coates, Peterson, and Perry 1982). Part of that world, of course, is conveyed symbolically through the mass media. The lyrics of popular music, films, MTV and television, and magazines all portray sexual experience as attractive and cost free. The sexual standards of popular culture inevitably are channeled through the media to the social world of adolescents, affecting their attitudes and actions.

Adolescents' sexual behavior resembles the behavior of their peers and, even more, perceptions of their peers' sexual experience. In the National Survey of Children, a nationwide study of youth carried out in 1981, 47 percent of the fifteen- and sixteen-year-olds who said that they had many sexually experienced friends were nonvirgins as compared to 10 percent who said that few or none of their friends were sexually experienced (see Furstenberg, Moore, and Peterson 1985). Of course, teenagers, females in particular, project their own experiences to their friends, and they may also be more likely to select friends who have experiences similar to their own; but their actions are sometimes regulated by the behavior of their close friends (Billy, Rodgers, and Udry 1981). The adolescent's desire to be accepted by

peers may encourage some to engage in early intercourse.

Peer influence can be controlled in part by parents (Fox 1981). Families may be able to choose to live in neighborhoods or to send their children to schools where early intercourse is not the norm. Families with more economic resources can exercise much greater control over their teens' behavior while poorer parents, especially poor blacks, are at a great disadvantage in selecting areas that decrease the risk of early sexual activity. Parents who effectively supervise their children may be able to restrict the opportunity for early intercourse. Children are at greater risk of early sexual activity if they live in a single-parent family or if they are unsupervised in the afternoons and evenings (Zelnik, Kantner, and Ford 1981; Moore, Simms, and Betsey 1984).

Parents may also restrict early coitus by explicit appeals to their children to delay intercourse. The evidence on the effect of parental communication about sexual matters is mixed, partly because most parents avoid extensive discussions about sexual matters (Thornberg 1975). Parents who have close relations with their children may be more effective in getting them to conform to parental expectations, which typically discourage early sexual experience. Parents who communicate more easily and openly with their adolescents may also discourage them from being overly dependent on peers. And, there is a widespread belief supported only by inconsistent evidence that more open communication encourages sexually active teens to use contraception (Fox, Fox, and Frohardt-Lane 1982; Furstenberg et al. 1983). Newcomer and Udry (1984) have challenged the belief that parents exert much influence on their teenagers' sexual behavior through social communication. They contend that a generational link exists because of two inheritable biological traits: the age of menarche affects the timing of intercourse and fecundity affects the probability of pregnancy. Thus, girls resemble their mothers' fertility pattern because they share biological characteristics that shape the probability of early intercourse and risk of pregnancy.

Use of Contraception Among Sexually Active Adolescents

Rates of sexual activity among teens in the United States are not notably higher than rates in several countries in Western Europe. Yet the incidence of pregnancy and childbearing in the United States, especially among younger teens, exceeds the level of most other industrialized nations (Westoff, Calot, and Foster 1983; Jones et al. 1985). This is partly due to poor contraceptive use among American youth. Case studies conducted by the Alan Guttmacher Institute suggest that American youth are exposed to mixed messages about contraception and that birth control services are not effectively delivered to the teenage population (Jones et al. 1985).

Consider the case of the typical teenage female as she enters her sexual career. In all likelihood, she has never had any explicit or extensive discussions with her parents about the pros and cons of sexual activity, her responsibilities if she does become sexually active, the procedure for obtaining birth control, and the advantages or disadvantages of different methods. (If the teenager is a male, he is probably even less likely to have received adequate sexual socialization from his family.) If she has received sexual information in school, she has probably been supplied with some facts about human reproduction, descriptions of sexually transmitted diseases, and some general discussion about values in human relationships; this information was probably taught as a brief unit in a health or biology course.

Our hypothetical adolescent, like most of her peers, probably feels confused and very ambivalent about becoming sexually active. Consequently, her first experience of intercourse is not planned or clearly foreseen. She probably did not discuss birth control with her partner. Afterward, she almost certainly will conceal the occurrence from her parents though she may confide in a close friend. Particularly if she is in her early teens, she may not have intercourse again in the next month, and she is likely to continue to have sexual relations only on an episodic basis for some time.

This teenager may know about methods of birth control, she may even know the location of a local birth control clinic, but she may have also heard that "pills are dangerous to use," that "parents must give their permission," or that "you go through an embarrassing examination" if you visit a clinic. If she has a family doctor, she probably has not seen that person for some time and does not feel comfortable acknowledging that she is sexually active or asking her parents for advice. For all of these reasons, our typical adolescent takes no action until a year or so later, sometimes only after she has missed her period. At this point, she may make a hurried call to the local clinic, tell her parents, or seek help from a private physician. If she is lucky, it is not too late.

If her pregnancy scare turns out to be a false alarm and she receives birth control, the scenario continues. Whether she enters a clinic or receives private services, she is likely to be provided with oral contraceptives. If her parents and friends do not know that she is sexually active, she must take the pills on the sly. Although she has been told to call back the clinic or her doctor if she experiences any physical side effects, she remains fearful about the effects of the pill. If she experiences any symptoms, she is probably just as likely to stop taking the pill as she is to seek assistance. Especially if she is having intercourse only occasionally, she may decide not to take the pill on a daily basis. She is reluctant to think of herself as the kind of girl who is prepared to have sex. Besides, if she has sex only once or twice a month, she believes that her risks of becoming pregnant are small. She may begin skipping the pill occasionally and gradually discontinue use. Or she may lose her pill

supply and never get around to going back to the clinic. And so, our typical teenager who has been equipped with contraception is once again at risk of becoming pregnant.

Most but not all teenagers follow this scenario. Over half of all teenagers do not use contraception the first time they have sexual relations, and the majority do not practice birth control regularly thereafter (Zelnik and Shah 1983). Most teenagers who use clinic services have been sexually active for a year or more before their initial visit (Zabin, Kantner, and Zelnik 1979). About a third of the teens who come to clinics do not return for the required follow-up visits (Shea, Herceg-Baron, and Furstenberg 1984). One study that followed up clinic attenders found that, after they first received birth control, only 40 percent used contraception every time they had intercourse over a fifteen-month period (Furstenberg et al. 1983).

Not surprisingly, teenagers who experience physical side effects from birth control are more likely to stop. Also, teenagers who have sex only occasionally and are not in steady dating relations are less likely to practice contraception faithfully. Several studies have shown that teenagers who come from better-educated families and who, themselves, have higher educational ambitions are better contraceptors (Moore, Simms, and Betsey 1984).

Some attempts have been made to develop a psychological profile of poor contraceptors. In general, it is not easy to identify psychological characteristics associated with ineffective use of birth control. High-risk takers, as might be expected, are prone to discontinuation, but many other standard psychological attributes have low or no predictive ability to distinguish continuous users from dropouts (Mindick and Oskamp 1982). Even reasonably well-motivated and psychologically robust teenagers will be imperfect users given the problems we describe. Many adults face the same difficulties and react similarly. The most widely used method of contraception among adults in their thirties is sterilization (Bachrach 1984). Presumably mature adults resort to sterilization because they have many of the same apprehensions and problems with contraception that teenagers do. The difference is that teens do not have the option of sterilization. Most sexually active teens eventually practice contraception, and the majority use it regularly if not absolutely consistently. Zelnik and Kantner (1978) estimate that without the practice of contraception, 680,000 additional teenage pregnancies would occur each year.

Contraceptive services for teens are relatively novel. It was not until 1970 and the passage of Title X—legislation that provided subsidized family planning services for low-income women—that access to contraception for unmarried minors became widely available. But the provision of contraceptive services for the young has remained controversial. Funding cuts have forced cutbacks in the expansion of family planning programs designed to reach the young. Political, economic, and social influences have discouraged innovative and aggressive programs and have required ser-

vice providers to adopt a low profile.

Compared to many European countries, the United States has adopted a timid and reactive approach to contraceptive services. Many critics of family planning programs believe that providing birth control to teens promotes sexual activity. While there is no evidence for this contention, and some evidence to the contrary, it is an assertion that is not easily dismissed by empirical data. Present policy seems to be a compromise course, permitting but not promoting contraception.

The Resolution of Pregnancy

Close to 1.1 million teenagers become pregnant each year, about two-fifths of them below the age of eighteen. The vast majority of teenage pregnancies are unintended. In the Zelnik and Kantner survey, less than a fourth of the teens indicated that their pregnancy was planned; most were initially upset when the pregnancy occurred. These expressions of sentiment are consistent with the figures on abortions. Among women under the age of eighteen, nearly one of every two pregnancies is voluntarily terminated (Henshaw et al. 1985). If abortion services were easier to obtain, the proportion would, no doubt, be even higher. Moreover, many teenagers who did not want to become pregnant elect to have the child because they disapprove of abortion. A common response in one study that asked teenagers about their attitudes toward abortion was "It's not fair to make the baby pay for the mother's mistake" (Fursten-berg 1976).

Only a small fraction of whites and an even smaller fraction of blacks use adoption as a way of avoiding early parenthood. By all accounts this proportion has been declining in recent decades, especially among whites. No doubt the availability of abortion is a factor. Also, as adoptions have decreased, the practice may receive less peer group and family encouragement. Among blacks there was never a large "market" for formal adoptions, though many teens, in fact, allow their child to be informally adopted by relatives or friends (Hill 1977; Stack 1974).

With the rise of marriage age and the growing tolerance for out-of-wedlock childbearing, "shotgun" weddings have all but disappeared among black teenagers and diminished sharply among whites (O'Connell and Rogers 1984). The sixteen-year-old pregnant girl who would have wed a generation ago now reasons that her seventeen-year-old boyfriend is in no position to support the child and estimates that she will do a lot better by finishing school and deferring marriage. The evidence that we present later suggests that she may well be right. Moreover, rising rates of divorce have blurred the distinction between unmarried and previously married parents; they are lumped together under the common rubric of single parents. Thus, many pregnant teenagers are willing to forestall or forego marriage altogether.

Some claim that the availability of welfare discourages marriage and may even encourage some adolescents to begin early childbearing. There is little evidence, however,

that more generous welfare payments deter marriage or promote earlier parenthood. Most empirical tests of this hypothesis find that the direct link between welfare and family formation among the very young is weak or nonexistent (Placek and Hendershot 1974; Furstenberg 1976; Moore and Burt 1982).

Few teenagers who have children believe that welfare will provide adequate support. Most expect to work and probably overestimate their ability to find steady employment. The majority look to their immediate family for temporary relief. And most studies of the accommodation to early parenthood show that parents of teenage childbearers do, in fact, shoulder much of the economic burden. A major reason young black women are able to keep children is that their parents and siblings frequently share the childrearing responsibilities. The availability of public assistance may contribute to the support furnished by the extended family, but parents seem to be willing to lend assistance whether or not they receive welfare supplements (Furstenberg and Crawford 1978; Presser 1980; Kellam et al. 1982).

The Consequences of Childbearing

Existing research has consistently shown that early childbearing reduces the life chances of women to achieve their educational goals. Teenage mothers are much more likely to drop out of high school, even when compared to peers of similar socioeconomic backgrounds and academic aptitude (Card and Wise 1981). How much educational decrement is due to childbearing, itself, and how much is due to lower academic commitment and competence is still an open question (Rindfuss, St. John, and Bumpass 1984; Hofferth and Moore 1979). It seems likely that if childbearing could be postponed, many young mothers would achieve more school than they otherwise do, although some would find other reasons to discontinue their education.

A generation ago, pregnancy was grounds for expulsion from school. As school systems have become more accommodating to young mothers, more have remained in school (Mott and Maxwell 1981). Still, a large proportion cannot handle the dual responsibilities of being a mother and a student. Some of these women eventually return to school or obtain a degree by passing a high school equivalency test (GED). A seventeen-year follow-up of a sample of young mothers in Baltimore revealed that about one woman in six completed high school in her twenties or early thirties. This result suggests that some of the shorter term follow-ups may underreport the educational achievement of teenage mothers and therefore overstate the difference between early and later childbearers, but even so the disparity in schooling level is significant (Furstenberg and Brooks-Gunn 1985).

Partly because of their educational deficit, teenage mothers are less likely to find stable and remunerative employment and are more likely to rely on public assistance than are women who begin childbearing later in life. Several studies have discov-

ered a significant difference in job status and income, which seems attributable to the timing of parenthood (Hofferth and Moore 1979; Card and Wise 1978; Trussel 1981). Again, that difference can be only partially explained by differences in socioeconomic background and abilities.

Many teenage mothers who use public assistance in their late teens to cope with the economic strains of early parenthood eventually return to work when their youngest children reach school age. In the Baltimore study, the proportion on welfare dropped substantially between the three-year and seventeen-year follow-up. Thus, the gap between early and later childbearers may diminish over time, especially when later childbearers drop out of the labor force to have children in their late twenties and early thirties. Nonetheless, most studies indicate that early childbearers will not achieve complete economic parity with women who postpone parenthood until they are adults.

A major reason for the residual difference is that later childbearers are more likely to enter stable marriages than women who have children in their early teens. Women who marry early in life have a much higher risk of divorce, especially if they marry as a result of pregnancy (Furstenberg 1976; McCarthy and Menken 1979). And many of those who delay marriage and elect to become single parents may never marry at all. Few married-coupled households live in poverty while more than a third of single-parent households are poor (Welniak and Fendler 1984).

We suspect that the payoff in postponing childbearing is significantly lower for blacks than whites. The labor market is dismal for young blacks; so, too, the opportunities for marriage. In economic terms, marriageable age is very late for blacks. Accordingly, many are willing to reverse the sequence of marriage and parenthood, deciding to have children before they marry (Moore, Peterson, and Furstenberg 1984). Because they can rely on family support, blacks often have children and remain in the parental household. If they are fortunate enough to have a mother, aunt, or older sister who will care for the child, they probably will return to school. Compared to whites, black women are much more likely to complete high school after becoming mothers (Mott and Maxwell 1981) and may, therefore, suffer relatively less disadvantage. After all, their peers who postpone parenthood have only modest prospects of entering a stable marriage, given the poor economic chances of black males in their early twenties. Still, evidence from the seventeen-year follow-up in Baltimore revealed that blacks who bear children in their teens are significantly less likely to be married and, therefore, less economically secure in later life than black women who postponed parenthood.

Another condition diminishing the difference between early and later childbearers is the availability of contraception and abortion. A generation ago, there was a wide difference in family size between women who began childbearing as teenagers and those who waited until their twenties. A difference still exists among recent cohorts but it is probably narrowing. Teenage parents generally do not want larger families than older childbearers, but they are at greater risk of having children in excess of their desires because of their early start. Increasingly, however, many are using contraception or abortion to limit their family size. In the Baltimore study, 20 percent of the sample with two or more children reported that they had aborted a pregnancy, and 64 percent reported that they were sterilized by the time of the seventeen-year follow-up. These young mothers may have been exceptionally well equipped to regulate their fertility because they all had access to family planning at the time of their initial pregnancy. Nonetheless, their receptivity to family planning services suggests that young mothers may recognize the necessity of limiting their family size to achieve some measure of economic well-being. An intriguing and important question, receiving little empirical attention, is why some young mothers manage the transition to parenthood successfully while others do not.

Most but not all partners of adolescent mothers are teenagers. Young fathers seem to be less adversely affected by early parenthood than young mothers (Card and Wise 1981). Men's educational and economic careers may not be directly influenced by the occurrence of an early birth unless they drop out of school to marry their pregnant partner. Relatively few are now required or even requested to take that step.

A large proportion of fathers never acknowledge fatherhood. In the Baltimore study, a much lower proportion of adolescent males report that they have ever impregnated a woman than females report ever having been pregnant (Furstenberg and Brooks-Gunn 1985). Pregnant teenagers report that they informed their partner. Apparently, a substantial minority of fathers refuse to admit their responsibility or refuse to accept the obligations fatherhood implies. Qualitative evidence collected from fathers indicates that many doubt their capacity to provide support and are ill prepared to lend emotional support to the mother or parental nurturance to the child.

The minority of fathers who become involved are generally in more committed relationships with the mother or in a better position to furnish economic aid to the child. Approximately a quarter of the Baltimore fathers living outside the home and known to be alive continued to see their child on at least a weekly basis five years after the delivery. A sixth of the biological fathers living outside the home were still as involved in raising the child at the seventeen-year follow-up. Never-married fathers generally were no less active in child rearing than the previously married men. In either case, only a small minority of fathers played an important role in supporting or raising the children, though they remained significant figures to the children so long as they retained at least occasional contact (Furstenberg and Talvitie 1979).

One clinical study that examined family dynamics following pregnancy discovered that fathers frequently were seen as competitors by the parents of the adolescent girl. Having to choose between an insecure relationship with a male and a secure one with the family, most teenage mothers opted to cut ties with the father (Furstenberg 1980; Stack 1974). Teenage mothers typically elect to remain with their family during the transition to parenthood, but the limited data available suggest that co-residence is temporary for most young mothers. In the Baltimore study, the majority left the parental household when they were ready to marry or have a second child, or when they became self-supporting. By the seventeen-year follow-up, fewer than one in ten were residing with a parent, and many of these women had returned to the family of origin after a marital separation.

A great deal of variation exists in the styles of parental collaboration between the young mother and her immediate family, regardless of whether or not the mother continues to reside with her parents. At one extreme, the grandmother assumes major responsibility for child rearing and the mother and child become quasi siblings. At the other extreme, the grandmother and other relatives are supportive figures but the mother assumes the primary responsibility for child care. The weight of evidence suggests that collaborative child care in general works to the benefit of both the mother and child (Kellam, Ensminger, and Turner 1977; Baldwin and Cain 1980). Children have more favorable developmental outcomes when the mother is not the sole parent figure. Presumably the skill and support of a more experienced figure, usually the grandmother, provides an on-site mentor for the young mother.

Consequences of Early Childbearing upon Children's Development

Only a handful of studies have been conducted on the relationship of early parenthood to child development, and most of these are confined to the period of infancy and early childhood (Baldwin and Cain 1980; Brooks-Gunn and Furstenberg 1985). However, the limited evidence, based largely on the Collaborative Perinatal Project (Marecek 1979), suggests that children in the preschool and early school years born to teenage mothers are at a developmental disadvantage compared to children born to older mothers. Small but consistent differences in cognitive functioning between offspring of early and later childbearers appear in preschool and continue into elementary school (Broman 1981; Marecek 1979, 1985). These decrements are, interestingly, observed in the sons but not the daughters of early childbearers. Larger effects are reported for psychosocial than cognitive development. For example, children of teenage mothers, as early as the infant years, are rated as being more active and as possessing less self-control. By preschool, they are rated as more aggressive as well. Again, these differences in children of early and late childbearers are characteristic of boys but not girls (Broman 1981; Marecek 1985). Such cognitive and psychosocial differences may set the stage for later school and social difficulties.

By adolescence, school achieve-ment among the offspring of adolescent mothers is markedly lower. For example, in the Baltimore study and in the National Survey of Children, about half the adolescents born to teenage mothers had repeated a grade. In comparison, only 20 percent of those adolescents born to later childbearers in the National Survey of Children had repeated a grade (Brooks-Gunn and Furstenberg 1985). School misbehavior, an indication of disinterest and learning problems, also is twice as high in adolescents whose mothers were teenagers at their birth than in those whose mothers were older.

The question still remains, What factors account for these differences? The strongest empirical evidence involves the adverse social and economic effects of early parenthood on children. Teenage mothers are generally more likely to be poor and less educated; their children are likely to grow up in disadvantaged neighborhoods, attend low-quality schools, and experience high rates of family instability. To the extent that teenage parenthood elevates the risks of these events occurring, it definitely contributes to the likelihood of unfavorable outcomes. However, child differences do not entirely disappear when family background is held constant (Broman 1981). One reason may involve the higher likelihood of residing in a single-parent household, if one has a teenage parent. All family members may benefit by having a number of adults in the household; for teenagers, lack of support may be especially devastating. Thus, children of teenagers may be especially at risk when their mothers separate from their family of origin or when they alter a preexisting household arrangement.

Over and above the residential and economic instability associated with early childbearing, teenage parents may be less experienced or less adequate in their parenting. However, we have little information on teenagers' parental practices with the exception of their treatment of infants. Few differences between teenage and older mothers have been found; however, one that has, vocalization, may be directly linked to depressed cognitive scores in preschool and childhood (Field 1981; Sandler, Vietze, and O'Connor 1981). Practitioners expect a higher incidence of child abuse, learning disabilities, delinquency, and sexual promiscuity among children of teenage parents, but the empirical record is very unclear. It remains for researchers to establish whether, how much, and why early childbearing complicates the development of children. Equally important is learning how some children manage to escape these risks.

Strategies: Intervention, Prevention, Amelioration, and Rehabilitation

If there is little consensus on why teenage childbearing is a problem, it follows that there is little agreement on what to do about it. In large part, prescriptions for action follow from a diagnosis of the situation. In one camp are the traditionalists who see the problem as moral breakdown in the family and the solution as restitution of the social order. In another are reformers who accept if not welcome many of the family changes and want to institutionalize them by building new supports for the contemporary family. Somewhere in the middle are pragmatists who are less certain about the desirability or inevitability of change but who are prepared to accommodate to the current reality. Each of these constituencies favors a somewhat different response to early childbearing though often there is a blurring of the lines on certain policies. We shall consider several major intervention strategies.

Postponing Sexual Activity

Conservatives have long argued that the most effective strategy for preventing early childbearing is to encourage delay of sexual activity until adulthood, preferably until marriage. Most advocates of family planning have countered that such a strategy is ineffective and potentially counterproductive. They contend that teenagers will continue to have sex but will be unprepared to use contraception because of a greater reluctance to acknowledge their sexual activity, (Kenney, Forrest, Torres 1982).

The Office of Adolescent Pregnancy provides funding for programs to delay the onset of sexual activity (Society for Research in Child Development 1984). The strategy is to discourage teenagers from engaging in sex much as they are discouraged from smoking or using alcohol and drugs. If teenagers are often ambivalent and uncertain about making the transition to nonvirginity, some may well respond to an appeal to delay. But it is not clear that a limited school-based program can compete effectively with many of the more important influences of the media, neighborhood, or peer group. As yet, little evidence supports this approach.

There is, of course, great variety in the aims and content of sex education programs, and thus it is difficult to reach any general conclusions about the effects of such programs. A recent comprehensive evaluative study concluded that sex education programs did increase short-term knowledge and, in some instances, affected attitudes about sexuality and heterosexual relations. It could not, however, demonstrate that sex education programs influenced the behavior of adolescents. Programs did not seem to raise or to lower the level of sexual activity, promote more effective contraceptive use, or decrease the incidence of pregnancy (Kirby 1984). Many of the interventions studied were not aimed at affecting behavior and were too limited in scope to anticipate such change. Skeptics will surely say that short-term evaluations of short-term programs will at best show short-term effects. But if these model programs do not affect behavior, then sex education, by itself, is not likely to be a powerful instrument in pregnancy prevention.

While program evaluations have not produced much evidence for a strong impact on behavior, two separate surveys that asked adolescents if they had received sex education did find more encouraging results. In one survey, younger teens who reported classroom instruction were less likely to have had intercourse (Furstenberg, Moore, and Peterson 1985). In the other survey, they were as sexually active as students who had not received sex education but they were more likely to practice contraception (Zelnik and Kim 1982). None of these studies confirms the impression of critics of sex education that school-based programs promote sexual activity among the young.

Contraceptive Programs

Advocates of family planning programs contended for many years that greater access to family planning by teens would have a marked impact on the rate of pregnancy and childbearing among adolescents. Birth control became more available to teenagers during the 1970s, but the incidence of teenage pregnancy and childbearing remained high. This result may be caused by many sexually active teenagers finding their way to services too late, using contraception ineffectively, or shying away from the most reliable methods. Programs have not been very successful in overcoming many obstacles to effective use. Consequently, among younger teens only the most highly motivated practice birth control consistently. Inconsistent use is better than nothing, and given infrequent sexual patterns, many teenagers manage to avoid pregnancy with the help of contraception and a certain amount of luck.

The greater availability of contraception may reenforce a more tolerant climate toward nonmarital sexual behavior as some argue, but it would be difficult to demonstrate any direct influence of contraceptive programs on teenage sexual behavior. The growth of contraceptive programs was a response to rather than a precipitant of changing patterns of behavior among the young. Rates of pregnancy and childbearing began to rise in the early 1970s before contraception was widely available to teens. In any case, it seems unlikely that many teenagers decide to become sexually active because of contraception because few avail themselves of it before beginning to have sex.

Despite a decade of experience with contraceptive programs for adolescents, we still do not know much about how to make them more effective. In the past, family planning programs tried to tailor clinics to suit youthful tastes—providing rock music in the waiting room, offering rap sessions, or employing peer counselors. None of these measures had much effect on clinic continuation or contraceptive compliance. Teenagers are probably attracted to many of the same standards that appeal to adults seeking contraception: convenience, confidentiality, competence, and humane treatment. Whether teenagers need more than that is not firmly established though one study has shown that they respond well to authoritative advice (Nathanson and Becker 1985). They may, for example, require aggressive outreach to get them into programs and more support to continue.

A small number of school-based contraceptive programs have been developed in the past few years. This seems like a promising approach for providing easy access, reasonable confidentiality (when the programs offer general health services as well), and an efficient means of follow-up. Whether these programs work better than clinics situated in planned parenthood affiliates, hospitals, and health centers, or services provided by private physicians, is not yet known. Some evaluations of alternative programs, such as school-based health clinics, are currently underway.

We suspect that no single model is likely to appeal to all teenagers. Adolescents have diverse needs depending on age, gender, ethnicity, locality, and personality. A system where contraceptive services were in oversupply, where there was competition for clients, and where there was some overlap and redundancy might produce the best results. We are far from developing such a system. Cross-national studies suggest that there are many different approaches to delivering contraception to young people (Jones et al. 1985). The lesson to be learned from these international comparisons is that given a reasonable amount of societal commitment, young people can and will use contraception. The United States seems to be something of an exception, perhaps because we have not yet accepted the reality of premarital sex among young people.

Abortion Services

So long as adolescents are sexually active and use contraception with difficulty or not at all, pregnancy rates will remain high. In 1981, 1.3 million teenagers between the ages of fifteen and nineteen became pregnant. Almost four in ten of these pregnancies were ended by an abortion. After *Roe v. Wade*, the Supreme Court decision that eliminated most barriers to legalized abortion, the incidence of abortion among teens, as well as among older women, rose sharply. In the past few years, however, rates have leveled off and may even be declining as financial and political obstacles to abortion have increased.

Of all age groups, except for women over forty, teens have the highest ratio of abortions to pregnancies. In 1981 teens obtained 28 percent of all abortions (Henshaw et al. 1985). Despite their frequent use of abortion, teens, especially those under eighteen, face special problems in obtaining abortions. Younger teens may deny the symptoms of pregnancy, or even fail to recognize them, and consequently delay action until it is too late to obtain a first-trimester abortion. Lack of resources may also restrict access; many teenagers cannot or will not ask their family for help and are reluctant to approach the father of the child who may not support their decision to have an abortion. Desire to keep the pregnancy confidential hampers their ability to get economic assistance and social support for terminating the pregnancy. Finally, teenagers not living near an abortion facility may find it difficult to locate and travel to a service outside of their immediate community. Most counties in the United States, especially nonmetropolitan areas in the middle of the country, do not offer local services. Abortion rates for teenagers in New York, Massachusetts, and the District of Columbia are about three times the rate for teenagers living in Utah, Mississippi, or West Virginia.

Adoption Services

Only a small percentage of teens who decide to bear children give them up for adoption. Most estimates suggest that it is fewer than one out of ten. Adoption has become less popular as adolescents have either elected abortion or single parenthood. It is not well understood why adoption has become less socially acceptable.

Under the current administration, the Office of Adolescent Pregnancy has vigorously promoted adoption as an alternative to abortion or single parenthood for teenagers. Efforts have been made to provide more information to pregnant teens about this alternative and to make it financially easier for teens to bear children for subsequent adoption. While it is too soon to evaluate the success of these efforts, it appears that most teenagers are unwilling to bring a pregnancy to term if they are not prepared to keep their child.

Formal adoptions are especially rare among black teens. In the past, the demand for black infants was small. In addition, the black community was strongly committed to providing assistance to young mothers. When parents could not provide support, relatives and friends often stepped in to provide temporary foster care and sometimes informal adoption. This practice continues today. Black children of teenage mothers are more likely to be raised in part by grandparents, uncles and aunts, or quasi kin (Stack 1974; Hill, 1977).

Services for Teenage Parents

Beginning in the late 1960s, a wide variety of health and welfare services were developed for teenage parents and their children. Such services included prenatal and postnatal medical care, family planning services, day care, and educational and vocational counseling and programs aimed at preventing school dropout and increasing job experiences. These services now are often packaged together in comprehensive programs. It is assumed that programs that address a range of needs will be more efficient and effective in attracting teens and sustaining their involvement.

Regrettably, these comprehensive service programs have not been carefully evaluated. Klerman and Jekel (1973), in an assessment of one of the first such programs, concluded that the impact of the intervention did not seem to last any longer than the program. So long as teenagers received services, they seemed to benefit from the assistance provided; but when services were discontinued, teenagers experienced multiple adjustment problems.

The Baltimore study had similar findings. A hospital-based family planning and medical care program had modest effects in preventing second pregnancies, but the results did not persist. The services, provided during pregnancy, often did not address the needs of the young mothers in the year or two after delivery. Other interventions aimed at keeping adolescent parents in school have encountered similar limitations. Educational counseling or services during pregnancy do not seem to deter dropout significantly unless services continue postpartum.

The most ambitious evaluation of a treatment program to date was carried out under the auspices of the Manpower Demonstration Research Corporation. Project Redirection offered comprehensive services to severely disadvantaged pregnant teens and young mothers in four cities. In addition to a wide variety of services, community volunteers met on a regular basis with the participants. A careful evaluation was designed to compare the outcomes of teens served compared to counterparts in other cities not being served by comprehensive programs. A twelve-month follow-up showed that on a wide range of measures, the participants in Project Redirection were faring better than the members of the comparison group. They were more likely to be in school, more likely to have had work experience, and less likely to have become pregnant again a year later. Moreover, almost all the recruits to Project Redirection remained in the program, indicating their willingness to make use of the educational and vocational training. The results of the twenty-four-month follow-up were less favorable. As soon as teens left the program, ordinarily between twelve and eighteen months after their admission, they behaved almost identically to the comparison group. A substantial proportion discontinued their schooling and became pregnant again. The program seemed to have the greatest positive impact on the most disadvantaged youth in the study, but even among this group the impact was modest (Polit, Kahn, and Stevens 1985).

The literature on service program evaluations is limited, but some lessons can be drawn from the existing data. First, serving adolescent parents is a formidable challenge to providers. Teenage mothers, not to mention teenage fathers, generally have a large number of educational and economic deficits. The most competent and highly motivated can make use of regular programs, but the majority require intensive interventions with varied remedial services. Even well-delivered comprehensive programs will not appeal to many adolescent parents. A large number of teen parents will not have the commitment or the ability to remain in school and care for their children at the same time. On-site daycare will help some mothers, but others are not willing to use childcare outside the home and will only accept help from relatives.

No single program will appeal to all teen mothers. Most teen parents are prepared to continue in school but many are not. The school-resistant may accept vocational training or classes to prepare for a GED, though some young mothers are not eligible for special educational programs until they are older. One of the greatest difficulties in providing occupational training to adolescent parents is that so few teens can expect to find remunerative employment. Data from the seventeen-year follow-up in Baltimore showed that many teen mothers did not begin to work at a regular job until they were in their early or late twenties. At this point, many mothers were able to find employment and leave welfare. Significantly, educational and family planning services that the Baltimore teens received during pregnancy and just after delivery did have a noticeable impact on reducing their chances of being on welfare and having three or more children later in life.

In sum, our reading of the data is that for teenage parents, programs are probably worthwhile, but they are likely to have only a modest impact in ameliorating the consequences of early parenthood. But this is truly an area where an ounce of prevention is worth a pound of cure.

Implications for Programs and Policy

Primary prevention programs aimed at delaying sexual activity or promoting more effective contraceptive use are relatively new. Existing programs of sexual education have not as yet demonstrated their capacity to change the sexual practices of adolescent youth. The programs may be too little and may occur too late; however, it is equally plausible that they, like many other preventive programs directed at adolescent populations, are not forceful enough to alter peer-supported behavior. To do so requires sharper norms defining appropriate and inappropriate age range for teenagers to initiate sexual activity. Were such norms to exist, younger adolescents might be discouraged from engaging in intercourse as they are from using alcohol or drugs.

Family planning programs have had only modest success in preventing unwanted pregnancies. They could be more effective if they were openly supported by the larger society. At present they still have a secretive and sometimes intimidating image that deters adolescents from using them. In countries where premarital sexual activity is widely accepted, youth seem to be willing to use contraception more responsibly. American society will have to abandon the goal of premarital chastity, at least among older adolescents, to increase contraceptive compliance. To do so requires the adoption of a more open policy toward family planning: promoting contraceptive advertisements in the mass media, working with family physicians to encourage contraceptive practice among the sexually active, building a more extensive network of easily accessible contraceptive services, and other similar measures.

Contraception will remain difficult to use for young people. No methods other than the pill or condom are well suited to the irregular and unpredictable sexual patterns typical in the adolescent population. The pill and IUD may have undermined the use of the condom and discouraged males from assuming contraceptive responsibility. It is not obvious what concrete measures might be taken to promote greater responsibility on the part of males. Programs that have attempted to involve males have not had notable success in recruiting partcipants (Clark, Zabin, and Hardy 1984; Scales and Beckstein 1982).

Abortion remains a measure of last resort for many teenagers. It is increasingly less accessible for the very young and the very poor. If present restrictive policies toward abortion continue, we can expect to see a modest decline in the rate of abortions and perhaps a rise in the rate of unintended births among adolescents. We do not view adoption as a realistic alternative to abortion. The great majority of young people who are persuaded to bring their pregnancies to term are likely to have strong misgivings about adoption.

We briefly reviewed programs designed to ameliorate the impact of early childbearing. While it is too soon to give a definitive assessment of these services, the preliminary evidence suggests that they have only a modest impact on the lives of participants. Some teens will benefit from the assistance provided, but these programs are too limited in scope and duration to offset the disadvantages associated with premature parenthood for both young mothers and their offspring.

Given this bleak prognosis, we return to an earlier point. Preventive strategies are undoubtedly cheaper and probably more effective, but they are also imperfect. But even if we make modest inroads in the incidence of early childbearing, the gain can be considerable. If early childbearing begins to decline, social sanctions against adolescent parenthood may rise; this could have an additional dampening effect on the rate. In order for this "snowball effect" in public opinion to occur, local communities that currently regard early childbearing as inevitable, if undesirable, will have to assume greater responsibility for changing the social definition of adolescent childbearing. Recently, the Children's Defense Fund has undertaken a program of community education about the adverse effects of teenage parenthood. And the Girls Clubs have launched a campaign to prevent premature parenthood. These actions may signal a willingness of community-based organizations to participate in primary prevention efforts. Like early marriage, teenage parenthood may, in communities where it is presently tolerated, be treated with greater public opprobrium. The challenge is to alter opinion without eliminating services to those who do become pregnant.

Our survey of existing strategies for reducing the rate of early childbearing or ameliorating its negative consequences offers little comfort to policymakers who are searching for a quick fix. We believe that many of the existing programs are constructive, but they must be strengthened or extended in order to make more of a difference. The lack of systematic evaluation of existing services is a serious deterrent to making wise decisions about which programs should be retained and expanded and which should be dropped or radically altered.

In the 1970s there was a good deal of experimentation but few of the innovative efforts survived, in part because it was difficult to distinguish the successes from the failures. A clear lesson can be drawn from this experience for practitioners who want to address the problems associated with adolescent fertility in the 1980s. Social scientific theory and methods must be used more effectively to assess the value and the viability of both preventive and ameliorative services. If we are correct that different teens will benefit from different types of interventions at different points in the life course, the need for careful evaluation becomes all the more evident. The spirit of fiscal caution in the 1980s is a dangerous development to the extent that promising and potentially productive programs are stifled. But it could have one saluatory feature if it resulted in a more deliberate attempt to increase the payoff of existing programs.

Acknowledgments

This chapter draws on research supported by a grant from the Commonwealth Fund. The authors are grateful for the assistance of Laura Blakeslee and Julia Robinson in preparing the manuscript and for the critical review by Cheryl Hayes and Richard Lincoln.

References

Alan Guttmacher Institute. 1981. *Teenage pregnancy: The problem that hasn't gone away.* New York: Alan Guttmacher Institute.

Bachrach, Christine A. 1984. Contraceptive practice among American women, 1973–1982. *Family Planning Perspectives* 16(6):253–259.

Baldwin, Wendy, and Virginia S. Cain. 1980. The children of teenage parents. *Family Planning Perspectives* 12(1):34–43.

Billy, John O., Joseph Lee Rodgers, and J. Richard Udry. 1981. Adolescent sexual behavior and friendship choice. Carolina Population Center, University of North Carolina, Chapel Hill.

Broman, Sarah H. 1981. Longterm development of children born to teenagers. In *Teenage parents and their offspring*, ed. K. Scott, T. Field, and E. Robertson. New York: Grune and Sratton.

Brooks-Gunn, Jeanne, and Frank F. Furstenberg, Jr. 1985. Antecedents and consequences of parenting: The case of adolescent motherhood. In *The origins of nurturance*, ed. Allen D. Fogel and Gayle F. Melson. Hillsdale, N.J.: Lawrence Erlbaum Associates.

Card, Josefina J., and Lauress L. Wise. 1981. Teenage mothers and teenage fathers: The impact of early childbearing on the parents' personal and professional lives. In *Teenage sexuality, pregnancy, and childbearing*, ed. Frank F. Furstenberg, Jr., Richard Lincoln, and Jane Menken. Philadelphia: University of Pennsylvania Press.

Center for Disease Control. 1978. Teenage fertility in the United States, 1960, 1970, 1974: Regional and state variation and excess fertility. Atlanta: Public Health Service.

Chilman, Catherine S. 1983. *Adolescent sexuality in a changing American society: Social and psychological perspectives for the human services professions*, 2d ed. New York: John Wiley and Sons.

Clark, Samuel D., Jr., Laurie S. Zabin, and Janet B. Hardy. 1984. Sex, contraception, and parenthood: Experience and attitudes among urban black young men. *Family Planning Perspectives* 16(2):77–82.

Coates, Thomas J., Anne C. Peterson, and Cheryl Perry. 1982. *Promoting adolescent health: A dialog on research and practice.* New York: Academic Press.

Collaborative Perinatal Study. 1984. Adolescent pregnancy and childbearing: Rates, trends, and research findings. Washington, D.C.: National Institute of Child and Human Development. Includes Adolescent childbearing today and tomorrow, updated statement prepared for U.S. Senate Human Resources Committee, June 14, 1978, by Wendy Baldwin.

Degler, Carl N. 1980. *At odds: Women and the family in America from the revolution to the present.* New York: Oxford University Press.

Dryfoos, Joy. 1982. The epidemiology of adolescent pregnancy: Incidence, outcomes, and interventions. In *Pregnancy in adolescence: Needs, problems, and management*, ed. Irving R. Stuart and Carl F. Wells. New York: Van Nostrand Reinhold.

Field, Tiffany. 1981. Early development of the preterm offspring of teenage mothers. In *Teenage parents and their offspring*, ed. K. Scott, T. Field, and E. Robertson. New York: Grune and Stratton.

Fox, Greer Litton. 1981. The family's role in adolescent sexual behavior. In

Teenage pregnancy in a family context: Implications for policy, ed. Theodora Ooms. Philadelphia: Temple University Press.

Fox, Greer Litton, Bruce Fox, and Katherine Frohardt-Lane. 1982. Fertility socialization. In *The childbearing decision,* ed. Greer Litton Fox. Beverly Hills: Sage Publications.

Frank, Daniel B. 1983. *Deep blue funk and other stories: Portraits of teenage parents.* Chicago: Ounce of Prevention Fund.

Furstenberg, Frank F., Jr. 1976. *Unplanned parenthood: The social consequences of teenage childbearing.* New York: Free Press.

————. 1980. Burdens and benefits: The impact of early childbearing on the family. *Journal of Social Issues* 36(1):64–87.

Furstenberg, Frank F., Jr., and Jeanne Brooks-Gunn. 1984. Antecedents and consequences of teenage parenthood: Young mothers, fathers, and their children. Grant proposal submitted to the Robert Wood Johnson Foundation.

————. 1985. Adolescent mothers in later life. Report submitted to the Commonwealth Fund.

Furstenberg, Frank F., Jr., and Albert G. Crawford. 1978. Family support: Helping teenage mothers to cope. *Family Planning Perspectives* 10(6):322–333.

Furstenberg, Frank F., Jr., Roberta Herceg-Baron, Judy Shea, and David Webb. 1984. Family communication and teenagers' contraceptive use. *Family Planning Perspectives* 16(4):163–170.

Furstenberg, Frank F., Jr., Richard Lincoln, and Jane Menken, eds. 1981. *Teenage sexuality, pregnancy, and childbearing.* Philadelphia: University of Pennsylvania Press.

Furstenberg, Frank F., Jr., Kristin A. Moore, and James L. Peterson. 1985. Sex education and sexual experience among adolescents. Working draft, transcript.

Furstenberg, Frank F., Jr., Judy Shea, Paul Allison, Roberta Herceg-Baron, and David Webb. 1983. Contraceptive continuation among adolescents attending family planning clinics. *Family Planning Perspectives* 15(5):211–217.

Furstenberg, Frank F., Jr., and Kathy Talvitie. 1979. Children's names and paternal claims: Bonds between unmarried fathers and their children. *Journal of Family Issues* 1(1):31–57.

Grabill, Wilson H. 1976. Premarital fertility. In *Current population reports,* series P-23, no. 63. U.S. Department on Commerce, Bureau of the Census. Washington, D.C.: Government Printing Office.

Henshaw, Stanley K., Nancy J. Binkin, Ellen Blaine, and Jack C. Smith. 1985. A portrait of American women who obtain abortions. *Family Planning Perspectives* 17(2):90–96.

Hill, Robert B. 1977. *Informal adoption among black families.* Washington, D.C.: National Urban League.

Hofferth, Sandra L. 1984. Kin networks, race, and family structure. *Journal of Marriage and the Family* 46(4):791–806.

Hofferth, Sandra L., and Kristin A. Moore. 1979. Early childbearing and later economic well-being. *American Sociological Review* 44:784–815.

Jones, Elise F., Jacqueline Darroch Forrest, Noreen Goldman, Stanley K. Henshaw, Richard Lincoln, Jeannie I. Rosoff, Charles F. Westoff, and Deirdre Wulf. 1985. Teenage pregnancy in developed countries: Determinants and policy implications. *Family Planning Perspectives* 17(2):53–63.

Kellam, Sheppard G., Rebecca G. Adams, C. Hendricks Brown, and Margaret E. Ensminger. 1982. The long-term evolution of the family structure of teenage and older mothers. *Journal of Marriage and the Family* 44(3):539–554.

Kellam, Sheppard G., Margaret E. Ensminger, and R. Jay Turner. 1977. Family structure and the mental health of children: Concurrent and longitudinal community-wide studies. *Archives of General Psychiatry* 34:1012–1022.

Kenney, Asta M., Jacqueline D. Forrest, and Aida Torres. 1982. Storm over Washington: The parental notification proposal. *Family Planning Perspectives* 14(4):185–197.

Kinsey, Alfred C., Wardell B. Pomeroy, Clyde E. Martin, and Paul H. Gebhard. 1953. *Sexual behavior in the human female*. Philadelphia: W. B. Saunders.

Kirby, Douglas. 1984. *Sexuality education: An evaluation of programs and their effects*. Santa Cruz: Network Publications.

Klerman, Lorraine V., and James F. Jekel. 1973. *School-age mothers: Problems, programs, and policy*. Hamden, Conn.: Linnet Books.

McAnarney, Elizabeth R., and Corinne Schreider. 1984. *Identifying social and psychological antecedents of adolescent pregnancy: The contribution of research to concepts of prevention*. New York: William T. Grant Foundation.

McCarthy, James, and Jane Menken. 1979. Marriage, remarriage, marital disruption and age at first birth. *Family Planning Perspectives* 11(1)21–30.

Marecek, Jeanne. 1979. Economic, social, and psychological consequences of adolescent childbearing: An analysis of data from the Philadelphia collaborative perinatal project. Final Report to National Institute of Child and Human Development.

———. 1985. The effects of adolescent childbearing on children's cognitive and psychosocial development. Typescript.

Mindick, Burton, and Stuart Oskamp. 1982. Individual differences among adolescent contraceptors: Some implications for intervention. In *Pregnancy in adolescence: Needs, problems, and management*, ed. Irving R. Stuart and Carl F. Wells. New York: Van Nostrand Reinhold.

Moore, Kristin A., and Martha R. Burt. 1982. *Private crisis, public cost: Policy perspectives on teenage childbearing*. Washington, D.C.: Urban Institute Press.

Moore, Kristin A., James L. Peterson, and Frank F. Furstenberg, Jr. 1984. Starting early: The antecedents of early premarital intercourse. Presented at Population Association of America Meetings, Minneapolis.

Moore, Kristin A., Margaret C. Simms, and Charles L. Betsey. 1984. Choice and circumstance: Racial differences in adolescent sexuality and fertility. Draft project report. Washington, D.C.: Urban Institute.

Mott, Frank L., and Nan L. Maxwell. 1981. School-age mothers, 1968 and 1979. *Family Planning Perspectives* 16(6):287–292.

National Center for Health Statistics. 1985. Advance report of final natality statistics, 1983. *Monthly Vital Statistics Report* 34, no. 6, supp. DHHS Pub. No. (PHS)85-1120. Hyattsville, Md: Public Health Service.

Nathanson, Constance A., and Marshall H. Becker. 1985. The influence of client-provider relationships on teenage women's subsequent use of contraception. *American Journal of Public Health* 75(1):33–38.

Newcomer, Susan F., and J. Richard Udry. 1984. Mothers' influence on the sexual behavior of their teenage children. *Journal of Marriage and the Family* 46(2):477–485.

O'Connell, Martin, and Carolyn C. Rogers. 1984. Out-of-wedlock births, premarital pregnancies, and their effect on family formation and dissolution. *Family Planning Perspectives* 16(4):157–162.

Petchesky, Rosalind Pollack. 1982. *Abortion and woman's choice: The state, sexuality, and the conditions of reproductive freedom.* New York: Longman.

Placek, Paul J., and Gerry E. Hendershot. 1974. Public welfare and family planning: An empirical study of the "brood sow" myth. *Social Problems* 21(5): 658–673.

Polit, Denise, Janet Kahn, and David Stevens. 1985. *Project redirection: Conclusions on a program for pregnant and parenting teens.* New York: Manpower Demonstration Research Corporation.

Presser, Harriet B. 1980. Sally's corner: Coping with unmarried motherhood. *Journal of Social Issues* 36(1):107–129.

Rains, Prudence and Mors Rains. 1971. *Becoming an unwed mother: A sociological account.* Chicago: Aldine/Atherton.

Rindfuss, Ronald R., Craig St. John, and Larry L. Bumpass. 1984. Education and the timing of motherhood: Disentangling causation. *Journal of Marriage and the Family* 46(4):981–984.

Sandler, Howard, Peter Vietze, and Susan O'Connor. 1981. Obstetric and neonatal outcomes following intervention with pregnant teenagers. In *Teenage parents and their offspring,* ed. K. Scott, T. Field, and E. Robertson. New York: Grune and Stratton.

Scales, Peter, and Douglas Beckstein. 1982. From macho to mutuality: Helping young men make effective decisions about sex, contraception, and pregnancy. In *Pregnancy in adolescence: Needs, problems, and management,* ed. Irving R. Stuart and Carl F. Wells. New York: Van Nostrand Reinhold.

Shea, Judy A., Roberta Herceg-Baron, and Frank F. Furstenberg, Jr. 1984. Factors associated with adolescent use of family planning clinics. *American Journal of Public Health* 74(11):1227–1230.

Society for Research in Child Development. 1984. Adolescent pregnancy. *Washington Report* 1(2):1–11.

Stack, Carol B. 1974. *All our kin: Strategies for survival in a black community*. New York: Harper and Row.

Thornberg, Hershel D. 1975. Adolescent sources of initial sex information. In *Studies in adolescence: A book of readings in adolescent development*, ed. Robert E. Grinder. New York: Macmillan.

Thornton, Arland, and Deborah Freedman. 1983. The changing American family. *Population Bulletin* 38(Oct.):4.

Trussell, James. 1981. Economic consequences of teenage childbearing. In *Teenage sexuality, pregnancy, and childbearing*, ed. Frank F. Furstenberg, Jr., Richard Lincoln, and Jane Menken. Philadelphia: University of Pennsylvania Press.

U.S. Department of Commerce. Bureau of the Census. 1983a. Marital income and poverty status of families and persons in the United States, 1983. In *Current population reports*, series P-20, no. 385. Washington, D.C.: Government Printing Office.

———. 1983b. Marital status and living arrangements, March 1983. In *Current population reports*, series P-20, no. 389. Government Printing Office, Washington, D.C.

———. 1984. Childspacing among birth cohorts of American women, 1905 to 1959. In *Current population reports*, series P-20, no. 385. Washington, D.C.: U.S. Government Printing Office.

U.S. Department of Health and Human Services. 1980. Trends and differentials in births to unmarried women: United States, 1970–1976. In *U.S. national vital statistics*, series 21, no. 36. Publication No. (PHS) 80-1914. Washington, D.C.: Government Printing Office.

Welniak, Edward J., and Carol Fendler. 1984. Money income and poverty status of families and persons in the United States, 1983 (advance data from the March 1984 *Current population survey*). In *Current population reports*, series P-60, no. 145. U.S. Department of Commerce, Bureau of the Census. Washington, D.C.: Government Printing Office.

Westoff, Charles F., Gerard Calot, and Andrew D. Foster. 1983. Teenage fertility in developed nations, 1971–1980. *Family Planning Perspectives* 15(3): 105–110.

Zabin, Laurie Schwab, John F. Kantner, and Melvin Zelnik. 1979. The risk of adolescent pregnancy in the first months of intercourse. *Family Planning Perspectives* 11(4):215–222.

Zelnik, Melvin, and John F. Kantner. 1978. Contraceptive patterns and premarital pregnancy among women aged 15–19 in 1976. *Family Planning Perspectives* 10(3):135–142.

———. 1980. Sexual activity, contraceptive use and pregnancy among metropolitan area teenagers, 1971–1979. *Family Planning Perspectives* 12(5):230.

Zelnik, Melvin, John F. Kantner, and Kathleen Ford. 1981. *Sex and pregnancy in adolescence*. Sage Library of Social Research, no. 133. Beverly Hills: Sage.

Zelnik, Melvin, and Young J. Kim. 1982. Sex education and its association with teenage sexual activity, pregnancy, and contraceptive use. *Family Planning Perspectives* 14(3):117–126.

Zelnik, Melvin, and Farida K. Shah. 1983. First intercourse among young Americans. *Family Planning Perspectives* 15(2):64–70.

Chapter 16

Health Problems and Policy Issues of Old Age

Carroll L. Estes and
Philip R. Lee

Social policy affecting the aged and their health is growing in importance as the number of elderly increases, the burden of illness in old age persists, and the costs of providing health care continue to rise rapidly. For most of this century, the population aged sixty-five and older has been increasing at a rate more rapid than that of the U.S. population as a whole; four-generation families are becoming a common experience in American life (U.S. Congress, Senate 1984a). From 1960 to 1980, the population aged sixty-five years and over increased from 16.7 million (9 percent) to 25.9 million (11 percent of the population)—a 55 percent increase. During the same period, the number of those aged seventy-five to eighty-four rose 65 percent while the number of those over eighty-five rose 174 percent. By the year 2000, the percentage of elderly seventy-five years and over will continue to increase more rapidly than the percentage of those aged sixty-five to seventy-four. The former group will increase from the current 38 percent to 45 percent of the elderly population (Rice and Feldman 1983). More older people in our society are living to advanced ages. A critical question is whether they will encounter a growing burden of illness and disability as suggested by Rice and Feldman (1983), Schneider and Brody (1983), Myers and Manton (1984), and Verbrugge (1984), or whether their health will be better than that of earlier generations because of life-style and other changes as suggested by the work of Fries (1980, 1983, 1984) and Fries and Crapo (1981).

Over the past twenty years, the proportion of elderly people living below the poverty level has been substantially reduced. The aged also have more access to health care services. Yet, a host of problems remain. There are large disparities in income among the elderly; millions face a growing financial burden due to increasing out-of-pocket health care expenditures; community-based health and social services intended to supplement family care provided for the functionally dependent and chronically ill are not readily available; housing is a growing problem for the poor elderly; and many are socially isolated and live lives of quiet desperation.

The range of problems and the growing importance of the elderly in social and political arenas have been key factors in the growth of Social Security and pensions and in the development of an "aging enterprise" of professionals, agencies, institutions, and organizations of elderly to meet the social, housing, health care, and other needs of the elderly (Estes 1979).

In this chapter, we do not attempt to discuss some of the broader issues (e.g., military spending versus social spending; tax policies or the federal deficit) that directly affect the policy choices to be made as we approach the year 2000. Our focus here is on four areas: health and well-being of older persons; income and housing issues affecting the elderly; financing, organization, and delivery of long-term health care services; and health care cost-containment.

Health and Well-Being of Older Persons

Declining mortality rates across the entire lifespan and changing fertility rates are the major factors contributing to the proportionate increase in the population aged sixty-five years and older in the United States. Patterns of morbidity and mortality in the United States have changed dramatically during the twentieth century. Life expectancy at birth rose from forty-seven years in 1900 to sixty-eight years in 1950 (U.S. Department of Health and Human Services, Health Care Financing Administration 1980). This dramatic increase in longevity was the result of the sharp decline in infant mortality and the reduction in mortality from communicable diseases affecting mainly infants, children, and young adults. While life expectancy at birth increased dramatically between 1900 and 1950, life expectancy at age sixty-five increased by only two years (from 11.9 to 13.9 years). Between 1950 and 1982 life expectancy at age sixty-five increased from 13.9 to 16.8 years. There was a 3.8-year increase for women and a 1.6-year increase for men during this period (Waldo and Lazenby 1984). The overall death rate for the elderly fell 29 percent during the period 1950–1982, falling much more rapidly for women than for men (Waldo and Lazenby 1984). Most of the decline in mortality among the elderly has resulted from reductions in heart disease, cerebrovascular disease, and stroke (National Center for Health Statistics 1982, 34).

A critical question for the elderly, for health care providers, and for health-policy makers is the impact of this rapid decline in mortality on morbidity and disability among the elderly and on their need for and utilization of health and social services. The problem has been clearly defined by Rice and Feldman (1983): "Changes in levels of morbidity, in therapies and technologies, in the availability and cost of care, in social and economic conditions, will contribute to patterns and levels of utilization of medical care services, as will mortality rates and changes in the age structure of the population. Some of these factors will have to increase utilization while others may decrease it." One aspect of debate has focused on whether or not the future burden of illness in a growing elderly population suggests a greater drain on health and long-term-care resources than is predictable from projections of present patterns of utilization and expenditures (Rice and Feldman 1983; Gruenberg 1977; Manton 1982; Schneider and Brody 1983; Myers and Manton 1984; and Verbrugge 1984). Of particular import may be the burdens imposed by multiple chronic conditions—a problem that increases with advancing age and that limits activity and increases bed disability days, physician visits, and short-stay hospital care (Rice 1985). These views about the growth of morbidity and the decline of mortality contrast with those of Fries (1980, 1983, 1984), who has suggested that a compression of morbidity and a rectangularization of the mortality curve are likely to occur as life expectancy approaches the normal biological life span, which he estimates to be approximately eighty-five years.

The major causes of illness and limitation of activity among the elderly are injuries, chronic diseases, and stress-related conditions, including hypertension, suicide, alcoholism, and drug misuse. Today, the common association between old age

and physical decline in health is attributed primarily to chronic arthritis, heart disease, hearing and vision impairments, and hypertension (U.S. Congress, Senate 1983a). Alzheimer's disease, depression, and alcoholism are also major problems.

While a higher proportion of older than younger persons are afflicted by one or more chronic conditions, a majority of older persons continue to enjoy good health (U.S. Department of Health and Human Services, Health Care Financing Administration 1981). The need for assistance, however, increases with advancing age. For example, the percentage of persons extremely limited by chronic conditions is 6.2 percent among forty-five to sixty-four-year-olds, 14.4 percent for sixty-five to seventy-four-year-olds, and 33 percent for those eighty-five and older (U.S. Department of Health and Human Services, Health Care Financing Administration 1981). In the aggregate, older persons, particularly women and minorities with low incomes and lower educational levels, have a higher incidence of chronic diseases and disability (Butler and Newacheck 1981). Rural elderly also report a greater number of days per year of restricted activity (U.S. Congress, Senate 1982). In view of the lower income and educational levels of the rural elderly, this finding is not surprising.

In addition to the burden of illness and disability, income and social factors are important in determining whether an elderly person will be confined to a nursing home (Kane and Kane 1982; Butler and Newacheck 1981). It is estimated that for every nursing home resident, three people of equal functional impairment live in the community. Many functionally impaired elderly can be cared for at home largely because of services provided by family members, usually a spouse or adult offspring. Widows and widowers are five times more likely to be institutionalized than married persons; those elderly who were never married, divorced, or separated may have up to ten times the rate of institutionalization of married individuals (Butler and Newacheck 1981). Social support networks between elderly persons, relatives, and friends have been found to have a positive effect on patients' mental functioning and were a buffer between decline and risk of institutionalization (Wan and Weissert 1981). These findings emphasize the need to develop an adequate base of social support for the elderly through family, friends, and organized community services.

Income and Housing: Keys to the Health and Well-Being of the Elderly

Income

A large body of research identifies the link between income and health as measured by longevity, disability, and chronic illness (Luft 1978). Income is clearly a vital element in determining health status. Social security, the primary source of postretirement income for the majority of the elderly, thus becomes a critical element in national health policy. Although national policies related to the prevention of impoverishment in old age date to the Social Security Act of 1935, only recently have income maintenance policies been viewed as a cornerstone of health policies for the elderly (Ball 1981). It is clear from mortality and morbidity data as well as from numerous studies of health care utilization and cost that an important link exists between health and economic well-being. Thus, assessing the economic status of older persons is an important component of health policy planning for the elderly, but this task has become complex and controversial. Multiple factors such as labor market experience, education, marital status, family-member death, chronic or acute illness onset, and Social Security and tax policies combine to create differing effects at particular points in the life cycle.

Of the total income for persons aged sixty-five and over in the United States in 1980, 43 percent was obtained from Social Security, 18 percent from other retirement pensions, 15 percent from interest on savings, and 16 percent from earnings (U.S. Congress, Senate 1983a). The Social Security program (Old-Age, Survivors and Disability Insurance —OASDI) benefits 36 million persons, including not only the 25.5 million individuals who are over sixty-five years of age but also another 10.5 million individuals who are younger, retired, disabled, or survivors and dependents. Social Security benefits are generally low—in August 1985 the average monthly benefit for retired men was $521 and $399 for retired women, $518 for disabled men and $370 for disabled women, and $307 for aged widowers and $419 for aged widows (U.S. Department of Health and Human Services, Social Security Administration 1985).

The Supplemental Security Income (SSI) program, passed in 1972 and implemented in 1974, was significant in providing a guaranteed minimum income for the deserving poor who were aged, blind, or disabled. The program federalized state welfare payments and instituted national standards of income and resources. The federal SSI benefit has a cost-of-living adjustment (COLA) each year. States can supplement the basic federal SSI payment if they wish. Nationally, there are about 4.0 million beneficiaries, and most of the aged receiving SSI are very poor and very old women. However, to be eligible for SSI requires extreme poverty and almost no assets. The national income floor maintained by SSI provides an annual income that in 1982 was 71 percent of the poverty line for an aged individual (Trout and Mattson 1984).[1]

Social Security income for retired persons has been increasingly important in protecting the elderly from the adverse consequences of periodic swings in the economy, which have resulted in four recessions in the past twelve years. The prevalence of poverty among the elderly population in the early 1960s was reduced from 25 percent to 14 percent by the late 1970s, a reduction due largely to the adjustment of Social Security benefits to inflation. Yet inflation in the late 1970s still had a substantial effect on many of those living at the margin of poverty: the poverty rate increased from 14 percent in 1978 to 15.7 percent in 1980. During the recession of 1981–1982, for the first time, poverty rates among the general population rose rapidly and exceeded the elderly poverty rate.

Whether the aged are faring as well or better than younger Americans has become a salient issue at a time of government retrenchment in social domestic spending. Consequently, needy groups have found it more difficult to compete for scarce public resources. Research that measured per capita family income found that the average incomes of the aged and nonaged are about equal. However, if one measures the income of families or households, "aged unrelated individuals, who account for 33 percent of all aged persons, have under three-fifths of the income of nonaged unrelated individuals" (Grad 1984, 17).

While 1982 census data indicate a decline in elderly poverty (now 14.6 percent, or 3.6 million older adults), the pervasive and unrelenting experience of poverty among elderly blacks and Hispanics, and among many elderly whites, cannot be ignored. Minorities experience two to three times the poverty rate of whites, with 35.6 percent of aged blacks and 38.2 percent of Hispanics, as compared to 12.4 percent of aged whites, living at extreme levels of poverty in 1982. Moreover, the elderly living alone have a poverty rate of 27.1 percent (U.S. Congress, Senate 1983a).

The face of poverty is not only minority, it is female. Almost half (49 percent) of the elderly white single women and 80 percent of the elderly black single women live at or near the poverty level (Women's Equity Action League 1985). Half of the aged poor are widows or women who never married, who live alone (Orshansky

1979; Leadership Council of Aging Organizations 1983). The prevalence of poverty among older women reflects earlier social and economic inequities. Labor market experience in low-wage industries, pay inequities, interrupted employment patterns, and divorce are factors that will continue to adversely affect the economic well-being of future generations of retired women (O'Rand 1983).

The disparity between the worst-off elderly (those 14.7 percent with incomes less than $4,000 per year) and the best-off elderly (those 12 percent with incomes of $25,000 or more per year) corresponds to life-long conditions and opportunities. A great deal of advocacy effort and legislative policy in entitlement and discretionary programs are directed toward the poorest group, while tax policy aids the higher-income group. In between the extremes of income distribution is another equally important group known as the near poor. The aged surpass every other group at the near-poor levels. If the near poor (125 percent or 150 percent of current poverty criteria) are considered, the profile of poverty in old age rises dramatically (Lehrman 1980). For example, 21 percent of white elderly are at or below 25 percent of the 1982 poverty level ($6,465 per year), compared to 51.6 percent of black elderly and 40.9 percent of Hispanic elderly (U.S. Department of Commerce, Bureau of the Census 1983). These near-poor individuals are particularly relevant to health policy considerations because they are the least likely to be assisted by Social Security retirement programs and are the most likely to be

affected by increased cost-sharing in the Medicare program and to draw on the resources of Medicaid when ill.[2]

Housing Policies

The majority of today's elderly own homes, and the market value of these homes has recently increased substantially. Over 90 percent of the total value of the housing stock owned and occupied by those over age sixty-five years is homeowner equity. However, the resource of home ownership can be quickly and unexpectedly threatened with the onset of chronic illness requiring long-term social and medical maintenance costs. Even with the combined resources of home ownership, Medicare, and supplemental private health coverage (e.g., Medigap insurance), a broad sector of middle- and low-income retired persons are inadequately protected from the potentially catastrophic costs of severe chronic disease or injury.

Retirement often reduces disposable income by one-half to one-third, making the availability of affordable housing an important consideration. Older Americans pay a larger proportion of their incomes for rent than do other age groups. Approximately 2.3 million elderly households spend over 35 percent of their incomes on housing. Forty-one percent of elderly renters with incomes below poverty level spend over 45 percent of their incomes on housing (U.S. Congress, Senate 1983a).

Experience often has borne out the essential linkages between living arrangements, adequate income, and long-term-care needs (Wan, Odell, and Lewis 1982). Yet a comprehensive policy has not been formulated, and housing remains an essential but largely ignored dimension of long-term care (Meltzer, Farrow, and Richman 1981). Overall, public policy has fostered a piecemeal approach to housing needs, which ranges from large urban public housing projects to incentives for a privately developed and publicly financed nursing home industry.

The importance of relating housing to long-term care is often realized too late, when the functional independence of an individual has been threatened and families can no longer cope. Indeed the multi-billion-dollar nursing home industry has functioned as a substitute for the lack of adequate income, suitable low-cost housing, and community social supports (Scanlon, Difederico, and Stassen 1979).

The federal role in housing has addressed, to some extent, the needs of the severely disadvantaged. In addition to federally subsidized housing for low-income households (U.S. Public Law 93-383, 1974; sec. 8, Housing and Community Development Act), there is federal financing of housing construction for older persons (sec. 202) and grants to public housing authorities to provide nutritional meals and supportive services to partially impaired elderly and handicapped persons (U.S. Public Law 95-557, 1978; Congregate Housing Services Act; U.S. Congress, Senate 1983a). Under the Reagan administration, however, federal housing policy relies more on the existing housing supply and the use of vouchers rather than on construction of new feder-

ally subsidized housing units (Zais, Struyk, and Thibodeau 1982).

Board and care is another option in the housing market; for many it is an important resource in the long-term-care continuum. The term refers to the provision by a nonrelative of food, shelter, and some protective oversight and personal care that is generally nonmedical in nature (McCoy 1983). Variously called residential care facilities, domiciliary care homes, adult foster care homes, small group and community residences, these facilities include approximately 300,000 boarding homes and 30,000 board-and-care homes in the United States; they house approximately 1.5 million residents (U.S. Department of Health and Human Services, Office of the Inspector General 1982). The growth of the board-and-care industry in the past fifteen years is due largely to public reimbursement through the federal Supplemental Security Income (SSI) program or state supplemental payments for low-income aged, blind, and disabled persons.

Private sector supportive housing options include expensive life care agreements covering a comprehensive range of health, social, and housing needs; varying types of board-and-care facilities; and single-room occupancy hotels for independent living. Some private sector congregate housing options are attractive to proprietary interests because of the increasing numbers of frail elderly.

Life care is an option for financially secure elderly persons interested in a living arrangement that provides a full range of accommodations, including congregate housing, personal care, and nursing facilities. Residents generally move from one level to another as their needs change. Historically, life care retirement communities have utilized basically a prepaid long-term-care insurance plan to help capitalize this full range of housing options. Ideally the resident needs $200,000 in assets and a $20,000 yearly income in order to subscribe to a full life care agreement (Hambrook 1984).

Another recent development is the continuing-care community, a fee-for-service arrangement that increases in cost as one moves from one level of support to another. Tax-exempt bonds and real estate tax shelter arrangements have traditionally financed the estimated three hundred to six hundred communities in the United States now housing over one-hundred thousand older adults (depending on the definition used).

Other options such as accessibility modifications, accessory apartments, home-sharing arrangements, and home equity conversion plans have developed without any support from the public sector. For the approximately 10 million elderly who own their homes without any mortgage, the home equity conversion plan is a potential source of income for the purchase of supportive services or long-term-care insurance. The nation's first long-term mortgage program, one type of equity conversion, gives the borrower monthly loan advances that do not have to be repaid until the borrower dies, sells the home, or reaches age one hundred (Alpha Centerpiece Report 1984). Unfortunately, the number of people who could substantially benefit from home equity conversion programs has probably been overestimated. Careful analyses have shown that only about 20 percent of elderly homeowners could obtain as much as $2,500 per year in extra income from a standard conversion plan (Struyk 1986).

Financing, Organization, and Delivery of Health and Long-Term-Care Services

Current health care financing and social service programs for the elderly involve all levels of government as well as the private sector. At the federal level, Medicare provides health insurance coverage of hospital and physician services for most individuals aged sixty-five and over, for disabled persons under age sixty-five who meet certain criteria, and for those suffering from end-stage renal disease. There are 27 million elderly and 3 million disabled eligible beneficiaries on Medicare. Of the total Medicare expenditures for 1984 ($63.1 billion dollars), almost three-quarters was spent on hospital services (70 percent) and one-quarter on physician services (23.1 percent). Medicare expenditures were negligible in covering nursing homes (less than 1 percent) and less than 3.1 percent in covering home health care in fiscal year 1984 (U.S. Congress, Senate 1985). Medicare does not cover long-term care, out-of-institution drugs, dental care, eyeglasses, hearing aids, and other important health services for the elderly.

Because the federal government plays a dominant role in the payment for hospital and physician services for the elderly, its reimbursement policies have been important in driving costs upward. The critical policy objective of Medicare and Medicaid was to assure access to "mainstream" medical care for the elderly and the poor. To guarantee provider acceptance, Congress required that payment to hospitals would be made on the basis of their costs, determined after the care was provided. Physicians were paid on the basis of their usual, customary, and reasonable charges under Medicare and on the basis of a fixed fee scale under Medicaid. These policies held for almost twenty years, in spite of steadily rising costs that exceeded the consumer price index by a wide margin and rapidly increasing Medicare and Medicaid expenditures.

One immediate consequence of the implementation of Medicare, which had a significant impact on costs, was the dramatic increase in the use of short-stay hospital services by the elderly. There was, initially, an increase in both the rate of admission and the length of stay. After 1967 the average length of stay for the elderly began to decline, but the admission rate continued to increase (U.S. Department of Health and Human Services, Health Care Financing Administration 1980). Surgical rates also increased dramatically. In 1965 there were 6,554 operations for every 100,000 persons aged sixty-five and older; in 1975 there were 15,483 operations for every 100,000 persons aged sixty-five and older—an increase of over 100 percent (Kovar 1977). The use, outside the hospital, of prescrip-

tion drugs, an item not covered by Medicare, rose even more rapidly during this period (Lee 1980).

Although the number of hospital admissions and surgical procedures per 100,000 elderly rose dramatically, the use of physicians' services outside the hospital by the elderly changed relatively little. There was an increase in the use of physicians' services by the poor elderly and a decrease by the nonpoor, with the overall average remaining close to 6.5 visits per year for 1965 through 1978 (U.S. Department of Health and Human Services, Health Care Financing Administration 1980).

The increased utilization of hospital services by the elderly and the gradually increasing number of elderly were factors affecting the rapid increase in Medicare expenditures. These factors were relatively minor, however, when compared to the impact of general inflation and the additional price increases by hospitals and physicians, and the increased complexity of care provided. Although the rise in hospital costs has been the focus of policymakers' attention, the costs of physician services have risen even more rapidly since the enactment of Medicare (Etheridge and Merrill 1984).

An issue of growing concern to both patients and policymakers has been the cost of medical care during the last year of a person's life. During 1978, 1.9 million people died in the United States; of these, 1.3 million were Medicare enrollees (Lubitz and Prihoda 1983). These 1.3 million represented only 5.2 percent of Medicare enrollees but accounted for 28.2 percent of Medicare expenditures. The

Medicare program spent an average of $4,527 on enrollees in their last year of life, an amount 6.2 times the $729 spent on enrollees who did not die in 1978. For those who died, expenditures were also greater during the year prior to their death, but not as great as in the last year of life. In the last year of life, expenses increased as death approached: 30 percent of the expenditures were made during the last thirty days of life and 46 percent in the last sixty days (Lubitz and Prihoda 1983).

Although Medicare has been the most important source of payments for hospitals and physicians caring for the elderly since 1965, it is limited in scope of benefits and reimbursement policies required to meet the needs of the chronically ill and disabled elderly. The cost of care, that is, the full range of services addressing the health, personal, and social needs, is borne by both the private (the elderly themselves and their families) and the public sectors, including Supplementary Security Income (SSI), Medicare, and Medicaid. The Social Services Block Grant and Older Americans Act programs, which support the nonprofit voluntary agencies at the local level, are a vital part of the long-term-care picture in the community, but they garner considerably less public resources than the strictly medically defined long-term-care service.

State policy, because of the decentralization of policies relative to Medicaid and social services, has become a major factor determining the scope, structure, and availability of long-term care. The result has been a variety of approaches, in part dependent

on the fiscal condition of the states. The recession of 1981–1982 and the subsequent economic recovery have affected states quite differently; as a result, the resources available for public programs at the state level varies markedly (Estes, Newcomer, and Associates 1983).

Three developments are of great importance in the organization of health and long-term-care services if the needs of the chronically ill and disabled elderly are to be met effectively: (1) the need to better link and integrate acute-care and long-term-care services in the community; (2) the need to strengthen ambulatory care, community-based services (e.g., adult day care, congregate meals, senior centers), and in-home services and to reduce the emphasis on inpatient care in hospitals and nursing homes; and (3) the need to recognize the benefits (as well as the limits) and potential roles of family members and other sources of social support, including the full spectrum of nonprofit community agencies serving the elderly.

There have been many positive professional and community efforts (largely demonstration projects) directed toward a more comprehensive and humane long-term-care policy. Koff (1982) envisions a long-term-care system in which institution-based and community-based services are integrated and appropriately utilized in a "continuum of care." In contrast to this ideal, there is generally no systematic link between the myriad health and social services that have emerged as alternatives to institutionalization; nor is there a systematic link between the acute and chronic care systems (Vogel and Palmer 1983).

In addition to the changes in financing and organization that are needed, the effective care of the elderly requires changes at the clinical level. Clinical care, whether provided by physicians, nurses, dentists, or other health professionals, must take account of the behavioral and social factors, as well as of the biological and medical factors that contribute to morbidity among the elderly. This biopsychosocial approach was described by Engle (1977) and has recently been applied to the elderly. From this perspective, the functional status of the elderly would be affected by the biological, social, and psychologic changes. All of these factors must be considered in patient care, and they require a more broader approach than is customary for most physicians. Physicians can no longer isolate themselves in an office-based practice or in a hospital and expect to fully meet the needs of elderly patients with multiple social as well as medical needs. Linkages with the range of services essential to the care of the disabled, chronically ill elderly will be required.

Linkage is also needed between levels of care—primary, secondary, and tertiary—as well as between acute and long-term care. One approach to the better integration of acute and long-term care could be through the expansion of health maintenance organizations (HMOs). HMOs could encompass the full spectrum of social and health (and long-term care) needs, including home care, ambulatory care (including adult day care, congregate meals), and nursing home care, on a prepaid capitation basis to control costs (Diamond and Berman 1981). Called social health maintenance organizations (SHMOs), these new types of prepaid plans not only place providers at risk and change incentives (as do HMOs), they also have the potential for redesigning both the delivery and financing of long-term care.

Another linkage model that has emerged focuses on those in greatest need of medical and social services and provides a comprehensive range of services, primarily in the home and in the community. An example of such a model of comprehensive care for the very frail, sick, and disabled elderly is On Lok in San Francisco. Here, medical, nursing, and social services, physical, occupational, and recreational therapy, counseling, congregate meals, housing, transportation, respite care, and in-home services are provided by a single agency. For a patient population of over three hundred, all of whom were eligible for nursing home admission, it has been possible to meet the patients' needs in a humane, compassionate, and cost-effective manner. The physician and all other health professionals involved are team players, adjusting their respective roles to the patients' needs.

The emerging hospital model of acute and long-term care involves a "vertical" integration of traditional hospital inpatient services, with ambulatory care, home care, and nursing home care. Whether this approach will further fragment community-based care and whether it is the most cost-effective use of community resources remain to be seen.

These changes in health and long-term care will not be possible without substantial changes in medical, nursing, pharmacy, and dental education. Today's entering medical and nursing students particularly, as well as many of those in the other health professions, will spend an increasing part of their professional lives dealing with chronic illness and functional disability in their elderly patients. To do their jobs well, their education and training will need to place more emphasis on chronic diseases, aging, management of chronic disability, prevention and rehabilitation, and social and behavioral factors in health and disease.

Health Care Cost-Containment

The 1980s have brought a dramatic shift in health care and health care policies that promise to have a major impact in the care of the elderly. During the past decade the federal and state governments and the private sector have attempted a variety of regulatory and market strategies to slow the rapidly rising costs of health care. Early in the 1970s President Richard Nixon introduced wage and price controls to fight rapidly increasing inflation. These controls were retained in the health sector after they were removed for most of the economy. Wage and price controls were followed by an increased emphasis at the state level on health planning and control of capital expenditures by hospitals, the stimulation of

market forces and the encouragement of health maintenance organizations, fee schedules for physicians, reimbursement controls for nursing homes, and voluntary hospital cost-containment. In spite of these efforts, costs continued to rise rapidly through the 1970s and into the 1980s. Most of the efforts to control costs had little, if any, impact, and the growth of technology and the rapid increase in physician supply contributed to increased costs.

Procompetitive, antiregulatory, and prodecentralization (New Federalism) policies received increased emphasis after Ronald Reagan's election in 1980. The enactment of the Omnibus Budget Reconciliation of 1981, the Tax Equity and Fiscal Responsibility Act (TEFRA) of 1982, and the Social Security Amendments of 1983 was intended to create basic changes in Medicare and Medicaid policies, for the first time since their enactment in 1965. These policy changes, combined with rapid growth of HMOs in the private sector and increasing competition among physicians and hospitals for patients, set the stage for major changes in health care financing.

In 1981 provisions in the Omnibus Reconciliation Act (U.S. Public Law 97-35, 1981) reduced the federal Medicaid budget from the levels expected by the states; but the states were given greater flexibility to operate their programs. States were permitted to reduce eligibility for specific subgroups and services and were no longer required to use the Medicare cost-based hospital reimbursement formula in the Medicaid program. Thus, a costly, inflationary system that paid hospitals for services (that had already been provided) could be replaced by a prospectively determined payment system.

More important, the most significant policy shift since the enactment of Medicare occurred in 1983 with the change from retrospective cost-based reimbursement to prospective payment system for hospitals. Public Law 92-21 (the Social Security Amendments of 1983) changed the Medicare reimbursement to a prospective payment system based on a classification system known as diagnosis-related groups or DRGs.

Under the DRG prospective system, the critical factors in determining the Medicare payment for hospitals will no longer be costs but principal diagnosis, presence or absence of secondary diagnosis, patient age, patient sex, and the presence or absence of a surprise procedure. Initially, payment to the hospitals will be based on their historic costs (75 percent) and a regional cost factor (25 percent). Over four years all hospitals will be moved to a nationally determined rate per discharge. This fixed-price payment by case provides incentives for the hospitals to reduce their actual costs. What effects this system will have on payers, providers, and patients remains to be seen (Vladeck 1984). Key questions for the elderly under the DRG system are what its impact will be on the availability of needed hospital care and what the anticipated increased demand for in-home services will be as patients' length of hospital stay is reduced and they are discharged from hospitals earlier than in the past.

States have taken a number of steps to reduce Medicaid expenditures.

Seven states (New York, Maryland, Massachusetts, New Jersey, Wisconsin, Maine, and West Virginia) have adopted state systems of all-payer regulation of hospital costs instead of attempting simply to reduce Medicaid expenditures. These systems may include Medicare and Medicaid as well as private health insurance payments. During the past decade, experiences of states with hospital cost-control regulation, particularly all-payer regulation, indicates that this approach has been more effective than any other in controlling hospital cost increases (Biles, Schram, and Atkinson 1980; Coelen and Sullivan 1981).

A number of states (e.g., California, Utah, Texas, Arizona) have stressed the price-competitive, market-reform ideology, following three general strategies: (1) increased consumer cost-sharing; (2) the development of competitive health care systems that can contract on a capitation basis (e.g., health maintenance organizations); and (3) prospective pricing of hospital services, with contracts through Medicaid and private health insurance that limit consumer choice.

That the priority of the states is on cost savings rather than system reform is perhaps best understood in light of the fiscal condition of state governments, their own taxpayer reforms and revenues, fluctuations in the national economy (from inflation to severe recession, to recovery in recurring cycles), and uncertainty regarding future federal and state roles in health care for the elderly and the poor. To date, most states and federal cost-containment efforts have focused on hospital cost-containment through controls on utilization and reimbursement.[3] Physicians are likely to be the next target of cost-containment efforts, particularly in the Medicare program. The focus will be on physicians' fees, not on structural reforms.

Partly because Medicare, given its exclusive focus on older persons, has always commanded the primary attention of interest groups for the aging, and partly because Medicaid is fragmented within its federal-state structure into more than fifty programs, the significance of the Medicaid program for the aging has not been sufficiently appreciated. What happens to the Medicaid program at the state level in the next several years is likely to have major implications for recent efforts to develop a continuum of care. What happens at the state level in terms of both health care competition and regulation, and how effective these strategies prove to be in controlling health costs, is likely to determine whether the resources needed for more comprehensive services will be available.

Long-term-care costs remain a concern but have had a lower priority because the expenditure levels were well below those for hospitals and physicians. A wide range of options have been discussed, but there are few signs of the fundamental shift in service provision that many had hoped for—the substitution of lower-cost community-based services for high-cost hospital and nursing home services (Wood and Estes 1985). Many community-based home health and social services depend not only on Medicare and Medicaid reimbursement but on federal funding and federal-state matching funds to maintain services, particularly to the low-income elderly. The development of appropriate community-based home health and social services has traditionally rested within the private, nonprofit sector. It is this sector that appears to face a large proportion of cutbacks in public monies, which were initiated with the 1981 federal policy changes (Wood and Estes 1983). Recently, the proprietary sector has begun to provide in-home services (e.g., nursing, nutrition) because of changes in Medicare reimbursement that have made this segment of the long-term care continuum a potentially profitable market.

Conclusion

Research is needed to develop an understanding of the limits and the potential of an enlightened health and aging policy; it is also needed to disentangle the effects of disease from those of physiological or biological aging, and these from the effects of social, economic, and political factors and forces. As this chapter has discussed, the achievement of health is dependent upon a complex web of interactions among biological, behavioral, sociocultural, and environmental factors (McKeown 1976; Cassell 1976; Lee and Franks 1980). It is possible and important to construct policies that recognize the determinants of health and that foster healthy aging.

During the past twenty years public policies, particularly Social Security, Supplementary Security Income, Medicare, and Medicaid have made a substantial contribution to the health, well-being, and care of older

Americans. To achieve further gains a vital federal role is essential in health, income, housing, and long-term-care policies. An efficient and equitable health policy for the elderly must strive to achieve four goals: (1) Social Security and Supplemental Security Income, with levels adequate to assure that no elderly individuals or families live on a below-poverty income; (2) housing policies that meet the diverse needs of a heterogeneous older population, including provisions to meet the needs of the elderly for independent living and nursing home care if required; (3) policies and strategies that strengthen family and informal social support systems without undue hardship on the systems (and particularly on working women); and (4) an age-integrated health care and social service strategy that includes universal entitlement and comprehensive benefits, including long-term care with effective cost-control.

To improve efficiency requires an effective means to control the rapidly rising costs. This can best be accomplished through a strategy that includes both regulation and market reform, particularly payer regulation of hospitals as well as regulation of physician fees and nursing home costs at the state level; added incentives to health maintenance organizations and other competing health plans that offer comprehensive services on a capitation rather than fee-for-service basis; and incentives for less institutional care and more appropriate community-based, noninstitutional services.

Policymakers must be concerned not only with cost containment but with equity as well. An equitable allocation and distribution of the nation's health care resources require a vital federal leadership role in health and aging policies. As state and local governments, employers, and private insurance companies across the country devise ways to meet the countervailing demands of taxpayers, health providers, and the public needing health care, we believe that long-range comprehensive reform will best be achieved by concerted national leadership rather than by the piecemeal development of either policies based on market reforms and price competition or Medicare and Medicaid cost-containment strategies adopted independent of all other mechanisms of health care payment.

The situation is critical from all viewpoints—payers, providers, and the public. To serve the needs of the nation's population, including the elderly, a long-range and multigenerational perspective that will achieve an equitable as well as an efficient use of the nation's resources is needed. An intergenerational agenda is needed on health policies. National policies must provide the framework for both public and private action in order to continue to improve the health of the nation at a price we can all afford.

Acknowledgment

The authors gratefully acknowledge the assistance of Lenore E. Gerard in the preparation of this chapter.

Notes

1. This is still only a minimal amount of money. For example, while the maximum monthly benefit for an individual in 1983 was $304 per month, the average monthly benefit was less than $160 per month. States can and do supplement the federal benefit — in amounts ranging from a low of $20 to a high of $340. In three states (Alaska, California, and Massachusetts), supplementary payments actually raise the SSI levels above the national poverty index (Trout and Mattson 1984).

2. Escalating health care costs and budget cuts have significantly raised the proportion of costs personally shouldered by older Americans. In 1980 the nation's elderly used 13 percent of their income for health care; by 1984 this amount had risen to 15 percent — more than before Medicare and Medicaid began in 1965. By 1988, and under 1 current law, the elderly are projected to spend 17.5 percent of their income on health care of $2,194 per elderly person (U.S. Congress, House of Representatives 1985.) Out-of-pocket health care expenses are disproportionately borne by households incomes under $5,000 (U.S. Congress, Budget Office 1983).

3. Nursing home reimbursement policy has been one major state cost-containment method. In an attempt to control costs, there has been great variation among the states' attempts to control the number of nursing home beds. The number of nursing home beds per 1,000 residents aged sixty-five and older varies from 21.2 in Arizona to 93.2 in Minnesota (Harrington and Swan 1985); the expenditures for nursing home care tend to reflect these differences in bed supply.

References

Alpha Centerpiece Report. 1984. Long-term care alternatives: Innovations in financing chronic care for the elderly. Bethesda, Md.

Ball, M. 1981. Rethinking national policy on health care for the elderly. In *The geriatric imperative*, ed. A. R. Somers and D. R. Fabian. New York: Appleton-Century-Crofts.

Belloc, N. B., and L. Breslow. 1972. Relationship of physical health status and health practices. *Preventive Medicine* 1:409–421.

Berkman, L. F. 1985. The relationship of social networks and social support to morbidity and mortality. In *Social support and health*, ed. S. Cohen and S. L. Syme. New York: Academic Press.

Berkman, L. F., and L. Breslow. 1983. *Health and ways of living*. New York: Oxford University Press.

Biles, B., C. J. Schram, and J. Atkinson. 1980. Hospital cost inflation under state rate-setting programs. *New England Journal of Medicine* 303(12): 664–668.

Bovbjerg, R. R. 1984. *Medicaid in the Reagan era.* Washington, D.C.: Urban Institute.

Butler, L. H., and P. W. Newacheck. 1981. Health and social factors affecting long-term care policy. *Policy options in long-term care,* ed. J. Meltzer, F. Farrow, and H. Richman. Chicago: University of Chicago.

Butler, R. N., and M. I. Lewis. 1982. *Aging and mental health.* 3d ed. St. Louis, Mo.: Mosby.

Cassel, J. 1976. The contribution of the social environment to host resistance. *American Journal of Epidemiology* 104(2):107–123.

Coelen, C., and D. Sullivan. 1981. An analysis of the effects of prospective reimbursement programs on hospital expenditures. *Health Care Financing Review* 2(3):1–40.

Crystal, S. 1982. *America's old age crisis.* New York: Basic.

Diamond, L. M., and D. E. Berman. 1981. The social/health maintenance organization: A single entry, prepaid, long-term delivery system. In *Reforming the long-term care system,* ed. J. Callahan and S. S. Wallace. Lexington, Mass.: Lexington Books, D. C. Heath & Co.

Engel, G. L. The need for a new medical model: A challenge for biomedicine. *Science* 196(428):129–134.

Estes, C. L. 1979. *The aging enterprise.* San Francisco: Jossey-Bass.

Estes, C. L., R. J. Newcomer, and Associates. 1983. *Fiscal austerity and aging.* Beverly Hills, Calif.: Sage.

Etheredge, L., and J. C. Merrill. 1984. Medicare: Paying the physician. Washington, D.C., Urga Urban Institute. Typescript.

Fisher, C. 1980. Differences by age groups in health care spending. *Health Care Financing Review* 1(4):65–90.

Fries, J. F. 1980. Aging, natural health, and the compression of morbidity. *New England Journal of Medicine* 303:130–135.

————. 1983. The compression of morbidity. *Milbank Memorial Fund Quarterly: Health and Society* 61:397–419.

————. 1984. The compression of morbidity: Miscellaneous comments about a theme. *Gerontologist* 24(4):354–359.

Fries, J. F., and L. M. Crapo. 1981. *Vitality and aging: Implications of the rectangular curve.* San Francisco: W. H. Freeman.

Fuchs, V. R. 1984. Though much is taken: Reflections on aging, health, and medical care. *Milbank Memorial Fund Quarterly: Health and Society* 62(2):143–166.

Gibson, R. M., D. R. Waldo, and K. R. Levit. 1983. National health expenditures, 1982. *Health Care Financing Review* 5(1):1–31.

Grad, S. 1984. *Income of the population 55 and over, 1982.* U.S. Department of Health and Human Services, Social Security Administration. Washington, D.C.: Government Printing Office.

Gruenberg, E. M. 1977. The failures of success. *Milbank Memorial Fund Quarterly: Health and Society* 55(1):3–24.

Hadley, J. 1982. *More medical care, better health?* Washington, D.C.: Urban Institute.

Hambrook, A. 1984. Panel discussion on architectural issues and marketing techniques. Laventhol and Horwath First Annual Lifecare–Continuing Care Retirement Center Symposium. San Francisco, Calif.

Harrington, C., R. Newcomer, and C. L. Estes, and Associates. 1985. *Long term care of the elderly.* Beverly Hills, Calif.: Sage.

Harrington, C., and J. H. Swan. 1984. Medicaid nursing home reimbursement policies, rates, and expenditures. *Health Care Financing Review* 6(1): 39–49.

———. 1985. Institutional long term care services. In *Long term care of the elderly: Public policy issues,* ed. C. Harrington, R. Newcomer, C. Estes, and Associates. Beverly Hills: Sage.

Kane, R. A., and A. L. Kane. 1982. Long-term care: A field in search of values. In *Values and long-term care.* Lexington, Mass.-Heath.

Koff, T. H. 1982. *Long-term care: An approach to serving frail elderly.* Boston: Little, Brown.

Kovar, M. G. 1977. Elderly people: The population 65 years and over. In *Health United States, 1976–1977.* National Center for Health Statistics. Washington, D.C.: Government Printing Office.

Leadership Council of Aging Organizations. 1983. The administration's 1984 budget: A critical view from an aging perspective. Washington, D.C.

Lehrman, R. 1980. Poverty statistics serve as nagging reminder. *Generations: Journal of the Western Gerontological Society* 4(1):17.

Lee, P. R. 1980. Health policy issues for the aged and challenges for the 1980's. *Generations* 4(1):38–40, 73.

Lee, P. R., C. L. Estes, L. LeRoy, and R. J. Newcomer. 1982. Health policy and the aged. In *Annual review of gerontology and geriatrics,* vol. 3, ed. C. Eisdorfer. New York: Springer Publishing.

Lee, P. R., and P. E. Franks. 1980. Health and disease in the community. In *Primary care,* ed. J. Fry. London: William Heinemann Medical Books.

Lindeman, D. A., and A. Pardini. 1983. Social services: The impact of fiscal austerity. In *Fiscal austerity and aging,* ed. C. Estes, R. J. Newcomer, and Associates. Beverly Hills: Sage.

Lubitz, J., and R. Prihoda. 1983. Use and costs of Medicare services in the last years of life. In *Health: United States and prevention profile,* pp. 71–77. U.S. Department of Health and Human Services, Public Health Service, National Center for Health Statistics. Hyattsville, Md.: Government Printing Office.

Luft, H. S. 1978. *Poverty and health: Economic causes and consequences of health problems.* Cambridge, Mass.: Ballinger.

McCoy, J. L. 1983. Overview of available data relating to board and care and care homes and residents. U.S. Department of Health and Human Services. Unpublished memo.

McKeown, T. 1976. *The role of medicine: Dream, mirage, or nemesis.* London: Nuffield Provincial Hospital Trust.

Manton, K. C. 1982. Changing concepts of morbidity and mortality in the elderly population. *Milbank Memorial Fund Quarterly: Health and Society* 60(2):183–244.

Meltzer, J., F. Farrow, and H. Richman, eds. 1981. *Policy options in long term care.* Chicago: University of Chicago Press.

Myers, G. C., and K. C. Manton. 1984. Compression of mortality: Myth or reality? *Gerontologist* 24(4):346–353.

National Center for Health Statistics. 1982. *Health. United States, 1982.* DHHS Publication No. (PHS) 83-1232. Washington, D.C.: Government Printing Office.

Newcomer, R. J., M. P. Lawton, and T. Byerts, eds. 1985. *Housing an aging society.* New York: Van Nostrand Reinhold.

New York State Office on Aging. 1983. *Medicare: Analysis and recommendations for reform.* Albany, N.Y.: State Office on Aging.

O'Rand, A. M. 1983. Women. In *Handbook of the aged in the United States,* ed. E. Palmore. Westport, Conn.: Greenwood Press.

Orshansky, H. 1979. Statement in U.S. House Select Committee on Aging, Hearing on poverty among America's aged. August 9. Washington, D.C.: Government Printing Office.

Rice, D. 1985. Personal communication.

Rice, D. P., and J. J. Feldman. 1983. Living longer in the United States: Demographic changes and health needs of the elderly. *Milbank Fund Memorial Quarterly: Health and Society* 61(3):362–396.

Scanlon, W., E. Difederico, and M. Stassen. 1979. *Long-term care: Current experience and a framework for analysis.* Washington, D.C.: Urban Institute.

Schneider, E. L., and J. A. Brody. 1983. Aging, natural death, and the compression of morbidity: Another view. *New England Journal of Medicine* 309:854–856.

Struyk, R. J. 1986. Future housing assistance policy for the elderly. In *Housing an aging society,* ed. R. J. Newcomer, M. P. Lawton, and T. Byerts. New York: Van Nostrand Reinhold.

Trout, J., and D. R. Mattson. 1984. A 10-year review of the Supplemental Security Income program. *Social Security Bulletin* 47(1):3–24.

U.S. Congress. Budget Office. 1983. *Changing the structure of Medicare benefits: Issue and options.* Washington, D.C.: Government Printing Office.

———. House of Representatives. Committee on Ways and Means. 1985. *Background material and data on programs within the jurisdiction of the committee.* Washington, D.C.: Government Printing Office.

———. Select Committee on Aging. 1985. *The president's 1986 budget.* Washington, D.C.: Government Printing Office.

———. Senate. Special Committee on Aging. 1982, 1983a, 1984a, 1985. *Developments in aging: 1981, 1982, 1983, 1984.* Washington, D.C.: Government Printing Office.

———. 1983b. Hearings on life care communities: Promises and problems. Washington, D.C.: Government Printing Office.

————. 1984b. *Older Americans and the federal budget: Past, present, and future.* Washington, D.C.: Government Printing Office.

U.S. Department of Commerce. Bureau of the Census. 1983. Money income and poverty status of families and persons in the United States, 1982. Washington, D.C.: Government Printing Office.

U.S. Department of Health and Human Services. Health Care Financing Administration. 1980. *Ten years of short-stay hospital utilization and costs under Medicare: 1967, 1976.* Office of Research, Demonstrations, and Statistics. Washington, D.C.: Government Printing Office.

————. 1981. *Long term care: Background and future directions.* Washington, D.C.: Government Printing Office.

————. Office of the Inspector General. 1982. *Board and care homes: A study of federal and state actions to safeguard the health and safety of board and care residents.* Washington, D.C.: Government Printing Office.

————. Social Security Administration. 1984a. *Social Security bulletin: Annual statistical supplement, 1980.* Washington, D.C.: Government Printing Office.

————. 1984b. Social security in review. *Social Security Bulletin* 47(2):1.

————. 1985. *Monthly benefit statistics program data: Old-age, survivors, disability, and health insurance.* Washington, D.C.: Government Printing Office.

U.S. Public Law 93-383. 1974. Housing and community development act of 1974 (as amended). Washington, D.C.: Government Printing Office.

U.S. Public Law 95-557. 1978. Congregate housing services act of 1978 (as amended). Washington, D.C.: Government Printing Office.

U.S. Public Law 97-34. 1981. Economic Recovery Tax Act of 1981. Washington, D.C.: Government Printing Office.

U.S. Public Law 97-35. 1981. Omnibus Reconciliation Act of 1981. Washington, D.C.: Government Printing Office.

U.S. Public Law 97-248. 1982. Tax Equity and Fiscal Responsibility Act of 1982. Washington, D.C.: Government Printing Office.

Verbrugge, L. 1984. Longer life but worsening health? Trends in health and mortality of middle aged and older persons. *Milbank Memorial Fund Quarterly: Health and Society* 62(3):475–519.

Vladeck, B. C. 1984. Medicare hospital payment by diagnosis-related groups. *Annals of Internal Medicine* 100(4):576–591.

Vogel, R. J., and H. C. Palmer, eds. 1983. *Long term care: Perspectives from research and demonstrations.* Baltimore, Md.: U.S. Health Care Financing Administration.

Waldo, D. R., and H. C. Lazenby. 1984. Demographic characteristics and health care use and expenditures by the aged in the United States, 1977–1984. *Health Care Financing Review* 6(1):1–29.

Wan, T. T. H., B. F. Odell, and D. T. Lewis. 1982. *Promoting the well-being of the elderly: A community diagnosis.* New York: Haworth Press.

Wan, T. T., and W. G. Weissert. 1981. Social support networks, patient status, and institutionalization. *Research on Aging* 3(2):240–256.

Women's Equity Action League (WEAL). 1985. Facts on Social Security. Washington, D.C.: WEAL.

Wood, J. B., and C. L. Estes. 1983. The private nonprofit sector and aging. In *Fiscal austerity and aging*, ed. C. L. Estes, R. J. Newcomer, and Associates. Beverly Hills: Sage.

———. 1985. Private, nonprofit organizations and community-based long term care. In *Long term care of the elderly: Public policy issues*, ed. C. Harrington, R. Newcomer, and C. Estes and Associates. Beverly Hills: Sage.

World Health Organization. 1948. Test of the constitution of World Health Organization. *Official Records* 2:100.

Zais, J. P., R. J. Struyk, and T. Thibodeau. 1982. *Housing assistance for older Americans*. Washington, D.C.: Urban Institute.

Part IV

Prevention and Caring

Chapter 17

The Detection and Modification of Psychosocial and Behavioral Risk Factors

Stanislav V. Kasl

There is little doubt that the sociopolitical climate within the United States Public Health Service in the last decade has led to the identification of a strong health promotion, disease prevention agenda (Green, Wilson, and Bauer 1983). The Office of the Assistant Secretary for Health issued a number of publications between 1978 and 1981 that dealt with health promotion. The 1980 report entitled *Promoting Health, Preventing Disease: Objectives for the Nation* (U.S. Department of Health and Human Services, Office of the Assistant Secretary for Health 1980) defined a very ambitious set of goals (frequently stated in quantitative terms), falling into three categories: (1) preventive health services, such as high blood pressure control and family planning; (2) health protection, such as toxic agent control and accident prevention; and (3) health promotion, such as smoking, nutrition, and physical fitness.

The specific goals listed in *Promoting Health* suggest that biomedical technology would not play a dominant role; furthermore, the goals appear to be coordinated to existing technology and do not particularly presuppose the need for technological innovation in the basic biomedical sciences. The goals are particularly concerned with broad, nonspecific risk factors that are strongly linked to social and political institutions as well as to psychosocial characteristics of individuals and their primary social settings. The relevant technology for detecting and, particularly, for modifying these environmental and sociobehavioral risk factors must presumably come primarily from the social and behavioral sciences. What specifically are the relevant technologies and how many are already in place are clearly some of the major uncertainties growing out of *Promoting Health.* This is particularly true of the last section of the report, which deals, in part, with control of stress. Given the immense difficulties in establishing the etiological role of stress in disease or in identifying effective public health strategies for reducing stress on a national scale, one must wonder if popular preoccupation with stress, rather than a large body of scientific data, had led to the inclusion of this particular goal in the national agenda.

Another uncertainty that grows from the report, although not the subject of this chapter, is whether the executive and legislative branches of the federal government possess the political will and fortitude to implement, with dollars and legislation, any recommendations of the *Promoting Health* agenda. It is clear (e.g., Glasunov et al. 1983; McGuire 1984) that comprehensive and integrated programs of prevention/promotion need to include institutional strategies and participation of legislative/governmental bodies. Unfortunately, it is quite possible that the health promotion/disease prevention agenda of the USPHS is merely a harmless window dressing, developed in isolation from other federal agencies and without any real political backing.

This chapter will examine two issues that arise, broadly speaking, out of the prevention/promotion orientation: (1) What is the accumulated evidence regarding psychosocial and behavioral risk factors for disease and disability, particularly those that cut across different health outcomes and are not specific to one class of outcomes (such as cardiovascular disease, cancer, and mental illness, which are considered in other chapters of this book)? The discussion includes a consideration of research strategies for the detection of such risk factors. (2) What is our current understanding of the various techniques for modifying such risk-factors and what are the prospects for successful or unsuccessful application of such techniques? In this discussion, epidemiologic theory and methods will be used to provide an organizing and unifying framework. Epidemiology is seen as the best single framework when discussing etiologic evidence and risk-factor modification issues in a health policy framework (e.g., Morris 1975; Terris 1980).

A Conceptual Framework

One starting point is a schema (admittedly both hypothetical and idealized) of stages in the development of disease. Such stages would include: (1) asymptomatic status, risk factor(s) absent; (2) asymptomatic status, risk factor(s) present; (3) subclinical disease susceptible to detection; (4) initial symptom experience; (5) initial event; (i.e., diagnostic criteria for a disease are met); (6) course of disease (repeat episodes. residual disability, etc.), either as a natural course or as modified by treatment; (7) institutionalization; (8) mortality (case fatality).

Given this disease development schema, we can graft onto it a corresponding classification of health promotion/disease prevention activities, for example: (1) prevent initiation of adverse health habits or prevent exposure to environmental risk; (2) reduce (eliminate) existing adverse health habits or remove exposure; (3) promote detection of (silent) biological risk factors; (4) reduce biological risk factors by altering adverse health habits or by promoting acceptance of appropriate biomedical intervention; (5) promote early detection of subclinical disease or early response to symptoms; (6) once clinical disease is present, promote recovery and prevent repeat episodes (exacerbation) by enhancing likelihood of behaviors still pertinent at this stage (such as appropriate health behavior or adherence to rehabilitative or health-maintaining regimens).

The above schema is compatible with other typologies and classifications, such as concepts of primary-secondary-tertiary prevention in public health (e.g., Mausner and Bahn 1974), Suchman's (1965) stages of illness and medical care, the health behavior–illness behavior–sick role behavior continuum (Kasl and Cobb 1966), and Green's (1984) typology of health-related behaviors. The schema also helps us locate more precisely new concepts, such as the notion of at-risk role (Baric 1969), that are from

time to time introduced into this broad domain. Of course, the disease development schema cannot be equally helpful across different diseases, particularly for diseases of unknown etiology and conditions for which effective treatment has not been identified. However, it does have a number of advantages. Above all, it encourages us to be systematic and comprehensive, and it can organize our knowledge as well as define the scope of our ignorance. Furthermore, it helps us to better understand and analyze trends in illness and disability, as they might be indexed by a variety of indicators from mortality data to behavioral data (Wilson and Drury 1984). Thus mortality trends cannot tell us at what point(s) in the disease development the change is taking place, while risk-factor trends do not reveal whether changes in incidence of new events, repeat episodes, or case fatality will follow (Gillum, Blackburn, and Feinleib 1982). The developmental schema can also sensitize us to the fact that varying dynamics may characterize different stages. For example, a review of the recent evidence about the health belief model (Janz and Becker 1984) suggests that some components of the model (e.g., "perceived barriers") may be influential throughout the range of development, while others may be more narrowly involved (e.g., "perceived susceptibility" for initiating preventive health behaviors, and "perceived benefits" for maintaining selected treatment-related behaviors). In general, the broad evidence better supports the proposition that factors relating to incidence (initial event) of disease are different from those that affect course and outcome of disease, rather than the proposition that a same set of factors will be involved in both (e.g., Kasl 1983).

The disease development schema is also a crucial framework for understanding possible risk-factor dynamics. Because this chapter concentrates on psychosocial and behavioral risk factors, the major issue is how the (established) biological risk factors and the psychosocial variables relate to each other in the overall etiological picture. The most common objective is to show that the psychosocial risk factor is independent of the effect of the preexisting biological risk factors and that it contributes unique variance to the prediction after the biological risk factors have entered the prediction equation first. This characterizes the data analysis strategies of such well-known psychosocial epidemiology studies as Framingham (e.g., Haynes, Feinleib, and Kannel 1980), the Western Collaborative Group Study (Brand et al. 1976), and the Israeli Ischemic Heart Disease Project (e.g., Medalie and Goldbourt 1976). It is important to realize, however, that this analysis strategy does not pin down the specific role of psychosocial risk factors unless the study design itself zeroes in on small steps in the disease development schema. Thus, when one studies the recurrence of myocardial infarction (MI) among subjects who have had a first MI, the role of behavior Type A as a risk factor (Powell and Thoresen 1985) and the consequences of altering Type A behavior (Friedman et al. 1984) can be pinned down rather well. Incidentally, in such an analysis the biologi-

cal predictors for which one adjusts first are normally some indicator of disease severity, such as the Peel index for grading severity of infarction, as well as the traditional risk factors. But showing that coronary heart disease (CHD) mortality differences by marital status are not accompanied by corresponding differences in levels of cardiovascular risk factors (Weiss 1973), does not narrow down by much the number of ways in which marital status could affect this most distal indicator, CHD mortality. And, similarly, the observation that regional and urban-suburban differentials in U.S. CHD mortality are not explained by differentials in risk-factor levels (Kleinman et al. 1981) again leaves many interpretative options open.

When a potential psychosocial risk factor is predictive of a health status outcome but this contribution to prediction disappears when biomedical predictors are introduced first, we need the disease development schema to help us understand whether we are dealing with a spurious association or a situation in which the psychosocial variable antedates the biological predictor in a developmental sequence. For example, the apparent health benefits of church attendance (Comstock and Partridge 1972) were interpreted as spurious when later refined analysis (Comstock and Tonascia 1977) suggested that prior health status differences were influencing both church attendance and health status outcomes. But if the apparent benefits of initiating vigorous exercise on CHD vanish when one adjusts for changes in blood pressure, total cholesterol, and high-density lipoproteins (e.g., Froelicher 1981; Haskell 1984), we would not consider the role of exercise as spurious but rather would view the biological changes as mediating between onset of exercise and later CHD. Of course, definitive interpretations may not always be possible. For example, in a longitudinal study of elderly community residents we may find that health status outcomes such as hospitalization or death are not predicted from the major marital status categories (married and widowed) once one adjusts for health status differences at inception. This could be because marital status is unimportant, or because we are dealing with a self-selection effect, that is, the elderly widowed in good health remarry (e.g., Helsing, Szklo, and Comstock 1981). Also, the health benefits of being married could have taken place prior to the start of the study (i.e., as an earlier unstudied and undocumented influence on health status), and no additional benefits accrued during the period of study follow-up.

An Overview of Psychosocial and Behavioral Risk Factors for Disease

Epidemiology is conventionally defined as the study of the distributions and determinants of states of health in human populations (e.g., McMahon and Pugh 1970; Susser 1973). Psychosocial or social epidemiology has no conventional definition

(e.g., Last 1983), but its common usage suggests that it deals specifically with psychosocial determinants of (physical) states of health (e.g., Graham and Reeder 1979; Syme 1974). The term *behavioral epidemiology* is sometimes used (e.g., Sexton 1979) when one wishes to highlight the study of specific behaviors and their influence on health outcomes; prominent among these behaviors are the so-called health habits, such as smoking, alcohol consumption, exercise, and so on.

Biological risk factors are characteristically specific to a single disease category. Thus hyperuricemia is a risk factor for gout (Cobb 1971); but its risk-factor status for other health outcomes, notably heart disease, remains dubious (Report 1984). Similarly, serum cholesterol seems primarily linked to coronary heart disease; its link to other outcomes, such as cancer, is at best suggestive (Feinleib 1981). Blood pressure may be an exception to this generalization about specificity of biological risk factors since it may relate to total mortality and specific cancer mortality (Conti, Farchi, and Menotti 1983; Khaw and Barrett-Connor 1984), thus transcending its traditional status as a cardiovascular risk factor.

Psychosocial and behavioral risk factors, on the other hand, are more likely to relate to a variety of health outcomes. Certainly, the major research themes in this area, those dealing with stress and social support, illustrate the expectation that a diversity of health outcomes will be involved and should be studied. And even those risk factors whose original formulation ties them closely to one disease, such as Type A behavior and coronary heart disease, are coming to be viewed more broadly, and linkages to other health outcomes are being explored (e.g., Woods and Burns 1984; Woods et al. 1984). The broad formulations that exist in social epidemiology (e.g., Antonovsky 1979; Cassel 1976; Lindheim and Syme 1983) are, in part, attempts to capture at the theoretical level this apparent broad effect of psychosocial risk factors.

However, it is not clear that psychosocial variables have such broad nonspecific effects on diverse health outcomes and that they require broad theoretical formulations. In many instances we are dealing with psychosocial variables at a much higher level of aggregation and abstraction, compared to the biological factors; possibly, only for that reason do the effects appear broad and "nonspecific." Consider a small example: various specific dietary constituents, such as specific vitamins or specific trace elements, may have very specific physiologic and disease consequences. However, if exposure to these constituents is aggregated under the broad umbrella concept of, "dietary intake," the health consequences of such exposure would be correspondingly broad and diverse. Among the psychosocial variables, socioeconomic status is an example of a high-level construct that very likely encompasses a great variety of specific exposures and risk factors which, when aggregated rather than identified and distinguished, appear to produce broad nonspecific effects, an appearance of generalized susceptibility (e.g., Syme and Berkman 1976). From the viewpoint of social science theory

building, socioeconomic status is an appropriate and useful construct; it reflects accurately the organization of social reality and packages together suitable elements. However, from the perspective of understanding etiology of disease processes, it may be too nonspecific, too heterogenous. It may drive us to high-level theorizing involving other broad constructs, such as social disorganization and domination-subordination (Cassel 1974) that remain far removed from biological mechanisms of disease causation, thus failing to illuminate them.

Major concepts that currently dominate psychosocial epidemiology, primarily stress and social support—social networks, would appear vulnerable to the same criticism as socioeconomic status: they are very broad concepts that invite very general theoretical formulations about underlying processes. This may remove us too far from the many separate and discrete underlying mechanisms of disease causation and make it more difficult to identify the points in the overall causal matrix which are optimal in thinking about prevention and intervention.

The research evidence on psychosocial risk factors for disease is difficult to organize in any systematic fashion since there is no conceptual framework that investigators have been following to test an interrelated set of hypotheses, or even to build up evidence in a systematic fashion. Members of the task force on Social Determinants of Human Health, as part of a Fogarty conference on preventive medicine in the United States (Hinkle et al. 1976), proposed a general framework for different categories of determinants, including exposure to risk factors, exposure to medical care system, differential susceptibility, social change, habits, and customs. The relevance of such a general framework for specific diseases may be variable; for example, this classification may be more useful for organizing the evidence for cancer (e.g., Levy 1983) than for heart disease (e.g., Jenkins 1982). A recent NHLBI (National Heart, Lung, and Blood Institute) conference on the measurement of psychosocial risk factors in cardiovascular disease (Ostfeld and Eaker 1985) implicitly organized the evidence into the following categories: (1) socioeconomic factors, (2) personality variables (traits), (3) behavior Type A, anger, and hostility, (4) social support and social networks, (5) chronic and acute environmental stressors, and (6) acute physiological reactivity. (Behavioral variables reflecting health habits were judged to fall outside the scope of the conference).

From a historical perspective, it is possible to see the study of psychosocial risk factors for disease being initially dominated by psychosomatic medicine and its emphasis on specific intrapsychic conflict and personality traits, and on few selected diseases (Lipowski 1976; Weiner 1977). However, as the perspectives of the social and behavioral sciences as well as epidemiology and public health intruded upon this research domain, the study of psychosocial risk factors broadened to include social-environmental factors and behavioral variables linked to health habits and medical care (Kasl 1977). A concomitant broadening was the shift from a focus on

etiology (onset of new illness) to interest in the whole spectrum of health status changes (course, treatment, and recovery) and the rejection of the notion that the "psychosomatic" perspective was applicable only to a few selected diseases. The current interest in stress (acute and chronic), and social support and networks, is a perfect embodiment of the spirit of broadening the perspective from a concern with personal traits and characteristics to a concern with environmental characteristics and the interaction of the two in a rich causal matrix. Unfortunately, from the perspective of conceptual and operational clarity, this "perfect embodiment" may in fact be an obstacle since we seem to have latched onto broad concepts that not only combine the personal and environmental processes but threaten to destroy the boundaries between the two.

The recent Institute of Medicine volume *Stress and Human Health* (Elliott and Eisdorfer 1982) notes emphatically that very few studies examine all three components in the general paradigm: stressor → biological mechanism or reaction → health status change. Rather, most studies omit the intervening step or only deal with the first link in the chain. The latter set is not the focus of this chapter, but one general comment is appropriate in this context. The combined evidence from such studies, which generally are referred to as acute physiologic reactivity, shows that they do not provide the missing link to disease outcomes (e.g., Krantz and Manuck 1985; Steptoe 1984). This situation occurs for several reasons, the literal one being that if the studies do not include disease outcomes, any link to such outcomes is not established but only, at best, plausibly inferred. Nor is the result due to many studies being done in laboratory settings, thus making the real-life analogue to the experimental stressors difficult to determine. Two other reasons seem to be involved. First, the biological variables included in the reactivity studies often do not have a clear-cut status as predictors of disease outcomes, that is, as established risk factors; this is true, for example, for indicators of endocrine function. Thus a recent review of variability of plasma lipids in response to emotional arousal (Dimsdale and Herd 1982) revealed that free fatty acids were much more reliably sensitive to a variety of psychosocial exposures and manipulations compared to triglycerides and cholesterol; unfortunately, it is doubtful that free fatty acids play a role in the underlying disease process for heart disease, atherogenesis. Second, it is unclear when we can legitimately extrapolate from acute reactivity and expect persistent elevation of a biological marker in response to chronic exposure. For example, a review of the evidence on chronic responses to stress (Rose 1980) revealed many instances in which the endocrine responses (particularly cortisol), though sensitive to acute stressors, undergo extinction when the individuals are re-exposed to those stressors or are exposed to chronic stressors. Rose's own data from the study of air traffic controllers (Rose et al. 1982) suggest that persistent responding to chronic exposures may be a function of individual differences and be pres-

ent only in a subset of individuals; it may not be inherent to the chronic characteristics of the environmental stimulus. Results consistent with the implications drawn from Rose's review were obtained in a study of male blue-collar workers losing their jobs because of a permanent shutdown (Cobb and Kasl 1977; Kasl 1982). A number of biological markers, such as blood pressure, cholesterol, and uric acid, showed reliable increases during the four to six weeks before and the four to six weeks after plant closing. However, when the comparison involved longer periods of unemployment (four to six months), the findings revealed that the still-unemployed men returned to "baseline" levels, similar to the decline for men who had become re-employed by that time.

Selected Findings on Psychosocial and Behavioral Risk Factors for Disease

In the few pages devoted to this topic it is not possible to do justice to the large literature on psychosocial and behavioral risk factors for disease. The discussion and commentary will be necessarily selective. My primary goal is to identify research themes and strands of evidence that have public health and clinical relevance; that is, the variables are worth our attention and they lend themselves to prevention/intervention/modification efforts.

If one uses a pragmatic classification schema and admittedly somewhat imprecise labels, one can organize the research material into the following areas: (1) stress—(a) chronic stressors, (b) acute stressors, individual events or exposure, and (c) acute stressors, aggregated undifferentiated amalgams of "sums" of events; (2) diverse traits, states, attitudes, and beliefs; (3) social support and network relationships; and (4) health habits—smoking, alcohol and dietary consumption, and physical activity. (Not included are research areas, such as social class, paths to medical care, and behaviors in the health care setting, that are relevant in terms of the disease development schema enunciated earlier but are, in fact, covered elsewhere in this volume.)

It is worth noting that my classification system is highly compatible with the contents of various self-administered forms for health risk appraisal that have become such popular gimmicks in the for-profit health promotion setting. Thus, one might suspect that this listing has convergent validity. However, responsible investigators have uniformly condemned such health hazard/health risk appraisal instruments as unscientific (e.g., Fielding 1982a; Schoenbach, Wagner, and Karon 1983; Vogt 1981; Wagner et al. 1982)—not just because the client-supplied data on risk factors are an inadequate proxy for clinical examination and laboratory data but also because the whole scientific base for risk predictions is quite fragmentary and insufficient. This suggests that the quality and quantity of evidence may be such that action/intervention programs cannot be confidently derived.

With respect to stress, a number of recent reviews provide the reader with a sense of the field (e.g., Cooper 1983; Craig and Brown 1984; Elliott and Eisdorfer 1982; Goldberger and Breznitz 1982; Henry 1982; Kasl 1984a, 1984b; McQueen and Siegrist 1982; Sterling and Eyer 1981). This list can be easily enlarged if one also wishes to consider focused reviews of specific health outcomes such as cancer and heart disease (e.g., Cox and McKay 1982; Eliot, Buell, and Dembroski 1982; Haney 1980; Jenkins 1982; Levy 1983; Morrison and Paffenbarger 1981; Ostfeld and Eaker 1985; Sklar and Anisman 1981). It is commonplace to warn the reader that stress is a term that resists agreed-upon definition and usage: it refers to stimulus conditions, to responses or outcomes, or to the whole process linking the two. A further warning is that there are no agreed-upon indicators—disease outcomes, biological parameters, behavioral or psychological processes—that could be used as unique criteria denoting presence or absence of stress.

Stress research is perhaps at its clearest when it deals with health consequences of specific events or environmental exposures that represent specific transitions. Thus, for example, the evidence regarding bereavement is reasonably clear (e.g., Helsing, Szklo, and Comstock 1981; Jacobs and Douglas 1979; Jacobs and Ostfeld 1977; Osterweis, Solomon, and Green 1984; Parkes 1972): bereavement is associated with increased mortality (especially for men) for a variety of causes, with reduced immunocompetence, with higher levels of psychophysiological symptoms, with greater distress, and with higher rates of health care utilization. The evidence concerning retirement is unusually clear, showing a high level of agreement: studies consistently fail to document adverse health effects of this major life transition (e.g., Kasl 1980; Minkler 1981; Rowland 1977; Satariano and Syme 1981), and the recent research findings (e.g., Ekerdt et al. 1983) are consistent with the earlier reviews. Of course, the health consequences of other specific events are more difficult to study and thus yield less than conclusive evidence. The picture of health effects of economic instability and unemployment (e.g., Brenner and Mooney 1983; Catalano and Dooley 1983; Colledge 1982; Dooley and Catalano 1984; Horwitz 1984; John, Schwefel, and Zöllner 1983; Kasl 1982; Spruit 1982) is very much muddled: evidence from ecological analyses of business cycle fluctuations and yearly mortality rates at the national level have suggested powerful effects on deaths from a variety of causes, while longitudinal epidemiological studies of individuals have had difficulty documenting prolonged physiological effects that would have suggestive health consequences. Cross-level analyses have not reconciled these findings but have instead suggested the operation of several distinct causal pathways and much variability of impact, depending on the setting (e.g., urban versus rural) and sociodemographic characteristics of individuals.

When stress research examines the health consequences of exposure to "stressful life events" in general, and when exposure is indexed by one or another of the popular measures (e.g., Holmes and Rahe 1967) that represent an undifferentiated aggregation of many events, then the evidence becomes unclear, untrustworthy, and invites dismissal on numerous methodological grounds. (For a discussion of some of these methodological points, see Dohrenwend and Dohrenwend 1981; Kasl 1984c; Schroeder and Costa 1984.) Consequently, the frequently observed (weak to moderately strong) association between reported exposure to higher numbers of stressful life events (SLE) and poorer health for a variety of causes must be viewed with extreme skepticism when one or more of the following alternative explanations is plausible: (1) the SLE measure indexes the same concept (poor health or poor functioning) as does the "dependent" variable; (2) presence of poor health influences reporting of SLEs or reporting biases are shared by both instruments for assessing SLEs and health status, particularly since many "events" have a vague or unknown objective referent; (3) high scores on the SLE instrument reflect a personal characteristic (trait, self-selection factor) that is the underlying factor in the observed association with health status. Given these concerns, the best rule seems to be to pay attention primarily to studies that use a longitudinal design and carry out careful statistical adjustments for necessary covariates, including prior symptoms or health status. Such studies, it turns out, obtain generally discouraging results (e.g., Billings and Moos 1982; Goldberg and Comstock 1976; Kobasa, Maddi, and Courington 1981; McFarlane et al. 1983; Rundall 1978; Williams, Ware, and Donald 1981). And we must remember that even if a sound research design encourages the interpretation that the SLE measure is indeed a risk factor for adverse health-status changes, we still need to pin down the proper interpretation of the SLE measure: does it truly index differential exposure to SLEs, or is the underlying variable something else, such as a stable neurotic trait (e.g., Costa et al. 1982; Costa and McCrae, 1985)?

Stress research studies concerned with chronic stress and physical health status concentrate heavily on the work setting, a topic covered by another chapter in this volume. Chronic stressors related to other major roles, especially in the family, are typically concerned with psychological distress and mental health outcomes (e.g., Holahan and Moose 1981; Ilfeld 1982; Pearlin and Johnson 1977). However, analyses of physical health outcomes in relation to status characteristics, particularly education, of spouse pairs (e.g., Haynes, Eaker, and Feinleib 1983; Suarez and Barrett-Connor 1984) are reasonably interpreted within a framework of marital status inconsistency, a presumptive chronic stressor. Interest in status inconsistency among social epidemiologists has waxed and waned over the years, and the evidence remains promising though spotty (e.g., Graham and Reeder 1979; Jenkins 1976; Kasl and Cobb 1969; Shekelle, Ostfeld, and Paul 1969). Evidence for effects of chronic stress on physical health might also be sought in enduring environmental exposures, such as aspects of the residential environment or specific conditions such as noise (Evans 1982; Hinkle and Lor-

ing 1977; Jones and Chapman 1984; Moos 1979). However, here a more precise conceptualization of stress would come in quite handy since it is far from clear why linkages between physical parameters and biomedical outcomes need to be interpreted by postulating the existence of a "stress" process. For example, a positive association between rates of some infectious diseases and residential crowding (Cox et al. 1982) should lead us to speculate about stress only if we have grounds to believe that some simpler explanation, such as greater opportunity for the spread of an infectious agent, is inadequate. Environmental exposures that are primarily psychological, such as threat of residential crime among the elderly (Goldsmith and Goldsmith 1976) or fear of nuclear accident or of exposure to radiation (Goldhaber, Staub, and Tokuhata 1983; Houts et al. 1984) are better seen in the stress framework than are exposures to noise, heat, and pollution (Evans 1982).

After stress, the second most common current topic among investigators interested in psychosocial risk factors for disease is the combined topic of social support—social networks. Because of a number of recent reviews and overviews, this topic is readily accessible (e.g., Berkman 1984; Broadhead et al. 1983; Cohen and Syme 1985; Wallston et al. 1983). Accessibility, however, does not mean that a set of summarizing conclusions is possible. In fact, the field is in an awkward transition stage, moving from (a) a grand formulation that primarily served to alert us to some nonbiological health-status influences, found in a loose set of variables reflecting the nature of the relation of the individual to significant others, to (b) a substantial fractionation of concepts, multiplicity of measures, search for plausible mechanisms, and a very slow accumulation of replicated evidence. The enormous richness of conceptual distinctions and measures available or proposed (Bruhn and Phillips 1984; Cohen and Syme 1985; House 1981; House and Kahn 1985), while fully appropriate at this stage, makes it difficult to evaluate the promise of the evidence and to detect any converging trends in concepts and measures. Methodological concerns raised earlier in connection with global indexes of stressful life events are fully applicable here as well.

Within psychosocial epidemiology, the 1979 publication on social networks (Berkman and Syme 1979) may be credited with reviving a long dormant interest in marital status/social isolation/social participation. The results, more fully analyzed in a later publication (Berkman and Breslow 1983), reveal that the social networks index—a simple composite of marital status, contacts with friends and relatives, church membership, and group membership—is related to mortality during a nine-year follow-up. This higher mortality among those with fewer social ties is independent of the effects of many covariates, including prior health status, health practices, and sociodemographic factors. Individuals with fewer social ties had also more adverse health status changes over the follow-up period, again adjusted for the necessary covariates. That the effects of this index were independent

of many covariates should not blind us to the fact that the quantity of social ties is a dimension richly embedded in a matrix of other important variables: individuals with more social ties are of higher social class, have a higher life satisfaction, have better health habits, and have a history of lower residential mobility.

Other investigators have been inspired to examine predictors of mortality in their data sets, but it is difficult to speak of replication since the predictors—some measure of network attachments or relationships—as well as the crucial covariate, prior health status, differ greatly. Thus Blazer's (1982) strongest predictor was "perception of social support," a highly subjective index of, among other things, feelings of loneliness and not being understood by anyone. Analyses of the Tecumseh data (House, Robbins, and Metzner 1982) also revealed a few predictors of survival: for men, being married and having a higher level of social relationships; for women, attending church and spending less time watching television. However, analyses of data from the Honolulu Heart Program (Reed et al. 1983) failed to replicate the observed cross-sectional association, in a longitudinal analysis of incidence (new cases), between several social network scales and CHD in Japanese men living in Hawaii. Furthermore, no interaction was observed; that is, those in the highest categories of biological risk were neither more likely nor less likely to be "protected" by network dynamics. Later analyses of incidence of stroke, cancer, and all diseases combined (Reed, McGee, and Yano

1984) also failed to establish a link to social network indicators.

Other variables that have been used in social epidemiological analyses of health outcomes bear a strong conceptual link to the social network dynamics. These include history of residential mobility (e.g., Metzner, Harburg, and Lamphiear 1982) and indexes of cultural and social assimilation in cross-cultural research (e.g., Reed et al. 1982). In fact, the whole literature on the health impact of migration (Kasl and Berkman 1983) could be usefully re-examined from the perspective of recent social network/social support formulations. One of the unsettled issues is, When does attachment to culture and people of origin protect from disease, while attachment to culture and people of host country increase disease risk? When is the situation reversed?

Another unsettled issue is the relative role, in the whole etiological picture, of objective network conditions versus subjective reactions. Thus Berkman and Breslow (1983) observe that marital status, but not marital adjustment, were predictive of survival. Similarly, the Tecumseh data (House, Robbins, and Metzner 1982) revealed no predictive power due to subjective satisfaction with social relationships. On the other hand, the Blazer (1982) results favored the most subjective index in the prediction of mortality. Any speculations about how to "promote social bonding" (Rook 1984) must await clarification of this issue.

Survival analyses continue to be useful but we now need more studies in the medical care setting where smaller segments of the disease development spectrum can be examined more intensively. A recent report on the influence of marital status on survival after myocardial infarction (Chandra et al. 1983) finds nothing new but represents a most convincing analysis to date, since excellent statistical adjustments for biomedical covariates (especially history and clinical complications) were possible. Now we need information on the process itself so we can illuminate the actual dynamics of marital status in such survival.

A consideration of stress and social support covers the bulk of the research on psychosocial risk factors for disease. Other psychosocial variables (states, traits, attitudes) that have been examined cannot rival the interest that stress and social support have generated; only Type A behavior in relation to CHD has accumulated a critical mass of evidence. Unfortunately, since the rather optimistic 1981 review of evidence (Review Panel 1981), the Type A picture has become considerably muddier because of negative findings from several major U.S. clinical trials and non-U.S. epidemiologic studies (Matthews 1985; Siegel 1984). We have studies of atherosclerosis (angiography), incidence, recurrence, survival, and intervention; we also have a variety of measures of Type A, on different populations, looking at different clinical endpoints (angina, myocardial infarction, sudden death, etc.). Because of inconsistent results, all the work seems somewhat inconclusive, including attempts to better conceptualize the essential pathogenic component of this broad construct. Negative evidence, such as failure to predict survival after myocardial infarction (Case et al. 1985), could result from the specific measure of Type A used, the specific subject population studied, or an erroneous hypothesis conjectured—that Type A does not really predict survival after a heart attack.

Other psychosocial variables may be designated as "promising" at this stage: (1) anger and hostility (Chesney, Rosenman, and Goldston 1985; Matthews 1985; (2) hardiness, sense of control, and related constructs (Kobasa, Maddi, and Kahn 1982; Seeman and Seeman 1983); (3) self-rated or subjective health (Kaplan and Comacho 1983; Mossey and Shapiro 1982); (4) religiousness and church membership (Berkman and Breslow 1983; House, Robbins, and Metzner 1982; Zuckerman, Kasl, and Ostfeld 1984); (5) depression, particularly as it relates to course of illness and survival (Kasl 1983; Siegel 1985).

The final set of variables we will consider briefly fall into the category of health habits or health practices. Smoking will not be included in the discussion because of the easily accessible documentation of its adverse health effects (e.g., U.S. Department of Health and Human Services, Office on Smoking and Health 1982; Report 1984) and because of its coverage in the cancer and cardiovascular disease chapters of this volume. Similar reasons justify my omission of the general issue of diet, or the intake of specific nutrients. Of course, this topic is more controversial than the smoking evidence. I shall discuss briefly the issues of exercise, alcohol and coffee consumption, and general indicators of overall health habits.

The reader should realize that unlike the previous evidence on general psychosocial risk factors, where the research is still struggling with the quality of the epidemiologic evidence, the data on health habits are more likely to generate a different type of issue, for example, Do we know how to intervene effectively? and Will intervention have the expected health benefits? These issues are discussed in the next section of this chapter.

The benefits of exercise or high levels of physical activity are found primarily in the cardiovascular area (Froelicher 1981; Haskell 1984). Thus exercise induces favorable changes in risk factors, such as plasma lipids and blood pressure (Haskell 1984; Ibrahim, 1983; Paffenbarger et al. 1983). However, it is possible that benefits will not be seen in young adolescents (Dwyer et al. 1983) or that they will be hard to detect in naturalistic longitudinal observations on adults who initiate exercising for a variety of reasons (Yamamoto, Yano, and Rhoads 1983). With respect to disease outcomes, the evidence favors the conclusion that exercise lowers the risk of fatal and nonfatal CHD (e.g., Paffenbarger and Hyde 1984; Salonen, Puska, and Tuomilehto 1982), but comprehensive reviews reveal that about 40 percent of studies find no association (LaPorte et al. 1984). The value of exercise in cardiac rehabilitation seems beyond a reasonable doubt (Froelicher 1981). Levels of physical activity may also be related to other health outcomes, such as colon cancer (Garabrant et al. 1984) and osteoporosis (Kottke, Caspersen, and Hill 1984). Doubt has been expressed about psychological benefits of habitual aerobic exercise (Hughes 1984), and studies with positive findings suggest only weak effects (Goldwater and Collins 1985). Also some recent evidence shows that high levels of aerobic fitness may act as a buffer against adverse health consequences of high levels of stressful life events (Kobasa, Maddi, and Puccetti 1982; Roth and Holmes 1985). The overall picture, then, is promising but not entirely clear; greater precision in measuring fitness and quantifying the full spectrum of activities should clarify the picture further (LaPorte et al. 1984; Paffenbarger and Hyde 1984).

The data on alcohol consumption in relation to CHD strongly support the notion that moderate alcohol consumption has a protective effect on CHD morbidity and mortality (Kozarevic, Demirovic et al. 1982; Kittner et al. 1983; Marmot 1984; Yano, Reed, and McGee 1984). Heavy alcohol consumers may have higher CHD mortality (e.g., Fraser and Upsdell 1981), but the evidence is far from consistent (Marmot 1984). However, there are other social and medical consequences of heavy alcohol consumption, such as stomach cancer (Gordon and Kannel 1984) or breast cancer (Lê et al. 1984), and a policy of advocating increased alcohol consumption remains unacceptable. Nondrinkers do have generally higher morbidity and mortality rates (e.g., Gordon and Kannel 1984; Kittner et al. 1983; Marmot 1984), but self-selection factors (e.g., preexisting disease-causing abstention) and possible measurement problems (e.g., selective denial) make it difficult to understand such an association. Alcohol

consumption presents a mixed picture with respect to cardiovascular risk factors: it increases CHD risk because of its effect on blood pressure (Kozarevic, Racic et al. 1982; McQueen and Celentano 1982), but lowers CHD risk because of its effect on high-density lipoprotein cholesterol (Barrett-Connor and Suarez 1982).

Data on *coffee* consumption have begun to suggest a possible link to some cancers, especially bladder (e.g., Marrett, Walter, and Meigs 1983; Snowdon and Phillips 1984), but the evidence at present is limited and not particularly consistent, especially in the cardiovascular area (Report 1984).

The predictive power of general self-report measures of health habits, such as the Health Practices Index developed for the Alameda County study (Berkman and Breslow 1983), is dependent not only upon the actual role of the separate component "practices" (e.g., exercise, smoking, obesity) in health outcomes but also upon the accuracy of self-reports. For example, self-assessments of overweight status seem to have an adequately high level of association with objective measurements (Stewart and Brook 1983), while self-assessments of fitness seem to have almost no validity (Optenberg et al. 1984). Reports of other practices, such as smoking, can in principle be quite accurate, but motivational issues related to the purposes for which the data are collected can easily undermine such accuracy.

The collective evidence on such health habit indexes (Berkman and Breslow 1983; Branch and Jette 1984; Metzner, Carman, and House 1983;

Wingard, Berkman and Brand 1982) favors the conclusion that such measures are useful in predicting morbidity and mortality. Consistent data are obtained for self-reports of cigarette smoking, relative weight, and physical activity as predictors; there is also consistency in that eating breakfast and snacking lightly between meals have no predictive power. Sleeping regularly seven to eight hours a night is not consistently related; alcohol use is not measured quite consistently across studies, but it appears that high alcohol consumption increases the risk of adverse outcomes. The one study dealing with the elderly (Branch and Jette 1984) found no predictors of mortality for men and only smoking status for women; however, the covariate adjustments included only a subjective measure of health status, which is inadequate and may lead to overcorrection, in view of the previously cited data on self-rated health. There is also some evidence that among black women, the predictive power of health practices may be the weakest (Berkman and Breslow 1983).

The Alameda County data also reveal that more favorable health practices are found among whites, those of higher social class, and those with richer social network connections. More favorable health practices are also related to higher levels of preventive health care, to higher life satisfaction, and to fewer feelings of isolation, depression, and personal uncertainty. The predictive power of the practices is, of course, tested after adjustment for these and other covariates; however, as in the case of the index of social networks, we are dealing with a predictor richly embedded in a matrix of other influences or correlates.

Implications of the Evidence for Modification of Risk Factors

Since the evidence on effects of smoking is so overwhelming and the benefits of successful interventions (prevent initiation or promote cessation) are so unalloyed, a discussion of efforts and strategies with regard to control of smoking permits a "pure case" analysis of social science issues. These issues may be generic to other health habits or psychosocial risk factors, but they become muddied by controversies over the adequacy of basic evidence regarding causation of disease via the risk factor.

Control of smoking has been approached from a variety of perspectives, including public policy, medical, psychological, and social (Benfari and Ockene 1982; Breslow, 1982; Kuller et al. 1982; Syme and Alcalay 1982). These writings, plus excellent overviews of the field (particularly Pechacek and McAllister 1980) permit several conclusions: (1) A number of (very likely) highly effective strategies of control remain beyond our reach because of various sociopolitical realities; these include prohibition or restriction of smoking, regulation of distribution, heavy taxation, and restrictions on advertising. (2) Knowledge of disease consequences of smoking is widespread, and stepped-up public information efforts appear unwarranted. (3) Modest declines in smoking rates continue, especially among adolescents (Malley, Bachman, and Johnston 1984). (4) Smoking cessation outcomes are similar across a variety of programs and approaches—initial, dramatic reduction in smoking followed by high rates of recidivism, so long-term abstention rates are only about 20 to 25 percent. Successful maintenance strategies have not been worked out. (5) The medical care setting is not particularly effective, unless severe illness is present or there is imminent danger from continuation of smoking (Pederson 1982). (6) Predictors of successful long-term cessation reside not in program characteristics but in preexisting participant variables: high expectation of success, fewer cigarettes smoked at entry, long periods of previous abstinence, and ease of prior cessation attempts (Ockene et al. 1982). (7) Prevention of initiation of smoking is considered the superior public health strategy. Unfortunately, most prevention strategies only change attitudes but fail to deter smoking. School-based prevention strategies perhaps need to concentrate on high-risk individuals—those who have recently begun to smoke and those with peer and family models who smoke (Flay, et al. 1985). (8) Over 90 percent of individuals who quit smoking during the last twenty years or so did so on their own. We do not know how to maximize this process or what self-help strategies, which smokers most often request (e.g., instructional booklets for self-monitoring), are most attractive and effective.

Some self-help strategies, such as advertising and then sending out leaflets (Davis, Faust, and Ordentlich 1984) may not be very successful but can be very cost-effective.

The above summary of efforts to control smoking includes many points applicable to other health interventions as well. For example, high recidivism is also characteristic of programs dealing with exercise (Dishman 1982; Serfass and Gerberich 1984), weight loss (Foreyt, Goodrick, and Gotto 1981), and alcohol problems (Room 1984). Dietary changes can be maintained over a longer period of time (e.g., Reeves et al. 1983), but participants in such programs may be rather self-selected (Hollis et al. 1984). Another similarity with smoking is that successful features of exercise or weight loss programs are not clear, and thus no one particular program can be strongly advocated (Forety, Goodrick, and Gotto 1981; Oldridge 1982). There is ample room for inventiveness and exploration of new strategies, such as creating a weight loss competition among work-based groups (Brownell et al. 1984). The importance of preprogram efficacy expecations, as with smoking, comes through in many other studies as well (e.g., Hollis et al. 1984; Jeffery et al. 1984; Kaplan, Atkins, and Reinsch 1984), but we do not know how to move from a theoretical recognition of the importance of this dimension to a successful intervention technique (McReynolds, Green, and Fisher 1983). Unlike the smoking studies, studies of healthy life-styles have provided little reliable information on how many people initiated various other healthy life-styles or what motivated them; nor have such studies provided information on reasons for various secular trends, such as the decline in cholesterol levels (Hershcopf et al. 1982).

Life-style interventions are, of course, conducted in specific settings: the workplace appears to be the most common one (Brennan 1982; Fielding, 1982b, 1984; Pomerleau 1983), but others include the community (Farquhar 1978; Nash and Farquhar 1980; Winkelstein and Marmot 1981), the clinic or other health care setting (Syme 1978), or, more rarely, the family (Baranowski 1982) or congregate housing unit, such as those for the elderly (Pickard and Collins 1982). Given this diversity of settings, it is difficult to understand why investigators have not paid more attention to the nature of the specific setting, and its dynamics, in order to develop more powerful intervention strategies that might maximally exploit the possibly unique dynamics of each setting (Andreoli and Guillory 1983). This criticism is particularly applicable to workplace research where cost-effective access to target individuals and vague references to social support systems are the only factors explicitly mentioned.

The large clinical trials conducted in the last decade, such as HDFP (Hypertension Detection and Follow-up Program Cooperative Group 1979), LRC (Lipid Research Clinic Program 1984), and MRFIT (Multiple Risk Factor Intervention Trial Research Group 1982), are enormously expensive, and their findings have been, in some sense, disappointing. Thus there is urgency in the need to understand better the specific dynamics of the intervention settings and to design more powerful interventions. However, other benefits might accrue as well. For example, further analyses of the HDFP data (Hardy and Hawkins 1983) revealed that the health benefits of "stepped-up care" over "referred care" were greater than could be accounted for by treatment variables, such as medication status and changes in blood pressure; thus there seemed to be nonspecific (psychosocial?) benefits of being in the intervention group. On the other hand, the MRFIT results (Stallones 1983) showed CHD mortality benefits in the "special intervention" group that, compared to "usual care" group, were much less than could be expected on the basis of differential changes in cholesterol, blood pressure, and cigarette smoking; thus in the second instance, there seemed to be nonspecific benefits of being in the "control" group. The difference between the two studies is intriguing. A better understanding of the dynamics of the intervention setting might illuminate other important issues: When should we expect adverse effects of labeling, that is, detection of silent elevated risk factors (Johnston et al. 1984; Polk et al. 1984)? Why do compliers on placebo often have better health outcomes than noncompliers on placebo, or even noncompliers on medication (Epstein 1984)? How are perceptions of risk factors and susceptibility altered by the different interventions in the different settings (Weinstein 1984).

In concluding this section I wish to note that it would be difficult, and really premature, to expand this discussion of modification of risk factors to include the psychosocial risk factors reviewed earlier, that is, stress, social support, behavior Type A, and so on. There are two major reasons for this: (1) The etiological evidence, that is, the causal role of these risk factors in disease onset or exacerbation, is very uneven and incomplete. Furthermore, we do not understand underlying specific mechanisms, and we are often unsure if the detected risk factor is more than an indicator variable of an undescribed underlying cause, in which case modifying it might have no benefits. (2) Intervention techniques for some classes of variables, such as social support/social networks, are hardly in place (Cohen and Syme 1985), while for others, such as Type A, the work is still in early stages (Powell 1984). For stress management, on the other hand, a plethora of techniques is available (Jacob and Chesney 1984; Goldberger and Breznitz 1982; Murphy 1984). But these techniques have been tried on only a short-term basis with only proximate or intermediate outcomes (that is, not health status benefits). Furthermore, the public health acceptability of these techniques is likely to be quite low in an outreach intervention; long-term adherence is likely to be worse. And, of course, stress management does not address at all the issue of environmental modification.

Conclusion

The strong health promotion/disease prevention agenda of the past decade leads to a need to examine critically the evidence with respect to psychosocial and behavioral risk factors that may contribute to disease onset or exacerbation. Ideally, we need to know: What are these risk factors? How can we monitor them, that is, identify persons or groups at high risk and determine how they came to be at high risk? How can we alter these risk factors and what are the consequences of such modifications?

This chapter outlined a conceptual framework, a disease development schema, that helps us organize the evidence pertinent to these questions. Studies of stress, social support—social networks, diverse traits/states/attitudes, and several health habits were reviewed. The evidence is uneven, and confident answers to the above questions cannot be offered as yet. Thus, for example, in spite of the large volume of research on stress and social support, essential evidence that translates into a set of clear-cut health promotion/disease prevention activities is simply not available. We do not know what indicators of stress or support would bring us the closest to the underlying disease etiology dynamics, and thus reveal the optimal point for intervention; nor do we have intervention strategies that are documented to have high public health acceptability, are associated with long-term changes, and have the expected health benefits. Only the domain of health habits leads to reasonable conclusions regarding their status as risk factors, the probable health benefits of their modification, and the existence of intervention techniques of reasonable promise. Establishing long-term maintenance of altered life-styles and understanding better the dynamics of "spontaneous" life-style changes would seem to be the two highest priorities for further work on health habits.

References

Andreoli, K. G., and M. M. Guillory. 1983. Arenas for practicing health promotion. *Family and Community Health* 5:28–40.

Antonovsky, A. 1979. *Health, stress, and coping.* San Francisco: Jossey-Bass.

Baranowski, T., P. R. Nader, K. Dunn, and N. A. Vanderpool. 1982. Family self-help: Promoting changes in health behavior. *Journal of Communication* 32:161–172.

Baric, L. 1969. Recognition of the "at risk" role: A means to influence health behavior. *International Journal of Health Education* 12:24–34.

Barrett-Connor, E., and L. Suarez. 1982. A community study of alcohol and other factors associated with the distribution of high density lipoprotein cholesterol in older vs. younger men. *American Journal of Epidemiology* 115:888–893.

Benfari, R. C., and J. K. Ockene. 1982. Control of cigarette smoking from a psychological perspective. *Annual Review of Public Health* 3:101–128.

Berkman, L. F. 1984. Assessing the physical health effects of social networks and social support. *Annual Review of Public Health* 5:413–432.

Berkman, L. F., and L. Breslow. 1983. *Health and ways of living.* New York: Oxford University Press.

Berkman, L. F., and S. L. Syme. 1979. Social networks, host resistance, and mortality: A nine-year follow-up study of Alameda County residents. *American Journal of Epidemiology* 109:186–204.

Billings, A. G., and R. H. Moos. 1982. Stressful life events and symptoms: A longitudinal model. *Health Psychology* 1:99–117.

Blazer, D. G. 1982. Social support and mortality in an elderly community population. *American Journal of Epidemiology* 115:684–694.

Branch, L. G., and A. M. Jette. 1984. Personal health practices and mortality among the elderly. *American Journal of Public Health* 74:1126–1129.

Brand, R. J., R. H. Rosenman, R. I. Sholtz, and M. Friedman. 1976. Multivariate prediction of coronary heart disease in the Western Collaborative Group Study compared to the findings of the Framingham Study. *Circulation* 53:348–355.

Brennan, A. J. J., ed. 1982. Worksite health promotion. *Health Education Quarterly* 9 (supp.):5–91.

Brenner, M. H., and A. Mooney. 1983. Unemployment and health in the context of economic change. *Social Science and Medicine* 17:1125–1138.

Breslow, L. 1982. Control of cigarette smoking from a public policy perspective. *Annual Review of Public Health* 3:129–151.

Broadhead, W. E., B. H. Kaplan, S. A. James, E. H. Wagner, V. J. Schoenbach, R. Grimson, S. Heyden, G. Tibblin, and S. H. Gehlbach. 1983. The epidemiologic evidence for a relationship between social support and health. *American Journal of Epidemiology* 117:521–537.

Brownell, K. D., R. Y. Cohen, A. J. Stunkard, M. R. J. Felix, and N. B. Cooley. 1984. Weight loss competitions at the work site: Impact on weight, morale, and cost-effectiveness. *American Journal of Public Health* 74:1283–1285.

Bruhn, J. G., and B. V. Phillips. 1984. Measuring social support: A synthesis of current approaches. *Journal of Behavioral Medicine* 7:151–169.

Case, R. B., S. S. Heller, N. B. Case, A. J. Moss, and the Multicenter Post-Infarction Research Group. 1985. Type A behavior and survival after acute myocardial infarction. *New England Journal of Medicine* 312:737–741.

Cassel, J. 1974. An epidemiological perspective of psychosocial factors in disease etiology. *American Journal of Public Health* 64:1040–1043.

———. 1976. The contribution of the social environment to host resistance. *American Journal of Epidemiology* 104:107–123.

Catalano, R., and D. Dooley. 1983. Health effects of economic instability: A test of economic stress hypothesis. *Journal of Health and Social Behavior* 24:46–60.

Chandra, V., M. Szklo, R. Goldberg, and J. Tonascia. 1983. The impact of marital status on survival after an acute myocardial infarction: A population-based study. *American Journal of Epidemiology* 117:320–325.

Chesney, M. A., R. H. Rosenman, and S. E. Goldston, eds. 1985. *Anger and hostility in behavioral medicine.* New York: Hemisphere.

Cobb, S. 1971. *The frequency of rheumatic diseases.* Cambridge: Harvard University Press.

Cobb, S., and S. V. Kasl. 1977. *Termination: The consequences of job loss.* HEW Publication No. (NIOSH) 77-224. Cincinnati: National Institute for Occupational Safety and Health.

Cohen, S., and S. L. Syme, eds. 1985. *Social support and health.* New York: Academic Press.

Colledge, M. 1982. Economic cycles and health: Towards a sociological understanding of the impact of the recession on health and illness. *Social Science and Medicine* 16:1919–1927.

Comstock, G. W., and K. B. Partridge. 1972. Church attendance and health. *Journal of Chronic Diseases* 25:665–672.

Comstock, G. W., and J. A. Tonascia. 1977. Education and mortality in Washington County, Maryland. *Journal of Health and Social Behavior* 18:54–61.

Conti, S., G. Farchi, and A. Menotti. 1983. Coronary risk factors and excess mortality from all causes and specific causes. *International Journal of Epidemiology* 12:301–307.

Cooper, C. L., ed. 1983. *Stress Research.* Chichester, England: Wiley.

Costa, P. T., Jr., J. L. Fleg, R. R. McCrae, and E. G. Lakatta. 1982. Neuroticism, coronary artery disease, and chest pain complaints: Cross-sectional and longitudinal studies. *Experimental Aging Research* 8:37–44.

Costa, P. T., Jr., and R. R. McCrae. 1985. Hypochondriasis, neuroticism, and aging: When are somatic complaints unfounded? *American Psychologist* 40:19–28.

Cox, T., and C. McKay. 1982. Psychosocial factors and psychophysiological mechanisms in the aetiology and development of cancers. *Social Science and Medicine* 16:381–396.

Cox, V. C., P. B. Paulus, G. McCain, and M. Karlovac. 1982. The relationship between crowding and health. In *Advances in environmental psychology*, vol. 4: Environment and Health, ed. A. Baum and J. E. Singer. Hillsdale, N.J.: Erlbaum.

Craig, T. K. J., and G. W. Brown. 1984. Life events, meaning, and physical illness: A review. In *Health care and human behaviour*, ed. A. Steptoe and A. Mathews. London: Academic Press.

Davis, A. L., R. Faust, and M. Ordentlich. 1984. Self-help smoking cessation and maintenance programs: A comparative study with 12-month follow-up by the American Lung Association. *American Journal of Public Health* 74:1212–1217.

Dimsdale, T. E., and J. A. Herd. 1982. Variability of plasma lipids in response to emotional arousal. *Psychosomatic Medicine* 44:413–430.

Dishman, R. K. 1982. Compliance/adherence in health-related exercise. *Health Psychology* 1:237–267.

Dohrenwend, B. S., and B. P. Dohrenwend, eds. 1981. *Stressful life events and their contexts.* New York: Prodist.

Dooley, D., and R. Catalano. 1984. The epidemiology of economic stress. *American Journal of Community Psychology* 12:387–409.

Dwyer, T., W. E. Coonan, D. R. Leitch, B. S. Hetzel, and R. A. Baghurst. 1983. An investigation of the effects of daily physical activity on the health of primary school students in South Australia. *International Journal of Epidemiology* 12:308–313.

Ekerdt, D. J., L. Baden, R. Bossé, and E. Dibbs. 1983. The effect of retirement on physical health. *American Journal of Public Health* 73:779–783.

Eliot, R. S., J. C. Buell, and T. M. Dembroski. 1982. Bio-behavioral perspectives on coronary heart disease, hypertension, and sudden cardiac death. *Acta Medica Scandinavica* 660 (supp.):203–213.

Elliott, G. R., and C. Eisdorfer, eds. 1982. *Stress and human health.* New York: Springer.

Epstein, L. H. 1984. The direct effects of compliance on health outcome. *Health Psychology* 3:385–393.

Evans, G. W., ed. 1982. *Environmental stress.* New York: Cambridge University Press.

Farquhar, J. W. 1978. The community-based model of life style intervention trials. *American Journal of Epidemiology* 108:103–111.

Feinleib, M. 1981. On a possible inverse relationship between serum cholesterol and cancer mortality. *American Journal of Epidemiology* 114:5–10.

Fielding, J. E. 1982a. Appraising the health of health risk appraisal. *American Journal of Public Health* 72:337–340.

———. 1982b. Effectiveness of employee health improvement programs. *Journal of Occupational Medicine* 24:907–916.

———. 1984. Health promotion and disease prevention at the worksite. *Annual Review of Public Health* 5:237–265.

Flay, B. R., K. B. Ryan, J. A. Best, K. S. Brown, M. W. Kersell, J. R. d'Avernas, and M. P. Zanna. 1985. Are social-psychological smoking prevention programs effective? The Waterloo Study. *Journal of Behavioral Medicine* 8:37–59.

Foreyt, J. P., G. K. Goodrick, and A. M. Gotto. 1981. Limitations of behavioral treatment of obesity: Review and analysis. *Journal of Behavioral Medicine* 4:159–174.

Fraser, G. E., and M. Upsdell. 1981. Alcohol and other discriminants between cases of sudden death and myocardial infarction. *American Journal of Epidemiology* 114:462–476.

Friedman, M., C. E. Thoresen, J. J. Gill, L. H. Powell, D. Ulmer, L. Thompson, V. A. Price, D. D. Rabin, W. S. Breall, T. Dixon, R. Levy, and E. Bourg. 1984. Alteration of type A behavior and reduction in cardiac recurrences in postmyocardial infarction patients. *American Heart Journal* 108:237–248.

Froelicher, V. 1981. Can exercise prevent coronary heart disease? *Washington Public Health* 2(2):9–12.

Garabrant, D. H., J. M. Peters, T. M. Mack, and L. Bernstein. 1984. Job activity and colon cancer risk. *American Journal of Epidemiology* 119:1005–1014.

Gillum, R. F., H. Blackburn, and M. Feinleib. 1982. Current strategies for explaining the decline in ischemic heart disease mortality. *Journal of Chronic Diseases* 35:467–474.

Glasunov, I. S., V. Grabauskas, W. W. Holland, and F. H. Epstein, 1983. An integrated programme for the prevention and control of noncommunicable diseases. *Journal of Chronic Diseases* 36:419–426.

Goldberg, E. L., and G. W. Comstock. 1976. Life events and subsequent illness. *American Journal of Epidemiology* 104:146–158.

Goldberger, L., and S. Breznitz, eds. 1982. *Handbook of stress.* New York: Free Press.

Goldhaber, M. K., S. L. Staub, and G. K. Tokuhata. 1983. Spontaneous abortions after the Three Mile Island nuclear accident: A life table analysis. *American Journal of Public Health* 73:752–759.

Goldsmith, J., and S.S. Goldsmith, eds. 1976. *Crime and the elderly.* Lexington, Mass.: Lexington Books.

Goldwater, B. C., and M. L. Collis. 1985. Psychologic effects of cardiovascular conditioning. *Psychosomatic Medicine* 47:174–181.

Gordon, T., and W. B. Kannel. 1984. Drinking and mortality: the Framingham Study. *American Journal of Epidemiology* 120:97–107.

Graham, S., and L. G. Reeder. 1979. Social epidemiology of chronic diseases. In

Handbook of medical sociology, ed. H. E. Freeman, S. Levine, and L. G. Reeder. Englewood Cliffs, N.J.: Prentice-Hall.

Green, L. W. 1984. Modifying and developing health behavior. *Annual Review of Public Health* 5:215–236.

Green, L. W., R. W. Wilson, and K. G. Bauer. 1983. Data requirements to measure progress on the objectives for the nation in health promotion and disease prevention. *American Journal of Public Health* 73:18–24.

Haney, C. A. 1980. Life events as precursors of coronary heart disease. *Social Science and Medicine* 14A:119–126.

Hardy, R. J., and C. M. Hawkins. 1983. The impact of selected indices of antihypertensive treatment on all-cause mortality. *American Journal of Epidemiology* 117:566–574.

Haskell, W. L. 1984. Exercise-induced changes in plasma lipids and lipoproteins. *Preventive Medicine* 13:23–36.

Haynes, S. G., E. D. Eaker, and M. Feinleib.1983. Spouse behavior and coronary heart disease in men. Prospective results from the Framingham Heart Study, 1. Concordance of risk factors and the relationship of psychosocial status to coronary incidence. *American Journal of Epidemiology* 118: 1–22.

Haynes, S. G., M. Feinleib, and W. B. Kannel. 1980. The relationship of psychosocial factors to coronary heart disease in the Framingham study, 3: Eight-year incidence of coronary heart disease. *American Journal of Epidemiology* 111:37–58.

Helsing, K. J., M. Szklo, and G. W. Comstock. 1981. Factors associated with mortality after widowhood. *American Journal of Public Health* 71: 802–809.

Henry, J. P. 1982. The relation of social to biological processes in disease. *Social Science and Medicine* 16:369–380.

Herschcopf, R. J; D. Elahi, R. Andres, H. L. Baldwin, G. S. Raizes, D. D. Schocken, and J. D. Tobin. 1982. Longitudinal changes in serum cholesterol in man: An epidemiologic search for an etiology. *Journal of Chronic Diseases.* 35:101–114.

Hinkle, L. E., Jr., B. P. Dohrenwend, J. Elinson, S. V. Kasl, A. McDowell, D. Mechanic, and S. L. Syme. 1976. Social determinants of human health. *Preventive medicine USA.* New York: Prodist.

Hinkle, L. E., Jr., and W. C. Loring, eds. 1977. *The effect of the man-made environment on health and behavior.* DHEW Publication No. (CDC) 77-8318. Washington, D.C.: Government Printing Office.

Holahan, C. J., and R. H. Moose. 1981. Social support and psychological distress: A longitudinal analysis. *Journal of Abnormal Psychology* 90: 365–370.

Hollis, J. F., G. Sexton, S. L. Connor, L. Calvin, C. Pereira, and J. D. Matarazzo. 1984. The Family Heart Dietary Intervention Program: Community response and characteristics of joining and nonjoining families. *Preventive Medicine* 13:276–285.

Holmes, T. H., and R. H. Rahe. 1967. The social readjustment rating scale. *Journal of Psychosomatic Research* 11:213–218.

Horwitz, A. V. 1984. The economy and social pathology. *Annual Review of Sociology* 10:95–119.

House, J. S. 1981. *Work stress and social support.* Reading, Mass.: Addison-Wesley.

House, J. S., and R. L. Kahn. 1985. Measures and concepts of social support. In *Social support and health,* ed. S. Cohen and S. L. Syme. New York: Academic Press.

House, J. S., C. Robbins, and H. L. Metzner. 1982. The association of social relationships with mortality: Prospective evidence from the Tecumseh Community Health Study. *American Journal of Epidemiology* 116:123–140.

Houts, P. S., T. W. Hu, R. A. Henderson, P. D. Cleary, and G. K. Tokuhata. 1984. Utilization of medical care following the Three Mile Island crisis. *American Journal of Public Health* 74:140–142.

Hughes, J. R. 1984. Psychological effects of habitual aerobic exercise: A critical review. *Preventive Medicine* 13:66–78.

Hypertension Detection and Follow-up Program Cooperative Group. 1979. Five-year findings of the Hypertension Detection and Follow-up Program. *Journal of the American Medical Association* 242:2562–2571.

Ibrahim, M. A. 1983. In support of jogging. *American Journal of Public Health* 73:136–137.

Ilfeld, F. W., Jr. 1982. Marital stressors, coping styles, and symptoms of depression. In *Handbook of stress: Theoretical and clinical aspects,* ed. L. Goldberger and S. Breznitz. New York: Free Press.

Jacob, R. G., and M. A. Chesney. 1984. Stress management for cardiovascular reactivity. *Behavioral Medicine Update* 6(4):23–27.

Jacobs, S., and L. Douglas. 1979. Grief: A mediating process between loss and illness. *Comprehensive Psychiatry* 20:165–174.

Jacobs, S., and A. Ostfeld. 1977. An epidemiological review of the mortality of bereavement. *Psychosomatic Medicine* 39:344–357.

Janz, N. K., and M. H. Becker. 1984. The health belief model: A decade later. *Health Education Quarterly* 11(1):1–47.

Jeffery, R. W., W. M. Bjornson-Benson, B. S. Rosenthal, R. A. Lindquist, C. L. Kurth, and S. L. Johnson. 1984. Correlates of weight loss and its maintenance over two years of follow-up among middle-aged men. *Preventive Medicine* 13:155–168.

Jenkins, C. D. 1976. Recent evidence supporting psychologic and social risk factors for coronary disease. *New England Journal of Medicine* 294:987–994, 1033–1038.

―――. 1982. Psychosocial risk factors for coronary heart disease. *Acta Medica Scandinavica* 660 (supp.):123–136.

John, J., D. Schwefel, and H. Zöllner, eds. 1983. *Influence of economic instability on health.* Berlin: Springer-Verlag.

Johnston, M. E., E. S. Gibson, C. W. Terry, R. B. Haynes, D. W. Taylor, A. Gafni, J. I. Sicurella, and D. L. Sackett. 1984. Effects of labelling on income, work, and social function among hypertensive employees. *Journal of Chronic Diseases* 37:417–423.

Jones, D. M., and A. J. Chapman, eds. 1984. *Noise and society.* Chichester, England: Wiley.

Kaplan, G. A., and T. Comacho. 1983. Perceived health and mortality: A nine-year follow-up of the Human Population Laboratory cohort. *American Journal of Epidemiology* 117:291–304.

Kaplan, R. M., C. J. Atkins, and S. Reinsch. 1984. Specific efficacy expectations mediate exercise compliance in patients with COPD. *Health Psychology* 3:223–242.

Kasl, S. V. 1977. Contributions of social epidemiology to studies in psychosomatic medicine: Summarizing discussion. In *Advances in psychosomatic medicine,* vol. 9, ed. S. V. Kasl and F. Reichsman. Basel, Switzerland: S. Karger.

———. 1980. The impact of retirement. In *Current concerns in occupational stress,* ed. C. L. Cooper and R. Payne. Chichester, England: Wiley.

———. 1982. Strategies of research on economic instability and health. *Psychological Medicine* 12:637–649.

———. 1983. Social and psychological factors affecting the course of disease: An epidemiological perspective. In *Handbook of health, health care, and the health professions,* ed. D. Mechanic. New York: Free Press.

———. 1984a. Chronic life stress and health. In *Health care and human behaviour,* ed. A. Steptoe and A. Mathews. London: Academic Press.

———. 1984b. Stress and health. *Annual Review of Public Health* 5:319–341.

———. 1984c. When to welcome a new measure (editorial). *American Journal of Public Health* 74:106–108.

Kasl, S. V., and L. Berkman. 1983. Health consequences of the experience of migration. *Annual Review of Public Health* 4:69–90.

Kasl, S. V., and S. Cobb. 1966. Health behavior, illness behavior, and sick role behavior. *Archives of Environmental Health* 12:246–266, 531–541.

———. 1969. The intrafamilial transmission of rheumatoid arthritis, 6: Association of rheumatoid arthritis with several types of status inconsistency. *Journal of Chronic Diseases* 22:259–278.

Khaw, K.T., and E. Barrett-Connor. 1984. Systolic blood pressure and cancer mortality in an elderly population. *American Journal of Epidemiology* 120:550–558.

Kittner, S. J., M. R. Garcia-Palmieri, R. Costas, Jr., M. Cruz-Vidal, R. D. Abbott, and R. J. Havlik. 1983. Alcohol and coronary heart disease in Puerto Rico. *American Journal of Epidemiology* 117:538–550.

Kleinman, J. C., V. G. DeGruttola, B. B. Cohen, and J. H. Madans. 1981. Regional and urban-suburban differentials in coronary heart disease mortality and risk factor prevalence. *Journal of Chronic Diseases* 34:11–19.

Kobasa, S. C., S. R. Maddi, and S. Courington. 1981. Personality and constitution as mediators in the stress-illness relationship. *Journal of Health and Social Behavior* 22:368–378.

Kobasa, S. C., S. R. Maddi, and S. Kahn. 1982. Hardiness and health: A prospective study. *Journal of Personality and Social Psychology* 42:168–177.

Kobasa, S. C., S. R. Maddi, and M. C. Puccetti. 1982. Personality and exercise as buffers in the stress-illness relationship. *Journal of Behavioral Medicine* 5:391–404.

Kottke, T. E., C. J. Caspersen, and C. S. Hill. 1984. Exercise in the management and rehabilitation of selected chronic diseases. *Preventive Medicine* 13:47–65.

Kozarevic, D., J. Demirovic, T. Gordon, C. T. Kaelber, D. McGee, and W. J. Zukel. 1982. Drinking habits and coronary heart disease: The Yugoslavia cardiovascular disease study. *American Journal of Epidemiology* 116:748–758.

Kozarevic, D., Z. Racic, T. Gordon, C. T. Kaelber, D. McGee, and W. J. Zukel. 1982. Drinking habits and other characteristics: The Yugoslavia cardiovascular disease study. *American Journal of Epidemiology* 116:287–301.

Krantz, D. S., and S. B. Manuck. 1985. Measures of acute physiologic reactivity to behavioral stimuli: Assessment and critique. In *Measuring psychosocial variables in epidemiologic studies of cardiovascular disease,* ed. A. M. Ostfeld and E. Eaker. NIH Publication No. 85-2270. Washington, D.C.: Government Printing Office.

Kuller, L., E. Meilahn, M. Townsend, and G. Weinberg. 1982. Control of cigarette smoking from a medical perspective. *Annual Review of Public Health* 3:153–178.

LaPorte, R. E., L. L. Adams, D. D. Savage, G. Brenes, S. Dearwater, and T. Cook. 1984. The spectrum of physical activity, cardiovascular disease, and health: An epidemiologic perspective. *American Journal of Epidemiology* 120:507–517.

Last, J. M., ed. 1983. *A dictionary of epidemiology.* New York: Oxford University Press.

Lê, M. G., C. Hill, A. Kramar, and R. Flamant. 1984. Alcoholic beverage consumption and breast cancer in a French case-control study. *American Journal of Epidemiology,* pp. 350–357.

Levy, S. M. 1983. Host differences in neoplastic risk: Behavioral and social contributors to disease. *Health Psychology* 2:21–44.

Lindheim, R., and S. L. Syme. 1983. Environments, people, and health. *Annual Review of Public Health* 4:335–359.

Lipid Research Clinic Program. 1984. The Lipid Research Clinics coronary primary prevention trial results. *Journal of the American Medical Association* 251:351–364, 365–374.

Lipowski, Z. J. 1976. Psychosomatic medicine: An overview. In *Modern trends in psychosomatic medicine,* vol. 3, ed. O. Hill. London: Butterworths.

McFarlane, A. H., G. R. Norman, D. L. Streiner, and R. G. Roy. 1983. The process of social stress: Stable, reciprocal, and mediating relationships. *Journal of Health and Social Behavior* 24:160–173.

McGuire, W. J. 1984. Public communication as a strategy for inducing health promoting behavioral change. *Preventive Medicine* 13:299–319.

McMahon, B., and T. F. Pugh. 1970. *Epidemiology: Principles and methods.* Boston: Little, Brown.

McQueen, D. V., and D. D. Celentano. 1982. Social factors in the etiology of multiple outcomes: The case of blood pressure and alcohol consumption patterns. *Social Science and Medicine* 16:397–418.

McQueen, D. V., and J. Siegrist. 1982. Social factors in the etiology of chronic disease: An overview. *Social Science and Medicine* 16:353–367.

McReynolds, W. T., L. Green, and E. B. Fisher, Jr. 1983. Self-control as a choice management with reference to behavioral treatment of obesity. *Health Psychology* 2:261–276.

Malley, P. M., J. G. Bachman, and L. D. Johnston. 1984. Period, age, and cohort effects on substance use among American youth, 1976–82. *American Journal of Public Health* 74:682–688.

Marmot, M. G. 1984. Alcohol and coronary heart disease. *International Journal of Epidemiology* 13:160–167.

Marrett, L. D., S. D. Walter, and J. W. Meigs. 1983. Coffee drinking and bladder cancer in Connecticut. *American Journal of Epidemiology* 117:113–127.

Matthews, K. A. 1985. Assessment of Type A, anger, and hostility in epidemiologic studies of cardiovascular disease. In *Measuring psychosocial variables in epidemiologic studies of cardiovascular disease*, ed. A. M. Ostfeld and E. Eaker. NIH Publication No. 85-2270. Washington, D.C.: Government Printing Office.

Mausner, J. S., and A. K. Bahn. 1974. *Epidemiology: An introductory text.* Philadelphia: W. B. Saunders.

Medalie, J. H., and U. Goldbourt. 1976. Angina pectoris among 10,000 men, 2: Psychosocial and other risk factors as evidenced by a multivariate analysis of a five-year incidence study. *American Journal of Medicine* 135:811–817.

Metzner, H., W. J. Carman, and J. S. House. 1983. Health practices, risk factors, and chronic disease in Tecumseh. *Preventive Medicine* 12:491–507.

Metzner, H. L., E. Harburg, and D. E. Lamphiear. 1982. Residential mobility and urban-rural residence within life stages related to health risk and chronic disease in Tecumseh, Michigan. *Journal of Chronic Diseases* 35:359–374.

Minkler, M. 1981. Research on the health effects of retirement: An uncertain legacy. *Journal of Health and Social Behavior* 22:117–130.

Moos, R. H. 1979. Social-ecological perspectives on health. In *Health psychology*, ed. G. C. Stone, F. Cohen, and N. E. Adler. San Francisco: Jossey-Bass.

Morris, J. N. 1975. *Uses of epidemiology.* London: Churchill Livingstone.

Morrison, F. R., and R. A. Paffenbarger, Jr. 1981. Epidemiological aspects of biobehavior in the etiology of cancer: A critical review. In *Perspectives on behavioral medicine*, ed. S. M. Weiss, J. A. Herd, and B. H. Fox. New York: Academic Press.

Mossey, J. M., and E. Shapiro. 1982. Self-rated health a predictor of mortality among the elderly. *American Journal of Public Health* 72:800–808.

Multiple Risk Factor Intervention Trial Research Group. 1982. Multiple Risk Factor Intervention Trial: Risk factor changes and mortality results. *Journal of the American Medical Association* 248:1465–1477.

Murphy, L. R. 1984. Occupational stress management: A review and appraisal. *Journal of Occupational Psychology* 57:1–15.

Nash, J. D., and J. W. Farquhar. 1980. Applications of behavioral medicine to disease prevention in a total community setting: A review of the three community study. In *The comprehensive handbook of behavioral medicine, vol. 3: Extended applications and issues*, ed. J. M. Ferguson and C. B. Taylor. New York: Spectrum Publications.

Ockene, J. K., R. C. Benfari, R. L. Nuttall, I. Hurwitz, and I. S. Ockene. 1982. Relationship of psychosocial factors to smoking behavior change in an intervention program. *Preventive Medicine* 11:13–28.

Oldridge, N. B. 1982. Compliance and exercise in primary and secondary prevention of coronary heart disease: A review. *Preventive Medicine* 11:56–70.

Optenberg, S. A., D. R. Lairson, C. H. Slater, and M. L. Russell. 1984. Agreement of self-reported and physiologically estimated fitness status in a symptom-free population. *Preventive Medicine* 13:349–354.

Osterweis, M., F. Solomon, and M. Green, eds. 1984. *Bereavement: Reactions, consequences, and care.* Washington, D.C.: National Academy Press.

Ostfeld, A. M., and E. Eaker, eds. 1985. *Measuring psychosocial variables in epidemiologic studies of cardiovascular disease.* NIH Publication No. 85-2270. Washington, D.C.: Government Printing.

Paffenbarger, R. S., Jr., and R. T. Hyde. 1984. Exercise in the prevention of coronary heart disease. *Preventive Medicine* 13:3–22.

Paffenbarger, R. S., Jr., A. L. Wing, R. T. Hyde, and D. L. Jung. 1983. Physical activity and incidence of hypertension in college alumni. *American Journal of Epidemiology* 117:245–257.

Parkes, C. M. 1972. *Bereavement: Studies of grief in adult life.* New York: International Universities Press.

Pearlin, L. I., and J. S. Johnson. 1977. Marital status, life strains, and depression. *American Sociological Review* 42:704–715.

Pechacek, T. F., and A. L. McAlister. 1980. Strategies for the modification of smoking behavior. Treatment and prevention. In *The comprehensive handbook of behavioral medicine, vol. 3: Extended applications and issues*, ed. J. M. Ferguson and C. B. Taylor. New York: Spectrum Publications.

Pederson, L. L. 1982. Compliance with physician advice to quit smoking: A review of the literature. *Preventive Medicine* 11:71–84.

Pickard, L., and J. B. Collins. 1982. Health education techniques for dense residential settings. *Educational Gerontology* 8:381–393.

Polk, B. F., L. C. Harlan, S. P. Cooper, M. Stromer, J. Ignatius, H. Mull, and T. P. Blaszkowski. 1984. Disability days associated with detection and treatment in a hypertension control program. *American Journal of Epidemiology* 119:44–53.

Pomerleau, O. F., ed. 1983. The University of Connecticut Symposium on employee health and fitness. *Preventive Medicine* 12:597–719.

Powell, L. H. 1984. The Type A behavior pattern: An update on conceptual, assessment, and intervention research. *Behavioral Medicine Update* 6 (4):7–10.

Powell, L. H., and C. E. Thoresen. In press. Behavioral and physiological determinants of long-term prognosis after myocardial infarction. *Journal of Chronic Diseases.*

Reed, D., D. McGee, J. Cohen, K. Yano, S. L. Syme, and M. Feinleib. 1982. Acculturation and coronary heart disease among Japanese men in Hawaii. *American Journal of Epidemiology* 115:894–905.

Reed, D., D. McGee, and K. Yano. 1984. Psychosocial processes and general susceptibility to chronic disease. *American Journal of Epidemiology* 119: 356–370.

Reed, D., D. McGee, K. Yano, and M. Feinleib. 1983. Social networks and coronary heart disease among Japanese men in Hawaii. *American Journal of Epidemiology* 117:384–396.

Reeves, R. S., J. P. Foreyt, L. W. Scott, R. E. Mitchell, J. Wohlleb, and A. M. Gotto, Jr. 1983. Effects of low cholesterol eating plan on plasma lipids: Results of a three-year community study. *American Journal of Public Health* 73:873–877.

Report of Inter-Society Commission for Heart Disease Resources. 1984. Optimal resources for primary prevention of atherosclerotic disease. *Circulation* 70(1):155A–205A.

Review Panel on Coronary Prone Behavior and Coronary Heart Disease. 1981. Coronary-prone behavior and coronary heart disease: A critical review. *Circulation* 63:1199–1215.

Rook, K. S. 1984. Promoting social bonding: Strategies for helping the lonely and socially isolated. *American Psychologist* 39:1389–1407.

Room, R. 1984. Alcohol control and public health. *Annual Review of Public Health* 5:293–317.

Rose, R. M. 1980. Endocrine responses to stressful psychological events. *Psychiatric Clinics of North America* 3(2):251–276.

Rose, R. M., C. D. Jenkins, M. Hurst, J. A. Herd, and R. P. Hall. 1982. Endocrine activity in air traffic controllers at work, 2: Biological, psychological, and work correlates. *Psychoneuroendocrinology* 7:113–123.

Roth, D. L., and D. S. Holmes. 1985. Influence of physical fitness in determining the impact of stressful life events on physical and psychological health. *Psychosomatic Medicine* 47:164–173.

Rowland, K. F. 1977. Environmental events predicting death for the elderly. *Psychological Bulletin* 84:349–372.

Rundall, T. G. 1978. Life change and recovery from surgery. *Journal of Health and Social Behavior* 19:418–427.

Salonen, J. T., P. Puska, and J. Tuomilehto. 1982. Physical activity and risk of myocardial infarction, cerebral stroke and death: A longitudinal study in Eastern Finland. *American Journal of Epidemiology* 115:526–537.

Satariano, W. A., and S. L. Syme. 1981. Life changes and disease in elderly populations. In *Aging: Biology and behavior*, ed. J. L. McGaugh and S. B. Kiesler. New York: Academic Press.

Schoenbach, V. J., E. H. Wagner, and J. M. Karon. 1983. The use of epidemiologic data for personal risk assessment in health hazard/health risk appraisal programs. *Journal of Chronic Diseases* 36:625–638.

Schroeder, D. H., and P. T. Costa, Jr. 1984. Influence of life event stress on physical illness: Substantive effects or methodological flaws? *Journal of Personality and Social Psychology* 46:853–863.

Seeman, M., and T. E. Seeman. 1983. Health behavior and personal autonomy: A longitudinal study of the sense of control in illness. *Journal of Health and Social Behavior* 24:144–160.

Serfass, R. C., and S. G. Gerberich. 1984. Exercise for optimal health: Strategies and motivational considerations. *Preventive Medicine* 13:79–99.

Sexton, M. M. 1979. Behavioral epidemiology. In *Behavioral medicine: Theory and practice*, ed. O. F. Pomerleau and J. P. Brady. Baltimore: Williams and Wilkins.

Shekelle, R. B., A. M. Ostfeld, and O. Paul. 1969. Social status and incidence of coronary heart disease. *Journal of Chronic Diseases* 22:381–394.

Siegel, J. M. 1984. Type A behavior: Epidemiologic foundations and public health implications. *Annual Review of Public Health* 5:343–367.

———. 1985. Personality and cardiovascular disease: Prior research and future directions. In *Measuring psychosocial variables in epidemiologic studies of cardiovascular disease*, ed. A. M. Ostfeld and E. Eaker. NIH Publication No. 85-2270. Washington, D.C.: Government Printing Office.

Sklar, L. S., and H. Anisman. 1981. Stress and cancer. *Psychological Bulletin* 89:369–406.

Snowdon, D. A., and R. L. Phillips. 1984. Coffee consumption and the risk of fatal cancers. *American Journal of Public Health* 74:820–823.

Spruit, I. P. 1982. Unemployment and health in macro-social analysis. *Social Science and Medicine* 16:1903–1917.

Stallones, R. A. 1983. Mortality and the Multiple Risk Factor Intervention Trial. *American Journal of Epidemiology* 117:647–650.

Steptoe, A. 1984. Psychophysiological processes in disease. In *Health care and human behaviour*, ed. A. Steptoe and A. Mathews. London: Academic Press.

Sterling, P., and J. Eyer. 1981. Biological basis of stress-related mortality. *Social Science and Medicine* 15E:3–42.

Stewart, A. L., and R. H. Brook. 1983. Effects of being overweight. *American Journal of Public Health* 73:171–178.

Suarez, L., and E. Barrett-Connor. 1984. Is an educated wife hazardous to your health? *American Journal of Epidemiology* 119:244–249.

Suchman, E. A. 1965. Stages of illness and medical care. *Journal of Health and Human Behavior* 6:114–128.

Susser, M. 1973. *Causal thinking in the health sciences: Concepts and strategies of epidemiology.* New York: Oxford University Press.

Syme, S. L. 1974. Behavioral factors associated with the etiology of physical disease. A social epidemiological approach. *American Journal of Public Health* 64:1043–1045.

———. 1978. Life-style interventions in clinic-based trials. *American Journal of Epidemiology* 108:87–91.

Syme, S. L., and R. Alcalay. 1982. Control of cigarette smoking from a social perspective. *Annual Review of Public Health* 3:179–199.

Syme, S. L., and L. F. Berkman. 1976. Social class, susceptibility, and sickness. *American Journal of Epidemiology* 104:1–8.

Terris, M. 1980. Epidemiology as a guide to health policy. *Annual Review of Public Health* 1:322–344.

U.S. Department of Health and Human Services. Office of the Assistant Secretary for Health. 1980. *Promoting health, preventing disease: Objectives for the nation.* Washington, D.C.: Government Printing Office.

———. Office on Smoking and Health. 1982. *The health consequences of smoking: Cancer. A report of the surgeon general.* Publication No. DHHS (PHS) 82-50179. Washington, D.C.: Government Printing Office.

Vogt, T. M. 1981. Risk assessment and health hazard appraisal. *Annual Review of Public Health* 2:31–47.

Wagner, E. H., W. L. Berry, V. J. Schoenbach, and R. M. Graham. 1982. An assessment of health hazard/health risk appraisal. *American Journal of Public Health* 72:347–352.

Wallston, B. S., S. W. Alagna, B. M. DeVellis, and R. F. DeVellis. 1983. Social support and physical health. *Health Psychology* 2:367–391.

Weiner, H. 1977. *Psychobiology and human disease.* New York: Elsevier.

Weinstein, N. D. 1984. Why it won't happen to me: Perceptions of risk factors and susceptibility. *Health Psychology* 3:431–457.

Weiss, N. S. 1973. Marital status and risk factors for coronary heart disease: The United States Health Examination Survey of Adults. *British Journal of Preventive and Social Medicine* 27:41–43.

Williams, A. W., J. E. Ware, Jr., and C. A. Donald. 1981. A model of mental health, life events, and social supports applicable to general populations. *Journal of Health and Social Behavior* 22:324–336.

Wilson, R. W., and T. F. Drury. 1984. Interpreting trends in illness and disability. *Annual Review of Public Health* 5:83–106.

Wingard, D. L., L. F. Berkman, and R. J. Brand. 1982. A multivariate analysis of health-related practices. A nine-year mortality follow-up of the Alameda County study. *American Journal of Epidemiology* 116:765–775.

Winkelstein, W., Jr., and M. Marmot. 1981. Primary prevention of ischemic heart disease: Evaluation of community interventions. *Annual Review of Public Health* 2:253–276.

Woods, P. J., and J. Burns. 1984. Type A behavior and illness in general. *Journal of Behavioral Medicine* 7:411–415.

Woods, P. J., B. T. Morgan, B. W. Day, T. Jefferson, and C. Harris. 1984. Findings on a relationship between Type A behavior and headaches. *Journal of Behavioral Medicine* 7:277–286.

Yamamoto, L., K. Yano, and G. G. Rhoads. 1983. Characteristics of joggers among Japanese men in Hawaii. *American Journal of Public Health* 73: 147–152.

Yano, K., D. M. Reed, and D. L. McGee. 1984. Ten-year incidence of coronary heart disease in the Honolulu Heart Program: Relationship to biologic and lifestyle characteristics. *American Journal of Epidemiology* 119: 653–666.

Zuckerman, D. M., S. V. Kasl, and A. M. Ostfeld. 1984. Psychosocial predictors of mortality among the elderly poor: The role of religion, well-being, and social contacts. *American Journal of Epidemiology* 119:410–423.

Chapter 18

Health and the Workplace

James S. House and
Eric M. Cottington

N ow is an opportune time to write about health and the workplace. The period since World War II has seen two major scientific and social movements toward promoting health and preventing disease in the workplace. The first has peaked and declined, and we are in the midst of the second. Each movement has had unique causes and consequences; each has emphasized an important aspect of the total problem of health and the workplace. We first sketch the essential elements of these two movements, their unique strengths and weaknesses, and then move to a broader consideration of how and why the workplace is central to societal efforts at health promotion and disease prevention. Here we focus on a topic that has not been sufficiently addressed in either of the two major movements but that is particu-larly germane to our own interests, to the changing nature of work in our so-ciety, and to this volume on the rele-vance of social science to health—the impact of the psychosocial work environment on health.

Shifting Bases of Concern

The Occupational Safety and Health Movement

The traditional basis for concern with health and the workplace was to im-prove occupational safety and health, that is, to reduce the incidence of in-juries, illnesses, and deaths attribut-able to occupational causes. Both scientific and social concern with oc-cupational safety and health grew with the process of industrialization, with workers or their representatives providing major impetus. Government was increasingly drawn into the issue—first at local and state levels and then nationally—to adjudicate disagreements between workers and employers over what constitutes unsafe or unhealthful working conditions, whether injuries or illnesses are "work related," and how much employers and their insurers are liable for the costs incurred by victims of work-related injury or illness.

The development of this "occupational safety and health movement" peaked in the late 1960s (as did many parallel environmental and social welfare movements) with the passage of the Coal Mine Health and Safety Act of 1969 and the Occupational Safety and Health Act of 1970. The OSH Act sought to "assure safe and healthful working conditions for working men and women." It created the National Institute of Occupational Safety and Health to research standards for safe and healthy working conditions, and the Occupational Safety and Health Administration within the Department of Labor to establish, promulgate, promote, and enforce standards. (See Ashford 1976 for an overview of the sources and consequences of the OSH Act, especially its failings as well as it accomplishments.)

The occupational safety and health movement (and the OSH Act) had several distinctive emphases. First, it focused on *occupational* safety and health, those aspects of health that were directly work related. Second, it focused on the work *environment* as the major source of occupational health problems and hence as the major target for interventions to improve occupational health. Third, it focused on *physical, chemical,* and *biological* factors as the major environmental determinants of occupational health. Only secondarily was attention paid to the social environment of the workplace or the psychology and behavior of workers as independent factors in occupational health.

The occupational safety and health movement succeeded in identifying a wide variety of physical, chemical, and biological sources of occupational injury and illness, ranging from inadequate safety shielding of machinery to exposure to coal and cotton dust, infectious agents (Janis and Garibaldi 1983), asbestos (Selikoff, Hammond, and Churg 1968), and chemical carcinogens (Doll 1981). Control and reduction of workplace exposures to such agents as asbestos, cotton dust, and vinyl chloride has reduced the incidence of cancer and respiratory diseases (Ashford and Andrews 1983). Precise determinants of economic impact are difficult, but asbestos exposure regulations have saved between $164 and $652 million annually (Lasagna, Wordell, and Hansen 1978). Ashford and Andrews (1983, 895) conclude that the "prevailing view is that environmental, health and safety regulation can produce highly positive net benefits to society." However, the economic and social costs of such regulations have also produced a reaction among those who bear such costs, principally employers. This reaction, coupled with a decline in the political ascendancy of labor and the Democratic party as well as with increasing economic problems in the private and public sector, has led to a decline in the strength of the occupational safety and health movement and the rise of the workplace health promotion movement.

The Workplace Health Promotion Movement

The burgeoning cost of health care in our society has fostered a new basis of concern with health and the workplace. Because our health insurance system is largely organized and financed through the workplace, employers pay about one-half of our societal health care bill. As a result, for example, $500 of the cost of each vehicle manufactured by Chrysler in 1982 went to cover health care costs (Fielding 1984; Rosen 1984). Employee health costs, more broadly defined to include absenteeism and loss of productivity, have been estimated as high as 25 percent of most employers' payrolls.

Employers and health insurers (including government), then, have a vital and material interest in improving the health of workers and reducing health care costs. The increasing role of the workplace in health care delivery, as in employer- or occupation-based HMOs, is beyond the scope of this chapter. The rapid proliferation of employer health promotion and employee assistance programs is, however, central to our concern with the role of the workplace in promoting health and preventing disease (Fielding 1984; "Millions Spent in Efforts to Keep Employees Well" 1984). These programs involve some combination of efforts at smoking cessation, weight control and better nutrition, increase of exercise levels, control of alcohol and substance abuse, stress-management techniques, personal counseling, and perhaps screening for risk factors of cardiovascular diseases or cancer. These programs are grounded in growing scientific evidence (e.g., Berkman and Breslow 1983; Ostfeld, chap. 8, this volume) and policy conviction (Lalonde 1974; U.S. Department of Health and Human Services 1979, 1980) that individual health behaviors and habits are a major cause of general mortality and morbidity in our society.

The major thrusts of this work-
The major thrusts of this workplace health promotion movement differ significantly from those of the occupational safety and health movement, which it superseded. First, the workplace health promotion movement focuses on general health and disease, not just on those aspects of health and disease that are directly work related. Indeed, there is a strong tendency to neglect or even deny the impact of the work environment on health and to view the workplace as a site for dealing, preventively or therapeutically, with health problems, the etiologies of which are assumed to be largely *non*-work-related. Employers and insurers are trying to counteract or mitigate the impact, on organizational functioning and employer-based health insurance systems, of unhealthy life-styles (including ways of adapting to stress) that employees have developed prior to or outside their worklife. Second, the workplace health promotion movement focuses on the individual, rather than on the

environment, as the major source of health problems and hence as the major target for interventions to improve health in the workplace or elsewhere (Berkman and Breslow 1983; Castillo-Salgado 1984).

Growing evidence suggests that workplace health promotion programs can be effective in reducing smoking, controlling hypertension, reducing obesity, and increasing exercise levels (Fielding 1984; Rosen 1984), possibly more effective than similar programs outside of work (Alderman and Davis 1980; Fielding 1982). Much of the current evidence, however, derives from company reports; rigorous evaluation studies are generally lacking. Most important, we as yet have little basis for inferring that the changes in health behavior produced by workplace health promotion programs, with the possible exception of smoking cessation programs, are sufficiently large and sustained to produce significant changes in morbidity and mortality, much less reductions in health care expenditures and other costs or gains in productivity that would make them clearly cost-effective (Fielding 1984).

Toward a More Comprehensive Approach

The occupational safety and health and workplace health promotion movements have focused on important and complementary aspects of the overall problem of health and the workplace. Nevertheless, a more comprehensive approach toward health and the workplace is needed.

This approach should recognize and retain the strengths of each movement, using the complementary strengths of one to compensate for the limitations of the other, while also taking into account factors neglected by both of these movements.

The traditional concern of the occupational safety and health movement with creating a more healthful working environment must be reaffirmed. An increasing majority of adults of working age spend one-third to one-half of their waking hours at work. For many, the work environment is the single environment in which they spend the most time, even more time than in the home. On the basis of sheer exposure, the work environment must be considered a major potential influence, for better or worse, on the health of working-age adults. While the traditional focus on the physical-chemical-biological environment remains important, the number of potentially hazardous physical-chemical-biological agents is enormous and new ones are emerging every day. One must be concerned not only with individual substances but also with potential interactive combinations (Ashford 1976). Public sanitation, which has mimimized exposure to a wide range of harmful biological, physical, and chemical agents, has contributed more to improved public health in the last two centuries than the identification and elimination of particular bacteria, viruses, or toxins. Similarly, general workplace sanitation—minimizing exposure to agents and situations not known to be benign—is likely to be the most rapid and cost-effective route to reducing adverse health effects of the physical-chemical-biological environment.

We cannot fully understand the health effects of the work environment without also understanding the health impact of individual attributes and the larger environment in which people live. Thus the workplace health promotion movement has provided a useful complement to the occupational safety and health movement. The former movement has taken a "wholistic" view of health, recognizing that a wide range of health habits and behaviors, which characterize individuals both at work and outside of work, are significant determinants of morbidity and mortality and important potential modifiers of the impact of health hazards at work and outside of work.

Yet to view individuals as able to control all aspects of their health and health behavior, as health promotion efforts do in many instances, is essentially to "blame the victim" (Castillo-Salgado 1984). Efforts to reduce smoking, for example, must recognize the powerful role of cigarette manufacturers and advertisers in promoting smoking, the role of organizations in condoning it, and the role of social and environmental stresses and influences in individuals' lives in promoting or maintaining it. At a minimum, the work environment must be made supportive of health promotion efforts. This has been done in some successful workplace health promotion programs, such as that at Johnson and Johnson where "alteration of the work environment, such as establishment of a company smoking policy, changing the food in the company cafeterias, and building exercise facil-

ities, is considered an integral and essential part of the program" (Fielding 1984, 251).

The Role of the Psychosocial Environment

The psychosocial work environment —largely neglected by both the occupational health and safety and workplace health promotion movements —should, on a variety of grounds, be an increasingly important component of any comprehensive effort at workplace health promotion. First, the changing nature of work is continually increasing the importance of the psychosocial work environment. The occupational health and safety movement's concern with the physical-chemical-biological work environment developed in an era when agriculture, extraction of natural resources, manufacturing, and rail transportation were the major industries in our society. The shift away from such blue-collar agricultural and industrial work toward white- and pink-collar professional, managerial, and clerical work constitutes a major societal trend. Even in the blue-collar sector, mechanization and automation have made work environments more "professional" and "technical" in nature. The most significant aspects of work environments are therefore increasingly psychosocial—the level and scheduling of work loads, interpersonal relationships, responsibility for people and property, conflicts between work and nonwork life. These changes and the development of a world economy have increased the prevalence and perhaps impact of psychosocial stressors such as job insecurity and loss, and technological and organizational change.

Second, the psychosocial work environment affects both health promotion and occupational health and safety. As noted earlier, the psychosocial environment both furthers and impedes efforts at health promotion. For example, occupational stress may increase the incidence and prevalence of poor health behavior while social support may increase the effectiveness of efforts at health promotion (Caplan, Cobb et al. 1980; Caplan, Harrison et al. 1980). A small but growing body of theory and evidence also suggests that psychosocial stress can exacerbate the impact of a variety of physical, chemical, and biological hazards (Cassel 1976; House et al. 1979; Pasmore and Friedlander 1982).

Third, concern with the psychosocial work environment leads naturally into a concern with health effects of the psychosocial environment outside of work and the increasingly important interaction between sources of stress at work and outside of work. As women, and also men, increasingly have work as well as family responsibilities, the importance of the relation between work and nonwork factors grows in relation to health (Haynes and Feinleib 1980; Haw 1982).

Fourth, the psychosocial work environment is amenable to the types of broad environmental changes that can reduce the prevalence and incidence of a wide range of health problems. The impact of most psychosocial factors are not disease specific (Cassel 1976; Berkman and Breslow

1983). The psychosocial factors discussed below—demanding work, control, social support, and participation—are amenable to organizational interventions that can affect a wide variety of workers.

Finally, the known physical-chemical-biological and health behavior risk factors, which have until now been the focus of research and interventions regarding health and the workplace, can account for only a small portion of the variation in major health outcomes. Marmot and Winkelstein (1975) demonstrated, for example, that the major risk factors of heart disease—smoking, blood pressure, and cholesterol—explain only a small portion of the total variation in the incidence of heart disease. They pointed to psychosocial factors as promising additional variables predicting heart disease; subsequent research discussed later in this chapter has confirmed their intuition.

Health Effects of the Psychosocial Work Environment

Kasl (1981, 682) has aptly characterized much of the data on the health effects of psychosocial aspects of work as "fragmentary . . . difficult to replicate and subject to multiple etiological interpretations." Nevertheless, we see a growing convergence of evidence from cross-sectional, retrospective, and prospective field studies, as well as limited experimental studies on animals and humans. This evidence suggests that several key psychosocial characteristics of the work environment have a substantial impact on health behaviors, morbidity, and even mortality: (1) job demands or pressures, (2) personal control, and (3) social support (cf. reviews by Cooper and Payne 1978; Cottington and House, in press; Holt 1982; House 1974a, 1974b, 1981; Kahn 1981a; Kasl 1974, 1978, 1982). These three psychosocial aspects of work are linked more or less directly to a fourth factor—participation in decision making—which has not been so explicitly linked with health outcomes but which is both a major focus of current efforts at organizational change and a major potential mechanism for modifying levels of job demands, personal control, and social support. Thus, our discussion will first review the theoretical and empirical basis for the impact of job demands, personal control, and social support on health and health behavior; then we will consider how these variables may be modified via changes in participation as well as in other organizational processes.

Job Demands and Health

A large number of studies have found associations between health or health behaviors and job demands or pressures, including excessive workload, responsibility or requirements for vigilance, and interpersonal or role conflicts either at work or between work and nonwork roles or activities (Caplan, Harrison et al. 1980; Holt 1982; House et al. 1979; Jenkins 1971, 1976; Kasl 1978, 1982). The unique effects of particular job de-

mands or pressures are not easily identified from these studies since different types of pressures tend to cluster within jobs or classes of workers. Studies using more "objective" indexes of job demands and pressures often compare workers in different occupations that differ simultaneously on a variety of potential stressors. Air traffic controllers and foremen, for example, have been shown to have higher rates of health problems than other workers (Cobb and Rose 1973; Rose, Jenkins, and Hurst 1978; Pflanz 1971; Susser 1967). They also appear simultaneously to have higher levels of workload, responsibility, and interpersonal or role conflicts. Studies using measures of different types of perceived job demands (workload, responsibility, role conflict, etc.) find moderate to high positive correlations among these measures (e.g., Caplan, Harrison et al. 1980; House et al. 1979) and generally find multiple demands or pressures related to a given health outcome.

These results are subject to two methodological reservations. First, the observed associations tend to be strongest and most consistent when self-reported job demands are associated with self-reported health problems, especially symptoms of psychological disorder, and become weaker as the measure of health becomes more objective (e.g., blood pressure). Second, the vast bulk of the research is cross-sectional or retrospective. These two factors make the causal interpretation of many studies quite ambiguous, as Kasl (1978, 1981, 1982) and others have observed. Poor health may affect the type of job a person has or the way a person perceives the job, rather than vice versa; or reports of poor health and job demands may reflect an underlying psychological malaise.

More compelling are prospective studies in which job demands or pressures are used to predict changes in health status. Good prospective evidence on psychosocial job demands and health has begun to be published only in the last five to ten years. The emerging evidence is, however, increasingly compelling and consistent with prior cross-sectional and retrospective research. Karasek, Theorell, and associates have reported prospective as well as cross-sectional and retrospective evidence linking psychosocial job demands to coronary heart disease (CHD) morbidity and mortality in several populations of Swedish workers (Karasek et al. 1981; Theorell 1982). In a ten-year prospective study in Belgium, Kittel, Kornitzer, and Dramaix (1980) found a 50 percent higher incidence of CHD among employees of a private bank characterized by greater competitive pressure and organizational change than among employees of a more stable and less pressured public bank.

Analyses by Haynes, Feinleib, and Kannel (1980) of the Framingham Heart Study found a questionnaire measure of Type A behavior, comprised heavily of questions about work-related demands and pressures, to be a significant predictor of the incidence of CHD, over and above the effects of conventional risk factors such as smoking, blood pressure, and cholesterol.[1] Ruberman et al. (1984) found that life stress (including a significant occupational component) and social isolation increased subsequent mortality among male survivors of myocardial infarction.

The chronicity of job demands appears to be crucial to their health effects. For there to be substantial effects on physical morbidity to mortality, job demands and pressures must be sustained over a long enough time period for the long-term etiologic processes of chronic diseases to operate. In a ten-year prospective analysis of a cohort of adults in the Tecumseh Community Health Study, House et al. (in press) found that a single subjective assessment of job demands was not predictive of mortality from all causes. In a subset of men on whom a second assessment was available about two years later, however, those who both times reported elevated job demands were three times as likely to die in the succeeding decade as men whose level of job demands was reported low both times or elevated only one time. This relationship held even after adjustment for a wide range of other social and biomedical risk factors of mortality.

In many of the studies just reviewed, evidence for the existence of job demands comes from workers' reports and hence may reflect not only the external work environment but also the way workers respond to it. As discussed more fully later, further research is needed to better understand the extent to which reports or perceptions of job demands are a function of environmental conditions, individual characteristics, or the interaction among them. Experimental and quasi-experimental studies on humans and animals, however, show marked psychological, behavioral, and physiological effects of experimentally induced, objective stressors such as workload, responsibility, and conflict with others. In experiments with humans, the induced stressors are necessarily limited in their duration. The outcomes studied are not diseases per se but changes in psychological, physiological, or behavioral variables (e.g., blood pressure, catecholamine excretion, stomach acid levels, anxiety, behavioral disorganization) which, if prolonged, could constitute or produce serious disease outcomes (Sales 1969; Williams 1975; Levi 1981). In some animal studies, however, the intensity and duration of the stressors is sufficient to produce serious disease outcomes (e.g., hypertension, ulcers) and even death (Brady 1958; Weiss, 1970).

Only a limited number of studies have looked explicitly at how work and nonwork demands and pressures combine to influence health. Studies of shiftwork as well as other research identify conflict between the demands of major nonwork and work roles as a form of stress with consequences for health (Mott et al. 1965; Tasto and Colligan 1978; House et al. 1979). Studies of working women sometimes, though not always, find poorer health among those who also have significant child-rearing responsibilities (Cottington and House, in press). As the number of women, and especially the number of mothers of young children, in the labor force continues to grow, we need more research on the effects of the work environment on the health of women and on the interplay between work and nonwork factors in the health of both men and women.

Personal Control, Social Support, and Health

Two additional psychosocial aspects of work appear to have important health consequences. These variables—personal control of the work process or environment and social support—are of interest not only because they appear to directly affect health, but also because they may help to reduce levels of job demands or to buffer or mitigate the impact of job demands on health. The evidence on the relation of these variables to health is newer and less extensive than in the case of job demands, but the results are still compelling.

Sutton and Kahn (1984) have reviewed a wide variety of laboratory and field studies suggesting that if individuals have greater ability to "predict, understand or control" events in their organizational environment, they will experience less organizational stress or be less adversely affected by it. The work of Karasek, Theorell, and associates (Karasek et al. 1981; Theorell 1982) has focused on how the combination of job demands *and* control (or what the researchers term "decision latitude") affects health. Their cross-sectional, retrospective, and prospective studies all indicate that lack of control over one's work process and environment constitutes an additional risk factor for cardiovascular disease. They also suggest, though less conclusively, that lack of control exacerbates the impact of job demands on morbidity and mortality (cf. Kasl 1981).

Indirect evidence of the importance of control over one's work environment comes from studies of the effects of personality dispositions. Kobasa, Maddi, and Zola (1983) have studied a personal disposition, which they term hardiness, in which a sense of control over one's environment is a major component. They find that hardiness buffers the impact of job demands on self-reported health problems. Although Kobasa, Maddi, and Zola view hardiness as a personality trait, aspects of it such as a sense of control are likely to respond to current environmental constraints as well as to earlier experience that is formative of personality. Thus, this research, and similar work showing that a general sense of mastery or control can mitigate the effects of more general life stress on health (e.g., Pearlin et al. 1981), is consistent with the notion that occupational conditions that enhance workers' sense of mastery or control can be beneficial to health.

Students of occupational stress, and of stress more generally, have in the last decade focused increasing attention on social support as a potential mechanism that can simultaneously improve health, reduce stress, and buffer the impact of stress on health. Both the definition and measurement of social support are multifaceted (cf. House 1981; House and Kahn 1985; Cohen and Syme 1985). At a minimum, social support refers to the quantity of relationships with significant other people such as family and friends. In this sense, extreme lack of support is social isolation. The term *support* also generally denotes or connotes certain qualitative functions served by such relationships. Specifically, supportive relationships provide a person with information, instrumental assistance, and, most important, emotional support—a sense that others care about and understand him or her and are ready, willing, and able to help in times of need.

A number of large cross-sectional studies have found that perceived support from work supervisors and co-workers is associated with lower levels of perceived work stress and better self-reported physical and mental health. In these studies social support also buffered the impact of occupational stress on health (House and Wells 1978; Karasek, Triantis, and Chaudhary 1982; LaRocco, House, and French, 1980; Winnubst, Marcellissen, and Kleber 1982), although such buffering effects are not always found. (See Cohen and Wills 1985; House 1981; LaRocco, House, and French 1980; and Williams and House 1985 for a review and discussion of the patterning and meaning of these results.) The relative importance of supervisors and co-workers as sources of support varies with occupational conditions. Where co-workers are readily available sources of support, they tend to be more important; where workers have no co-workers or can not communicate easily with them, supervisors are more consequential (LaRocco, House, and French 1980; Williams and House 1985).

Prospective studies have also shown that supportive relationships with work supervisors or co-workers reduce the incidence of coronary heart disease. In the Israel Ischaemic Heart Disease Project involving ten thousand men aged forty and over, Medalie et al. (1973a, 1973b) found a higher five-year incidence of angina pectoris among men who reported lack of appreciation and feelings of hurt in their relationships with supervisors and co-workers. Similarly, in the Framingham Heart Study, female clerical workers with nonsupportive bosses had a higher incidence of coronary heart disease and cerebrovascular disorders than female clericals with supportive bosses (Eaker and Feinleib 1983; Haynes and Feinleib 1980). These results are consistent with other prospective studies that have found the absence or relative lack of significant social ties to be a major risk factor for mortality over and above other known risk factors in general populations (Berkman and Syme 1979; House, Robbins, and Metzner 1982) as well as among the aged (Blazer 1982) and those who have experienced myocardial infarctions (Ruberman et al. 1984).

All of the work cited here has been published in the last half-dozen years. Yet it is impressively consistent in documenting the ability of social support both at work and outside of work to reduce stress, improve health, or buffer the impact of stress on health. As with control, the results of these field studies of "real-life" situations are reinforced by parallel findings from experimental studies of both animals and humans (House 1981).

Implications and Applications

Existing evidence is quite compelling that high job demands and low levels of personal control and social support are at work are deleterious to health; new evidence is still accumulating. Where comparative evidence is available, the effects of these variables on mortality in prospective studies generally approximate or exceed the effects of major biomedical risk factors, which are the targets of current health promotion programs at the workplace and outside (cf. House et al., in press, for relevant data from the Tecumseh Health Study; Ruberman et al. 1984 for data on a population with CHD). Thus, it is reaonsable to expect that reducing job demands and increasing personal control and social support at work can have effects on overall morbidity and mortality commensurate with reductions in other risk factors. Changes in these psychosocial variables are also likely to improve employees' job satisfaction, reduce absenteeism and turnover, and perhaps have other positive effects on organizational functioning. Thus, the potential benefits of changes in these psychosocial variables, for health and overall individual and organizational functioning, are considerable.

Why then are we not making major efforts in the United States to improve the psychosocial work environment as a means of promoting health? There are a number of potential reasons. First; job demands, personal control, and social support all inherently involve an interaction between the nature of individuals and the nature of their environment. How demanding a job is depends not only on the nature of the job but on the nature of the person. Similarly, whether a worker experiences a sense of control or social support on the job is a function of the nature of both the job environment and the worker.

This insight sometimes leads to the conclusion that problems of job demands, worker control, or social support—which are often generically termed job stress—are largely individual problems, and that we have no evidence that the work environment is responsible for these problems. This conclusion is simply not true. Some of the evidence reviewed above uses quite objective, environmental definitions of job demands, control, and support (e.g., occupational differences or the presence or absence of social ties). Although much of the evidence is based on more subjective self-report measures, we know that these reports vary significantly and consequentially by occupations and industries, by objective job conditions within occupations and industries, and with changes in a given work environment (House 1980; Katz and Kahn 1978; Kahn 1981a). We do not yet understand in any precise way the relative contribution of the individual and the environment to the creation of job demands, worker control, and social support. This is a critical area for future research, with important practical implications. We do know that the environmental contribution is substantial and that a single environmental change can affect a large number of individuals, whereas efforts to change individual dispositions or behaviors often require much more intensive, individually focused efforts. Thus, environmental changes can improve health and are likely to be cost-effective, provided we can produce the desired changes.

This brings us to a second potential reaason for a relative lack of visible efforts to improve the psychosocial work environment as a means of improving health. Do we know how to modify the psychosocial work environment in ways that can reduce deleterious job demands and enhance personal control and social support and thus improve health? The answer is yes and no—the same answer that could be given to the question, Do we know how to modify health behavior or the physical-chemical environment in the workplace and thus improve health? Evidence indicates, for example, that workplace health promotion can reduce smoking or increase exercise levels. We do not yet have clear evidence that these changes in health behavior affect enough individuals for a long enough time to produce significant long-term improvements in health or reductions in health care costs. The same could be said about many physical, chemical, or biological hazards.

Considerable evidence from the general literature on organizations shows that job demands, personal control, and social support vary across work environments and can be changed in response to changes in these environments. Both the technology and organization of the work environment significantly affect these and other responses of workers to their work setting. Blauner (1964) documented the powerful impact of technology; he found that as the mechanization and capital intensity of production technology increased from craft production through machine tending and assembly-line production, the control of workers over their work process and their level of social integration and intrinsic involvement at work declined. However, further capitalization and mechanization in the form of automated or continuous process production reversed these deleterious effects and enhanced control, social integration, and intrinsic work involvement. Subsequent research confirms Blauner's findings (e.g. Shepard 1977; Haddad, House, and Jackman 1985). Haddad, House, and Jackman (1985), also found that various objective and perceived job demands vary by technology.

Thus, technology and technological changes constitute one means of modifying social support, worker control, and job demands. Obviously, such changes are large and expensive and unlikely to be made solely for health reasons. The impact of technology on job demands, social support, worker control, and health should be considered, however, when options for technological change are considered. This has been and is being done in Scandinavian countries where, for example, conventional automobile assembly-line technology has been modified in new auto and engine plants to allow groups of workers to cooperate in a set of assembling operations, hence increasing worker control and social integration and reducing the stress of monotonous, machine-paced work (cf. Katz and Kahn 1978, chap. 17; Gardell 1981; Eketorp 1981). We know of no systematic evidence on the health effects of such change. Given the rapid rate of technological change for many industries, the opportunity exists in this country to design technology to enhance worker control and social integration, to reduce certain kinds of job demands, and to evaluate the health impact of such changes.

Even with technology fixed, work organization can be modified to affect levels of control, support, and job demands. The classic examples of this process are the Tavistock Institute Studies of "sociotechnical systems." In both British coal mines and Indian textile mills it was possible without changing technology to reorganize the work process so that groups of workers cooperated in carrying out a set of jobs, each of which had formerly been performed by a single worker. The result was increased worker control and social integration and decreased monotony and perhaps job demands (Emery and Trist 1960). A limited range of organizational experiments in the United States shows similar results (Kahn 1981b, 31–33). The Tavistock studies and most, though not all, subsequent studies found that the organizational changes also improved productivity.

No simple set of procedures can be applied in all work settings to modify control, support, or job demands. Any intervention must be tailored to the occupations, industries, or work sites involved. In the case of control and support, however, a set of simple principles characterize most successful interventions. For control, these include delegating authority from higher to lower levels, increasing the range of skills and activities of each worker, and increasing shared group decision-making. For support, the keys are to reduce social and physical isolation, promote group interaction and train workers, especially supervisors and managers, to be supportive in their interactions with others. The training is the same that might be given to improve group functioning and supervision generally; the attributes that research has found to characterize good supervisors, especially participative supervisors, are precisely those that would make supervisors supportive and promote supportive behavior among co-workers (House 1981, chaps. 5, 6; Likert 1961; Redding, 1972; Jablin 1979).

Methods for reducing job demands are necessarily more complex, since the concept of job demands is more multifaceted than that of control or even support. And the environmental factors that can produce or mitigate demands are likely to be more variable across situations. Before undertaking any change or intervention program it is important to assess the need for change. For example, we ought to assess levels of control and support across workers, jobs, and work settings before deciding where, when, and how to intervene, just as we ought to know levels of smoking, blood pressure, or alcohol and substance abuse before formulating health promotion programs. This assessment is even more crucial in the case of job demands, since the nature of the demands and the ways of modifying them will be somewhat unique in each situation. Even if the generic problem is the same in different situations, the nature and sources of it will vary. Workloads or role conflicts on an automobile assembly line and in a hospital are likely to be very different, though each setting may have high levels of both types of demands.

Efforts should be made to determine through surveys or objective ratings the level and nature of job demands in different parts of a work setting, then to develop ways of modifying the particular aspects of the

work environment or process to reduce demands, and finally to evaluate the outcome. Pasmore and Friedlander (1982) illustrate how this was done in their action research project, which sought to reduce the level of muscle and joint injuries (tenosynovitis) in a manufacturing plant. Interviews and surveys conducted by a worker study group identified job stress and tension as a major source of the problem; the study group also identified potential solutions, including biomechanical changes in the work process, greater avenues for worker-management cooperation, and improved supervisor training. In other settings, reallocation or reorganization of workloads and responsibilities, improved methods for communicating and adjudicating conflicting demands, or other changes may be appropriate.

The process described by Pasmore and Friedlander is similar to that used in Japanese, European, and American programs to increase worker participation and involvement, whether termed quality circles, quality of work life, employee involvement, or something else (Amsden 1983). Thus increased employee participation, and interaction among workers and with management, in determining the goals and means of the work process emerges as a common theme in efforts to modify job demands, worker control, and social support. Understanding the relations among these variables is a major task for future research, including some in which we are involved; but a tentative formulation is now possible as shown in figure 18.1.

Participation is seen as directly

FIGURE 18.1.

A model of the relationships among participation, support, control, demands, and health in the workplace.

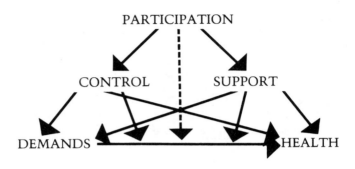

influencing worker control and social support. An employee who works with others in determining the goals and means of the work process should have an enhanced sense of individual (or collective) control and support. Both the degree of control over the work environment and the supportiveness of fellow workers and management can directly influence health as previously noted. Yet both can also indirectly influence health by directly affecting the level of job demands or modifying its relationship to health. For instance, employees with greater control over how their work is done may develop more efficient processes that reduce high levels of workload. Or increased support from fellow workers and management may help lower the amount of responsibility or role conflict the worker perceives. Finally, control and support may modify the relationships between job demands and health by making the individual better able to cope with a particular job demand. In sum, figure 18.1, while tentative, suggests that participation can play a major role in the prevention or alleviation of work-related health problems.

The major reason that more efforts have not been made to modify the psychosocial work environment as a means of improving health is that those in a position to make such modifications, including government, management, the medical profession, and sometimes even unions, have not encouraged and have often resisted such efforts. The contrast between the experimentation and intervention of the United States and Scandinavian countries is striking. As noted earlier and described more fully elsewhere (e.g., Gardell and Johansson 1981), in the Scandinavian countries, especially Sweden and Norway, mod-

ifying the psychosocial work environment to improve health and well-
being has increasingly become a
priority of labor, government, and
management, to the point where legislation is directed at increasing
worker participation and improving
the psychosocial work environment.
This move cannot reflect a difference
in access to information or research.
Rather it reflects a different political
balance. Just as the occupational
safety and health and workplace
health promotion movements in this
country have waxed or waned in response to the activities of relevant interest groups, efforts to modify the
psychosocial work environment to
improve health are also a function of
the degree to which employers, workers, insurers, government, and the
medical profession choose to act on
the basis of existing knowledge.

Integrating Research and Applications

Having just argued that the uses made
of scientific research are as much or
more a function of political factors
than of the nature of the research base
itself, let us close by suggesting that
research could still be used to better
inform applications and interventions and that such interventions
could make a valuable contribution
to research. Resources for improving
health in the workplace are limited.
Policymakers and health professionals must choose among courses of action, trying to find ones that are most
cost-effective. Such choices could be
made more intelligently if we had a
better information system for moni-

toring the health of workers and relating it to the nature of, or changes in,
workers and their work environment.

The United States has traditionally
had, at best, a haphazard system for
monitoring morbidity and mortality
in specific occupations and industries
at the level of work sites, employers,
broad occupational groups, states, or
the nation as a whole. Comprehensive national data on mortality by occupation have been assembled only at
intervals of twenty to thirty years,
and sometimes only on a partial basis
(House 1976). Few if any employers or
employee groups (e.g., unions) systematically monitor the morbidity
and mortality of their total workforce, much less of different subgroups of workers.

Decision makers need answers to
two kinds of questions. First, what
are our biggest health problems in
terms of their human and economic
costs? The answer requires knowing
the number and nature of health
problems in a population. Major problems will be those that are severe or
life threatening even if limited in
prevalence, (e.g., angiosarcoma in
plastics and chemical workers) or
those that are less severe but widespread (e.g., tenosynovitis in the plant
studied by Pasmore and Friedlander).
A health monitoring system can provide such answers and provide them
at an early point. Currently, such
problems are recognized only when
the economic or mortality costs become patently excessive.

Second, decision makers also need
a means for evaluating the cost-effectiveness of various interventions
to improve health or reduce disease.
A health monitoring system provides

an ongoing baseline and follow-up mechanism for evaluating specific interventions on a broad range of criteria. The relative short-term and long-term impact of different health promotion programs or work environment changes can only be compared if we have baseline and follow-up measures of health for both treated and untreated populations.

Finally, both researchers and decision makers need new ideas on the causes and consequences of workplace health problems. These ideas could be generated by linking up a health monitoring system with information on the nature and perception or experience of different psychosocial and physical work environments and with different workplace-based preventive and therapeutic health programs.

Because our health insurance and pension system is largely employer based, it should be possible to monitor employee health, at least at the level of work sites and organizations or insurers, by using existing data on employee health care utilization and associated diagnoses. Care must be taken to guard the anonymity of individual employees. What is of interest are differences in the prevalence and incidence of different kinds of health problems in groups of employees defined by their occupation, work site, specific work environment, or combinations thereof. Where there is reason to believe that specific health hazards may exist, more intensive monitoring may be necessary via surveys, risk-factor screening, or even medical exams. Again, such information may already be collected for other reasons (e.g., periodic physicals to determine fitness for specific jobs).

The Kaiser-Permanente health care system provides an example of the use of health care utilization data for research purposes. For instance, a recent study by Friedman (1983) examined the incidence of cryptococcosis (a rare, yet fatal disease) in over one million subscribers to the Kaiser-Permanante Medical Care Program in northern California during a ten-year period. These data indicated that the commonly accepted features of cryptococcosis, based on clinical reports (i.e., a disease of white males between thirty and fifty years of age), were not confirmed. The Ruberman et al. (1984) study cited earlier similarly used records of a health insurance group. These data sources could equally well be used for occupational epidemiology.

At levels above the work site or employer with a common health insurer, the monitoring problem becomes more complex. Systematic collection and utilization of death certificate data on last and usual occupations and industry would be a major step. The development of at least regional registries of cases of major diseases (e.g., CHD, stroke, cancer, accidental death, suicide, hospitalized psychiatric disorders), again coordinated with occupational data, would be very useful. Such registries are a major basis for research in Sweden (e.g., Theorell 1982).

Conclusion

This chapter has described a more effective and comprehensive approach to making the workplace a central element in health promotion and disease prevention. The foundation of this approach is a renewed focus on the role of the work environment in affecting health and health behavior, combined with the recognition that individual attributes and behavior can significantly condition these effects. Efforts aimed at creating a more healthful work environment should consider the total work environment, including its psychosocial aspects. By increasing employees' control of the work process and their social support and by reducing job demands, significant mental and physical health benefits should accrue. Innovations in the technology and organization of work and increased employee participation represent promising, effective ways to produce these desired psychosocial changes. An integral component of this approach is to develop and utilize a better information system for monitoring the health of workers, the changes in the nature of workers and their work environment, and the cost-effectiveness of various interventions to improve health or reduce disease.

Unfortunately, there is often a tendency among employers in both the private and public sector to view health as an individual problem, and to see efforts to monitor the health of workers or the healthfulness of the work environment as exposing the employer to risks and problems that could otherwise be avoided. Efforts are made to minimize the relevance of the work environment to health, both absolutely and relative to nonwork influences on health. Such a posture may appear cost-effective in the short run but can prove disastrous in the long run. Major asbestos producers are now threatened with bankruptcy for failing to detect and avoid, decades ago, the deleterious health consequences of asbestos exposure.[2] The legal system increasingly holds employers responsible for identifying and knowing latent health risks, warning workers of such risks, and taking timely and positive steps to reduce such risks (Baram 1984).

Baram (1984, 1165) has typified the two contrasting views of the role of employers in assessing the healthfulness of their work environments:

Many firms have viewed these [assessment] strategies as *defensive* options. . . . This view maintains the corporation's traditional position of responding to external developments such as litigation and regulatory activity. It tends to contain some costs, but to reduce few health risks. Some firms now view new assessment procedures as a *positive* opportunity for management to take the initiative at early planning and decision-making levels to prevent the generation of health risks and their economic consequences. This perspective entails a greater investment, but can put the firm out front on future problems to better prevent health risks and economic losses.

Baram argues that the latter "positive" view is more cost-effective in the long run as well as more defensible both legally and ethically. Finally, he notes that it enables "epidemiologists and other health scientists to efficiently structure valid scientific studies which will yield more useful and credible results" (p. 1166). As em-

ployers, health insurers, and govern- come for employers, employees and
ment have developed increasingly their unions or occupational associa-
comprehensive information systems tions, health practitioners, and re-
on the utilization of health services, searchers to collaborate on develop-
the incremental cost of developing ing comprehensive programs for
and maintaining a comprehensive monitoring and researching health
system for monitoring and research- in the workplace and improving
ing health and the work environment the healthfulness of the work envi-
has declined. In our view the time has ronment.

Acknowledgments

The authors are indebted to Robert Caplan, Wendy Fisher-House, R. Van Harrison, and Barbara Israel for comments on a previous draft, and to Marie Klatt
for preparing the manuscript and much of the bibliography.

Notes

1. The concepts and measures of Type A that were originated by Friedman
and Rosenman 1974 place heavy emphasis on work involvement and pressures. Thus the evidence of a prospective association of Type A with CHD incidence in general population groups in California (Rosenman et al. 1976),
Framingham (Haynes, Feinleib, and Kannel 1980), and Belgium (French-Belgian Collaborative Group 1982) may provide indirect support for the impact of
job demands on morbidity and mortality. More recent prospective studies of
populations with CHD or at high risk of CHD have failed to find a similar
effect. Nevertheless, Type A is now an acknowledged risk factor of CHD (National Heart, Lung, and Blood Institute 1981).

2. Our discussion cannot deal with those health consequences of work that
are external to the workplace—environmental pollution or product liability,
for example. But similar arguments can be made for monitoring research and
attempting to modify the external health consequences of the workplace.
Again, short-run avoidance of such concerns can bring disastrous long-run
consequences.

References

Alderman, M. H., and T. K. Davis. 1980. Blood pressure control programs on
and off the worksite. *Journal of Occupational Medicine* 22:167–170.

Amsden, D. M. 1983. Introduction to quality circles. In *Quality circles papers: A compilation*. American Society for Quality Control, Milwaukee, Wis.

Ashford, N. A. 1976. *Crisis in the workplace: Occupational disease and injury*. Cambridge: MIT Press.

Ashford, N. A., and R. A. Andrews. 1983. Impacts of occupational and environmental health and safety regulations. In *Environmental and occupational medicine*, ed. W. N. Rom. Boston: Little, Brown.

Baram, M. S. 1984. Charting the future course for corporate management of health risks. *American Journal of Public Health* 74(10):1163–1166.

Berkman, L. F., and L. Breslow. 1983. *Health and ways of living*. New York: Oxford University Press.

Berkman, L. F., and S. L. Syme. 1979. Social networks, host resistance, and mortality: A nine-year follow-up study of Alameda County residents. *American Journal of Epidemiology* 109(2):186–204.

Blauner, R. 1964. *Alienation and freedom*. Chicago: University of Chicago Press.

Blazer, D. G. 1982. Social support and mortality in an elderly community population. *American Journal of Epidemiology* 115(5):684–693.

Brady, J. V. 1958. Ulcers in "executive monkeys." *Scientific American* 199: 95–103.

Caplan, R. D., S. Cobb, J. R. P. French, Jr., R. V. Harrison and S. R. Pinneau, Jr. 1980. Job demands and worker health. ISR Research Report, University of Michigan, Ann Arbor.

Caplan, R. D., R. V. Harrison, R. V. Wellons, and J. R. P. French, Jr. 1980. Social support and patient adherence: Experimental and survey findings. ISR Research Report, Institute for Social Research, University of Michigan, Ann Arbor.

Cassel, J. 1976. The contribution of the social environment host resistance. *American Journal of Epidemiology* 102:107–123.

Castillo-Salgado, C. 1984. Assessing recent developments and opportunities in the promotion of health in the American workplace. *Social Science Medicine* 19(4):349–358.

Cobb, S., and R. M. Rose. 1973. Hypertension, peptic ulcer, and diabetes in air traffic controllers. *Journal of the American Medical Association* 244: 489–492.

Cohen, S. and S. L. Syme, eds. 1985. *Social support and health*. New York: Academic Press.

Cohen, S. and T. Wills. 1985. Stress, social support, and the buffering hypothesis. *Psychological Bulletin* 98:310–357.

Cooper, C. L. and R. Payne, eds. 1978. *Stress at work*. Chichester, England: John Wiley and Sons.

Cottington, E. M., and J. S. House. In press. Occupational stress and health: A multivariate relationship. In *Handbook of psychology and health*, ed. A. R. Baum and J. E. Singer. Hillsdale, N.J.: Erlbaum.

Doll, R. 1981. Avoidable cancer: Attribution of risk. *South African Cancer Bulletin* 25(3):125–146.

Eaker, E. D., and M. Feinleib. 1983. Psychosocial factors and the ten-year incidence of cerebrovascular accident in the Framingham Heart Study. *Psychosomatic Medicine* 45 (abstract).

Eketorp, S. 1981. Metallurgy in a social context. In *Working life*, ed. B. Gardell and G. Johansson. Chichester, England: John Wiley and Sons.

Emery, F. E., and E. L. Trist. 1960. Socio-technical systems. In *Management sciences models and techniques*, vol. 2. London: Pergamon Press.

Fielding, J. E. 1982. Effectiveness of employee health improvement programs. *Journal of Occupational Medicine* 24(11): 907–916.

———. 1984. Health promotion and disease prevention at the worksite. In *American review of public health*, vol. 5. Palo Alto, Calif.: Annual Reviews, Inc.

French-Belgian Collaborative Study Group. 1982. Ischemic heart disease and psychological patterns. *Advanced Cardiology* 29:25–31.

Friedman, G. D. 1983. The rarity of cryptococcossis in Northern California: The 10-year experience of a large defined population. *American Journal of Epidemiology* 117(2):230–235.

Friedman, M., and R. Rosenman. 1974. *Type A behavior and your heart*. New York: Knopf.

Gardell, B. 1981. Strategies for reform programmes on work organization and work environment. In *Working life*, ed. B. Gardell and G. Johansson. Chichester, England: John Wiley and Sons.

Gardell, B., and G. Johansson eds. 1981. *Working life*. Chichester, England: John Wiley and Sons.

Haddad, A., J. S. House, and M. Jackman. 1985. The impact of technology on industrial work and workers. Survey Research Center, University of Michigan, Ann Arbor. Typescript.

Haw, M. A. 1982. Women, work, and stress: A review and agenda for the future. *Journal of Health and Social Behavior* 23:132–144.

Haynes, S. G., and M. Feinleib. 1980. Women, work, and coronary heart disease: Prospective findings from the Framingham Heart Study. *American Journal of Public Health* 70:133–141.

Haynes, S. G., Feinleib, M., and W. B. Kannel. 1980. The relationship of psychosocial factors to coronary heart disease in the Framingham study, 3: Eight-year incidence of coronary heart disease. *American Journal of Epidemiology* 111:37–58.

Holt, R. H. 1982. Occupational stress. In *Handbook of health*, ed. L. Goldberger and S. Breznitz. New York: Free Press.

House, J. S. 1974a. Occupational stress and coronary heart disease: A review and theoretical integration. *Journal of Health and Social Behavior* 15: 12–27.

———. 1974b. Occupational stress and physical health. In *Work and the quality of life: Resource papers for "Work in America,"* ed. J. O'Toole. Cambridge: MIT Press.

———. 1976. Using health criteria in a system of indicators of the quality of employment. In *Measuring work quality for social reporting*, ed. A. J. Biderman and T. F. Drury. New York: Halstead Press.

————. 1980. Occupational stress and the physical and mental health of factory workers. Report on NIHM Grant No. 1R02MH28902. Research Report Series, Institute for Social Research, University of Michigan, Ann Arbor.

————. 1981. *Work stress and social support.* Reading, Mass.: Addison-Wesley.

House, J. S., and R. L. Kahn. 1985. Measures and concepts of social support. In *Social support and health*, ed. S. Cohen and S. L. Syme. New York: Academic Press.

House, J. S., A. J. McMichael, J. A. Wells, B. H. Kaplan, and L. R. Landerman. 1979. Occupational stress and health among factory workers. *Journal of Health and Social Behavior* 20:139–160.

House, J. S., C. Robbins, and H. M. Metzner. 1982. The association of social relationships and activities with mortality: Prospective evidence from the Tecumseh Community Health Study. *American Journal of Epidemiology*, 116: 123–140.

House, J. S., V. Strecher, H. L. Metzner, and C. Robbins. In press. Occupational stress and health among men and women in the Tecumseh Community Health Study. *Journal of Health and Social Behavior* (in press).

House, J. S., and J. A. Wells. 1978. Occupational stress, social support, and health. In *Reducing occupational stress: Proceedings of conference*, ed. A. McLean, G. Black, and M. Colligan. U.S. Department of Health, Education, and Welfare. HEW (NIOSH) Publication No. 78-140. Washington, D.C.: Government Printing Office.

Jablin, E. G. 1979. Superior-subordinate communication: The state of the art. *Psychological Bulletin* 86(6):1201–1222.

Janis, B., and R. A. Garibaldi. 1983. Occupational infections. In *Environmental and occupational medicine*, ed. W. N. Rom. Boston: Little, Brown.

Jenkins, C. D. 1971. Psychologic and social precursors of coronary disease. *New England Journal of Medicine* 284:244–255, 307–317.

————. 1976. Recent evidence supporting psychologic and social risk factors for coronary disease. *New England Journal of Medicine* 294: 987.

Kahn, R. L. 1981a. *Work and health.* New York: Wiley.

————. 1981b. Work and health: Some psychosocial effects of advanced technology. In *Working life*, ed. B. Gardell and G. Johansson. Chichester, England: John Wiley and Sons.

Karasek, R., D. Baker, F. Marxer, A. Ahlbom, and T. Theorell. 1981. Job decision latitude, job demands, and cardiovascular disease: A prospective study of Swedish men. *American Journal of Public Health* 71:694–705.

Karasek, R., K. P. Triantis, and S. S. Chaudhry. 1982. Coworker and supervisor support as moderators of associations between task characteristics and mental strain. *Journal of Occupational Behavior* 2:181–200.

Kasl, S. V. 1974. Work and mental health. In *Work and the quality of life*, ed. J. O'Toole, pp. 171–196. Cambridge: MIT Press.

———. 1978. Epidemiological contributions to the study of work stress. In Stress at work, ed. C. L. Cooper and R. Payne, pp. 3–48. New York: Wiley.

———. 1981. The challenge of studying the disease effects of stressful work conditions. *American Journal of Public Health* 71:682–684.

———. 1982. Chronic life stress and health. In *Health care and human behavior*, ed. A. Steptoe and A. Mathews. London: Academic Press.

Katz, D., and R. L. Kahn. 1978. *The social psychology of organizations*. 2d ed. New York: John Wiley and Sons.

Kittel, F., M. Kornitzer, and M. Dramaix. 1980. Coronary heart disease and job stress in two cohorts of bank clerks. *Psychotherapy and Psychosomatics* 34:110–123.

Kobasa, S. C., S. R. Maddi, and M. A. Zola. 1983. Type A and hardiness. *Journal of Behavioral Medicine* 6:41–51.

Lalonde, M. 1974. *A new perspective on the health of Canadians*. Ottawa, Canada: Ministry of Health and Welfare.

LaRocco, J. M., J. S. House, and J. R. P. French, Jr. 1980. Social support, occupational stress, and health. *Journal of Health and Social Behavior* 21: 202–218.

Lasagna, L., W. Wordell, and R. Hansen. 1978. Technical innovation and government regulation of pharmaceuticals in the U.S. and Great Britain: A report to the National Science Foundation. Rochester N.Y.: Center for the Study of Drug Development at the University of Rochester.

Levi, L. 1981. *Preventing work stress*. Reading, Mass.: Addison-Wesley.

Likert, R. 1961. *New patterns of management*. New York: McGraw-Hill.

Marmot, M., and W. Winkelstein, Jr. 1975. Epidemiologic observations on intervention trials for prevention of coronary heart disease. *American Journal of Epidemiology* 101(3):177–181.

Medalie, J. H., H. A. Kahn, H. A. Neufeld, E. Riss, U. Goldbourt. 1973a. Five-year myocardial infarction incidence, 2: Association of single variables to age and birthplace. *Journal of Chronic Disease* 26:329–349.

Medalie, J. H., M. Snyder, J. J. Groen, H. N. Neufeld, U. Goldbourt, and E. Riss. 1973b. Angina pectoris among 10,000 men. *American Journal of Medicine* 55:583–589.

Millions spent in efforts to keep employees well. 1984. *New York Times*, Oct. 14, p. 29.

Mott, P. E., F. C. Mann, Q. McLaughlin, and D. P. Warwick. 1965. *Shift work*. Ann Arbor: University of Michigan Press.

National Heart, Lung, and Blood Institute. 1981. Coronary-prone behavior and coronary heart disease: A critical review. *Circulation* 63:1199–1215.

Pasmore, W., and F. Friedlander. 1982. An action-research program for increasing employee involvement in problem solving. *Administrative Science Quarterly* 27:343–362.

Pearlin, L. I., M. A. Lieberman, E. G. Managhan, and J. T. Mullan. 1981. The stress process. *Journal of Health and Social Behavior* 22:337–356.

Pflanz, M. 1971. Epidemiological and sociocultural factors in the etiology of duodenal ulcer. In *Advances in psychosomatic medicine,* vol. 6: *Duodenal ulcer,* ed. H. Weiner. Basel, Switzerland: Karger.

Redding, W. C. 1972. *Communication within the organization: An interpretive review of theory and research.* New York: Industrial Community Council.

Rose, R. M., C. D. Jenkins, and M. W. Hurst. 1978. Air traffic controller health change study: A report to the FAA. Boston University, School of Medicine.

Rosen, R. H. 1984. Worksite health promotion: Fact or fantasy. *Corporate Commentary* 1:1–8.

Rosenman, R. H., R. J. Branc, R. I. Sholtz, and M. Friedman. 1976. Multivariate prediction of coronary heart disease during 8.5 year follow-up in the Western Collaborative Group Study. *American Journal of Cardiology* 37:903–910.

Ruberman, W., E. Weinblatt, J. D. Goldberg, and B. S. Chaudhary. 1984. Psychosocial influences on mortality after myocardial infarction. *New England Journal of Medicine* 311(9):552–559.

Sales, S. 1969. Differences among individuals in affective, behavioral, biochemical, and physiological responses to variations in workload. University Microfilms 69-18098. *Dissertation Abstracts International* 30:2407-B.

Selikoff, I. J., E. C. Hammond, and J. Churg. 1968. Asbestos exposure, smoking, and neoplasia. *Journal of the American Medical Association* 204:106.

Shepard, J. M. 1977. Technology, alienation, and job satisfaction. *Annual Review of Sociology* 3:1–21.

Susser, M. 1967. Causes of peptic ulcer: A selective epidemiologic review. *Journal of Chronic Disease* 20:435–456.

Sutton, R., and R. L. Kahn. 1984. Prediction, understanding, and control as antidotes to organizational stress. In *Handbook of organizational behavior,* ed. J. Lorsch. Cambridge: Harvard University Press.

Tasto, D., and M. Colligan. 1978. Health consequences of shift work. DHEW (NIOSH) Publication No. 78-154. Washington, D.C.: Government Printing Office.

Theorell, T. G. T. 1982. Review of research on life events and cardiovascular illness. *Advances in Cardiology* 29:140–147.

U.S. Department of Health and Human Services. 1979. *Healthy people: The surgeon general's report on health promotion and disease prevention.* Washington, D.C.: Government Printing Office.

———. 1980. *Promoting health/preventing disease: Objectives for the nation.* Washington, D.C.: Government Printing Office.

Weiss, J. M. 1970. Psychological factors in stress and disease. *Psychosomatic Medicine* 32:397–408.

Williams, D. R., and J. S. House. 1986. Social support and stress reduction.

In *Job stress and blue collar work*, ed. C. Cooper and M. Smith. New York: John Wiley and Sons.

Williams, R. B., Jr. 1975. Physiological mechanisms underlying the association between psychosocial factors and coronary disease. In *Psychological aspects of myocardial infarction and coronary care*, ed. W. D. Gentry and R. B. Williams. St. Louis, Mo.: C. V. Mosby.

Winnubst, J. A. M., F. H. G. Marcelissen, and R. J. Kleber. 1982. Effects of social support in the stressor-strain relationship: A Dutch sample. *Social Science and Medicine* 16:475–482.

Chapter 19

Coping and Social Supports
Their Functions and Applications

Leonard I. Pearlin and
Carol S. Aneshensel

The notions of coping and social supports have been widely incorporated into the language and thought of health professionals. Inevitably, as interest in the constructs grows, so does the number of answered questions about them. Their assessment, their effects on the well-being of people, their limitations, and their use as intervention tools are among the issues that are continually evaluated and reevaluated. This process is not made easier by the fact that different groups of professionals approach coping and social supports with different interests and assumptions. Indeed, a major goal of this chapter is to explicate these approaches, to delineate their distinctive features, and to call attention to their dynamic interconnections.

We shall treat in some detail three such approaches or, as we call them, paradigms. Briefly enumerated, one is the stress paradigm, usually employed in research into difficult life circumstances of community-based populations. Within the context of this paradigm, coping and social supports function as potential barricades to the stressful and health-threatening consequences of such circumstances as sudden life changes or chronic strains. A second paradigm focuses on health behavior, that is, habits and actions beneficial or inimical to well-being. Here, coping and supports are viewed as potential mechanisms for altering the antecedent risk behavior. The third paradigm begins with an existing illness and is primarily concerned with how coping and supports function either to alleviate the illness or to lessen adjustment problems stemming from the illness. Although these paradigms constitute different vantage points for viewing coping and supports, they are interrelated and, as we shall propose, can usefully be regarded as elements in a more inclusive and continuous process. The paradigms, the way each assumes coping and supports to function, and their interconnections will become clear in the course of the chapter.

It is unusual to deal with coping and social supports together, as we do here. They have different intellectual roots and involve quite different phenomena. Coping, of course, refers to the things people do in their own behalf to avoid or minimize the stress that would otherwise result from problematic conditions of life (Pearlin and Schooler 1978), particularly conditions that impose demands challenging to the resources of the individual (Lazarus 1966). Social supports represent the social resources one is able to call upon in dealing with such conditions. Despite these differences, the two concepts are alike in that they provide the health professional with the ability to explain variations in outcomes among persons sharing similar conditions. Thus, the stress researcher knows that persons exposed to equivalent hardships do not experience the same degree of stress, that attempts to alter risk behaviors do not meet with uniform success, and that efforts to ameliorate the impact of illness may work better for some than for others. In each instance, coping and social supports help explain why similar circumstances can have dissimilar consequences. Because of their potentially powerful roles in mediating outcomes and because they are so useful in explaining what would otherwise be inexplicable, these two concepts have become pivotal constructs in the work of health professionals. It is their common role that gives reason to treat them together in this chapter.

The Functions of Coping and Social Supports in the Stress Paradigm

Investigations into the harmful health consequences of stress have generally followed the basic paradigm illustrated in figure 19.1. The problematic life circumstances that give rise to stress and tax the individual's ability to respond are of two general types: events, usually of an undesirable and relatively abrupt nature, that result in discontinuity or change requiring readjustment; and persistent or continuing problems that occur within ongoing social roles. Although typically considered discretely, these two sources of stress are interrelated. Thus, life event change may lead to stress by altering the meaning of existing role strain, intensifying strain, or creating new strains within social roles (Pearlin et al. 1981). Role strains often present themselves insidiously and become relatively fixed and ongoing in daily experiences as chronic, low-key frustrations and hardships (Pearlin and Lieberman 1979).

Included in the broad spectrum of health outcomes that have been studied as consequences of these "naturalistic" stressors are emotional distress, physical morbidity, and mortality. Stressful experience has been regarded as contributing to specific health conditions such as heart disease (e.g. Jenkins 1976) or cancer (e.g., Schmale and Iker 1971), as well as to nonspecific morbidity, including common, relatively minor physical ailments such as colds, flu, or chronic pain (e.g., Aneshensel and Huba 1984) and psychological disorder. As emphasized in several recent overviews (Kasl 1984; Kessler, Price, and Wortman 1985; Thoits 1983), methodological problems plague this body of research and inhibit confidence in assertions about the etiological role of stress. These uncertainties notwithstanding, the weight of evidence indicates that stressful circumstances exert an influence on health and well-being (Bunney et. al. 1982). The magnitude of the harmful impact of stress, however, has consistently been shown to be modest in size. This has served to direct attention to those factors that exacerbate, ameliorate, or otherwise mediate the impact of stress on health and well-being, specifically to the role of coping and social supports.

There is something beguilingly presumptive in the labels *coping* and *social supports*. The very terms imply a built-in positive consequence. They suggest that when people behave in a manner we designate as coping, or that when people have social relationships we refer to as supportive, certain desirable effects are taking place. However, this is not necessarily the case. In their study of people who had lost a spouse or child, for example, Wortman and Lehman (in press) find that would-be supporters were commonly judged by the bereaved individuals to be unhelpful. The authors speculate that would-be supporters are occasionally ineffective because the victims' loss can lead to feelings of threat, vulnerability, and helplessness on the part of the supporters. There may be, additionally, some uncertainty and anxiety over appropriate behavior, which in turn impedes empathic responses.

These findings are but a modest illustration of the broad array of mechanisms, forms, and limiting conditions that are involved in the study of coping and social supports. To immerse ourselves in these issues would quickly take us beyond the scope of this chapter. Therefore, we shall confine ourselves to an examination of the consequences or, as we refer to them, the functions of coping and social supports. Following in part from earlier conceptualizations (Pearlin and Schooler 1978), four types of functions can be distinguished: (1) *prevention* of the stressful situation; (2) *alteration* of the stressful situation; (3) *changing the meaning* of the situation; and (4) *management of the symptoms* of stress. Within the context of the stress paradigm shown in figure 19.1, the functions of coping and social supports can be seen in relation to both the stressor and its effect on health. We shall describe each of these functions in turn.

Preventive Functions

Virtually nothing is known of how coping and supports protect health by

FIGURE 19.1.

The basic stress paradigm.

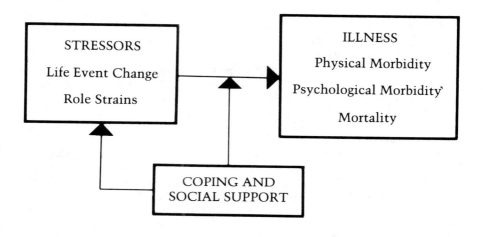

preventing stressful problems from surfacing in people's lives. Yet all of us have had occasion to wonder if certain friends and acquaintances are not "snakebitten"—living under a cloud, hounded by relentless misfortune—while others appear to sail through life untouched by serious difficulties. Such differences, of course, may very well be explained by differences in the basic circumstances and life chances of people, their emotional resources, and their involuntary random exposure to hardship. But can such differences also be explained by differences in coping repertoires and access to and use of supports? Perhaps, but we cannot be sure at this time. The reasons we cannot be certain involve the methods used to study coping and supports within the framework of the stress paradigm. Simply put, researchers typically begin to examine people's coping behavior and social supports *after* a health-threatening problem emerges. As a result, more is known of how people deal with problems than of how they avoid them.

Although we lack concrete information, it is possible to speculate about the preventive functions of coping and social supports. With regard to coping, we must recognize that there is a large class of potential health-threatening stressors whose occurrence can be forecasted far in advance of their actual appearance. We refer particularly to life-cycle transitions that can entail rather profound life change. Getting married, having children, launching them onto their own uncharted seas, entering grandparenthood, and retiring from work are such changes. These sorts of changes are remarkably free of lasting deleterious health consequences (Pearlin 1980). One explanation is their predictability: because these life-cycle changes are foreseeable, they permit long periods of anticipatory or preparatory coping. We cannot be sure, of course, whether anticipatory preparation actually prevents problems from arising or simply helps us deal with them once they do arise. We suspect that the avoidance of problems and the readiness to deal appropriately with them are both learned beforehand.

Successfully confronting a problem at one point can help prevent the recurrence of the same problem at a later point. Menaghan's (1982) longitudinal analysis of marital problems, which are closely associated with psychological depression, provides a good example. She found that people who coped effectively with marital problems were more likely to be free of such problems four years later than those coping with the same type of problems with less effective means. Thus, efficacious coping can have a double function. Not only does it reduce stress in the short run but it actually provides a preventive barricade against the future emergence of problems in that role area. Concomitantly, of course, the less successful people are in coping with existing problems, the more likely these problems will endure into or reappear in the future.

Social supports also have preventive functions. Indeed, supports may be more important to the prevention of health-related problems than coping. The most obvious way in which such functions would be accomplished is through the "wisdom" the group imparts to its members: the ability both to anticipate problems and, once recognized, to adopt appropriate avoidance strategies. Clearly, people acquire such abilities from others. Among the norms that we absorb from our membership and reference groups are those that define what is undesirable and should be avoided, what is acceptable but should be approached warily, and what should be actively sought after. Without being aware of it, we learn a litany of dos and don'ts that will presumably shield us from risk. On the other hand, the very supports that shield may also function to increase the exposure to stress and health risks. The more extensive one's social network, for example, the more likely one is to be touched by stressors occurring to others, such as, the death of a close friend. Similarly, to the extent that a person's reference groups engage in certain patterns of behavior, such as smoking or heavy drinking, pressures to conform to group standards can have harmful health effects.

The Alteration of the Problematic Situation

If stressors cannot be prevented or avoided, the next most desirable function of coping and social supports would seem to be modification of the situation (or one's behavior within it) in a way that eliminates or reduces its stress-producing properties. For example, if one is having problems at work, changing the problematic aspects of the work situation would be highly desirable. It is reasonable to suppose that this is a function that people would seek to maximize. With regard to coping, it is surprising that behavior serving this function does not appear particularly prominent in people's repertoires (Pearlin and Schooler 1978). One possible reason is that some problematic situations are recognized by people as intractable, as not meriting efforts to change them. Second, the source of one's stress may not always be apparent. We are capable of experiencing health-damaging stress without being certain of its origins; or, more likely, we attribute the stress to one situation while in reality it comes from another. Thus, coping may be misdirected. Third, one may decide not to act directly upon the situation because the action might trigger consequences one does not wish to face. A worker might ask his boss to eliminate dangerous job conditions but risk the possibility of being fired.

Coping actions intended to alter certain aspects of a situation are also quite capable of producing unintended and unwanted alterations, thus inhibiting efforts directed at change.

Social supports, perhaps more than coping, can actively function to change situations. They do so, we believe, largely through the exercise of what is usually referred to as instrumental (in contrast to expressive) support. Instrumental supports are those that broadly involve the giving of material help, assistance, or information (House 1981). One's network, of course, serves as a nexus for such support and can be used to change certain kinds of problematic situations. If someone is unemployed, for example, relatives, friends, or neighbors, functioning as a referral system for the person, may alert him to job opportunities. Or, short of helping him find a new job, they might ease the burden by providing loans, gifts of food, or other material goods. Of course, some stressful situations can no more be changed successfully by a support group than by the individual caught up in it. Nevertheless, the resources of support groups are potentially powerful instruments in altering the stressful properties of situations.

The Alteration of Meaning

Because many situations that eventually damage psychological and physical health are resistant to change, people engage instead in actions that change the meaning of the situation. The situation remains intact, but perceptions, beliefs, and knowledge are modified in a way that reduces its threatening or harmful qualities.

A number of cognitive and perceptual devices that neutralize the meaning of potentially stressful situations have been identified (Pearlin and Schooler 1978). For example, people often trivialize problematic situations, defining them as too unimportant to be painful or threatening. Since the importance that we assign to a situation influences the threat we feel when things go wrong, diminishing a situation's importance minimizes its threat. Another perceptual process entails the relegation of difficult situations to the commonplace and normal. If we can regard a marital problem, for example, as similar to the problems that our best friends also experience, we can explain our difficulties as a normative, to-be-expected set of experiences. Misery does not simply love company, misery is in active search of company and is often assuaged by it. Many other perceptual devices that people employ vary in form but perform the same function: they endow a situation with a meaning that reduces its stress-arousing qualities.

Along with coping, social supports also contribute importantly to the perceptual management of the threatening properties of stressful circumstances. A natural product of interaction in groups is the acquisition of norms, that is, shared ways of defining situations—appraising them as good or bad, desirable or undesirable —and of prescribing or approving modes of action and reaction. Thus, although an individual's experiences might be unique, the ways the individual assesses and acts upon them

may be a consequence of internalized group standards. The norms of membership and reference groups can legitimize and reinforce the perception of a situation as threatening, or they can help define the same situation as ordinary, trivial, fatalistically inexorable, or undeserving of concern, worthy only of being ignored. The objective properties of a situation often do not by themselves determine its threatening quality. Instead, people's normative aspirations, values, and ideologies shape perceptions and combine with the objective situation in giving rise to threat.

Evidence shows that support groups also mediate the stress process by helping the individual maintain a positive self-concept in the face of hardship (Pearlin et al. 1981). Here the group does not influence the perception of the situation as much as it influences the perception of the self in the situation. The support group, in effect, helps the individual maintain self-esteem and a sense of mastery by interpreting the stressful situation as one that does not reflect negatively on these prized elements of self. The maintenance of the self in difficult life situations is a crucial defense against stress.

Control of Stress Symptoms

A final function of coping and supports is seen in behaviors that control symptoms, particularly states such as anxiety and depression, keeping them within manageable bounds so that they do not overwhelm the individual. Folkman and Lazarus (1980) refer to this process to as emotion-focused coping, in contrast to that which is problem focused. Much of the popular understanding of coping relates to this function, as does the "stress management" industry that has evolved in recent years. One can turn to biofeedback or bird-watching, to meditation or massage, running or rebirth, drinking or daydreaming—indeed to virtually any activity that provides some relief either from awareness of problematic circumstances or from the tensions and other symptoms associated with them. Dealing effectively with symptoms of distress enables individuals to direct their attention to the important demands of their lives (Mechanic 1962). Based on current knowledge, it is not possible to identify techniques that are superior to others in providing relief. However, some that effectively control symptoms in the short run might very well have deleterious consequences in the long run. To take but one example, alcohol use may provide some immediate relief from symptoms of distress, but too much over too long a period can have a devastating impact on health (Aneshensel and Huba 1983; Pearlin and Radabaugh 1976).

How do social supports function for the control of symptoms? One way is by validating the individual's response to the stressor. Those confronting major life crises or persistent strains are often perplexed and frightened by their emotional and physiological arousal; open discussion of the problem and legitimization of these fears by others can be a critical factor in enabling the individual to manage distress and avoid being overwhelmed by it (Wortman and Lehman, in press). Much of what is called expressive support is provided through these kinds of exchanges. In addition, of course, social life itself is diversionary. The things that individuals do to relieve tensions are often done in groups; some stress management behaviors, in fact, require other people. Once more, then, we find that coping and social supports have striking parallel functions within the stress paradigm.

The Functions of Coping and Social Supports in the Health Behavior Paradigm

The distinguishing feature of the earlier stress paradigm (or model) is its concern with the etiological role of threatening or painful experience in the occurrence of illness. By contrast, a second paradigm—the health behavior paradigm—focuses more directly on what people do. Whereas the first considers life circumstances that people experience, the second is primarily concerned with actions directly connected to health outcomes. Although we refer to this as the health behavior paradigm, we shall incorporate in our discussion of it behavior that is damaging to health as well. We shall continue to explore the functions of coping and social supports, this time within the context of a distinctly different paradigm.

The diagrammatic representation of the health behavior paradigm in figure 19.2 is simple, but the relation-

FIGURE 19.2.
The health behavior paradigm.

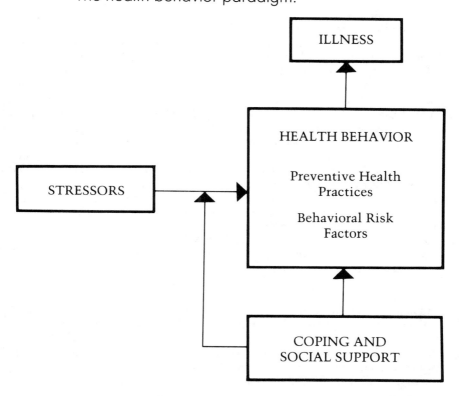

ships it encompasses can be quite complex and indirect. Thus, in a real sense, health behaviors can themselves be coping behaviors, functioning to promote health or avoid illness. To some extent, therefore, the distinction in figure 19.2 between these behaviors and coping is somewhat arbitrary. Nevertheless, it is a distinction worth keeping. While health behavior contributes to health directly, other modes of coping contribute indirectly. For example, one may cope successfully with work problems and in doing so avoid compulsive overeating, a risk behavior associated with illness. To reach a point where one is able to put aside health-damaging behaviors, one might first have to cope with the conditions leading to such behavior.

The behaviors that put health at risk are widely known but, nevertheless, widely practiced. For example, studies have systematically explored how certain aspects of an individual's daily patterns of living affect overall health status (Belloc and Breslow 1972; Belloc 1973; Wiley and Camacho 1980). Behaviors found to be related to concurrent and subsequent health status and to mortality include smoking, alcohol consumption, lack of physical exercise, insufficient or excessive hours of sleep, and over-eating. Although the threat of subsequent illness, particularly of heart disease or cancer, motivates many individuals to give up risk behavior such as smoking, or to engage in preventive health behaviors such as breast or testicular self-examination, many individuals continue to engage in a variety of behaviors that are harmful to their health or fail to take positive steps to improve their health. Although behaviors can serve a preventive function, the threat of subsequent illness has proved only partially effective in motivating individuals to engage in such behavior.

One paradoxical reason for persistent risk behavior is that several behaviors known to be inimical to health are also known to represent stress management strategies used in coping with current stressors. Thus, Holroyd and Lazarus (1982) suggest that coping may contribute to disease onset or progression, as when men at risk for coronary heart disease increase their smoking in response to stress, or when peptic duodenal ulcer sufferers increase their consumption of alcohol in response to work stress.

Similar relationships are well illustrated by alcohol consumption. A major motivation for drinking is self-medication of psychological distress. Segal, Huba, and Singer (1980), for instance, found that young adults used

alcohol because they were sad, depressed, anxious, or nervous. Similarly, Pearlin and Radabaugh (1976) found that economic strain, anxiety, and alcohol use are related, suggesting that alcohol may be used to cope. Thus, moderate levels of alcohol consumption have a stress-buffering function (Neff and Husaini 1982), but heavy drinking to cope with stressors is related to higher levels of distress (Bell, Keeley, and Buhl 1977; Woodruff et al. 1973). Aneshensel and Huba (1983) also report that while attempts to self-medicate a depressed mood through increased alcohol consumption may be effective in the short run, the long-term impact is a heightening of depressed affect. Therefore, the very behavior that represents coping in the context of a stress model can take the form of a behavioral threat to health in the health behavior model.

Health behaviors are intricately interwoven with the individual's social ties. Thus, while stress is related to increased alcohol use, supportive social ties are related to decreased levels of alcohol use over time (Aneshensel and Huba 1984). And, as Wortman (1984) suggests, supportive social ties may provide the necessary motivation to engage in and maintain health-promoting behaviors such as exercise or proper nutrition, or to adhere to medical regimens during illness.

Unfortunately, one's network of social support may induce negative as well as positive health habits. Thus, Berkman (1984) notes that individuals who have ties with persons who smoke cigarettes, drink alcohol, are physically active, or maintain certain dietary practices may follow the patterns set forth by their group simply to maintain group identity. Incidentally, results from longitudinal research also show that social network characteristics (marriage, contacts with extended family and close friends, church group membership, and other group affiliations) are associated with a decreased mortality risk independent of these health practices (Berkman 1984). Thus, while social networks may contribute to a decreased health risk through their impact on health behaviors, their relevance to health is more inclusive than their effects on health behaviors.

Coping and Social Supports in the Illness Behavior Paradigm

The health behavior model, then, treats illness as an outcome of behavior and focuses on how the precursors of illness can be modified or buttressed by coping and supports. In contrast, another approach, which we refer to as the illness behavior paradigm, begins with the illness and treats adjustment as the outcome. In effect, the illness, injury, disability, or distress is treated as the stressor, and recovery from it or adjustment to it are the desired outcomes. The outcomes, in turn, are influenced by what we designate as illness behaviors.

Illness behaviors refer to the "varying perceptions, thoughts, feelings, and acts affecting the personal and social meaning of symptoms, illness, disabilities and their consequences"

(Mechanic 1977). Within the context of this model, interest is in part directed to the influence of coping and social supports on actions such as symptom recognition, help seeking, health services utilization, compliance, and rehabilitative activity. These behavioral responses essentially define how a person adapts to illness (DiMatteo and Hays 1981; Mechanic 1972; Wortman 1984). While illness behaviors are distinct from the illness itself, the ways in which an individual responds to the threat of acute illness or to the demands of a chronic illness can be important determinants of the course of the illness and of the medical care received (Holroyd and Lazarus 1982).

Coping and supports have dual but interrelated roles in this paradigm. As can be seen in figure 19.3, they can be directed to the easing of the illness stressor and to the enhancement of recovery and adjustment. Of course, coping or supports that alleviate the health problem will presumably also speed recovery and alleviate adjustment problems. Correspondingly, improved adjustment can, in some instances, contribute to improved health. Moreover, as in the case of the health behaviors, the distinctions between illness behavior and coping are blurred in some instances because illness behaviors may themselves represent attempts to cope with the illness stressor.

There are many ways that people cope with illness, from compliance with medical regimens to engaging in wish-fulfilling fantasies (Felton and Revenson 1984). Thoughtful reviews of research and interventions that fit the illness behavior model are provided by Cohen and Lazarus (1980) and by DiMatteo and Hays (1981). As for coping with stress in general, responses to illness involve efforts to change the health problem itself or its meaning, or to reduce the symptoms of distress associated with it. Whatever the specific responses to illness may be, they probably follow a sequence beginning with recognition of the health problem, interpretation of its significance, evaluation of potential responses to it, and action directed at alleviating or adjusting to it.

One critical aspect of coping with illness concerns the decision to seek medical care. For similar symptoms or disorders, those experiencing psychological distress are more likely to seek care than those who are not distressed (Frerichs et al. 1982; Mechanic 1976; Tessler, Mechanic, and Dimond 1976). Mechanic (1977) describes to what extent help seeking may reflect a learned willingness to seek care or a sense of alarm and need for help. Of course, the complaint of an illness legitimizes seeking support

FIGURE 19.3.
The illness behavior paradigm.

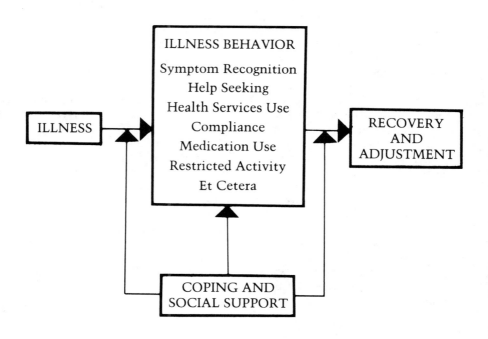

and reassurance from a physician, particularly among those who are receptive to the patient role (Mechanic 1972). The physician's ability to satisfy socioemotional needs in the health care encounter affects, in turn, the patient's satisfaction with medical care, compliance with treatment regimens, and the ultimate outcome of treatment (DiMatteo 1979).

The very nature of the illness may dictate behavioral responses to it and the readiness to seek medical care. Thus, the illness or injury may be an objective condition with a discrete onset, as typified by acute infectious disease, or it may be characterized by the gradual emergence of signs and symptoms that are not clearly defined or understood. The ambiguity or unfamiliarity with the symptoms associated with a general feeling of ill health can evoke a sense of threat and generate psychological distress. Such arousal can cause people to experience both a heightened discomfort and a heightened awareness of symptoms (Mechanic 1972). The recognition of symptoms and the appraisal of their meaning and seriousness can, in turn, have a major impact on the available options for coping with the illness (Mechanic 1977).

Unlike coping responses to many other types of stressors, changing the situation is the primary function of many coping responses to illness, from help seeking through compliance with medical regimens. There are some health problems, however, that because of their irreversibility are not responsive to such efforts. Certain kinds of hearing loss or spinal cord injury are instances of anatomical damage that cannot be corrected by our own coping efforts. In such

instances, the major coping efforts may be focused on adjustment to the health problem and on regulation of the emotional distress created by it.

Social supports have been found to be important determinants of adjustment to illness and disability. In the case of hearing loss, for example, the psychological adjustments of people with similar disabilities has been found to vary with the availability of supports (Frankel and Turner 1983). Similarly, Ben-Sira (1984) finds that emotional support from one's physician is the most sought-after but least attainable resource in alleviating emotional distress associated with chronic illness. In this connection, too, Wortman (1984) notes that uncertainties and fears of cancer sufferers are likely to result in enhanced need for social support throughout the course of diagnosis and treatment, but that intense anxieties and the stigma associated with the disease can cause difficulties in mobilizing the desired support. She notes that cancer is unique in its ability to elicit negative feelings in others, leading them to behave toward the cancer patient in ways that are unsupportive. Thus, social relationships become a source of stress rather than a source of support (Wortman 1984; Wortman and Lehman, in press).

DiMatteo and Hays (1981) similarly note that social support may have a negative impact on recovery from serious illness or injury. They describe how social support may interfere with compliance to medical regimens if the prescribed treatment goes against the values, beliefs, or patterns of conduct of the family. Furthermore, by being overprotective or anxious about the patient, social network members may contribute to a self-perception as an impaired person and impede the resumption of normal social role activity (DiMatteo and Hays 1981; Mechanic 1977).

A person's social network facilitates or discourages medical care contacts through the transmission of norms and values concerning medical care, the provision of knowledge about sources of care and their evaluation of the seriousness of the disorder, and assistance in overcoming logistical and financial barriers to obtaining health care (Berkman 1984; Lieberman 1982). This is particularly clear in decisions to seek psychiatric care. Here we see that persons experiencing emotional distress commonly discuss their problems with friends and relatives before seeking formal help. And persons are more likely to seek care if treatment is discussed during such lay consultation or if members of their network have had prior experience with psychiatric sources of care (Yokopenic, Clark, and Aneshensel 1983).

Interest in the illness behavior model sometimes involves the search for "naturalistic" uses of existing coping patterns and support resources, but in other instances, it involves the deliberate creation or manipulation of coping responses or social supports. Purposeful intervention is typically less interested in discovering coping repertoires or modes of support in general than it is in stimulating those particular mediators thought to be effective in reducing health problems and maladjustment. Forming self-help groups for people who suffer from a particular illness or disability, or encouraging people to acquire specific coping mechanisms such as an exercise regimen, are illustrations of the purposive use of this model.

The Stress Process: A Synthesizing Paradigm

In recent years it has become increasingly recognized that stress is not a happenstance result of transient circumstances but that it is quite predictable and orderly. Stress, moreover, is typically caused not by one factor but by multiple conditions that converge over time in the lives of people. These conditions include life events (such as illness events) and more enduring or chronic life strains (such as marital strife). The amalgam of multiple life problems that results in psychological or physical disorder has come to be referred to as the stress process (Pearlin et al. 1981). Because this approach takes into account constellations of interrelated problematic circumstances, it suggests more potential strategies than do other paradigms for maximizing the functions of coping and social supports. This will become clearer as we describe the stress process as illustrated in figure 19.4.

The three paradigms we have already presented are encompassed by the stress process orientation. That is, stressors are shown to be antecedents of illness and health behaviors; health behavior is shown to influence the risk of illness, and, moving from left to right, illness is shown to influence illness behavior and adjustment.

FIGURE 19.4.

The stress process paradigm.

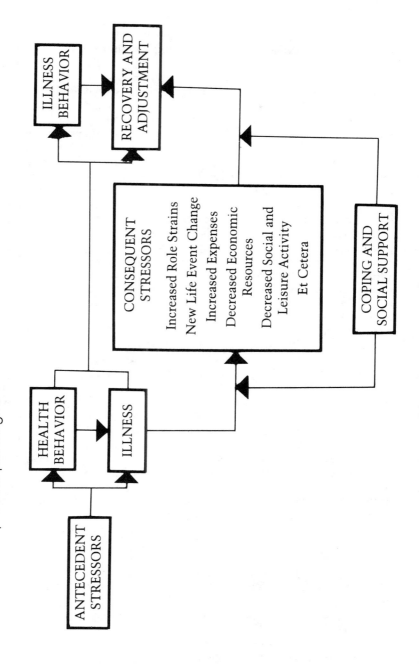

These relationships essentially reflect the models described earlier. Next—and really the crux of the stress process—the model assumes that a serious illness will spawn other serious life problems. Some of these strains are in social roles, such as in marriage, parenthood, and work. To illustrate, if someone has a myocardial infarction, it could create problems in sexual relations, in recreational activities, in employment and work performance, and so on. Serious illness may also lead to undesirable life events, as when the demands it places on the family result in divorce or separation (DiMatteo and Hays 1981). Similarly, because of an economic drain or an inability to work, the patient might experience a reduction in the economic resources needed to maintain social roles and to obtain treatment. In addition, the illness might result in a curtailment of leisure activities and social interactions. The point to be underscored is that illness, whether brought about by stress, by risk behavior, or by both, is itself capable of creating a cluster of consequent stressors.

Once created, each of these strains and problems now constitutes its own independent source of stress, capable of exacerbating adjustment problems and the illness itself. Thus, returning to our illustration, no longer would infarction be the sole, direct cause of psychological distress or other adjustment problems. Through the consequent stressors created by the illness, there might now be several indirect paths to distress as well.

Given that people usually have to confront constellations of problems and demands, it is incomplete and misleading simply to ask, for example, how people cope with an illness, at least one of serious proportions. The illness may now be but one element in a dense cluster of life problems, each calling on different coping responses, perhaps, and each mobilizing and using different support systems. Moreover, in coping with one of these problems, the person may exacerbate another. Responding to financial pressures, for example, a patient might return to work before it is medically advisable, or might postpone obtaining needed treatment. The model is complicated and difficult to capture within a single research effort or intervention program. Yet, it approximates the structural and experiential realities of people's lives, realities that can have profound consequences for well-being.

As the number of elements embodied in the conceptual model increase, the potential points of mediation by coping behavior and social supports expand commensurately. Previously we discussed how social supports and coping can function for the prevention or amelioration of illness and for the enhancement of adjustment to it. For simplicity, figure 19.4 does not reproduce these functions; instead, it highlights the additional tasks that are created by the potential emergence of consequent constellations of stressors. Thus, one major function of coping and supports within the context of the processual model is to limit the number, intensity, and density of problems that emanate from the illness. The more one is free to deal with the illness alone, without a host of surrounding problems and strains, the more recovery presumably will be facilitated. As the figure indicates, a second major task is presented when coping and ancillary supports fail to prevent or minimize consequent stressors; at this point they can function to reduce adverse illness behaviors and to enhance recovery and adjustment.

As health workers, our ultimate interest is in knowing how coping and social supports ease the adjustment problems related to a serious illness, hasten recovery, slow deterioration, or, perhaps, prevent future illnesses. To best achieve these goals, other problems clustering around the illness must also be recognized because often people are not free to deal with the illness alone but must also deal with its attendant strains and difficulties. The stress process model and its multiple implications may appear to be beyond the reach of the program planner and health professional. We submit, however, that it may be the most effective approach available for developing and applying clinical interventions. Workers responsible for helping people cope with a health problem have certainly had occasion to recognize the clustering of interrelated problems. As far as stress-related problems are concerned, one cannot promote health or deal with illness without taking into account the larger social psychological terrain of people's lives.

A final issue regarding the functions of coping and social supports is not readily apparent in the figure. It concerns the fact that the label of illness subsumes symptoms of both psychological distress and physical ailments. Symptoms of physical and psychological disorder tend to co-occur and to constitute a mutually reinforcing feedback cycle, with illness events leading to increased distress, and psychological distress leading to increased physical symptoms (Aneshensel, Frerichs, and Huba 1984). Psychological distress may be an inherent part of the physical ailment, it may be a reaction to learning that a disease is present, or it may be a manifestation of the social and psychological consequences surrounding various illnesses (Kathol and Petty 1981). The cycle of physical illness and psychological distress can also result from the impairment of the capacity to cope with needs and goals, the aggravation of previously unresolved intrapsychic conflicts, and the inability to meet sexual, social, and economic role demands (Lipowski 1975). The cycles of psychological and physical disorder, whatever their mutually reinforcing mechanisms may be, represent additional targets for mediation by coping and supports. Social supports and coping efforts directed at the cyclic sequelae of the illness may therefore also enhance emotional adjustment and prevent symptoms of distress from aggravating not only the illness but other problematic areas of functioning as well.

Conclusion

Coping and social supports, both as they normally exist in the repertoires and relationships of people and as they may be purposefully stimulated, have a potentially useful role in controlling illness, some of its etiological agents, and its consequences. Strategically employing them requires that we know the delicate interactions between several conditions: the social and psychological characteristics of the people involved, the kinds of problems they face, the kinds of coping resources and social supports at their disposal, and the kinds of outcomes that emerge. We must be aware both of the limitations of coping and supports and the limitations of our own current understanding of them. Otherwise, we will generate a set of expectations that can only be a source of disappointment.

Many life conditions that threaten health are simply not responsive to individual's coping efforts and social supports. Extreme economic deprivation, continued involuntary unemployment, entrapment in a depersonalizing job setting, and responsibility for young children as a single parent are a few examples of situations that may be stubbornly resistant, if not impervious, to coping efforts and social supports (Pearlin and Lieberman 1979). However, the efficacy of these mediators is regulated not only by the cleverness and resourcefulness of individuals but also by the nature of the problems that beset them. No preventive program will work if it simply prescribes or advocates certain modes of coping or uses of social supports without taking into consideration the specific problematic circumstances people confront. To stay afloat it is useful to know how to swim; but whether or not the ability to swim will keep us from drowning depends on whether we are struggling against a relentless

ocean tide or a toe cramp in a backyard pool. Enthusiasm about coping and social supports is misplaced if it rests on the expectations that they are universally efficacious in protecting health.

However useful coping and social supports are for some, they are unevenly distributed and leave many people exposed to health-threatening stress. Policies and programs at a collective level can compensate for the absence of adequate coping and supports at an individual level. Systematic health interventions may be much more dependable and effective than reliance on uncertain and sporadic individual coping and supports. Certain health risks and problems may be best approached as social problems rather than exclusively as problems to be solved at an individual level.

The ways we use coping and supports depend on whether we see the health problems in which we want to intervene as a result of other conditions we want to change or as the cause of subsequent problems we want to buffer. As we have argued, the implicit models and paradigms we adopt have a direct influence on how we judge coping and supports to be best employed. The stress process approach recognizes that serious life problems rarely occur singly; over time they generate constellations of problems. Consequently, interventions addressed only to health problems may overlook other problems that impede recovery, hinder adjustment, and perpetuate bad health and future risk behavior. The specialty of our interests as health workers and researchers should not obscure the functional unity to people's lives, making it unlikely that one can enjoy well-being in one aspect of life while under serious and continued stress in others.

The real problem we face in developing effective interventions is not that we are in danger of overcomplicating the issues but that, in ignoring the complexities, we shall continue to be less effective than we should like to be.

Acknowledgments

The authors' work was supported through their participation in the Consortium for Research Involving Stress Processes, funded by the W. T. Grant Foundation. Additional support came from the National Institute of Mental Health. The authors wish to thank Virginia Hansen for editorial assistance.

References

Aneshensel, C. S., and R. R. Frerichs, and G. J. Huba. 1984. Depression and physical illness: A multiwave, nonrecursive causal model. *Journal of Health and Social Behavior* 25:350–371.

Aneshensel, C. S., and G. J. Huba 1983. Depression, alcohol use, and smoking over one year: A four-wave longitudinal causal model. *Journal of Abnormal Psychology* 92(2):134–150.

————. 1984. An integrative causal model of the antecedents and consequences of depression over one year. In *Research in community and mental health*, ed. J. R. Greenley, 4:35–72. Greenwich, Conn.: JAI Press.

Bell, R. A., K. A. Keeley, and J. M. Buhl. 1977. Psychopathology and life events among alcohol users and nonusers. In *Currents in alcoholism*, ed. F. A. Seixas, 2:103–123. New York: Grune and Stratton.

Belloc, N. B. 1973. Relationship of health practices and mortality. *Preventive Medicine* 2:67–81.

Belloc, N. B., and L. Breslow. 1972. Relationship of physical health status and health practices. *Preventive Medicine* 1:409–421.

Ben-Sira, Z. 1984. Chronic illness, stress, and coping. *Social Science and Medicine* 18:725–736.

Berkman, L. F. 1984. Assessing the physical health effects of social networks and social support. *Annual Review of Public Health* 5:413–432.

Bunney, W., Jr., A. Shapiro, R. Adler, J. Davis, A. Herd, I. Kopin, D. Krieger, S. Matthyse, A. Stunkard, and M. Weissman. 1982. Panel report on stress and illness. In *Stress and human health*, ed. G. R. Elliott and C. Eisdorfer, pp. 255–321. New York: Springer Publishing.

Cohen, F., and R. S. Lazarus. 1980. Coping with the stresses of illness. In Health psychology, ed. G. Stone, F. Cohen, and N. E. Adler, pp. 217–254. San Francisco: Jossey-Bass.

DiMatteo, M. R. 1979. A social-psychological analysis of physician-patient rapport: Toward a science of the art of medicine. *Journal of Social Issues* 35:12–33.

DiMatteo, M. R., and R. Hays. 1981. Social support and serious illness. In *Social networks and social support*, ed. B. H. Gottlieb, pp. 117–148. Beverly Hills: Sage.

Felton, B. J., and T. A. Revenson. 1984. Coping with chronic illness: A study of illness controllability and the influence of coping strategies on psychological adjustment. *Journal of Consulting and Clinical Psychology* 52(3): 343–353.

Folkman, S., and R. S. Lazarus. 1980. An analysis of coping in a middle-aged community sample. *Journal of Health and Social Behavior* 21:219–239.

Frankel, B. G., and R. J. Turner. 1983. Psychological adjustment in chronic disability: The role of social support in the case of the hearing impaired. *Canadian Journal of Sociology* 8(3):273–291.

Frerichs, R. R., C. S. Aneshensel, P. A. Yokopenic, and V. A. Clark. 1982. Physical health and depression: An epidemiologic survey. *Preventive Medicine* 11:639–646.

Holroyd, K. A., and R. S. Lazarus. 1982. Stress, coping, and somatic adaptation. In *Handbook of stress: Theoretical and clinical aspects*, ed. L. Goldberger and S. Breznitz, pp. 21–35. New York: Free Press.

House, J. S. 1981. *Work stress and social support*. Reading, Mass: Addison-Wesley.

Jenkins, C. S. 1976. Recent evidence supporting psychologic and social risk factors for coronary disease. *New England Journal of Medicine* 294: 987–994, 1033–1038.

Kasl, S. V. 1984. Stress and health. *Annual Review of Pubic Health* 5:319–341.

Kathol, R. G., and F. Petty. 1981. Relationship of depression to medical illness: A critical review. *Journal of Affective Disorders* 3:111–121.

Kessler, R. C., R. H. Price, and C. B. Wortman. 1985. Social factors in psychopathology: Stress, social support, and coping processes. *Annual Review of Psychology* 36:531–572.

Lazarus, R. S. 1966. *Psychological stress and the coping process*. New York: McGraw-Hill.

Leiberman, M. A. 1982. The effects of social supports on responses to stress. In *Handbook of stress: Theoretical and clinical aspects*, ed. L. Goldberger and S. Breznitz, pp. 764–783. New York: Free Press.

Lipowski, Z. J. 1975. Psychiatry of somatic diseases: Epidemiology, pathogenesis, classification. *Comprehensive Psychiatry* 16:105–124.

Mechanic, D. 1962. *Students under stress: A study in the social psychology of adaptation*. New York: Free Press.

———. 1972. Social psychologic factors affecting the presentation of bodily complaints. *New England Journal of Medicine* 286:1132–1139.

————. 1976. Stress, illness, and illness behavior. *Journal of Human Stress* 2:29–40.

————. 1977. Illness behavior, social adaptation, and the management of illness: A comparison of educational and medical models. *Journal of Nervous and Mental Disease* 165:79–87.

Menaghan, E. 1982. Measuring coping effectiveness: A panel analysis of marital problems and coping efforts. *Journal of Health and Social Behavior* 23(3):220–234.

Neff, J. A., and B. A. Husaini. 1982. Life events, drinking patterns, and depressive symptomatology: The stress-buffering role of alcohol consumption. *Journal of Studies on Alcohol* 43:301–318.

Pearlin, L. I. 1980. The Life Cycle and Life Strains. In *Sociological theory and research*, ed. H. M. Blalock, pp. 349–360. New York: Free Press.

Pearlin, L. I., and M. A. Lieberman. 1979. Social sources of emotional distress. In *Research in community and mental health*, ed. R. Simmons, 1:217–248. Greenwich, Conn: JAI Press.

Pearlin, L. I., M. A. Lieberman, E. G. Menaghan, and J. T. Mullan. 1981. The stress process. *Journal of Health and Social Behavior* 22:337–356.

Pearlin, L. I., and C. W. Radabaugh, 1976. Economic strains and the coping functions of alcohol. *American Journal of Sociology* 82:652–663.

Pearlin, L. I., and C. Schooler. 1978. The structure of coping. *Journal of Health and Social Behavior* 19:2–21.

Schmale, A. H., and H. P. Iker. 1971. Hopelessness as a predictor of cervical cancer. *Social Science and Medicine* 5:95–100.

Segal, B., G. J. Huba, and J. L. Singer. 1980. *Drugs, daydreaming, and personality: A study of college youth.* Hillsdale, N.J.: Lawrence Erlbaum Associates.

Tessler, R., D. Mechanic, and M. Dimond. 1976. The effect of psychological distress on physician utilization: A prospective study. *Journal of Health and Social Behavior* 17:353–364.

Thoits, P. A. 1983. Dimensions of life events that influence psychological distress: An evaluation and synthesis of the literature. In *Psychosocial stress: Trends in theory and research*, ed. H. B. Kaplan, pp. 33–103. New York: Academic Press.

Wiley, J. A., and T. C. Camacho. 1980. Life-style and future health: Evidence from the Alameda County Study. *Preventive Medicine* 9:1–21.

Woodruff, R. A., Jr., S. B. Guze, P. J. Clayton, and D. Carr. 1973. Alcoholism and depression. *Archives of General Psychiatry* 28:97–100.

Wortman, C. B. 1984. Social support and the cancer patient: Conceptual and methodologic issues. *Cancer* 53(May 15 supp.):2339–2360.

Wortman, C. B., and D. R. Lehman. In press. Reactions to victims of life crises: Support attempts that fail. In *Social support: Theory, research, and application*, ed. I. B. Sarason and B. R. Sarason. The Hague: Martinus Nijhof.

Yokopenic, P. A., V. A. Clark, and C. S. Aneshensel. 1983. Depression, problem recognition, and professional consultation. *Journal of Nervous and Mental Disease* 171:15–23.

Chapter 20

Patient-Practitioner Relationships and Compliance with Prescribed Medical Regimens

Bonnie L. Svarstad

Until the past decade physicians showed little concern about whether patients complied with prescribed regimens because physicians prescribed a relatively small number of drugs, many of which were palliative in nature. However, physicians are now armed with an astonishing array of drugs that have a remarkable potential for reducing morbidity and mortality (Silverman and Lee 1974). For example, it is well documented that high blood pressure is a major cause of mortality and morbidity from stroke, heart failure, and kidney failure and that modern antihypertensive agents effectively reduce these risks (V.A. Cooperative

Study Group on Antihypertensive Agents 1967, 1970, 1972; Hypertension Detection and Follow-up Program Cooperative Group 1979). However, these studies were conducted under optimal conditions in the sense that patients were not allowed to enter the clinical trial if they were considered a poor risk for compliance; in other cases patients were exposed to programs specially designed to promote continued compliance with the prescribed regimens.

Unfortunately, this problem is not so easily solved in everyday medical practice. Patients cannot be disqualified because they are considered a poor risk for compliance, and most clinicians are practicing under conditions that were not designed for the promotion of compliance. As a result, studies have repeatedly shown that large numbers of patients drop out of treatment within one year, that many patients fail to take enough medication to achieve adequate blood pressure control, and that only 20 to 30 percent of known hypertensives are under good control (Haynes et al. 1982; Rudd et al. 1979; McKenney et al. 1973).

When this problem was first discovered, many practitioners responded with "awestruck disbelief" (Sackett and Haynes 1976). They also theorized that the problem was limited to certain patient populations and that compliance could be improved by providing general education about the disease and its treatment. Later studies showed, however, that general education often fails to resolve the problem (Sackett et al. 1975) and that low patient compliance is a significant problem across a wide range of diseases and in all socioeconomic groups, all age and educational levels, and all practice settings (Haynes, Taylor, and Sackett 1979). In fact, patient noncompliance is so prevalent that several authorities now regard it as one of the most significant problems facing medical practice today (Eraker, Kirscht, and Becker 1984).

In recent years theories of compliance behavior have become more sophisticated, and much has been learned about the various ways of improving it. Nevertheless, many intervention programs are less than fully effective, and the problem continues to be an enigma. As a result, an interdisciplinary group convened by the National Heart, Lung, and Blood Institute recently concluded that we must continue to seek a better understanding of the problem and better ways of managing it (Haynes et al. 1982). According to this group, research on the practitioner-patient relationship is one of the most promising new directions in improving compliance. Therefore, now is an appropriate time to review what is known about practitioner-patient relationships as they relate to patient compliance and to draw implications for clinical practice.

My purpose in this chapter is to discuss a number of communication strategies that have proven useful in improving compliance with prescribed regimens. However, before reviewing relevant studies in this area, I will clarify my assumptions about compliance and outline a theoretical framework for understanding the potential links between practitioner-patient communication and compliance.

Theoretical Framework

There are many different theories about the cause of noncompliance. For example, cognitively oriented psychologists emphasize the patient's inability to comprehend and remember what practitioners tell them to do (Ley 1977); whereas, other researchers emphasize the patient's lack of motivation. Proponents of the health belief model argue that compliance is related to patients' beliefs about their susceptibility to illness, the severity of their disease, the efficacy of treatment, and the benefits of therapy versus its negative aspects (Rosenstock 1974; Maiman and Becker 1974). Other theorists argue that compliance is related to patients' feelings of incompetence (Caplan et al. 1980), their unconscious fears and intrapsychic conflicts (Appelbaum and Gutheil 1980), their unmet expectations and dissatisfaction with the practitioner-patient relationship (Korsch, Gozzi, and Francis 1968; Davis 1968), and their lack of adequate environmental stimuli and positive reinforcement (Zifferblatt 1975).

My basic position is that none of these traditional approaches provides a complete picture. We need a broader perspective that places more emphasis on the quality of practitioner-patient communication. Therefore, I am proposing a new way of looking at compliance. This approach is called the health communication model because it suggests that compliance is primarily, though not entirely, determined by the nature and quality of practitioner-patient communication. The main components of this model are shown in figure 20.1.

My first assumption is that compliance requires comprehension and recall of the regimen as well as motivation to follow it (see arrows 1 and 2). This means that the practitioner's behavior is linked to the patient's compliance behavior in several ways. Practitioners can influence compliance by using more effective techniques for enhancing patient understanding and recall (arrow 3) and by using more effective ways of motivating the patient (arrow 4). The specific

techniques will be discussed in a later section of this chapter.

My second assumption is that patients experience a variety of problems and concerns that undermine their willingness and ability to comply. Therefore physicians must monitor patients' behavior, ask them about the problems they are having, and use other follow-up strategies that will be discussed later (arrow 5). These follow-up strategies serve several purposes. They increase practitioners' awareness of any misunderstandings patients may have, thereby enabling practitioners to clarify their directions (arrow 6). They increase practitioners' awareness of suspected adverse drug reactions and individuals' specific fears, doubts, and hesitations about the diagnosis and treatment, thereby enabling practitioners to individualize the regimen and resolve whatever problems or concerns are undermining the patient's desire to comply. In addition, they reinforce the importance of therapy, thereby directly effecting motivation (arrow 8).

It is beyond the purpose of this chapter to discuss the many other factors that can influence the communication-compliance process. However, it is important to recognize the characteristics of the treatment plan, the potential role of patient as well as practitioner differences, environmental factors, and other factors that are known to modify the effects of communication. Because some of these factors are not directly and consistently related to compliance, many researchers have dismissed them as irrelevant. However, previous work (Svarstad 1974) suggests that these factors influence the patient's readi-

FIGURE 20.1.
The health communication model.

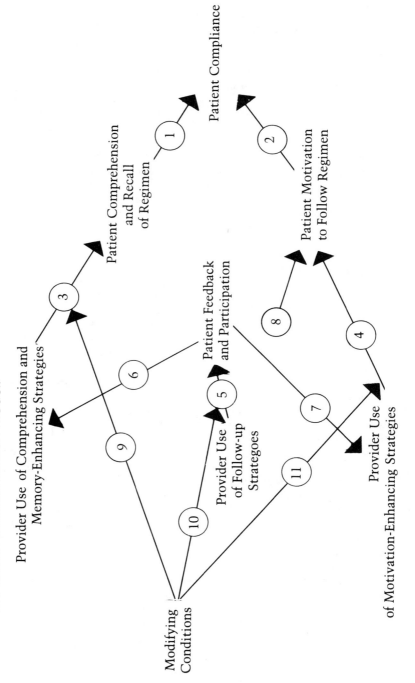

ness to learn (arrow 9), the patient's willingness to provide accurate feedback and to participate in the encounter (arrow 10), and the patient's receptivity to the practitioner's persuasive appeals and problem-solving efforts (arrow 11). Thus, we must continue to seek a better understanding of how these factors might facilitate or inhibit practitioner-patient communication.

Let us now turn to a review of the specific strategies that can be used to improve communication and compliance.

Strategies for Enhancing Patient Comprehension and Recall

The health communication model posits that there are at least seven ways of enhancing patient comprehension and recall of the regimen: providing more explicit directions, explaining the purpose or importance of therapy, supplementing oral counseling with written instructions, presenting information in categorical form, repeating important points, simplifying instructions, and providing consistent advice.

Explicit Directions

Providing more explicit directions is one way of enhancing the patient's comprehension of the specific regimen. It involves breaking the regimen down into its behavioral components and explicitly stating or spelling out what the patient is supposed to do in specific terms, thereby reducing the potential for misinterpretation.

An example of vague medication advice is "take one capsule every six hours." This statement includes the recommended dosage and dosage interval, but several points are unclear. Should the medicine be taken every six hours, regardless of how one is feeling? Or, should it be taken every six hours as needed for a particular symptom? Must it be taken every six hours around the clock or only during the waking hours? What should the patient do if side effects occur, if doses are forgotten, or if the symptoms disappear? How long should it be taken?

Several studies have shown that explicit directions can reduce, though not completely eliminate, patient misunderstanding and medication errors. Mazzullo, Lasagna, and Grinar (1974) asked patients to interpret ten prescription labels and found that many patients made errors when interpreting common instructions. For example, only 36 percent knew they were supposed to take four doses a day when instructed to take an antibiotic "every six hours." Many patients simply assumed that they were to take three doses a day because they thought of a "day" as eighteen hours of waking time and divided that time into three six-hour periods. They were less likely to make such errors when given more precise instructions.

Other researchers have studied

how physicians actually give prescription advice in various settings and discovered direct links between the explicitness or completeness of the provider's directions and patient comprehension of the drug regimen and between patient comprehension and compliance (Boyd et al. 1974; Hulka et al. 1976; Svarstad 1974, 1976). One of these studies involved direct observation and quantitative analysis of physicians' oral and written prescription directions (Svarstad 1976). The data showed that 17 percent of the drug orders were never discussed during the physician-patient encounter. Further analysis revealed that the physicians typically mentioned the drug name, the recommended dose, and number of times per day but that other parts of the drug regimen often were not discussed or written on the prescription label. The patient was explicitly told how long to take the drug in only 10 percent of the cases; in the majority of the cases there was no explicit statement about the dosage routine, that is, whether the drug was to be taken on an "as needed" or continuous basis. When the physicians were asked why they were not more explicit, they indicated that they had forgotten or that they had simply assumed that the patient would know. Actually, many patients were able to infer what the physician expected without receiving explicit instructions. However, those who received explicit instructions had a more accurate understanding of the regimen and a higher rate of compliance.

In addition to improving the patient's understanding of the regimen,

experimental studies suggest that specific instructions may facilitate greater recall and acceptance because patients view specific statements as more important than general statements (Ley 1977; Bradshaw et al. 1975; Kanouse and Hayes-Roth 1980). For example, one study examined the recall of dietary instructions by obese women. The women who were given general instructions such as "you must lose weight" recalled only 16 percent of the instructions; whereas, the women who were given specific instructions such as "you must lose ten pounds in weight" remembered 51 percent of the instructions.

Explanation of Purpose or Importance

Research in cognitive psychology suggests that people understand and remember best those items that have meaning and relevance for them (Kanouse and Hayes-Roth 1980). This suggests that a practitioner's recommendation will be easier to interpret and remember if the practitioner explains the purpose or stresses the importance of a recommendation.

Support for this notion is found in physician-patient communication studies, which show that patients who are given a brief explanation about the drug purpose have a better understanding of the drug function, which, in turn, enhances the patient's ability to interpret and recall the specific regimen (Hulka et al. 1976; Svarstad 1976). Stressing the importance of certain instructions also improves patient recall of medical advice, according to experiments by Ley (1972).

Written Reinforcement and Supplementation

Many studies have shown that health professionals can enhance patient knowledge and compliance by reinforcing and supplementing oral advice with written instructions and compliance aids. This reinforcement and supplementation can take several forms. For example, compliance with short-term antibiotic regimens has been significantly improved by pharmacists and physicians who supplement oral instructions with improved prescription labels and stickers (Lima et al. 1976), instruction cards (Madden 1973), one-page information sheets (Colcher and Bass 1972; Sharpe and Mikeal 1974; Gotsch and Liguori 1982), special drug packaging (Linkewich, Catalano, and Flack 1974), and an information sheet along with an illustrated calendar and a calibrated liquid measuring device to improve pediatric compliance with liquid antibiotics (Mattar, Markello, and Jaffe 1975).

Practitioners also can reduce confusion and noncompliance among patients who are taking two or more prescription medications for chronic conditions. For example, elderly patients who receive multiple drugs will generally have higher knowledge and compliance scores if their pharmacist or physician supplements oral counseling and traditional labels with a daily drug reminder chart, a medication calendar, or a special prescription container that shows exactly when each dose is to be taken (Ga-

briel, Gagnon, and Bryan 1977; Wandless and Davie 1977; Rehder et al. 1980; Martin and Mead 1982). Previous work also suggests that patients will have a more accurate recall of dosage changes and discontinued drugs if the physician provides a written list of the patient's current medications and their dosage schedules or encourages the patient to bring medication containers to the clinic so that labels can be kept up to date (Svarstad 1974).

Although written instructions and compliance aids can be effective in improving compliance, there are several caveats. First, no evidence suggests that these techniques can replace oral counseling. In fact, studies that do not include verbal review by a health professional usually fail to achieve the desired results (Morris and Halperin 1979). Second, there can be considerable differences in the nature and quality of written instructions and aids, the patients' needs and abilities, and the ways in which these techniques are used and evaluated. Thus, it is not surprising that providing written information about antibiotics results in varying degrees of success (Svarstad 1979) and that medication calendars, special prescription containers, and measuring devices occasionally produce mixed results (MacDonald, MacDonald, and Phoenix 1977; Eshelman and Fitzloff 1976; Crome, Akehurst, and Keet 1980; Ellison and Altemeier 1982). Third, it appears that written instruction improves compliance through its effects on patient knowledge and recall of the specific regimen. However, to my knowledge, it has not been shown to increase patient motivation to follow long-term drug therapies. This may explain why written reinforcement generally improves compliance with short-term regimens but is not sufficient for improving long-term compliance (Etzweiler and Robb 1972; Sackett et al. 1975; Clinite and Kabat 1976; Dwyer and Hammel 1978; Ehmke, Stehbens, and Young 1980).

Explicit Categorization

Another method of improving compliance is explicit categorization. This technique is based on psychological research that shows people remember best those items presented in clusters or categorical form (Ley 1977). It involves categorizing the advice to be given, announcing the name of each category, and repeating the category name before giving the advice or information in that category. For example, Ley (1980, 138) suggests that the clinician might end the visit by saying, "I am going to tell you what is wrong, what tests will be needed, what medications will be needed, what you must do. . . . First, what is wrong. You have. . . . Second, what tests will be needed. You will need . . ." and so on.

In an experimental study of general practice patients and normal subjects, Ley and his colleagues (1973) presented various types of medical advice and information in ordinary or explicit categorical form. They found the predicted differences in recall; the patients' mean recall of advisory statements increased from 28 percent to 65 percent with explicit categorization. Similar results have been re-

ported in other studies examining this method (Ley 1977, 1979).

Repetition

Another way of improving recall is to repeat those items that are likely to be misconstrued or forgotten. While this technique does not always have the predicted effect, the available studies generally show that it will result in a 20 to 30 percent improvement in patient recall of medical advice (Kupst et al. 1975; Ley 1979, 1980).

Simplification

Since patients often have difficulty understanding medical terminology, clinicians have been encouraged to avoid medical jargon when instructing patients (Korsch, Gozzi, and Francis 1968; Korsch and Negrete 1972). Practitioners also have been encouraged to use the method of simplification when preparing patient education materials. This technique involves using common words, shorter, words, and shorter sentences and has been demonstrated effective in improving patient recall and compliance with dietary and drug regimens (Ley 1977, 1980). For example, Ley and his associates (1976) developed easy, moderate, and difficult-to-read leaflets for psychiatric patients who were prescribed an antidepressant or a tranquilizer. They found that the easier leaflets were more effective in reducing noncompliance and that the difficult leaflets had no significant effect. In fact, patients who received the difficult leaflet made about the same number of medication errors as the patients who received no information.

Consistency of Advice

Most patients probably receive consistent advice from their providers. However, a few studies show that physicians do not always document their prescriptions in the medical record, and, as a result, patients occasionally receive several drugs from the same therapeutic class and duplicate prescriptions for the same drug (Malahy 1966; Bond and Monson 1984). Pharmacists also can contribute to noncompliance by not providing the correct amount of medication, omitting information that was provided by the physician, or making errors when typing the label (Mattar, Markello, and Jaffe 1975; Svarstad 1976). When pharmacists and physicians make an effort to minimize such problems, improved compliance is evident (Mattar, Markello, and Jaffe 1975; Bond and Monson 1984).

The Use of Multiple Strategies

To test the joint effects of various comprehension and memory-enhancing strategies, Svarstad (1976) developed a composite index for measuring the quality of physicians' oral and written instructions about medication. The index measured the explicitness of directions, the level of explanation about drug purpose, the amount of written reinforcement, and the degree of consistency between prescription forms and labels. As predicted, there was a positive association between the overall quality of instruction and the patient's understanding of the regimen as well as between the quality of instruction and the patient's compliance.

The joint effects of simplification, repetition, and explicit categorization were assessed in a study reported by Ley (1976). In this experiment obese patients were given a low carbohydrate diet guide and one of two leaflets that contained additional information regarding the diet. The experimental leaflet contained the same content as the control leaflet but was easier to read and included explicit categories and repetition. The patients who received the experimental leaflet lost almost two times as much weight as the patients who received the control leaflet.

Whether compliance can be improved by teaching practitioners to use various comprehension and memory-enhancing techniques has not been determined. However, there is some evidence that patient recall can be significantly improved by teaching practitioners to give more explicit advice, to stress the importance of advice, and to use repetition, explicit categorization, and simplification (Ley 1977).

Strategies for Enhancing Patient Motivation and Feedback

The health communication model suggests five general ways of enhancing patient motivation and feedback. They include positive inducements and reinforcement, positive expectations and direction, a participatory approach to negative patient feedback, compliance monitoring and follow-up, and friendliness or approachability.

Positive Inducements and Reinforcement

Social psychological research suggests that our behavior is, in part, determined by the value we place on a particular outcome and by our subjective estimate that a particular action will produce that outcome (Rosenstock 1974; DiMatteo and DiNicola 1982). The implication is that patients will be more motivated to follow a specific regimen if they are convinced that compliance will produce a specific outcome (e.g., improved health, praise, or a monetary reward) and if they place a high value on that outcome. Thus, practitioners should be able to improve compliance by providing information about the potential value or benefits of compliance, by sharing laboratory results and other data so patients can see how the regimen is helping them, or by providing other positive inducements and reinforcement.

Support for this hypothesis is found in a number of observational and experimental studies. For example, observational data indicate that the patient's personal physician can increase the patient's evaluation of the treatment plan and the rate of medication compliance by explaining the reason or potential value of therapy, providing feedback on the patient's therapeutic status, and emphasizing the importance or need for continuous therapy (Svarstad 1976). In a more controlled study, Inui, Yourtee, and Williamson (1976) found that physicians who were taught various strategies for altering patients' beliefs about the efficacy and benefits of treatment were more successful than control physicians. The patients of tutored physicians held more positive views about the regimen, were more compliant, and had better blood pressure control.

Other experiments have documented improved compliance after implementing special programs that include blood pressure monitoring and feedback by pharmacists and nurses (Wilber and Barrow 1969; McKenney et al. 1973, 1978; Alderman and Schoenbaum 1975), blood pressure monitoring by the patient (Haynes et al. 1976; Nessman, Carnahan, and Nugent 1980), monetary rewards and praise by a nonprofessional (Haynes et al. 1976), and home visits to increase family support and reinforcement (Levine et al. 1979). Contingency contracting also appears to be an effective method for enhancing compliance among hypertensive patients (Swain and Steckle 1981). This technique involves the formulation of a professional-patient contract that specifies a target goal and the rewards for achieving that goal.

While positive inducements and feedback have been shown effective, we must be cautious when applying the results of these studies. First, blood pressure monitoring techniques tend to fail when they are used in a mechanical way and no effort is made to change the patient's beliefs and behavior (Johnson et al. 1978).

Second, these techniques are particularly helpful during the first six months of treatment but do not add much after that time (Haynes et al. 1976; Stahl et al. 1984). Third, significant results can be obtained by involving the family and delegating certain responsibilities to nonhealth professionals who give monetary rewards and praise for complying with the regimen. However, the best results are obtained when a health care provider is closely involved and when the feedback or reinforcement is intrinsic to the treatment goal. For example, programs that involve blood pressure monitoring and feedback by the patient's personal physician, nurse, or pharmacist generally achieve blood pressure control for 70 to 90 percent of the patients in the experimental group (Takala, Niemela, and Rosti 1979; McKenney et al. 1973; Wilber and Barrow 1969; Nessman, Carnahan, and Nugent 1980; Stahl et al. 1984). Programs that rely on nonmedical professionals achieve blood pressure control for only 30 to 66 percent of the patients (Haynes et al. 1976; Levine et al. 1979). A final point is that treatment successes are generally lost when these techniques are no longer used by the practitioner (Wilber and Barrow 1969; McKenney et al. 1973; Dunbar, Marshall, and Hovell 1979). This suggests that continued interaction with a practitioner is a key factor.

Positive Expectations and Direction

Another social psychological principle is that people are more likely to take certain actions if they believe that someone in authority expects them to act in certain ways and if they believe that these expectations are legitimate or proper (French and Raven 1959; Raven, 1974). This implies that patients will be more compliant if clinicians state their expectations in a positive or directive manner as opposed to a permissive or nondirective manner.

Only a few studies have examined this hypothesis, but the results are fairly consistent. Compliance tends to be higher when practitioners take a directive as opposed to a nondirective or permissive approach (Davis 1968; Svarstad 1976; Nathanson and Becker 1985). Because these data appear inconsistent with the nondirective philosophy of practitioners who have begun to challenge traditional authoritarian models of patient care, researchers have been surprised when they found a positive correlation between the amount of direction and patient compliance (Nathanson and Becker 1985). However, the data are not as inconsistent as they appear. First, clinicians can be directive or speak with authority without being authoritarian (Quill 1983). That is, they can take a position and provide clear guidance without belittling and intimidating patients, ignoring patients' views, and using other authoritarian and threatening tactics. Second, stating one's expectations in a positive or directive manner is not enough. Patients still need to understand what they are supposed to do and to believe that the provider's expectations are legitimate or proper. Thus, the best results are found when clinicians provide good instructions, explain the rationale for therapy, and use their authority in a sparing or judicious manner (Svarstad 1976).

The Participatory Approach to Negative Feedback

Using the previously mentioned techniques, the physician can have a substantial impact on the patient's acceptance of the diagnosis and regimen. However, patients do not always agree with what they are told. There is considerable potential for conflict after the patient has gained more experience with the regimen (Davis 1968; Freidson 1970). As a result, practitioners are often confronted with explicit and subtle forms of "negative feedback" on a variety of issues. For example, patients will challenge the diagnosis, question the seriousness of their illness, or complain that the medication bothers them in some way. Others will appear discouraged and state that they are unable to comply. Still others will express uncertainty about the efficacy or safety of the regimen and become fearful or angry when the practitioner wants to increase the dosage, add another drug, or pursue more aggressive therapy.

There are at least four ways of responding to such negative feedback. They include the authoritarian, permissive, psychotherapeutic, and participatory approaches. Clinicians who adopt the authoritarian approach generally assume that patients' underlying fears, anxieties, and hesitations about treatment are clinically insignificant or trivial and that patients should either accept the regimen or find another practitioner. Thus, they respond to negative feedback by ignoring or dismissing many of the patient's complaints, demanding compliance, and becoming angry or hostile (Davis 1966; Svarstad 1976; Danziger 1981). Because these tactics are usually considered inappropriate, no experimental studies have evaluated their impact on compliance. However, observational studies have shown that ignoring the patient's fears and concerns about the regimen does not make them go away and that coercive tactics eventually lead to patient concealment and dissatisfaction, errors in clinical judgment, and a higher drop-out rate (Svarstad 1978).

Taking a permissive or lenient approach is also considered inappropriate by medical writers. Nevertheless, there are physicians who unwittingly adopt this approach in an apparent effort to maintain the patient's good will. According to Podell (1975), the practitioners who adopt this stance are highly attentive to the patient's reactions but do not make a concerted effort to assess and resolve the patient's primary concern. Instead, they defer the issue and hold off pursuing more aggressive and effective therapy. The patient stops protesting and remains in therapy, but the treatment goal is often sacrificed (Podell 1975).

The psychotherapeutic approach assumes that the patient's concerns about the regimen are largely psychological in origin. For example, psychodynamically oriented researchers argue that mentally ill patients resist therapy because they have unconscious fears and intrapsychic conflicts that lead to the denial of illness, distorted perceptions of the regimen, and negativistic struggles with the practitioner (Appelbaum 1977; Appelbaum and Gutheil 1980). Others have argued that patients with hypertension and other chronic illnesses resist therapy because they fear death and the loss of autonomy, are overwhelmed by anxiety, or lack confidence in their ability to control the illness. This has led to several studies examining the effectiveness of psychological support from a nurse (Caplan et al. 1976, 1980) and group or individualized counseling by a social worker (Levine et al. 1979; Webb 1980). Unfortunately, none of these interventions had a substantial effect on compliance rates.

Clinicians who adopt the participatory approach take a broader view of patient feedback and its role in the treatment process. They assume that patients not only have the right to question and complain but that negative feedback is a critical part of the communication and treatment process because it allows the practitioner to individualize or adjust the regimen and to resolve whatever physical, psychological, or social problems are interfering with the patient's desire to comply.

No experimental studies have elaborated and explicitly tested the participatory approach to negative feedback. But several experiments have indicated that patient feedback and adjustment of the regimen are very important elements in enhancing compliance. For example, compliance tends to be higher when the regimen is "tailored" to the patient's daily routine (Haynes et al. 1976), when patients are allowed to formulate or change their regimens within a medical protocol (Nessman, Carnahan, and Nugent 1980), and when patients are explicitly asked to identify the areas in which they would like some professional assistance (Swain and Steckel 1981).

Studies also show improved compliance when physicians and pharmacists make a concerted effort to identify and manage adverse drug reactions. For example, McKenney and his colleagues (1973) have suggested that hypertensive patients often experience adverse drug reactions and concerns that go "undetected, untreated, and unexplained" by physicians who may consider such reactions too mild or trivial to discuss with the patient. To improve this situation, they expanded the pharmacist's role in the long-term care given hypertensive patients. Patients in the study group were seen monthly by a clinical pharmacist who actively solicited patient complaints about the regimen and then used appropriate strategies for solving whatever problems a patient raised, regardless of their clinical significance or severity. The strategies depended on the patient's particular problem and included simple techniques such as acknowledging the legitimacy of the patient's problem, explaining why it occurred and how long it might persist, changing dosage intervals and times in order to make the regimen more tolerable, explaining how a patient can relieve orthostatic hypotension and other suspected adverse drug reactions, requesting laboratory tests to assist in the assessment of suspected adverse reactions, adjusting the regimen after consulting with the physician, and referring all moderate or severe reactions to the physician with recommendations for management and follow-up care. When these problem-solving strategies were combined with more explicit instructions and monitoring of compliance, there was a substantial improvement in patient compliance and blood pressure control.

A similar approach was taken by Bond and Salinger (1979). They showed that a clinical pharmacist working with a psychiatrist can have a substantial impact by carefully interviewing and helping schizophrenic patients solve their drug-taking problems. Rather than interpreting their patients' complaints as delusional perceptions or signs of denial, they viewed them as real problems that should be evaluated and managed by a knowledgeable practitioner. Using this approach, they were able to significantly reduce the incidence of side effects, the average recommended dosage, the number of patients requiring maintenance antiparkinsonian medication, and rehospitalization rates. Their conclusion was that previous workers had underestimated the role of the clinician in monitoring and adjustment of regimens and that "much of what has been interpreted in other reports as resistance to medication for psychodynamic reasons is, in part, based on factors such as overmedication and poor control of side effects" (pp. 502–503).

Compliance Monitoring and Follow-Up

One of the more effective ways of improving compliance is to increase the level of compliance monitoring. This involves checking the patient's compliance with previous advice and can take several forms. For example, one study found that compliance with drug regimens was higher in those cases where the physician conducted a thorough interview of the patient to determine exactly how the patient had been using the previously prescribed drugs (Svarstad 1976). Obtaining a compliance history is important for several reasons, as mentioned earlier. First, it is a fairly simple way of eliciting patient feedback and participation in the evaluation of the regimen, which, in turn, enables the physician to individualize the regimen and to resolve any misunderstandings or concerns that exist. Second, it is another way of reinforcing the practitioner's expectations and the importance of compliance. Third, close monitoring of drug use can be reassuring to patients who are fearful about multiple drug regimens or the long-term use of drugs. Some patients assume, for example, that physicians who ask detailed questions are more careful and, therefore, can be trusted.

Other effective ways of monitoring patient compliance include checking appointment records and recalling patients who do not show up (Alderman and Schoenbaum 1975; Takala, Niemela, and Rosti 1979), making home visits (Curry 1968; Wilber and

Barrow 1969; Hudson and Sbarbaro 1973), and monitoring serum drug levels (Lund, Jorgenson, and Kuhl 1964; Sherwin, Robb, and Lechter 1973; Eney and Goldstein 1976; Gundert-Remy, Remy, and Weber 1976).

Friendliness or Approachability

A final technique for enhancing the patient's motivation is to behave in a friendly or approachable manner. Theories of attitude change and communication suggest that this technique is important for several reasons. First, people tend to agree with someone they like or with someone with whom they have an emotionally satisfying relationship (McGuire 1973). Second, the rate of communication between two people tends to increase as their attitudes toward each other become more favorable (Newcomb 1953; Thibaut and Kelley 1959). This implies that patients may be more willing to accept advice from a friendly practitioner and that they may be more willing to express their fears and concerns to a practitioner who appears friendly or approachable.

Although the level of friendliness does not always correlate with compliance (Davis 1968), studies generally show an association between compliance and the affective tone of the practitioner-patient encounter. Expressions of negative feeling toward the patient are consistently related to low compliance; whereas, friendliness or approachability tends to be associated with higher rates of compliance (Davis 1968; Freemon et al. 1971; Svarstad 1976). Surveys also show a positive link between compliance and patients' perceptions of the practitioner's concern or interest in them as people (Nelson et al. 1975; Caplan et al. 1980).

Finally, some evidence indicates that patients are more willing to communicate with practitioners if practitioners give verbal and nonverbal cues that they are friendly or approachable. For example, patients have been shown to ask a higher number of questions if the physician greets the patient in a friendly manner, shows positive affect by smiling or laughing, allows the patient to speak without interrupting, and gives other signals that he or she is receptive to patient feedback and participation (Svarstad 1974).

The Use of Multiple Strategies

Several studies also show that compliance will be higher if one uses multiple strategies for enhancing patient motivation (Levine et al. 1979; Svarstad 1978). Perhaps the most detailed analysis was conducted by Svarstad (1978). This analysis involved the development of a standardized scale for scoring physicians' efforts to motivate their patients. Physicians were given positive points whenever they used a nonauthoritarian technique for motivating patients, including providing positive inducements or reinforcement, giving advice in a positive or directive manner, engaging in a high level of compliance monitoring, relating to the patient in an approachable manner, or using the participatory approach to negative patient feedback. Negative points were given when physicians used authoritarian techniques for managing negative patient feedback. As predicted, there was a positive association between compliance and the physician's use of nonauthoritarian strategies. When physicians used a high number of these techniques, they achieved patient compliance in 80 percent of the cases. Their rates of compliance were only 41 percent and 13 percent when they used a moderate or low number of strategies. These findings support the health communication model and suggest that research on the practitioner-patient relationship is indeed a promising new direction in improving compliance.

Conclusion

Clinical researchers and behavioral scientists have advanced a number of theories to account for noncompliance, and each of these theories has made a contribution to our understanding of the problem and better ways of managing it. However, noncompliance continues to undermine the effectiveness of antihypertensive therapy and other therapies that have a significant potential for reducing morbidity and mortality. Therefore, it is time to integrate what has been learned and to consider alternative approaches to the problem. To guide further work in this area, I have proposed the health communication model. This model has several advantages. First, it provides a more comprehensive view of the problem. It recognizes that noncompliance may be due to multiple causes, including lack of patient understanding and recall, lack of patient motivation, inadequate clinical supervision and problem solving, and dissatisfaction with the practitioner-patient relationship. Second, it calls attention to the full range of variables that can influence patient understanding and motivation, the interrelationships among these variables, and the dynamics of practitioner-patient communication. This type of schema is useful because it enables us to organize and evaluate existing theory and findings, to diagnose compliance problems, and to select interventions that are specifically designed to alleviate a particular type of compliance problem. A third advantage is that it integrates behavioral science principles and other concepts of quality care. It reminds us that modern drug technology is imperfect and that health professionals are practicing under conditions that were not designed for the promotion of compliance with long-term treatments. Improving compliance therefore requires much more than the dissemination of leaflets, the provision of socioemotional support, or the reinforcement of patient behaviors. It also requires a critical look at traditional ways of labeling prescription drugs and monitoring patient compliance and side effects, at the role of clinical expertise in adjusting regimens and resolving whatever problems are undermining the patient's desire to comply, and at new ways of utilizing nurses and pharmacists. The problem therefore presents new challenges and opportunities for health professionals, behavioral scientists, and policymakers.

References

Alderman, M. H., and E. E. Schoenbaum. 1975. Detection and treatment of hypertension at the work site. *New England Journal of Medicine* 293:65–67.

Appelbaum, P., and T. Gutheil. 1980. Drug refusal: A study of psychiatric inpatients. *American Journal of Psychiatry* 137:340–346.

Appelbaum, S. 1977. The refusal to take one's medicine. *Bulletin of the Menninger Clinic* 41:511–521.

Bond, C. A., and R. Monson. 1984. Sustained improvement in drug documentation, compliance, and disease control. *Archives of Internal Medicine* 144:1159–1162.

Bond, C. A., and R. Salinger. 1979. Fluphenazine outpatient clinics: A pharmacist's role. *Journal of Clinical Psychiatry* (Dec.):501–503.

Boyd, J. R., T. R. Covington, W. F. Stanaszek, and R. T. Coussons. 1974. Drug defaulting, part 2: Analysis of noncompliance patterns. *American Journal of Hospital Pharmacy* 31:485–491.

Bradshaw, P. W., P. Ley, J. A. Kincey, and J. Bradshaw. 1975. Recall of medical advice: Comprehensibility and specificity. *British Journal of Social and Clinical Psychology* 14:55–62.

Caplan, R. D., R. V. Harrison, R. V. Wellons, and J. R. P. French, Jr. 1980. *Social support and patient adherence: Experimental and survey findings.* Ann Arbor: Institute for Social Research, University of Michigan.

Caplan, R. D., E. A. R. Robinson, J. R. P. French, Jr., J. R. Caldwell, and M. Shinn. 1976. *Adhering to medical regimens: Pilot experiments in patient education and social support.* Ann Arbor: Institute for Social Research, University of Michigan.

Clinite, J., and H. Kabat. 1976. Improving patient compliance. *Journal of the American Pharmaceutical Association* 16:74–76, 85.

Colcher, I. S., and J. W. Bass. 1972. Penicillin treatment of streptococcal pharyngitis. *Journal of American Medical Association* 222:657–659.

Crome, P., M. Akehurst, and J. Keet. 1980. Drug compliance in elderly hospital in-patients: Trial of the Dosett box. *The Practitioner* 224:782–785.

Curry, F. J. 1968. Neighborhood clinics for more effective outpatient treatment of tuberculosis. *New England Journal of Medicine* 279:1262–1267.

Danziger, S. K. 1981. The uses of expertise in doctor-patient encounters during pregnancy. In *The sociology of health and illness*, ed. P. Conrad and R. Kern, pp. 359–376. New York: St. Martin's Press.

Davis, M. S. 1966. Variations in patients' compliance with doctors' orders: Analysis of congruence between survey responses and results of empirical investigations. *Journal of Medical Education* 41:1037–1048.

———. 1968. Variation in patients' compliance with doctors' advice: An empirical analysis of patterns of communication. *American Journal of Public Health* 58(Feb.):274–288.

DiMatteo, M. R., and D. D. DiNicola. 1982. *Achieving patient compliance.* New York: Pergamon Press.

Dunbar, J. M., G. D. Marshall, and M. F. Hovell. 1979. Behavioral strategies for improving compliance. In *Compliance in health care*, ed. R. B. Haynes, D. W. Taylor, and D. L. Sackett, pp. 174–190. Baltimore: Johns Hopkins University Press.

Dwyer, F. R., and R. Hammel. 1978. The impact of patient package inserts on essential hypertension. *Preventive Medicine* 7:64.

Ehmke, D. A., J. A. Stehbens, and L. Young. 1980. Two studies of compliance with daily prophylaxis in rheumatic fever patients in Iowa. *American Journal of Public Health* 70(11):1189–1193.

Ellison, R. S., and W. A. Altemeier. 1982. Effect of use of a measured dispensing device on oral antibiotic compliance. *Clinical Pediatrics* 21(11):668–671.

Eney, R. D., and E. Goldstein. 1976. Compliance of chronic asthmatics with oral administration of theophylline as measured by serum and salivary levels. *Pediatrics* 57:513–517.

Eraker, S. A., J. P. Kirscht, and M. B. Becker. 1984. Understanding and improving patient compliance. *Annals of Internal Medicine* 100:258–268.

Eshelman, F., and J. Fitzloff. 1976. Effect of packaging on patient compliance with an antihypertensive medication. *Current Therapeutic Research* 20:215–219.

Etzwiler, D., and J. Robb. 1972. Evaluation of programmed education among juvenile diabetics and their families. *Diabetes* 21:967–971.

Freemon, B., V. F. Negrete, M. Davis, and B. M. Korsch. 1971. Gaps in doctor-patient communication: Doctor-patient interaction analysis. *Pediatric Research* 5:298–311.

Freidson, E. 1970. *Profession of medicine.* New York: Dodd, Mead.

French, J. R. P., Jr., and B. Raven. 1959. The bases of social power. In *Studies in social power*, ed. D. Cartwright, pp. 607–623. Ann Arbor: Institute for Social Research.

Gabriel, M., J. P. Gagnon, and C. K. Bryan. 1977. Improved patient compliance through use of a daily drug reminder chart. *American Journal of Public Health* 67:968–969.

Gotsch, A. R., and S. Liguori. 1982. Knowledge, attitude, and compliance dimensions of antibiotic therapy with PPIs. *Medical Care* 20:581–595.

Gundert-Remy, U., C. Remy, and E. Weber. 1976. Serum digoxin levels in patients of a general practice of Germany. *European Journal of Clinical Pharmacology* 10:97–100.

Haynes, R. B., M. E. Mattson, A. V. Chobanian, J. M. Dunbar, T. M. Engebretson, T. F. Garrety, H. Leventhal, R. J. Levine, and R. L. Levy. 1982. Management of patient compliance in the treatment of hypertension: Report of the NHLBI working group. *Hypertension* 4(3):415–423.

Haynes, R. B., D. L. Sackett, E. S. Gibson, D. W. Taylor, B. C. Hackett, R. S. Roberts, and A. L. Johnson. 1976. Improvement of medication compliance in uncontrolled hypertension. *Lancet* (Jan. 12):1265–1268.

Haynes, R. B., D. W. Taylor, and D. L. Sackett, eds. 1979. *Compliance in health care.* Baltimore: Johns Hopkins University Press.

Hudson, L. D., and J. A. Sbarboro. 1973. Twice weekly tuberculosis chemotherapy. *Journal of American Medical Association* 223:139–143.

Hulka, B. S., J. C. Cassel, L. L. Kupper, and J. A. Burdette. 1976. Communication, compliance, and concordance between physicians and patients with prescribed medications. *American Journal of Public Health* 66:847–853.

Hypertension Detection and Follow-up Program Cooperative Group. 1979. Five-year findings of the Hypertension Detection and Follow-up Program, 1: Reduction in mortality of persons with high blood pressure including mild hypertension. *Journal of American Medical Association* 242:2562.

Inui, T. S., E. L. Yourtee, and J. W. Williamson. 1976. Improved outcomes in hypertension after physician tutorials: A controlled trial. *Annals of Internal Medicine* 84:646–651.

Johnson, A. L., D. W. Taylor, D. L. Sackett, C. W. Dunnett, and A. G. Shimizu. 1978. Self-recording of blood pressure in the management of hypertension. *Canadian Medical Association Journal* 119(Nov. 4):1034–1039.

Kanouse, D. E., and B. Hayes-Roth. 1980. Cognitive considerations in the design of product warnings. In *The Banbury Report, no. 6: Product labeling and health risks*, ed. L. A. Morris, M. B. Mazis, and I. Barofsky, pp. 147–164. Cold Spring Harbor Laboratory.

Korsch, B., E. Gozzi, and V. Francis. 1968. Gaps in doctor-patient communication, 1: Doctor-patient interaction and patient satisfaction. *Pediatrics* 42 (Nov.):855–871.

Korsch, B., and V. Negrete. 1972. Doctor-patient communication. *Scientific American* 227(Aug.):66–74.

Kupst, M. J., K. Dresser, J. L. Shulman, and M. H. Paul. 1975. Evaluation of methods to improve communication in the physician-patient relationship. *American Journal of Orthopsychiatry* 45:420.

Levine, D., L. Green, S. Deeds, J. Chwalow, R. Patternson Russell, and J. Finlay, J. 1979. Health education for hypertensive patients. *Journal of American Medical Association* 241(Apr. 20):1700–1703.

Ley, P. 1972. Primacy, rated importance, and recall of medical information. *Journal of Health and Human Behavior* 13:311–317.

———. 1976. Towards better doctor-patient communications: Contributions from social and experimental psychology. In *Communications in medicine*, ed. A. E. Bennet. London: Oxford University Press.

———. 1977. Psychological studies of doctor-patient communication. In *Contributions to medical psychology*, ed. S. Rachman, pp. 9–42. Oxford: Pergamon Press.

———. 1979. Memory for medical information. *Journal of Social and Clinical Psychology* 18:245–252.

———. 1980. Practical methods of improving communication. In *The Banbury Report, no. 6: Product labeling and health risks*, ed. L. A. Morris, M. B. Mazis, and I. Barofsky, pp. 135–146. Cold Spring Harbor Laboratory.

Ley, P., P. W. Bradshaw, D. Eaves, and C. M. Walker. 1973. A method for increasing patients' recall of information presented by doctors. *Psychological Medicine* 3:217–220.

Ley, P., V. K. Jain, and C. E. Skilbeck. 1976. A method for decreasing patient medication errors. *Psychological Medicine*, 6:599–601.

Lima, J., L. Nazarian, E. Charney, and C. Lahti. 1976. Compliance with short-term antimicrobial therapy. *Pediatrics* 57:383–386.

Linkewich, J. R., R. B. Catalano, and H. L. Flack. 1974. The effect of packaging and instructions on outpatient compliance with medication regimens. *Drug Intelligence and Clinical Pharmacy* 8:10–15.

Lund, M. R., S. Jorgenson, and V. Kuhl. 1964. Serum diphenylhydantoin (phenytoin) in ambulant patients with epilepsy. *Epilepsia* 5:51–58.

MacDonald, E. T., J. B. MacDonald, and M. Phoenix. 1977. Improving drug compliance after hospital discharge. *British Medical Journal* 2:618–621.

McGuire, W. 1973. Persuasion, resistance and attitude change. In *Handbook of communication*, ed. I. de Sola Pool, F. W. Frey, W. Schramm, N. Maccoby, and E. B. Parker, pp. 216–262. Chicago: Rand McNally.

McKenney, J. M., E. D. Brown, R. Necsary, and H. L. Reavis. 1978. Effect of pharmacist drug monitoring and patient education on hypertensive patients. *Contemporary Pharmacy Practice* 1(Fall):50–56.

McKenney, J. M., J. M. Slining, H. R. Henderson, D. Devins, and M. Barr. 1973. The effect of clinical pharmacy services on patients with essential hypertension. *Circulation* 48(Nov.):1104–1111.

Madden, E. E. 1973. Evaluation of outpatient pharmacy patient counseling. *Journal of American Pharmaceutical Association* 13:437–443.

Maiman, L., and M. Becker. 1974. The health belief model: Origins and correlates in psychological theory. *Health Education Monographs* 2(Winter): 336–353.

Malahy, B. 1966. The effect of instruction and labeling on the number of medication errors made by patients at home. *American Journal of Hospital Pharmacy* 23:283–292.

Martin, D. C., and K. Mead. 1982. Reducing medication errors in a geriatric population. *Journal of the American Geriatrics Society* 30:258–260.

Mattar, M. E., J. Markello, and S. J. Jaffe. 1975. Pharmaceutic factors affecting pediatric compliance. *Pediatrics* 55:101–108.

Mazzullo, J. V., L. Lasagna, and P. F. Grinar. 1974. Variations in interpretation of prescription instructions: The need for improved prescribing habits. *Journal of American Medical Association* 227:929–931.

Morris, L. A., and J. A. Halperin. 1979. Effects of written drug information on patient knowledge and compliance: A literature review. *American Journal of Public Health* 69:47–52.

Nathanson, C. A., and M. H. Becker. 1985. The influence of client-provider relationships on teenage women's subsequent use of contraception. *American Journal of Public Health* 75(Jan.):33–38.

Nelson, A., B. Gold, R. Hutchinson, and E. Benezra. 1975. Drug default among schizophrenic patients. *American Journal of Hospital Pharmacy* 32:1237–1242.

Nessman, D. G., J. E. Carnahan, and C. A. Nugent. 1980. Increasing compliance: Patient-operated hypertension groups. *Archives of Internal Medicine* 140(Nov.):1427–1430.

Newcomb, T. M. 1953. An approach to the study of communicative acts. *Psychology Review* 60:393–404.

Podell, R. 1975. *Physician's guide to compliance in hypertension.* West Point, Pa.: Merck and Co.

Quill, T. E. 1983. Partnerships in patient care: A contractual approach. *Annals of Internal Medicine* 98:228–234.

Raven, B. H. 1974. The comparative analysis of power and influence. In *Perspectives in social power*, ed. J. T. Tedeschi. Chicago: Aldine.

Rehder, T. L., L. K. McCoy, B. Blackwell, W. Whitehead, and A. Robinson. 1980. Improving medication compliance by counseling and special prescription container. *American Journal of Hospital Pharmacy* 37:379–385.

Rosenstock, I. 1974. Origins of the health belief model. *Health Education Monographs* 2:378.

Rudd, P., V. Tul, K. Brown, S. M. Davidson, and G. J. Bostwick, Jr. 1979. Hypertension continuation adherence. *Archives of Internal Medicine* 139:545–549.

Sackett, D. L., and R. B. Haynes, eds. 1976. *Compliance with therapeutic regimens.* Baltimore: Johns Hopkins University Press.

Sackett, D. L., R. B. Haynes, E. S. Gibson, B. C. Hackett, D. W. Taylor, R. S. Roberts, and A. L. Johnson. 1975. Randomized clinical trial of strategies for improving medication compliance in primary hypertension. *Lancet* 1:1205.

Sharpe, T. R., and R. L. Mikeal. 1974. Patient compliance with antibiotic regimens. *American Journal of Hospital Pharmacy* 31:479–484.

Sherwin, A. L., J. Robb, and M. Lechter. 1973. Improved control of epilepsy by monitoring plasma ethosuximide. *Archives of Neurology* 28:178–181.

Silverman, M., and P. Lee. 1974. *Pills, profits and politics.* Berkeley: University of California Press.

Stahl, S. M., C. R. Kelley, P. J. Neill, C. E. Grim, and J. Mamlin. 1984. Effects of home blood pressure measurement on long-term blood pressure control. *American Journal of Public Health* 74:704–709.

Svarstad, B. 1974. The doctor-patient encounter: An observational study of communication and outcome. Ph.D. diss., Department of Sociology, University of Wisconsin–Madison.

———. 1976. Physician-patient communication and patient conformity with medical advice. In *The growth of bureaucratic medicine. An inquiry into the dynamics of patient behavior and the organization of medical care*, ed. D. Mechanic, pp. 220–238. New York: John Wiley and Sons.

———. 1978. Doctor-patient communication. In *Patient education in the primary care setting,* ed. B. Currie, pp. 17–29. Proceedings of Second Conference on Patient Education in the Primary Care Setting, Madison, Wis.

———. 1979. Pharmaceutical sociology: Issues in research, education, and service. *American Journal of Pharmaceutical Education* 43:252–257.

Swain, M. A., and S. B. Steckel. 1981. Influencing adherence among hypertensives. *Research in Nursing and Health* 4:213–222.

Takala, J., N. Niemela, and J. Rosti. 1979. Improving compliance with therapeutic regimens in hypertensive patients in a community health center. *Circulation* 59:540–543.

Thibaut, J. W., and H. H. Kelley. 1959. *The social psychology of groups.* New York. John Wiley and Sons.

Veterans Administration Cooperative Study Group on Antihypertensive Agents. 1967. Effects of treatment on morbidity in hypertension: Results in patients with diastolic blood pressures averaging 115 through 128 mm Hg. *Journal of the American Medical Association* 202:1028.

———. 1970. Effects of treatment on morbidity in hypertension: Results in patients with diastolic blood pressures averaging 90 through 114 mm Hg. *Journal of American Medical Association* 213:1143.

———. 1972. Effects of morbidity in hypertension III: Influence of age, diastolic pressure, and prior cardiovascular diseases. Further analysis of side effects. *Circulation* 45:991.

Wandless, I., and J. W. Davie. 1977. Can drug compliance in the elderly be improved? *British Medical Journal* 1:359–361.

Webb, P. A. 1980. Effectiveness of patient education and psychosocial counseling in promoting compliance and control among hypertensive patients. *Journal of Family Practice* 10(6):1047–1055.

Wilber, J. A., and J. G. Barrow. 1969. Reducing elevated blood pressure: Experience found in a community. *Minnesota Medicine* 52:1303–1305.

Zifferblatt, S. M. 1975. Increasing patient compliance through the applied behavioral analysis. *Preventive Medicine* 4:173–182.

Chapter 21

Professional Responsibility and Medical Error

Charles L. Bosk

T he erosion of established authority; a loss of faith in progress; an increased appreciation of risk, uncertainty, and error; and a distrust of technological advance—these have all marked American society in the last quarter century. The medical profession, like all other major societal institutions, has been stirred by this shift in the prevailing cultural winds. How could it be otherwise? On a variety of fronts, from Congress to the courts to consumer groups, physicians find their old taken-for-granted autonomy challenged. These challenges range from public issues such as the cost of care and the distribution of physicians by specialty, by region, by gender, and by ethnic group, to such traditionally private concerns as the management of terminally ill patients and the care of critically ill neonates. At bottom, all of these concerns raise the same fundamental question, namely, Does the medical profession act in ways that represent broad collective interests or narrow self-interests?

Merely to raise the question in this way documents a significant shift in public perceptions of physicians. Not so long ago, the medical profession was presumed to act in the public good (Mechanic 1985). In the period immediately following World War II, funding for research, hospital expansion, and new technologies was rarely questioned, and even then, rarely denied. At a more personal level the intrusions of physicians—their pokings, dosings, probings, and cuttings—were assumed to do more good than harm by far. Competence was generally beyond dispute. Bad results served as reminders of the inevitable limits to medical practice. The physician, who was predominantly a white male, was a cultural hero—a symbol of what science coupled with compassion could accomplish.

A central element to the perception of the physician as a cultural hero was the dedication, conscientiousness, and selflessness medical work requires. The heroic vision of medical work celebrated individual achievement at the same time that it obscured common interests among physicians as members of the same occupation. To say that the herioc concept of the physician is now tarnished is to engage in serious understatement.

Interesting as this is, it is merely the background for my topic—medical errors and professional responsibility. My concern is to show how errors were treated under an older regime (and to a considerable extent are still treated today) as a private and individual matter and how they are now being transformed into a public and collective one. For that purpose I selectively review the literature on medical school, residency, and independent practice. The warrant for this is to see clearly how physicians learn to recognize errors, how they correct them, and how they treat their colleagues judged guilty of them. Some attention is paid in the literature to how controls might vary by practice setting (group versus solo practice, ambulatory versus hospital care), by speciality (surgery versus internal medicine versus psychiatry), or by type of community (urban versus rural). Nonetheless, an assumption governing most discussions of the topic was that social control was directed by physicians and that, whatever the shortcomings of this arrangement,

there was no viable alternative to it.

A whole host of changes in the organization of health care is affecting the dynamics of physician control identified in earlier studies reviewed in this essay (Starr 1983). As a result, medical error is now becoming a public and collective concern—its identification and treatment influenced by legislatures, courts, third-party payers, and managers as well as by physicians. Accordingly, this paper will also discuss the likely impacts of three changes in the context of health care on the management of physician error. These are (1) the growth of the number of physicians employed in organizational contexts in a buyer's market; (2) the increased surveillance by state medical boards and third-party payers; and (3) the impact of the malpractice risk on physician and hospital behavior.

The Definition of Error

Any discussion of social control in medicine must face the profound difficulty of defining what an "error" is. Two limitations are worth mentioning here. The first is the chronic uncertainty that inheres in medical practice (Davis 1960; Fox 1957). Only in the rare case can the physician say this patient has x and we must do y. Even when a patient certainly has x, this does not dictate treatment, which may vary according to the severity of x, the patient's age, the physician's "treatment philosophy," and the technology available in any practice setting. For some disorders, learned colleagues disagree over what is the treatment of choice. More often than not, physicians are compelled by the patient's pain, suffering, and downhill course to do something before all uncertainty is resolved. Not all actions that hindsight proves wrong are mistakes. To understand how social controls operate in the medical profession we must pay attention to how physicians draw the line between what is a reasonable treatment option, given the facts at hand, and what is an error. Below we shall consider how other actors—managers, lawyers, and insurance companies—apply different rules of thumb than do physicians.

The second limitation in defining error has to do with the variability in different specialities between the physician's action, on the one hand, and the patient's response on the other. In some areas of medicine where interventions are diffuse and relatively nonspecific, such as psychiatry, identifying a mistake is very difficult (Light 1980). In other areas, such as surgery, interventions are more precise, and presumably mistakes are easier to identify (Bosk 1979). Moreover, it is not just typical interventions that define with what ease or difficulty mistakes are labeled; practice setting is an important variable as well (Freidson 1975). For the physician's work to be suspect, it needs to be observable by others. The risk of being accused of serious "error" varies with surveillance (Coser 1961; Stelling and Bucher 1972). In the more traditional forms of practice, observability was minimal. As practice shifts to more collective forms, with greater centralization of record keeping and greater input among a variety of specialities, physician performance is becoming more observable both by colleagues and by others.

Error is a relative term. Its definition shifts with the context in which care is delivered. Rather than apply an absolute definition of error, we need to look at each stage of a physician's career and ask what performances are monitored and how; what kinds of conduct is blameworthy; and what kind of negative sanctions follow its discovery. By following this procedure for three stages of medical career—studenthood, residency, and practice, we develop a sense of how the profession imagines the ideal doctor and how it responds when the real diverges too sharply from the ideal. Further, we are then in a position to see how intramural definitions of care are altered by changes in the organization of care.

Social Control in Medical School

The socialization into the medical profession is one of the core topics in the social science literature on medicine. By socialization, sociologists mean that set of rites, rituals, and ordeals that transforms outsiders into insiders, that makes professionals out of laypersons. As important as this extended adult education is, the most potent social control that the medical profession exercises is in the selection of students. The competition for medical school admission is keen. In recent years the ratio of applicants to space has hovered around 2 to 1. Taking into account the surprisingly low attrition rate from medical schools —in 1979 less than 0.5 percent of the nation's 63,000 medical students permanently dropped out—which students are admitted plays a critical role in determining the character of the medical profession. Moreover, even though applications still exceed places available in medical school by a wide margin, applications to medical school have been decreasing in recent years. This decrease is an index of the declining glory in being a physician. At the same time, if this trend continues, it raises questions about how effective screening is as the primary mechanism of social control.

The selection criteria used by medical schools have been criticized for overvaluing "hard" measures of achievement, such as grades in science and Medical College Admission Test scores, and undervaluing "soft" measures of a student's fitness to be a physician, such as humanitarian concern—an admittedly difficult attribute to measure reliably. The emphasis on hard measures, combined with the surfeit of applicants, is said to create an unhappy competitive atmosphere on college campuses. This atmosphere allegedly often produces students who are intensely unempathic, aggressive, and less interested in patients than is necessary for compassionate caring. Even if one agrees that more attention needs to be paid to "soft" criteria in choosing medical students, a number of problems remain: Which soft measures? How reliable are they as predictors of performance? Beyond that lies another problem. Students are remarkably adept at inferring what the faculty wants to hear. How would admissions committees distinguish sincerely compassionate candidates from those merely presenting themselves consistent with desired criteria? These difficulties aside, there has been little systematic study of the undergraduate environment's impact on those who become medical students; this topic clearly deserves further exploration. I advance only a modest claim here; namely, the selection process rewards and reenforces little else but intellectual achievement. This is the first step in learning to think about the responsibilities of the doctor's work in a narrow technocratic rather than in a broader humanitarian frame.

What selection emphasizes, undergraduate medical school curricula reinforce. It is as if there are two curricula—one is public and shared; the other is private and personal. The public and shared curriculum involves the mastery of the body of cognitive knowledge that makes a physician. It is a world of tests, national boards, and universalistic measures. A major study of this phase of the medical curriculum is *Boys in White* by Becker et al. (1961). This study asks, How do students set the level and direction of their effort? The authors stress the importance of situational factors (as opposed to internalized values and norms) in influencing behavior. Not surprisingly, the faculty is the most critical situational factor in shaping the student response to medical school. Students structure their lives so that they can meet faculty demands. The idealism and altruism that are said to be part of medical work are extinguished as students meet the niggling demands of faculty. This pattern, found in the classroom experience of the preclinical years, follows students into the wards when they encounter patients for the first time. Students work hard when faculty are likely to notice or, more rarely, when such efforts benefit the student by expanding his or her clinical mastery. When these conditions are absent, students safely ignore their responsibilities—they "drylab" tests, make themselves scarce, and think nothing of leaving peers with extra work. In *Boys in White* the watchful eye of superordinate authority is the only effective social control. The closest analogy to *Boys in White* is an elementary school classroom. The teacher steps out and all decorum quickly deteriorates. While there is little reason to question the general findings of Becker and his associates, a major shortcoming of *Boys in White* is that it neglects to detail the variability in approach among medical students. Undoubtedly many students do only what is necessary to get by; others, however, strive to excel. How effort is distributed throughout a class varies. Factors that account for such variation are the internal disposition of students, their career aspirations, and the reward system employed by the medical school. Becker and his associates pay scant attention to any of those factors responsible for variations within a student group.

The other curriculum, the one that is private and personal, is detailed in the work of Renée C. Fox (1957, 1963, 1979). Fox's work begins with the premise that medical work involves

certain recurring existential or human conditions problems: problems of uncertainty, limitation, and emotional equipoise. The work itself is based on observations in settings quintessentially medical: the anatomy lab and the autopsy. Fox then analyzes the defense mechanisms that students develop to cope with the disturbing events that are part of medical work. Students learn to joke, intellectualize, and engage in probabilistic reasoning. In Fox's writings, social control becomes a matter of individual conscience and not omnipresent superordinate authority.

When joined, these works provide a rather complete view of how social controls operate during the student phase of a medical career. On the one hand, there is the cognitive body of materials to be mastered—the technical dimension of the doctor's work. Social controls are formal, explicit, and external. On the other hand, medical work has a moral or a normative dimension. Social control here is informal, implicit, and internal. Rather than the explicit and universal standards that mark the cognitive phase of the curriculum, one finds that behavior is reproached by allusion, parable, and mock-ironic jokes. Normative standards are very rarely an explicit part of the curriculum. More often than not they are a topic of structured silence. That is to say, it appears that there are topics about which physicians agree not to talk and that these topics comprise the psychologically most troubling aspects of medical work: intractable pain and suffering, physician impotence, and the frustrations built into the healer role. The general lesson here is that some parts of the doctor's work are public and accessible to control while others are private and should not be meddled with. This pattern continues throughout a physician's career.

Social Control in Residency

The major research on student socialization in medical school was completed during the 1950s. This emphasis is sensible if one considers where doctors were coming from and where they were going at the time. First recruits were a remarkably homogenous group, whatever variable—race, gender, class—one choses to measure. Beyond that, in the early 1950s the majority of physicians still considered themselves general practitioners, so there was a great similarity of occupational destination as well. In the 1950s when sociologists concentrated on the medical school, they had ample reason: this phase of schooling was the formative experience for a relatively homogenous group of recruits into a stable profession.

What was once the preserve of the profession as a whole has now become the province of residency. As occupational destinations have diverged, residency has replaced medical school as the summative statement of one's professional identity. Norms now crystallize around specialties. Residents learn what it is to be a physician by learning to think, act, feel like a specialist—be it a sur-geon, an obstetrician-gynecologist, a psychiatrist, or an internist.

If, on an individual level, residency shapes attitudes about care at a more macrolevel, residencies shape the overall structure of medical work, sorting the graduates of medical schools into the twenty-three diploma-granting specialities, and then sorting them again into niches within a specialty. Residencies provide different career opportunities for those within them. Some pave the way for academic careers by providing physicians with research training, funding sources, and contacts with research networks. Other residencies introduce younger physicians to an area's medical community and allow them to seek opportunities within a local market. In the short run, residency training determines what work one does, with whom, and under what conditions. In the long run, it is a substantial factor determining what kind of professional one becomes.

During training a resident learns a field's basic clinical problems, its treatment for them, and its philosophy of care. Beyond this, the resident learns a specialty's style, flavor, and way of doing things; the graduate medical student acquires the specialty's personality. Acquiring a specialty's personality has special significance for both teachers and students. For each it is evidence that a resident is making progress. On the one hand, residents use their clinical decisions as benchmarks to evaluate for themselves how well they exercise medical judgment. Residents who feel that they are not thinking about problems like their peers worry about the appropriateness of their career choice.

On the other hand, attending physicians find that residents who fail to absorb a specialty's approach "think wrong" about problems. Instances of "wrong thinking" by residents can be used by an attending to build a case that a resident lacks the intelligence, skills, or dedication needed to learn a specialty and that the resident should not be allowed to continue training. Further, attendings feel that residents who show good judgment are "our kind of people" and that "we can sleep well at night knowing that they are on call."

In residency training, learning is done under the pressure of time, through repetition, until responses become automatic. The educational philosophy that seems to guide the staffing of some residencies is that the less the coverage, the greater the clinical exposure, the more the learning. Given all this, mistakes in residency are seen as a regrettable but inevitable part of the baptism under fire that is house officer training.

All residents make mistakes. How residents manage error when it becomes manifest determines if the mistake is seen as innocent or blameworthy and if the resident develops a reputation as competent or negligent. An innocent mistake made by a competent resident has the following characteristics: the resident quickly recognizes the problem; the resident seeks appropriate help for it by informing the attending; the resident appears to have learned a "lesson" from the entire experience; and most important, the resident has not made the same mistake before on the same rotation. Errors with these characteristics are seen as part of the educational process. They allow attending

and resident to take the role of teacher and student respectively. The misadventure is reviewed retrospectively, the technical or judgmental error that led to the untoward result is identified, and a generalizable lesson is extracted from the whole sad experience.

A second type of error is seen as blameworthy. Such mistakes have the following characteristics: the resident failed to recognize a problem sufficiently early or attempted to cover the mistakes up; the resident failed to seek appropriate help; the resident failed to improve performance over successive trials; and the resident had made the same mistake previously, on the same service. Errors with these characteristics are not viewed as part of the ordinary educational process. Rather, they signal that a resident fails to possess the skills or honor the commitments that lifelong practice in a specialty requires. When such mistakes occur, attendings often approach residents, eager to punish. Public dressing-downs are not uncommon. Such action serves a number of purposes. It exacts a measure of retribution for the insult to the profession's integrity. At the same time, stern measures in the face of blameworthy error serve a general deterrent function; a warning is sent to more innocent residents about what to expect if they stand accused of blameworthy error.

Needless to say, residents fear being labeled as the kind of person who makes blameworthy errors. They dislike the everyday sanction of a public dressing-down and its attendant humiliation. But, more important, they fear more consequential sanctions of being blocked in their career by separation from a training program. Beyond that, residents fear being mislabeled. They are apprehensive that a small unrepresentative sample of their work will damn them forever and that, once labeled, all their work will go unnoticed.

Some features of the evaluation process make resident fears far from groundless. First, deciding whether a resident makes blameless or blameworthy mistakes is a clinical judgment based on the teaching faculty's observations and impressions of the resident in a limited period of time, usually one or two rotations. This clinical diagnosis is built on behavioral indicators, such as the resident's ability to accept criticism, his or her enthusiasm or pleasantness while meeting faculty demands, and his or her grooming. (Sometimes sloppiness is interpreted as a sign that an individual lacks the close attention to detail that medicine requires. At other times sloppiness is read as a lack of effort.)

Strikingly, this decision-making process has elements of a self-fulfilling prophecy. If a resident is considered trustworthy, monitoring is decreased and therefore deficiencies are less likely to be discovered. Conversely, if a resident is suspect, monitoring increases, thus increasing the probability that errors will be discovered. Errors so discovered confirm the suspicion that the resident is engaged in a pattern of behavior that is, arguably, negligent.

Another striking feature of the process is the apparently arbitrary nature of the paper record. In perusing the folders of residents in one training program that I studied, I found only one evaluation that mentioned a specific incident (Bosk 1979, 148–165). If this program's records are not unrepresentative, they reveal a potential problem in the social control system of residencies. On the one hand, residents who are dismissed from programs, without a paper record that justifies such an action, have a case that their "due process" rights have been violated. On the other hand, excessive documentation may create a work environment in which neither resident nor attending are comfortable. There is no gainsaying that balancing trust in a colleague's judgment with the resident's right to an impartial evaluation process is a complex issue. At the moment there is agreement on neither the process by which residents are evaluated nor on topics of that evaluation.

There is much ambivalence about how to deal with normative concerns in residency training. Bosk (1979) has found that normative mistakes are among the most serious that a resident can make. Yet those same physicians who find normative mistakes so calamitous when they are made by residents, disattend them when they are made by senior surgeons. What is labeled an indicator of "morals and ethics" for a resident is categorized a matter of "style, philosophy, and personality" in a senior physician. When training ends, an abiding concern for normative matters vanishes. What was proper surveillance of a resident is illegitimate meddling in the affairs of a peer. So, once training ends, a concern with normative matters is out of bounds. Such matters become private business, a topic of professional silence rather than debate. The visibility of normative matters in training serves a modeling function:

the community standards are publicly displayed and applied, but unevenly, only within the boundaries of a training institution and only upon residents. When training is completed, the resident is expected to have internalized the normative standards of the profession. Once this happens, problems are generally ignored.

That normative standards are taken seriously in residency and then disattended has great consequences for failing residents and the profession as a whole. First, most failing residents are able to secure positions in other training programs either within the same or in other specialties (Klineberg 1984). Thus residents can easily neutralize their failures by claiming that they were involved in a "personality conflict" or that the failing could not have been so serious or they would have been more seriously sanctioned. But, all things considered, they are still in training to be physicians. Just as significantly, that the profession as a whole tolerates in senior members what it punishes in junior members is a signal that these failings are not so serious to begin with. They need not concern physicians outside of residency too greatly. There are a few exceptions to this general rule, which we shall discuss later under the topic of impaired physicians.

Social Control in the Medical Career

Sociologists have easier access to academic settings than to any other site of medical practice. Moreover, student life is highly structured. It is safer to generalize across training institutions than across the whole diverse range of settings within which medicine is practiced. Nonetheless, studenthood is a small slice of a medical career. Physicians may practice thirty to forty years after leaving training. The social controls that are exercised over the course of a career deserve more attention than they have received to date.

Eliott Freidson has shown that physician sensitivity to social controls varies with the type of practice network. Freidson identified two distinct types: client- and colleague-dependent. Client-dependent physicians are by and large in solo practice. Consumer satisfaction rather than peer approval determines the economic survival of these professionals. This finding leads Freidson to suggest that where the two conflict, client-dependent physicians have an incentive to give professional standards somewhat short shrift. Colleague-dependent practice is a pole apart from the client-dependent type. Here, the physician's business depends upon referral from colleagues. As a result, doctors are responsive to the opinions and standards of peers. Freidson works from two principles. Where colleagues control rewards, they have an impact on the quality of practice. Where they do not, their opinions about what constitutes good practice can be safely ignored.

A second aspect of Freidson's work that bears on this discussion of medical error is his study (Freidson 1975) of social controls in a colleague-dependent network. In this setting, a comprehensive prepaid medical group, consumers who paid a yearly fee were provided a full range of services by salaried physicians whose credentials were above average. Freidson's site then afforded the opportunity to study social controls in the world of the HMO, a world that maximized the possibility of discovering errors:

> All physicians worked together in the same setting and saw the same patients, with a certain record system to which each physician would add his notes and which each physician could examine. Therefore, each physician's work could be more open to the examination of the others and each could be considerably more subject to the exercise of direct social control by the others than would be the case if they all worked separately scattered about in their individual offices. (P. 17)

All the preconditions for effective social control by peers of peers were present; what was lacking was an ongoing, efficient sanction system. There are several reasons for this situation. First, centralized records notwithstanding, colleagues knew little of one another's performance. The only direct knowledge was from episodic referrals, which most physicians felt were a too biased sample to draw hard conclusions. Most knowledge was gathered indirectly, its source being colleague gossip and patient complaints. Not surprisingly, there was considerable reluctance to base definitive action on this kind of unreliable hearsay testimony.

Next, there was considerable ambiguity about what was blameworthy error. The bright light test used by all physicians to identify and condemn unacceptable behavior was "gross and blatant" incompetence. As a result, blameworthy behavior was a rare event, the ceiling for it having been raised so high. Good reasons were found to explain and excuse straying from the norm. As a rule, errors and mistakes were occasion for correction rather than reproach. Another reason for the physician's reluctance to invoke formal sanctions was that they were limited and drastic. As a result such sanctions were more often threatened than applied. (As group practice evolves and becomes more standardized, it is likely that the range of available sanctions will expand. If this happens, the stress involved in physicians' disciplining errant colleagues will be lessened.)

The unavailability of formal sanctions led physicians to evolve an informal sanction system. Physicians complained to errant colleagues. If this failed to achieve results, a physician might take his complaints to his peers in the staff lunchroom. Sandwich sanctions present a risk to the complaining physician. Unless colleagues also have doubts about the target of the gossip, the complaining physician may be damned as overly perfectionist. Options are available to the offended physician who chooses not to subject a peer to lunchroom sanctions. Minimally, a physician can refuse favors to a colleague he deems unworthy. Maximally, he can organize a private boycott by refusing to refer patients to the offending colleague. Social controls that are private and personal predominate, despite the public and impersonal nature of the practice setting.

Freidson characterized the physician group he studied as a "delinquent subcommunity." By this phrase he meant that "its norms and practices were such as to both draw all members together defensively in a common front against the outside world of laity and, internally, to allow each his freedom to act as willed" (p. 244). Freidson's group seems to be the apotheosis of the socialization system described by Bosk. Individual conscience is the measure of all things; other sources of criticism are just so much meddling.

At a policy level, Freidson doubts that external controls over medical performance will ever be an adequate source of control. His work, in fact, demonstrates how easily physicians are able to neutralize and evade such control. As a result, Freidson argues that the best hope for improvement is an augmented collective spirit of service that permits the group to "both seek out and correct deviation without destroying discretion or commitment" (p. 258). How such a spirit is generated remains a mystery. Freidson's work, when added to the work on social controls, leads but to one conclusion: once formal licensing requirements are met, the profession abdicates its collective social control responsibilities to individual practitioners in all but cases of the most spectacular abuse.

Such a conclusion, however, needs softening. First, one needs to consider the growth of continuing medical education, a development that has taken place with the encouragement of the American Medical Association and the specialty boards. In 1978 half of all doctors spent $1,350 or more on accredited refresher courses. That such courses are tax deductible does not detract from the involvement of physicians in their own professional growth.

The second development is a recent intense interest in the "impaired physician." An awareness is growing in the profession of the costs of the ever-present stresses of medical work. "Impairment" is workplace injury to physicians. Alcoholism, drug addiction, the loss of psychic balance, the inability to make necessary concessions to advancing age—all these are defined as impairment. The concept of impairment medicalizes the deviance of physicians (Morrow 1984). This medicalization of deviance is not limited to the medical profession but has occurred in other societal domains as well. When the process is complete, deviance is a sickness that needs to be treated rather than an evil that needs to be punished. Most important, impairment allows physicians to manage social control problems in terms they are familiar with —the language of sickness—and in arenas they control—the domain of therapy.

While the concern with impairment is laudable, it also raises a number of concerns. Chief among these is, By what mechanisms are the impaired identified? There is no reason to believe that the rate of alcoholism, drug dependence, emotional instability, or whatever is any less among physicians than among the general population. However, the number of physicians who voluntarily come forward or who are brought to the notice of appropriate authorities is far fewer than any estimates one would make given base population. One problem then is how to channel those physicians who need help into appropriate programs. At the same time, we need to make sure that the blameless are not subject to harassment. In addition, problems of impairment are often those very conditions that physicians are not so successful in treating in the general population. If physicians are to participate in nonpunitive programs to meliorate their impairment, then these programs need careful monitoring and evaluation. Further, how the impaired are reintegrated into professional networks also needs careful consideration. Whatever one may say about impairment (for example, the most cynical may see such concerns as nothing more than an attempt to avoid more onerous external controls), the fact remains that the medical profession has taken the lead in a problem that is by no means limited to the medical profession. Much in the identification and treatment of impairment goes against the norm of colleague autonomy. How the tensions this creates are managed is a topic for further study.

Other Contexts, Other Controls

Physicians generally aver that the patient's best defense against error and incompetence is the individual practitioner's integrity and skill. Continuing medical education and state disciplinary boards are devices for monitoring and maintaining the ethic of individual self-regulation on which the profession rests. If physicians controlled the medical marketplace, this discussion of social control in medicine could end here. But the present conditions under which care is given and received and bought and sold, are more complex. Physicians have lost whatever exclusive claims they had to define the professional standard of error and responsibility. Medical error, waste, and incompetence is like health care itself: a whole parade of interest groups have a large stake in saying what it is and how it is managed. We shall consider below three stakeholders whose power to define errors has increased relative to physicians over the last ten years: (1) managers; (2) state regulatory agencies; and (3) patients who retain counsel.

Managers

There is growing recognition that a workforce problem exists in medicine. We have as a society more physicians than we need. Within this surplus, some regions are undersupplied and some specialities are understaffed. At the same time, care is costly, and these costs have risen faster than the general inflation rate. Both of these factors indicate that resources are being utilized inefficiently. Now to these two factors add a third: health care is increasingly an employee benefit. Rather than pay directly for health care, employees are typically enrolled in health care groups at work, either through third-party insurers or health maintenance organizations. This collectivization in the financing of health care has unsettled what we think of as ideal service. Emerging definitions stress economically efficient service both in the private sector where health care is an employee benefit and in the public sphere where it is a public cost. As a result, managers have gained a new ascendance in health care delivery.

What difference do managers make to medical definitions of error? If we assume that managers ration scarce resources, then it is easy to see how they become the official arbiters of what constitutes efficient service (Alper 1984). In order to make rational decisions by weighing costs and benefits, managers need data: What is the average length of stay following gallbladder surgery? How many elective arthoscopes does the average orthopedic surgeon perform? What is the most efficient procedure for a GI workup? Answering each of these questions involves compiling and aggregating practice profiles. A manager's routine activities threaten implicitly the medical profession's presumption that all colleagues finished with training participate equally in the ethic of skill and integrity. Managers make transparent what the profession would prefer to keep opaque: How each physician measures up against his peers. Physicians, of course, remain free to dispute managers' utilitarian definitions of efficiency.

To the degree that managers, not physicians, determine the bottom line, the balance of power in social control shifts away from physicians. The bottom line of manager removes some of the mystery from judgments of competence, some of the quality of "this is something only another physician can tell." One need not be a peer to recognize a statistical outlier. At the very least outliers need explanation. Persistent, repeated outliers deserve very close scrutiny. A world of such statistical precision and reliability, where the manager's bottom line tells the whole story, is, as any physician is quick to point out, nothing more than a managerial fantasy. Nonetheless, the point remains that managers push health-care-policy makers into making assessments of competence more standardized, more formal, and more objective. Further, the increased quantification of standards of care opens up the possibilities for recognizing a scale of competence that has many levels rather than the binary decision of skilled or incompetent. Physicians' salaries can then be tied to production; their activity can be limited to their own certified areas of procedural competence. Managers make the oversight of professional licensing as much an institutional as a professional concern. Controlling the resultant operational conflict is a critical policy issue. The trend has been to broaden the managers' stake in the outcome by recognizing the institution's liability in practice. Moreover, the oversupply of physicians allows managers to assert, with greater authority than was true when Freidson made his observations, the managerial standard of what is a mistake and how seriously it should be treated. With oversupply, there is little need to treat physicians with the care and circumspection due a scarce resource.

Managerial determinations of appropriate medical care are system centered. They are potentially in conflict with a patient-centered Hippocratic idea that requires the physician to "do something to help the patient" while pledging "to do no harm." The Hippocratic standard does not require that physicians consider the allocation of resources. Therefore, to the degree that managerial determinations are developed into treatment policies, discretion is removed from physicians. Whenever discretion is removed, physicians are freed to see their work in terms of its profane workaday rather than its sacred dimensions. Being a doctor becomes a matter of working at a job rather than laboring in a calling. When this change occurs, physicians have little incentive to act as advocates for any individual patient, and they increasingly frame decisions in terms of the good of the group. Moreover there is some ambiguity here about whose good is in question: Is it the sum of all patients, those who pay the pipers, or the pipers themselves?

Built into any increase in the managerial power in health care is the potential for conflict with medical authority. Each conflict inevitably focuses physicians on the fact that managers are in many domains the supervisory personnel. A fundamental question then becomes, What happens to the quality of physician work when autonomy is narrowed? When the physician recognizes that he or she is in the position of a worker? Surely physicians do not begin to act like assembly-line workers whose small acts of sabotage and larceny enliven an otherwise dull day? Since the residual autonomy vested in physicians is large, do they merely ignore this incursion and proceed as if the world of the clinic has not changed at all?

In the future, social controls in medicine will be largely determined by the unraveling of the following factors: Managers will have great influence as efforts are made to contain costs while maintaining quality. The influence of physicians will wane, partly because of oversupply and partly because of routinization of clinical care in the interest of efficiency. Inevitably physicians will, through this procedure, become proletarianized to a degree. The impact this will have on the profession's service ethic remains unclear. To what degree the medical profession adopts a "trade union" stance also is an open question (Marcus 1984). Further, these new political and practice arrangements may yield social control arrangements that look more like factory discipline in a union shop than professional self-regulation.

State Disciplinary Boards

States exhibit great variability in suspending and revoking medical licenses (Feinstein 1985). Some state boards take no action at all; others are quite aggressive. Many of these cases involve impaired physicians. Inactive states notwithstanding, it appears that oversight of medical performance is increasing. This increased surveillance includes prosecution for welfare chiseling (Medicare fraud and abuse), substance abuse, and sexual harassment of patients. All of this monitoring effects a greater willingness by the state to intrude on practice.

Social controls are likely to have a number of consequences. First, the awareness of increased surveillance is likely to encourage greater caution, circumspection, and even compliance with formal rules among physicians. Bentham once remarked that "the watchful eye of the public is the conscience of the statesman." Likewise, increased surveillance ups the ante for those physicians who might otherwise be tempted to commit acts of petty or grand larceny. Next, the public attention directed to the wrongs of physicians is a factor in eroding further the authority and trust extended to members of the profession. Each occasion of a physician publicly accused of wrongdoing makes the next case easier to imagine. All of this suggests that increased enforcement has built into it elements of self-fulfilling prophecy and deviance-amplifying effects. This effect is then likely to generate new regulations to handle problems whose dimensions turn out to be greater than originally expected. For example, in May 1985 Pennsylvania passed legislation making it easier to suspend physicians' licenses while disciplinary proceedings are progressing. Finally, the willingness to treat as criminal certain aspects of physician performance puts great pressure on the profession to step up its own social control mechanism, if only to avoid the good being stigmatized unfairly along with the unworthy.

Malpractice

The problems engendered by the malpractice crisis are worth a volume of their own. For the purposes of this chapter a few points need underscoring. Most important, malpractice actions are probably not an effective social control. Not all negligent errors by physicians have damages significant enough to pursue in a legal action. By the same token, not all serious damages are the result of a clearly negligent action by physicians although the courts often strain legal rules to allow injured patients to dip into the deep pocket of physicians' insurers.

Malpractice may not then be a very potent check on errant practice. To date, there is little reliable data on just how malpractice decisions affect the practice behavior of physicians. It is clear that the application of a broad standard of acceptable practice acts to deter involvement in technical areas outside one's competence, to spread risks through extensive consultation with colleagues, and generally to encourage caution.

To the degree that these defensive strategies involve more extensive procedures from a wide range of specialists, they push the cost of care upward. So it is possible that the problems of malpractice, when combined with the new managerial imperative, place physicians in a double bind (Stone 1985). This effect, however, can be considerably modified by the standard of care that the courts employ. If courts interpret "standard care" to be optimal treatment, then physicians' ability to cut costs is considerably compromised. However, if the courts interpret "standard care" as "reasonably affordable" procedures, then physicians can be judicially removed from the horns of this particular dilemma. Since the duty physicians owe to patients is a question for the judge and not the jury, this type of solution to the malpractice crisis is not beyond imagining.

On the one hand, the malpractice crisis points out how wide the gap is between physician and patient expectations of acceptable care. On the other hand, it indicates how little solidarity exists in the medical profession. Successful suits are not possible without expert witnesses. The breakdown of the "locality" rule for experts has demonstrated that physicians are more willing to testify against colleagues they need not work with daily. Malpractice situations show that the medical profession does not operate on the basis of a conspiracy of silence among like-minded professionals. Rather it documents the increased fragmentation and competing interests of physicians.

Conclusion

From this overview of social controls in medicine a few recurrent themes emerge. First, when viewing the internal dynamics of professional controls it appears that the vast majority of errors at all career stages are seen as blameless. Such errors are taken as opportunities to correct well-intended but wrong judgments or faulty techniques. There is much tolerance for such errors if for no other reason than that experience is a reliable teacher. A second type of error occurs which is rarely blameless. These errors are explained as the result of blatant and gross negligence, and are not tolerated. However, the standard for making them is set so high that they are rarely discovered. This is true for all levels of practice. However age, reputation, and rank provide older physicians protection against accusations of blameworthy error, protection that is not available to younger physicians. In general, the technical side of practice is monitored; the more subjective side of practice is considered personal and not subject to control.

As a result, in describing how responsibility is exercised in the face of medical error it is clear that the profession equates professional and individual controls. So long as the individual physician is responsible and conscientious, he or she is adequate. Where this is not the case, many small offenses to professional norms are tolerated without any collective response. A large outrageous offense often evokes a response. But between the saint and the moral cretin, there is a good deal of play in the system of social controls.

The professional standards for performance are quite forgiving, but they are not the only standards applied. Managers apply a criterion of efficiency quite different from that of physicians. State boards act punitively in areas that colleagues might ignore. Malpractice risk holds physicians accountable financially for negligent care. *Negligence* here is a judicially and not medically defined term. The general thrust of social controls is to hold physicians accountable to a wider range of interests with increasing societal power.

Within all of this change, there are some questions that the collectivity has yet to face. For example, there are few accurate estimates of how "perfect" we can expect medical care to be. Certainly there is no estimate of how much medical error is inevitable given the complexity of the work. That much said, it is clear that hierarchy and supervision exercise a potent constraining influence on individuals and that errors are fewer where they are present. Varieties of practice that provide more or less continuous supervision are likely to allow for the exercise of social control. Of course, at present physicians often define such forms of practice as punishment and do not generally welcome them. However, as the old forms of independent practice give way to new larger practice, this attitude will change. The key problem will then be sustaining a professional ethic of service in a bureaucratic setting hostile to it. How the problem is resolved depends to a large degree on how clearly competing interests are identified and resolved.

References

Alper, P. R. 1984. The new language of hospital management. *New England Journal of Medicine* 312(5):309–312.

Becker, H., B. Geer, E. Hughes, and A. Strauss. 1961. *Boys in white: Student culture in medical school.* Chicago: University of Chicago Press.

Bosk, C. 1979. *Forgive and remember: Managing medical failure.* Chicago: University of Chicago Press.

Coser, R. 1961. Insulation from observability and types of social control. *American Sociological Review* 26:28–39.

Davis, F. 1960. Uncertainty in medical prognosis. *American Journal of Sociology* 66:41–47.

Feinstein, R. J. 1985. The ethics of professional regulation? *New England Journal of Medicine* 312(12):801–804.

Fox, R. C. 1957. Training for uncertainty. In *The student physician*, ed. R. K. Merton, G. Reader, and P. Kendall, pp. 207–245. Cambridge: Harvard University Press.

———. 1979. The autopsy: Its place in the attitude learning of second-year medical students. In *Essays in medical sociology: Journeys into the field*, pp. 51–77. New York: John Wiley and Sons.

Fox, R. C., and H. Lief. 1963. Training for "detached concern" in medical students. In *The psychological basis of medical practice*, ed. H. Lief, V. Lief, and N. Lief, pp. 12–35. New York: Harper and Row.

Freidson, E. 1960. Client control and medical practice. *American Journal of Sociology* 65:374–382.

———. 1975. *Doctoring together.* New York: Elsevier.

Klineberg, J. 1984. Resident evaluation in internal medicine. Speech delivered at a meeting of American Board of Medical Specialties, Chicago, Ill.

Light, D. 1980. *Becoming psychiatrists.* New York: W. W. Norton.

Marcus, S. 1984. Trade unionism for doctors: An idea whose time has come. *New England Journal of Medicine* 311(23):1508–1511.

Mechanic, D. 1985. Public perceptions of medicine. *New England Journal of Medicine* 312(3):181–183.

Morrow, C. 1984. The medicalization of professional self-governance: A sociological approach. In *Social controls and the medical profession*, ed. J. Swazey and S. Scher, pp. 163–184. Boston: Eelgeschlager, Gunn and Hain.

Starr, P. 1983. *The social transformation of American medicine.* New York: Basic Books.

Stelling, J., and R. Bucher. 1972. Autonomy and monitoring on hospital wards. *Sociological Quarterly* 13:431–447.

Stone, A. A. 1985. Law's influence on medicine and medical ethics. *New England Journal of Medicine* 312(5):309–312.

Part V

Organization and Delivery of Health Services

Chapter 22

Payment Systems and Their Effects

William A. Glaser

Paying the doctor and the hospital have become perennial policy issues, dominating the headlines and absorbing much of the energy of governments worldwide. Every society's resources can be strained by rapidly increasing payments, and conflicts of interest over shares arise among powerful contestants.

Paying the Doctor

Health care has evolved paradoxically. In Europe and North America, the doctor began as a self-employed small businessman, while the hospital evolved from a charity sponsored by churches and voluntary associations. Doctors have always charged their patients, but hospitals have done so only during the last century. Doctors have always set fees covering both their personal income targets and their operating costs, while hospitals have usually earned no more than their costs. Many doctors have earned large incomes, but hospitals have constantly struggled to break even. Doctors have bought their own equipment and buildings from earnings, but hospitals traditionally have depended on charitable gifts and public grants.

The trend in the United States has been away from self-employed solo practice while preserving traditional payment methods. More than one-half of American office doctors now are organized in partnerships, and in single- or multispecialty groups. Fewer than one-half remain solo practitioners, and many individuals have become "professional corporations" to insulate themselves from financial risks and to take advantage of tax laws (American Medical Association 1984, 15). In contrast, European doctors have preserved the model of solo practice, having been guaranteed their costs and incomes by the official fee schedules of national health insurance.

Fee-for-Service

Methods. In nearly every developed country, the large majority of doctors have been paid like any other small businessman. They traditionally set a price for each service, with higher prices for the more time-consuming and the more resource-consuming procedures. The doctor was paid by the patient in cash or in kind. As medical practice became more complex, the services and fees became more varied. Left alone, each doctor preferred to set his own charges and manage his own finances. Competition might limit the range of fees in a community, but the more celebrated and more popular doctors could charge more.

The trend in Europe and Canada has been to standardize fees and make them public. Throughout the twentieth century, growing proportions of every population have been enrolled in official health insurance programs, either voluntarily or under compulsory social security laws. The revenue of the health insurance carriers has come from social security payroll taxes. Doctors would prefer to increase their charges without limit, while the sickness funds would prefer to use their monopoly power to offer very low fees or to hire doctors as salaried employees. The compromise has been fee schedules governing all doctors, all patients, and all sickness funds. The fee schedules are negotiated between medical associations and a collective bargaining unit from all the sickness funds. Doctors no longer bill patients, except in the voluntary, supplementary, and unregulated private practice; they bill the carriers. Usually doctors are not allowed to bill patients beyond the official rates paid by sickness funds (Glaser 1970, 1977).

Medical professionals everywhere resist the standardization, price controls, and scrutiny inherent in national health insurance, but everywhere they eventually surrender. Few doctors can survive financially outside statutory health insurance, since nearly the entire population takes advantage of its benefit packages. Doctors grudgingly accept the fee schedules and related rules as the price of a guaranteed high income.

The medical profession in the United States so far has preserved its financial independence by successfully fighting off enactment of general statutory health insurance. Instead, America has a mosaic of public and private payment programs, each with different rules covering the physician's fees (Showstack et al. 1979). Some third parties pay the doctor directly; these include Medicare (if the doctor agrees), Medicaid (if the doctor accepts such cases), and Blue Shield (in half the states). Most third-party arrangements indemnify the patient according to a benefit schedule, and the doctor can charge the patient more at his discretion; such third-party arrangements include Medicare (in two-thirds of the claims), Blue Shield (in half the states), and the many commercial insurance policies. As much as one-third of doctors' fees may be paid by patients out-of-pocket because doctors charge more than the insurance allowance or because the patient has limited medical care insurance (Freeland and Schendler 1984, 55). In other developed countries, few citizens lack coverage, and cost sharing by insured patients is small or absent.

Effects on the style of clinical practice. Since higher fees are earned for complex procedures (Burney et al. 1979, 68–69; Hsiao and Stason 1979), the doctor in theory has an incentive to perform more complex treatments, to substitute more technical for less technical work, and to adopt the newest methods. He is motivated to avoid primary care—particularly the elements of discussion and counseling in general practice, pediatrics, and geriatrics—in favor of the more technical specialties. American doctors are not controlled by strict fee schedules and can set fees sufficiently high to cover the costs of practice, the depreciation of equipment, and the repayment of debts.

Many influences besides financial incentives orient American medical practice toward advanced technical work. American medical schools attract students who already are highly interested in applied science, technology, and practical action (Coombs and Vincent 1971), and their curricula reinforce that viewpoint (Rezler 1974). Medical schools and teaching hospitals for both undergraduate and graduate medical education have the most advanced equipment, teach diagnosis by extensive testing, and encourage research to validate the newest methods (Lewis and Sheps 1983).

Highest prestige is associated with the most technically advanced clinical fields, such as the surgical subspecialties. The highest incomes are earned by the specialties using advanced equipment, namely, the surgical subspecialties with lower volumes and high unit fees, and several specialties that use productive equipment and staffing to generate very high volume at low unit fees (radiology, anesthesiology, and pathology) (Goldfarb 1981; American Medical Association 1983c). Therefore, in the United States many more physicians specialize than in other countries (American Medical Association 1983a, 15, 18; Mejia, Pizurki, and Royston 1979, 138). In the articles and advertisements in professional journals, in demonstrations at professional meetings, and in visits to hospitals, the large and dynamic medical equipment industry encourages doctors to investigate and routinely use the newest devices.

In the face of this formidable array of economic incentives, professional norms, and social influences, a serious problem is whether the medical profession can be induced to give enough attention to primary care, counseling, and services that depend primarily on cognitive skills. Fee-for-service is also used to pay for such services, but billings for nontechnical office visits and prolonged patient contacts yield lower incomes. A considerable policy literature and many demonstration projects search for methods of reorganizing medical practice. But the reformers shrink from abolishing fee-for-service in the surgical and technical specialties and shrink from substituting a flat-rate method that will place all specialties on the same footing.

Technically advanced acute care under American fee-for-service yields high incomes and prestige. But money alone does not dictate career choice. The highest incomes are earned by physicians in radiology and anesthesiology, but these areas attract only limited recruits since doctors prefer work that involves direct patient care as well as technical procedures (Lee 1984, 49–50).

Effects on distribution of services. Self-employed small businessmen, such as office-based doctors, serve customers who can pay. In the absence of methods to redistribute patients' purchasing power, the doctors who are more specialized, who offer more amenities in their practice, who come from higher classes, and who aim at higher incomes, seek a more affluent clientele. Doctors with less elaborate office amenities and less training have less prosperous patients. Doctors, and particularly specialists, cluster in the larger cities containing the largest numbers of paying patients.

National health insurance in Europe redistributes purchasing power among patients and reduces the link between social class and medical practice. Subscribers and taxpayers pay into sickness funds in relation to their incomes, patients are covered by high standard fees, and subscribers can visit the doctor without facing economic barriers. All doctors earn sufficient income to maintain adequate offices throughout the country. Some richer patients still visit urban specialists privately and pay cash or use private insurance to cover higher fees, but the average doctor receives standard rates for all or nearly all patients. Under national health insurance, the doctors' clinical decisions are much less affected by pecuniary incentives.

The United States has narrowed but not eliminated the differentials in fees paid by patients of different social classes and different regions. In contrast to statutory health insurance with standard rates applying to all payers, the United States has a mélange of different insurers covering different social groups and paying different fee levels. Patients insured by commercial companies and by Blue Shield executive plans provide the highest payments (when doctors bill the carriers) and can pay additional amounts in cash. Blue Shield's formula for "usual, customary, and reasonable" fees is more generous than that of Medicare. Doctors may feel defensive when refusing assignment under Medicare, but many try to charge more than Medicare's official rate; they cannot always extra-bill what they like, since elderly pensioners have limited incomes. Because so much of medical practice involves the elderly, doctors cannot avoid treating them, but generally doctors prefer a mix that includes more prosperous patients. The poor in America depend substantially on foreign-educated and foreign-born family doctors and usually must accept care by the salaried house staff when hospitalized. State Medicaid programs pay fees either by the Medicare formula or by low fee schedules, and therefore Medicaid recipients are less attractive to doctors. Few doctors practice in urban ghettoes and low-income rural areas. Poor persons without Medicaid and without cash —perhaps half of all persons below the official poverty line—must depend on the outpatient departments of hospitals, particularly municipal and rural public hospitals, where the medical care is given by salaried house staffs composed of junior doctors in training (Davidson 1980, esp. chaps. 6, 8; Davis and Schoen 1978; and Mitchell and Cromwell 1981).

The American method of deciding third-party fees perpetuates urban-rural differences rather than raising the levels in underdoctored areas. The calculations under the "usual, customary, and reasonable" methodology of Blue Shield and Medicare base current fees on the doctors' past charges and on the charges of other doctors in their area. Urban-rural differentials are perpetuated and steadily widen, since annual increases under Medicare are a constant percentage everywhere, representing the average increase in the cost of practice throughout the country. From the commercially insured patients—primarily city dwellers—the doctor can collect what he likes. Urban doctors' incomes remain higher because unit prices are higher, the volume of work is greater, and facilities support more expensive procedures (Burney and Gabel 1980; Cantwell 1979).

Effects on System Costs. Fee-for-service is believed to increase costs more than other payment systems do.

The doctor may be motivated to do more work, since income increases with volume. He is said to press for more technologically advanced and more expensive work, since his income rises with prices.

These hypotheses appear vindicated—if public policy permits the consequences. Developed countries using fee-for-service devote high proportions of their GNP to health, as in the United States, the Netherlands, Belgium, France, Germany, and Switzerland. However, the countries must be affluent. If a country's public policy is to spend much on health, it can do so even if doctors are salaried, as Sweden demonstrates (Maxwell 1981, chap. 3).

It is difficult to isolate the effects of fee-for-service from other factors that contribute to the same result. For example, a steady increase in use of diagnostic tests has been one of the most important reasons for the rapid growth of operating costs (Moloney and Rogers 1979). Testing has the financial advantage of yielding fees for the doctor and hospital without harming the patient. But other reasons for increases also exist, in addition to financial self-interest. Testing serves the widespread American medical philosophy of basing action on complete scientific knowledge. It also reduces the risk of lawsuits for malpractice.

Costs to the American system may not rise to their full potential. Instead of maximizing net income by the most profitable increases in both fees and work as demand grows, a long-term trend among doctors is to reduce their once burdensome hours and enjoy more leisure. They can accomplish this by raising fees—particularly by extra billing over third-party allowances—and pricing new procedures advantageously, so that they achieve a target income. While doctors' target incomes rise steadily, the system's total costs do not rise as high as they might under another theory, namely, the very high volume of a profit-maximizing medical profession. (The target income hypothesis and American evidence are in Feldstein 1983, chap. 9). Unlike a profit-maximizing business, American doctors until now have not seemed to organize their practices in the most efficient ways (Lee 1984). Germany spends a higher proportion of its GNP on doctors' services than America does because Germany's medical profession works longer hours, works more efficiently, and works more expensively.

Effects on Administration. An important reason for the enactment of statutory, universal, and standardized health insurance abroad is to make health finance stable and intelligible. Doctors and patients know the benefits and out-of-pocket payments in advance. Disputes and feelings of injustice are avoided. The population knows what it gets for its taxes.

The American health insurance system is so complex, heterogeneous, and changeable that the average American is very unclear about financing and benefits (Marquis 1983; Walden 1982). The Select Committee on Aging (U.S. Congress, House of Representatives 1978) found that salesmen can easily sell unnecessary and shallow insurance to the elderly. The payment of doctors is particularly confusing to patients since the American approach avoids standardization and rules in order to give maximum discretion to doctors. Under Medicare, a doctor is not required to accept assignment (i.e., forego extra billing) and can vary his practice with every bill, even with the same patient on successive days. Patients rarely know out-of-pocket payments in advance. Fees and out-of-pocket payments need not be the same, even for the same patient on successive visits, or for the same procedure by the same doctor on different visits. The patient gets unusually complicated bills from doctors, gets puzzling documents from third parties (either new bills or receipts reporting third-party payments to the doctor), and rarely understands them. For the same transaction with the doctor, the patient often has several third parties (such as Medicare and Medigap, Blue Shield and Major Medical), but he rarely can understand how they combine and how they may still leave him with out-of-pocket payments. A serious undercurrent in American health policy is discontent with fees and with an insurance system designed to please doctors.

To be paid in full, the American doctor for each procedure may have to bill both the patient (for out-of-pocket) and the patient's several third parties. To avoid financial uncertainty and administrative effort, doctors prefer to collect full payment from the patient and let the patient seek reimbursement from the insurance carrier (American Medical Association 1983b). However, fees are now so high that this sequence is unrealistic, and most doctors seem to delay final billing of patients until the patients have exhausted third-party re-imbursement. All this results in high administrative costs to doctors, delays, and many bad debts.

Standardization in European national health insurance is designed to be simple and cheap in administration, but the American method of paying doctors is expensive as well as turbulent. A very busy office, such as Blue Cross and Blue Shield of greater New York, must process over forty thousand claims forms per day. Each medical procedure results in several bills by the doctor to the patient's third parties and to the patient, plus reminders. Investigations of Medicaid have revealed erroneous double payments of both the original bill and the reminders, and double payments may be common among all payers. The administrative costs of third parties absorb 4.5 percent of all American health care costs (Gibson, Waldo, and Levit 1983, 7, 20), in addition to the administrative burdens on doctors, other providers, and patients. About 10 percent of the average doctor's fee for an office visit covers his administrative costs (Cromwell, Sloan, and Mitchell 1980).

Salary

Methods. Some reformers propose eliminating fee-for-service and the biases it generates toward acute care, higher costs, and administrative disorder. Since salaries are associated with employment in organizations or in medical groups, the proposal implies a shift from self-employment.

America's salaried doctors at present work in hospitals, medical schools, government agencies (for example, public health physicians), and other organizations. These units can be owned by private associations, by government, or by the doctors themselves. In health care organizations as well as establishments in other sectors, salaries are usually structured by rank and job title; they may or may not vary among the departments of the organization; the individual usually receives annual increases (or other periodic increases) for seniority. Contracts specify duties for certain lengths of time. Unlike most other employees of health care organizations, many hospital doctors are part time. The salary scale for the organization's doctors may be unique to that group; or the organization may follow a salary scale of a larger entity, such as the civil service of the government (Glaser 1970, chap. 4).

Usually salaried doctors do not receive their pay from the third parties that cover patient care, but the insurer or government Treasury pays the organization, and the organization pays the doctors. The doctors' pay is part of the organization's total budget.

Incentives from Salary. In theory, salaries should motivate doctors to give only the care patients need. Since the size of their incomes does not depend on the number of tasks —as under fee-for-service—clinical decision-making can be thorough and time consuming. Since incomes do not depend on the complexity of tasks—as under fee-for-service—salaried doctors in theory can give more supportive rather than technical care, they can diagnose by judgment rather than by overtesting. It is the organization rather than the doctor that owns expensive equipment. The doctor is under no pressure to overuse the equipment in order to amortize its purchase costs.

Salaried doctors are holders of ranks in an organization, and their rewards come from promotion and bonuses given by the management. Therefore, in theory they are motivated to cooperate with the policies of the organization and its owners, such as the containment of costs and the greater use of alternative delivery methods. If promotions and merit bonuses are given for better work, quality of care should improve. Thorough investigation and intellectual leadership should be rewarded; rapid and poor work should be discouraged. Research is rewarded.

Professional colleagueship in theory is promoted through similarity in rank and pay among different specialties. Wide gaps are avoided between those who earn much under fee-for-service (such as radiologists and surgeons) and those who earn much less (such as pediatricians and psychiatrists).

Salaries in theory induce doctors to fill jobs that do not pay fees, such as public health and medical administration. If the salaries are high enough, the doctors can forego outside private practice and are not on the lookout for potential private patients.

Trends. It is very difficult to assess the effects of salaries on medical practice in the United States because few salaried doctors provide primary and specialized care that is comparable to the work of self-employed fee-for-service doctors. Many salaried doctors work in hospitals as young house staff who help rather than compete with the attendings, who provide ambulatory care only to the indigent in OPDs, and who are studying as well as working. When they finish their salaried residencies they become typical office practitioners, usually paid by fee-for-service. Some salaried doctors are professors, researchers, and government administrators who provide little clinical care for patients during their salaried work time.

The total proportion of doctors on salary is slowly growing in the United States—52.6 percent of the total of 393,729 in late 1979—but some of the growth is due merely to the increase in the numbers of postgraduate students in residencies. The 52.6 percent includes 7.9 percent in salaried hospital jobs (most are not clinicians), 4.7 percent in the national government, and 8.6 percent in teaching, research, and administration (Kahn and Ortiz 1982).

Ten to 15 percent of all American doctors appear to be paid salaries for patient care, but actually they are not. They are members of the growing numbers of partnerships and groups that distribute their revenues by salaries during the year, and then distribute the balance by bonuses at the end of the year (Kahn and Ortiz 1982, 286). The partnerships, and all groups except HMOs, bill patients and third parties by fee-for-service in the traditional manner. Therefore, all these doctors are really paid by fee-for-service and are fully subject to fee-for-service incentives.

The tradition of open hospital staffs

paid by fees is deeply rooted in America, and both hospital doctors and office doctors resist the creation of closed and salaried hospital staffs. For example, the Hunterdon County Medical Center in New Jersey tried to work with closed-salaried staffs of full-time specialists without outside practices. The hospital billed third parties by fee-for-service, but the fees went into special funds that paid the doctors' salaries and bonuses. Office doctors could not treat their patients in the hospital but were required to refer them to the hospital specialists. The hospital doctors could not compete with the office doctors by building an extensive ambulatory practice. This organizational arrangement is typical in Europe. The designers of Hunterdon hoped it would become the model for high-quality, cost-effective, and disciplined hospital practice throughout America. But it did not spread, and the doctors eventually forced it to operate like all other hospitals. The hospital doctors demanded direct collection of each person's fees, not salaries, and demanded the right to provide ambulatory care to the community. The office doctors demanded admitting privileges. Hunterdon changed in order to survive. If it had not, the doctors could have destroyed it by inviting a for-profit chain to create a typical open-staff facility in competition (Wescott 1979).

Effects on Work and Costs. Because of the scarcity of salaried senior clinicians, the American literature contains few comparisons of salaried and fee-for-service practice and, therefore, few estimates of the effects of salary.

Instead, the literature describes many salaried programs, without evaluating them. (Even in Europe, it is difficult to identify the effects of salaried employment since it does not generate the numerous reports about work that are by-products of fee-for-service remuneration.)

Payment by salary is part of a larger organized system of care that may allow slower work or may press for speedier work, depending on conditions. It is the overall policy rather than the payment method alone that is essential. If an ambulatory care group pays its doctors by salary, without added bonuses for productivity, the doctors might work more slowly than if they personally earned item-of-service fees (Scheffler 1975). If the group has strong leadership, prefers ambulatory treatment to hospital referral, and gives promotions and bonuses to doctors who cooperate, the group does more work intramurally and refers less. These are the essential characteristics of many HMOs: revenue from prepaid annual subscription fees, payment of salaries to the doctors, strong management, and promotions to doctors who implement policy (Luft 1981). Under appropriate management and with rewards for good work, a full-time salaried hospital staff can be efficient and can give care of high quality (Roemer and Friedman 1971, esp. chap. 4).

Paying doctors by salary can result in higher or lower costs, depending on the administration of the system and on the bargaining power of the medical association. When European hospital doctors were persuaded to accept full-time salaries instead of fee-for-service—as in Sweden,

France, Germany, and several other countries—they were guaranteed very high rates, at least equal to their earnings from private practice. The junior doctors then demanded increases, so they ranked just below the senior doctors. Therefore, when a new system is installed, it is more expensive than the old and makes the entire medical profession at all ranks the best-paid occupation in the country. Each year, the medical association presses for increases so that the doctors' incomes remain above all other occupations (Glaser 1977, chap. 11, pp. 35–40).

Salaried doctors can practice expensively, if their own leaders and the public authorities fail to press for economies. Hospitals and health centers must buy the equipment and pay for the staff that the self-employed doctors previously covered from their fees. Free of personal responsibility for operating costs, salaried doctors can order all the tests and treatments that patients "need" and that they think might advance medical science. In the United States and Europe, the most expensive care is given by salaried doctors in teaching hospitals (examples in Glaser 1977, chap. 11, pp. 40–41; Culyer et al. 1978).

Paying the Hospital

Trends Abroad

The organization and payment of European and Canadian hospitals have become steadily more structured and standardized. The senior medical staffs in nonprofit and public hospitals are becoming full-time salaried. The nursing and domestic staffs have become secular, salaried, and unionized. Facilities planning has slowly grown to target capital grants and to regionalize hospitals. All countries have adopted cost reimbursement, prospective rates, and "all-payers methods" whereby each hospital provides the same benefits at the same rates for all third parties. Hospitals must submit detailed reports to sickness funds and to rate regulators about past and expected costs, and they must justify excessive items. The financing systems guarantee coverage of costs but not profits.

Hospitals are much more expensive than in the past because of higher wages, more sophisticated technical care, and more admissions due to aging of populations. Rising hospital costs have endangered the solvency of health insurance, and every country has struggled to reduce them. Rate regulation has steadily tightened. Global budgeting is now becoming common; after approving the hospital's expected costs for the coming year, sickness funds or government payers then grant the amount, requiring the hospital to perform all its work within the limit. By granting low increases each year, the payers hope to discourage unnecessary admissions and excessive stays.

Hospital doctors can use the nonprofit or public hospital to earn personal fees and increase their incomes if, as in Germany, the country's system allows them rights of private practice and use of some private beds. But the trend is toward full-time and salaried employment without private practice, as in France. Private practice by hospital doctors, where it continues, is being restricted in hours, numbers of private beds, and levels of fees. Therefore, the hospital doctors become members of nonprofit organizations and cease being entrepreneurs. Their salaries are generous but provide no incentives to use the hospital for personal gain and to raise operating costs. Private clinics still persist in substantial numbers in some European countries, where specialists without hospital appointments can build substantial private practices earning fees from both statutory health insurance and from private commercial health insurance.

Trends in the United States

The history and financial dynamics of American hospitals have been quite different. During the late nineteenth and early twentieth centuries, the American hospital industry resembled that of other countries: nonprofit and public hospitals were outnumbered by private clinics; doctors donated time to the hospitals as a professional duty and used their private clinics as workshops for earning fees; hospital patients could afford to pay the doctors little or nothing, and the doctors earned their incomes from office and clinic practice.

During the twentieth century, American nonprofit hospitals began to function like private clinics, for doctors in their localities. The European separation between hospital doctors and office doctors disappeared; American hospital medical staffs became "open" rather than

"closed." By now, 91.4 percent of all American doctors have admitting privileges in hospitals. Affiliated doctors have an average of admitting privileges in 2.3 hospitals (American Medical Association 1982; Gaffney and Glandon 1982, 55). When the office-based doctor hospitalizes a patient, he need not refer the patient to a member of a hospital staff; he can treat the patient without interruption before, during, and after hospitalization. The doctor's income from hospital patients can be very high. Because nonprofit hospitals operate like private clinics, American doctors do not need to maintain their own clinics, and the number of for-profit hospitals owned and managed by doctors has greatly diminished (Steinwald and Neuhauser 1970).

Every nonprofit and for-profit hospital is autonomous; each must find the money to survive. If a hospital loses market share to its competitors, it can go bankrupt. The key to survival and growth is pleasing doctors. Local physicians who bring many profitable cases are added to the staff. Affiliated doctors with many admissions get the new equipment, ancillary staffing, and prompt services they want. If a hospital does not give doctors what they want, they will take their admissions to one of their other affiliates, and the hospital will collapse.

Paying the American Hospital

The United States economy is one of free market competition and, unlike other countries, extends these principles into health care. Doctors compete with each other for patients and for facilities that will improve their services and increase their incomes. Hospitals compete with each other for doctors who will bring profitable referrals. Third-party insurers compete to increase their subscribers and restrain their costs. Unlike Europe, American third parties do not unite to standardize the payment rules and limit spending. The hospitals oppose standardization since costs not paid by one third party can be included in higher bills for others.

Methods. The result is great diversity and occasional change. Rate regulators in a few states (for example, New York, New Jersey, Maryland, and Massachusetts) have tried to standardize methods, but these states are still exceptions. In most of the country, each hospital is paid differently by various payers (Glaser 1984b):

Medicare. Until 1983 the national government reimbursed the costs of the patient per day in that hospital. Payment for that patient was calculated by multiplying the average Medicare per diem by that patient's length of stay (Beck 1984). After 1983, for each type of case (diagnosis-related groups or DRGs) the government paid a fixed sum calculated by national and regional average costs for each type of patient in all American hospitals (Grimaldi and Micheletti 1983).

Medicaid. The state government reimburses the costs of the average Medicaid patient per day in that

hospital, often defining allowable costs less generously than Medicare. Payment for that patient is a multiple of the Medicaid per diem and the patient's length of stay.

Blue Cross in one-half the states. The plan reimburses the costs of the average patient per day in that hospital, defined broadly. The amount sometimes is reduced by discounts negotiated between the plan and the hospital (Berman and Weeks 1982, chap. 6).

Blue Cross in the other half of the states. The plan pays for itemized services given that patient according to the hospital's schedule of charges. The charges are reduced by discounts negotiated between the plan and the hospital.

Commercially insured patients pay for itemized services according to the hospital's schedule of charges. The patient is reimbursed by the insurance carrier, or the carrier pays its share directly to the hospital. Individual commercial insurers have too small a market share in the hospital and are too competitive to negotiate discounts with hospitals. Their subscribers pay considerably more than the costs of their care.

Self-payers are billed for services according to the hospital's schedule of charges. The hospital collects whatever it can from the patient. Considerable numbers of bad debts result.

In America, hospitals' payment rates are decided by many methods:

Set unilaterally by payers. Medicare and Medicaid define the costs they will pay, and their field representatives screen each hospital's cost reports. The hospital associations try to revise the laws and regulations more generously by lobbying Congress and civil servants and by filing lawsuits.

Set unilaterally by the hospital. The charge schedule is written by each hospital freely, in order to maximize its revenue.

Negotiated. Each Blue Cross plan and each hospital negotiate over allowable costs or over acceptable charges.

Rate regulation by civil servants exists in several states. These arrangements vary in strictness and jurisdiction over numbers of payers. (New York, New Jersey, Massachusetts, Maryland, and Connecticut have been most persistent.) Since the nature and survival of rate regulation depend on the local political climate, some efforts have been started and repealed (Colorado and Illinois) (Glaser 1984a).

Effects of Various Units of Payment. The same hospital in the United States is paid in different units (i.e., daily average all-inclusive charges, item-of-service charges, DRGs, etc.) by different payers. It is very difficult to generalize about a particular unit in the American context because wide variations occur among hospitals and regions in administrative arrangements, in the strictness by payers and by government regulators (if any), in each hospital's total mix of payers, and in the motives and responses of occupational groups participating within

hospitals. However, the following paragraphs summarize high points of actual operations.

Per diem covering all allowable costs. Length of stay is not shortened. Doctors allow the patient to stay in a few extra days, if the patient and family wish. Hospital managers try to add items to the hospital's cost base, resulting in many disputes with payers. Large numbers of nurses, domestics, and junior doctors are hired. Each year's income (for the individual hospital) and costs (for the payer) exceed predictions because admissions and numbers of patient-days exceed predictions. Since profits are reimbursable in America, investor-owned hospitals prosper.

Per diem with limited definitions of allowable costs. Nonprofit and for-profit hospital managers avoid inpatients covered in this way. They try to refer such inpatients to public general hospitals. They may treat such a patient in the outpatient department, if the patient's ambulatory care insurance is more generous than his inpatient coverage or if the patient can be billed beyond his insurance coverage.

Itemized charges. Hospital managers install new equipment and hire technicians that can generate many procedures on the charge list, such as diagnostic tests and respiratory therapy. The hospital earns extra cash for amortization of debt and for other purposes. Hospital managers compete for doctors who can generate such work. Hospitals concentrate on cases that require short stays and that permit much work to be done in day care or in the OPD. Disputes between hospitals and some payers occur over the levels of charges. Middle-class patients who pay shares of these charges frequently complain. The poor leave many bad debts.

Case payments (diagnosis-related groups). Hospital managers try to specialize, attracting more admissions of cases they can treat cheaply and avoiding cases they treat more expensively than the peer-group average. Inpatients are admitted when they might be treated as well in the outpatient department. If a patient requires long hospitalization, the patient might be referred to programs managed by the hospitals and paid by different methods; such programs could include nursing homes, home care, and hospices. Higher turnover of patients occurs with more re-admissions. The cost base is reduced by restrictions on hiring, by resistance to wage increases, and by creation of fee-for-service medical practice plans for doctors who were previously salaried. Hospital managers compete to affiliate those doctors who generate profitable admissions. Managers work more closely with doctors to persuade the latter to write more profitable diagnoses, reduce length of stay, and refer expensive patients elsewhere.

Effects of Administrative Arrangements in the United States. Most states have no government regulation of hospital operating costs and very weak facilities planning. In the few states where rate regulation exists, it is usually permissive lest the hospital industry and medical association force its repeal. Therefore, hospital costs grow faster in the United States than in Europe. Annual increases in hospital spending relative to the general rate of inflation always fluctuate, but European countries now keep such increases close to inflation rates, while American hospital spending varies between 1.5 and 4.0 times the general inflation (Glaser 1984a).

An essential part of the system is self-financing of capital: payers accept as allowable costs interest, depreciation, and profits, and the managers can buy and amortize whatever new technology will please the doctors and keep the hospital competitive. Local governments underwrite bonds in the national bond market to help nonprofit hospitals raise funds for new construction, renovation, and new equipment. The hospitals pay off the bonds from increases in operating revenue. In America more than in any other country, because of the weakness of facilities planning and the self-financing of investment (Cohodes and Kinkead 1984), hospital owners and managers have more discretion in reorganizing and in adopting new programs.

Investor-owned hospital chains can self-finance as well, by mortgaging their assets or by issuing stock. As a result they grow by buying independent for-profit hospitals or impoverished public hospitals. These for-profit chains are nearly unique to America. In other countries, for-profit hospitals operate cautiously and have diminished in number. The American investor-owned chains attract much interest on Wall Street, and their national association (the Federation of American Hospitals) has become a very influential lobby in Washington (Gray 1983).

The lack of structure in U.S. hospital affairs permits greater innovation. New delivery methods—home care, day surgery, affiliated professional corporations, and so forth—are adopted in several places, are widely studied, and are quickly spread. In contrast, delivery methods change slowly in the more planned, regulated, and standardized countries of Europe. Because self-financing enables many hospitals to install and pay off the newest technology, the United States is the principal market for the world's medical equipment industry.

Limiting Costs

Since World War II, every developed country has reorganized its health care financing. At first the trends were expansionary. A nearly universal goal was access of all citizens to mainstream medicine, without financial barriers and without reliance on charitable services. Doctors were supposed to be guaranteed payment in full for all patients, at levels providing the best facilities. Hospitals were also supposed to receive payment in full so they could hire more employees, pay competitive wages, and constantly modernize their facilities. The changes succeeded in pouring more money into health care; by the

1980s, countries were devoting between 8 and 11 percent of GNP to health.

But the guardians of finance, the financial officers of government, worried about the rapid rise in payroll taxes in countries where health insurance was part of social security (most of Europe). Where government paid the providers (Great Britain, Scandinavia, and Canada), the financial officers worried about the rise in government expenditure and general taxes. The proponents of more spending were a formidable coalition, namely, the entire population of potential patients, the doctors, the hospitals, the unionized hospital workers, and the suppliers to the health industry. But the tax burden on employers was thought to discourage economic growth. Suddenly public policy priorities changed from expanding access and improving services to limiting costs. A struggle for power ensued between the financial officers and the proponents of growth and improvement. The policy instrument was control over reimbursement.

Parliamentary governmental systems are set up to make clear societal decisions. Universal entitlement had been decided by politicians and civil servants, and responsible decision-makers were in place in both government and in the national headquarters of third parties when problems needed remedy. Therefore, by the 1980s every European country and Canada had adopted collective cost-containment policies, such as strict rate negotiation with providers, rate regulation, or strict global budget grants to hospitals. The goal was to stop the growth of health's shares of GNP and of public budgets.

But the United States cannot adopt societal decisions. The country follows free market principles in public policy as well as in the economy. Nobody is in charge. Nobody is responsible for the economy. America expanded access and increased payments to providers not by a succession of societal decisions but through a variety of public and private programs, some lacking controls and expanding beyond anyone's expectations. As in other countries, financial squeezes were inevitably experienced, not by a single guardian of finance but by individual programs: first, by the state governments paying for Medicaid; then, by Blue Cross and by employers who bought its benefit packages; then, by private commercial insurers whose subscribers encountered cost shifting and extra billing by hospitals and doctors; finally, by national officials managing the Medicare trust funds.

During the Carter administration, America briefly considered a statutory all-payers system, with rate regulation for hospitals and fee schedules for doctors. But, Congress failed to enact the program. Instead of a single cost-containment policy imposed by the national government or by all the third parties, America seems to be developing multiple cost-containment policies, wherein each payer confronts each provider. Meanwhile, many cost-raising impulses remain in place, and doctors and hospitals will not limit their bills if they can avoid it. Other countries tend to freeze existing institutions under their nationwide and standard methods, but the profusion of new responses between payers and providers in America may evolve into something entirely new. The United States has always been a "demonstration laboratory" of entrepreneurial techniques, and the decentralized methods that have produced advanced medical services will now be tested to produce economy and efficiency as well.

References

American Medical Association. 1982. *SMS report.* Vol. 1, no. 11.

———. 1983a. *Physician characteristics and distribution in the U.S., 1982 edition.* Chicago: American Medical Association.

———. 1983b. Reports of the Council on Medical Service to the House of Delegates, D(A-83) and B(I-83).

———. 1983c. *SMS report.* Vol. 2, no. 4.

———. 1984. *Socioeconomic characteristics of medical practice.* Chicago: American Medical Association.

Beck, D. F. 1984. *Principles of reimbursement in health care.* Rockville, Md.: Aspen Systems Corporation.

Berman, H. J., and L. E. Weeks. 1982. *The financial management of hospitals.* 5th ed. Ann Arbor: Health Administration Press.

Burney, I. L., and J. R. Gabel. 1980. Reimbursement patterns under Medicare and Medicaid. In *Physicians and financial incentives*, ed. J. R. Gabel, pp. 11–14. U.S. Department of Health and Human Services, Health Care Financing Administration. Washington, D.C.: Government Printing Office.

Burney, I. L., G. J. Schieber, M. O. Blaxall, and J. R. Gabel. 1979. Medicare and Medicaid physician payment incentives. *Health Care Financing Review* 1:62–78.

Cantwell, J. R. 1979. Implications of reimbursement policies for the location of physicians. *Agricultural Economics Research* 31:25–35.

Cohodes, D., and B. M. Kinkead. 1984. *Hospital capital formation in the 1980s*. Baltimore: Johns Hopkins University Press.

Coombs, R. H., and C. E. Vincent, eds. 1971. *Psychosocial aspects of medical training*. Springfield, Ill.: Charles C. Thomas.

Cromwell, J., F. Sloan, and J. Mitchell. 1980. Physician administrative costs and Medicaid participation. In *Physicians and financial incentives*, ed. J. R. Gabel, pp. 35–44. Health Care Financing Administration, U.S. Department of Health and Human Services. Washington, D.C.: Government Printing Office.

Culyer, A. J., J. Wiseman, M. F. Drummond, and P. A. West. 1978. What accounts for the higher costs of teaching hospitals. *Social and Economic Administration* 12:20–30.

Davidson, S. M. 1980. *Medicaid decisions*. Cambridge, Mass.: Ballinger Publishing.

Davis, K., and C. Schoen. 1978. *Health and the War on Poverty*. Washington, D.C.: Brookings Institution.

Feldstein, P. J. 1983. *Health care economics*. 2d ed. New York: John Wiley and Sons.

Freeland, M., and C. E. Schendler. 1984. Health spending in the 1980s: Integration of clinical practice patterns with management. *Health Care Financing Review* 5:1–68.

Gaffney, J. C., and G. L. Glandon. 1982. The physician's use of the hospital. *Health Care Management Review* 7:49–58.

Gibson, R. M., D. R. Waldo, and K. R. Levit. 1983. National health expenditures, 1982. *Health Care Financing Review* 5:1–31.

Glaser, W. A. 1970. *Paying the doctor*. Baltimore: Johns Hopkins University Press.

———. 1977. The doctor under national health insurance: Foreign lessons for the United States. Unpublished report. Bureau of Applied Social Research, Columbia University.

———. 1984a. Hospital rate regulation: American and foreign comparisons. *Journal of Health Politics, Policy, and Law* 8:702–731.

———. 1984b. Juggling multiple payers: American problems and foreign solutions. *Inquiry* 21:178–188.

Goldfarb, D. L. 1981. Trends in physicians' incomes, expenses, and fees, 1970–1980. In *Profile of medical practice, 1981*, ed. D. L. Goldfarb, pp. 113–118. Chicago: American Medical Association.

Gray, B. H., ed. 1983. *The new health care for profit.* Washington, D.C.: National Academy Press.

Grimaldi, P. L., and J. A. Micheletti. 1983. *DRG update: Medicare's prospective payment plan.* Chicago: Pluribus Press.

Hsiao, W. C., and W. B. Stason. 1979. Toward developing a relative value scale for medical and surgical services. *Health Care Financing Review* 1:23–38.

Kahn, H. S., and P. Ortiz. 1982. The emerging role of salaried physicians. *Journal of Public Health Policy* 3:284–292.

Lee, R. H. 1984. The impact of changes in payment methods on the supply of physicians' services. In *Reforming physician payment: Report of a conference,* Institute of Medicine, pp. 44–62. Washington, D.C.: National Academy Press.

Lewis, I. J., and C. B. Sheps. 1983. *The sick citadel: The American academic medical center and the public interest.* Cambridge, Mass.: Oelgeschlager, Gunn and Hain.

Luft, H. 1981. *Health maintenance organizations: Dimensions of performance.* New York: John Wiley and Sons.

Marquis, M. S. 1983. Consumers' knowledge about their health insurance coverage. *Health Care Financing Review* 5:65–79.

Maxwell, R. 1981. *Health and wealth.* Lexington, Mass.: Lexington Books, D. C. Heath and Co.

Mejia, A., H. Pizurki, and E. Royston. 1979. *Physician and nurse migration.* Geneva: World Health Organization.

Mitchell, J. B., and J. Cromwell. 1981. Large Medicaid practices: Are they Medicaid mills? In *Issues in physician reimbursement,* ed. N. T. Greenspan, pp. 95–109. Health Care Financing Administration, U.S. Department of Health and Human Services. Washington, D.C.: Government Printing Office.

Moloney, T. W., and D. E. Rogers. 1979. Medical technology: A different view of the contentious debate over costs. *New England Journal of Medicine* 301:1413–1419.

Rezler, A. G. 1974. Attitude change during medical school: A review of the literature. *Journal of Medical Education* 49:1023–1030.

Roemer, M. L., and J. W. Friedman. 1971. *Doctors in hospitals: Medical staff organization and hospital performance.* Baltimore: Johns Hopkins University Press.

Scheffler, R. M. 1975. The pricing behavior of medical groups. *The Milbank Memorial Fund Quarterly: Health and Society* 53:225–240.

Showstack, J. A., B. D. Blumberg, J. Schwartz, and S. A. Schroeder. 1979. Fee-for-service physician payment: Analysis of current methods and their development. *Inquiry* 16:230–246.

Steinwald, B., and D. Neuhauser. 1970. The role of the proprietary hospital. *Law and Contemporary Problems* 35:818–827.

U.S. Congress. House of Representatives. Select Committee on the Aging.

498 William A. Glaser

1978. *Abuses in the sale of health insurance to the elderly.* Washington, D.C.: Government Printing Office.

Walden, D. C. 1982. Consumer knowledge of health insurance coverage. Unpublished report. National Center for Health Services Research, Washington, D.C.

Wescott, L. B. 1979. Hunterdon: The rise and fall of a medical Camelot. *New England Journal of Medicine* 300:952–956, 977–979.

Chapter 23

Economic Incentives and Constraints in Clinical Practice

Harold S. Luft

The American medical care system in the mid-1980s is undergoing major change. There is some shift away from regulatory strategies toward approaches intended to increase competition and use economic incentives and constraints to contain medical care costs. The implementation by Medicare, for example, of a prospective payment system in which hospitals will be paid a fixed sum of money for each patient according to diagnosis is seen by some as compromising quality of care and as an unprecedented intrusion of economics into clinical practice. Whether prospective payment will cause lower quality of care is an empirical question that will take years to answer. Economics has always been a factor in clinical practice; the new policies merely change the direction of the incentives.

Even if one can move beyond the rhetoric of the policy debates about what role economic incentives should have, economists and clinicians often still have major disagreements about the current importance of such incentives in clinical practice. The question at hand is actually rather narrow—to what extent do economic incentives and constraints influence physicians' clinical or patient care decisions? Note that the focus here is on the clinical decision, such as whether to order an X ray for an ankle injury. The production decision, whether the needed equipment should be leased or purchased, is much simpler. Most physicians would agree that economics may play a role in such situations, but patient outcomes are not affected by the choices. Physicians typically argue that economic incentives have little influence, except in a few obvious and distressing cases such as fee splitting and kickbacks, and furthermore, that economic incentives should have no place in clinical decisions. Physicians are more likely to recognize the existence of economic constraints because they are often visible, such as the inability of a financially strapped hospital to purchase up-to-date equipment, or the difficulties a physician faces when a patient's insurance coverage runs out. Economists, in contrast, argue that economic incentives have a major influence in clinical practice; some believe that expanding incentives and freeing physicians to use them would cure many ills of the medical care sector. Other economists think that a greater role of economic incentives could exacerbate current problems. Yet, while economists may disagree about how incentives should be used, there is little disagreement about their existence.

Models of Clinical Decision-Making

The usual medical model of decision making involves a complex, largely intuitive process whereby the physician considers signs, symptoms, and a variety of test results and, based upon scientific knowledge and clinical experience, arrives at a diagnosis and chooses the best treatment (Eddy 1982). The classic biomedical model usually presumes a single, potentially identifiable cause of a disease for which there is a single best treat-

ment. Only in recent years have some physicians recognized the existence of multiple factors in the causation of disease as well as the differences in some patients' responses to or preferences for alternative treatments for the same condition (McNeil et al. 1982). The traditional model implicitly places the physician in the role of a seeker of truth who must vigorously resist, for economic or other reasons, any deviation from the one right path. This model of behavior has other important implications. The physician is clearly in authority, and the patient must await the correct course of action. The authority of the physician also implies the responsibility for making the correct diagnosis and for choosing the correct treatment.

Diagnosis and treatment decisions often are not clear-cut, yet in practice, many physicians act as if things were clear-cut and develop "standard operating rules" or "clinical policies" that dictate what should be done (Eddy 1982). These clinical policies may be highly complex and contain numerous contingencies, such as the following: If signs A, B, and C are present, test X is negative, and there is no history of Y, the appropriate diagnosis is Q and the treatment is R. Furthermore, even when presented with the same clinical evidence, experienced physicians may often have different clinical policies and recommendations.

Some physicians argue for the explicit consideration of alternative treatments and the valuation of alternative outcomes (McNeil and Adelstein 1975; Pauker and Kassirer 1975). Most physicians, however, seem to avoid this approach, possibly because it is complex and requires analytic skills not taught in medical school, possibly because it highlights the uncertainties of the situation and forces the physician to confront choices explicitly. When faced with the need to make decisions, it is often more comfortable to believe that there is only one clearly correct choice rather than worrying that the path not chosen was really the better alternative.

In contrast to medical training, which emphasizes the rapid advances of scientific knowledge and the discovery of the single best course of treatment, economists are trained to believe that there are an infinite number of potential solutions to the problems of resource allocation, that selection should depend on individual preferences, and that the most efficient allocation of resources will be achieved if everyone pursues his or her own self-interest in a market economy. The difference in perspectives is implicit, rarely discussed or questioned, and so persuasive as to generally escape comment. In each instance the paradigms involve substantial simplifications and abstractions from reality (Kuhn 1970). Whether such abstractions pose a serious threat to their usefulness is beyond the scope of this chapter; however, the differences in worldview clearly affect the debate over the role of incentives in clinical practice.

Under the traditional medical model, the problem and its potential solution are dealt with independent of other factors. Moreover, although the physician is primarily concerned with the patient's clinical well-being, the evaluation of the best treatment is usually from the perspective of the physician rather than the patient. The extreme economic view is to include everything as part of the decision. For example, Grossman's model of the demand for health views the body as a machine that depreciates yearly until it breaks down and is overhauled (medical intervention) or scrapped (death) and for which preventive maintenance decisions are considered relative to other ways that the owner can spend his or her time and money (Grossman 1972, 1982). A simple example of the difference in perspectives can be seen in the use of the word *optimal* in the context of describing alternative treatments. Most clinicians use the term to describe the treatment that provides the greatest improvement (or chance of improvement) in health status, irrespective of cost. In contrast, most economists would include cost considerations in the evaluation of the alternatives. For example, a patient may consider optimal a slightly less efficacious, but much less expensive treatment because it would leave the family with a smaller financial burden. From the economist's perspective, physicians are like those auto mechanics who want to turn every ordinary family car into a luxury machine without considering whether the family would like to spend its time or money on something else.

The analogy to an auto mechanic may distress some physicians, but it incorporates the economist's recognition that many of the technical details of medicine are too complicated for patients to evaluate directly. Like most consumers who can determine whether a car is running better despite not understanding the complexities of auto repair, patients often can evaluate the results of medical care without understanding disease processes or therapeutic alternatives. The problem for the patient is finding someone to determine what is wrong, having the treatment choices identified and explained, and choosing the appropriate people to carry out the desired interventions. In this regard the economist views the ideal primary care physician as the patient's agent, providing the relevant information and selecting the appropriate specialists (Feldstein 1974; Pauly 1980). (Note the parallel to a trusted mechanic who can diagnose a transmission problem and then recommend a competent specialty shop to do the work.) A perfect physician-agent would lead the consumer to precisely the same decision as the consumer would have reached given all of the physician's expertise. This decision may well differ from traditional "best medical practice" or "optimal care" because the patient is likely to take into consideration the cost of the services, discomfort, the time involved in treatment, and other factors not usually part of choosing the best medical outcome.

Although the notion of a perfect agent is a very attractive theoretical concept, few perfect agents exist because of the conventional methods of organizing care and paying physicians. Often, diagnosis and treatment are difficult to separate, and much of the cost actually occurs in the diagnosis phase. In the dominant fee-for-service mode of payment, fees are heavily biased toward laboratory tests and diagnostic and therapeutic procedures in contrast to time spent talking with the patient (Schroeder and Showstack 1978; Showstack et al. 1979). The hypothetical "physician-as-perfect-agent" would be available and willing to spend time with the patient, investigate the problem, ponder the diagnosis, and calculate the alternatives. The best physician-agent would have no personal economic incentives either to encourage or discourage additional tests and procedures or to prefer one course of treatment over another. In practice, however, except for psychiatrists, fee-for-time arrangements for physicians are uncommon.[1] Furthermore, primary physicians are rarely only counselors, and even the diagnostic function involves many highly profitable tests.[2]

The crucial issue is not the method of paying the physician, whether fee-for-service, capitation, or salary, but the linkage between the physician as agent and the physician as provider. For instance, many medical school faculty are on a straight salary, yet they know that their department's revenues are dependent on fee-for-service billings and that a revenue shortfall will affect salaries, promotions, and perquisites. Similarly, the medical group in a health maintenance organization (HMO) may receive a capitation payment covering the annual primary care of its enrollees; but if the group orders too much hospital care, its share of the plan's net income will be smaller (Luft 1981). The incentives to provide services are reversed in some systems— fee-for-service has a bias toward more services, while the fixed budget of an HMO sets up a bias toward fewer services—but in each case economic factors are present that could influence clinical decisions. Whether physicians respond to such incentives is another question.

Incentives from the Perspective of the Physician and the Economist

The medical literature generally ignores the possibility of economic influences on clinical decisions. If the issue is discussed at all, it seems to be in terms of conscious behavior on the part of the physician. For instance, physicians in prepaid plans have identified as an advantage the fact that all their patients have comprehensive coverage, thus physicians need never be concerned that a proposed treatment would bankrupt the patient (Cook 1971). Clinicians in fee-for-service practice have mentioned being aware of the gross revenues associated with a procedure while making clinical recommendations. Most physicians, however, claim that economic incentives do not influence their patient care decisions. Similarly, when economic constraints are recognized, they are seen as impinging upon previously made decisions. For example, in the case of the patient who "clearly" should have a liver transplant but cannot afford one, economic constraints prevent a clinical decision from being carried out.

Economists take a different perspective, and, although their language may suggest conscious decision-making, they typically focus their attention on behavior and not-stated motives. If financial incentives would reward a certain behavior everything else being equal, and if the behavior is observed, the role of incentives is deemed empirically supported. In this type of analysis the economist typically ignores (or attempts to hold constant statistically) all but the economic variables such as prices and incomes. It is understood that in any particular case—clinical, personal, professional, or other—factors may be present and even dominant, but such factors are seen as essentially random. The clinician, in contrast, is trained to focus on precisely those noneconomic factors that the economist dismisses as random; the clinician will believe and argue that each case is handled individually, with attention only, or almost only, to the clinical problem. It may be the case that 95 percent of any decision is based on clinical factors and 5 percent on economic factors. The physician will believe that the economic factors are inconsequential; the economist will respond that if one examines many similar cases, abstracting from the random clinical factors, economics dominates and patterns emerge that cannot be explained by clinical factors.

Yet another difference in approach helps explain the different perceptions of the economist and the physician. The economist, for example, will ask whether, among one thousand individuals experiencing a given set of symptoms, those who have to pay for their care out of pocket are less likely to see a physician than those whose insurance will pay for the visit. In contrast, the physician focuses on those persons who come to the office for care. The physician notes that fees do not influence his or her patients, although the economist responds that fees will determine (at least in part) how many people decide to present themselves as patients.

Economists and clinicians also look for different things when examining data. In most instances the economist attempts to demonstrate a statistically significant effect of an economic variable. The interpretation of a significant finding is generally open to question on two grounds. The first is whether the observed correlation really implies causation or whether other, unobserved factors may be causing the measured relationship. The second is whether the statistically significant effect is substantively important. Large samples and sophisticated econometric models often allow very small effects to be measured, but such differences may be of no practical policy import. From the physician's perspective, subtle tendencies, regardless of the statistical significance or aggregate importance, are inconsequential unless one can identify clear instances in which the economic incentives can be shown to have led to an altered clinical decision. Thus, the examples of constraints are generally far more convincing to the physician.

Given the different orientations and tools, the physician's microscope and the economist's telescope, it is not surprising that the two cannot easily agree on what evidence is appropriate. Largely because physician-researchers have not considered the role of incentives a fruitful research area, much of the available evidence on the question uses the economist's approach of searching for tendencies across large numbers of cases.

Incentives and the Use of Technology

Some analysts suspect that the rapid growth in the use of medical technologies may stem not just from clinical efficacy but also from the high returns physicians receive by using such technology. It is estimated that a primary care internist can increase net income by a factor of almost three by prescribing a wide but not unreasonable set of tests (Schroeder and Showstack 1978). The term *not unreasonable* is a reflection that the use of such tests is sufficiently common to be almost standard practice; yet some clinicians argue that few of the tests are actually necessary (Griner et al. 1981; Martin 1982). Some diagnostic technologies, such as endoscopy and ultrasound during pregnancy, have been studied in detail. They are highly profitable, have proliferated rapidly, yet rarely result in a definitive change in treatment or outcome (Showstack and Schroeder 1981; Foltz 1984). Is this evidence of economic incentives influencing practice patterns? From the economist's perspective the answer is yes, but the clinician might quickly point to such factors as the low risk of the procedure and the importance of the reassurance it can provide to the patient (and the physician).

A study by Childs and Hunter (1972) of diagnostic X-ray use provides an example of the role of multiple factors in clinical patterns. They examined the use of X rays for persons under old-age assistance (thus controlling for income and insurance coverage). Patients of physicians who owned their own X-ray equipment (direct providers) were twice as likely to receive an X ray and were less likely to see a radiologist than were patients of physicians without such equipment. More important, patients of direct providers were much more likely to receive fluoroscopy alone and single-view chest films, procedures generally eschewed by radiologists as providing little useful information. The authors suggest that the "physician with X-ray apparatus, therefore, would be motivated to use that apparatus in order to amortize the capital costs as well as to produce income." They caution, however, that the ease of access may encourage more frequent use. One could argue that physicians who value X rays more highly (for clinical rather than economic reasons) would be more likely to use them more frequently and therefore would purchase the equipment. However, the frequent use of fluoroscopy and single-film studies suggests a lack of clinical sophistication. More recently, Danzon, Manning, and Marquis (1984) found a positive relation between volume of laboratory tests ordered by physicians for ambulatory patients and availability of the tests in-house. However, they could not determine whether accessibility (or profitability) caused more ordering, or more ordering made local control more desirable.

Technology use in hospitals has grown at a very rapid pace, perhaps more rapidly than in physicians' offices. In the last decade the hospital CT scanner and special care units have become almost ubiquitous, and other "little ticket" technologies have proliferated and added substantially to costs (Fineberg 1979; Moloney and Rogers 1979). Tracing the physician's incentives during the inpatient episode is more complex than for outpatient care. In many instances, both the hospital and the physician profit from the test; the hospital charges cover the test itself, such as an EKG, and the physician may charge a separate fee for interpreting the results. Sometimes the physician's fee is influenced by the patient's location; a hospital visit to a patient in intensive care may command a higher fee than a visit on the ward (California Medical Association 1975). Sometimes the primary care physician has no direct economic interest in additional tests, such as CT scans interpreted by radiologists. There can be indirect incentives, however, even without fee splitting. If a test can substitute for the primary physician's time and effort, that time can often be used to advantage elsewhere. Furthermore, if the hospital can profit from increased use of certain procedures, funds may be available to provide facilities and equipment physicians find attractive. Hospitals often can identify those physicians responsible for a large fraction of their revenues, and special efforts may be made to satisfy the demands of those physicians. Some direct evidence shows that ancillary costs in proprietary hospitals are significantly higher than in voluntary hospitals (Lewin, Derzon, and Margulies 1981). In California, ancillary services are used by proprietary hospitals as major profit centers (Blumberg 1979; Pattison and Katz 1983). What is less clear is whether and how physicians' clinical decisions are altered by proprietary hospitals.

Payment and Practice-Setting Incentives

Considerable evidence links the role of direct payment incentives and practice patterns. Physicians paid on a fee-for-service basis have a clear incentive to do more tests, procedures, and operations than those paid a fixed sum in salary or capitation. Bunker (1970) found that certain discretionary surgical procedures were performed twice as frequently per capita in the United States as in England and Wales. Although the difference in mode of payment—fee-for-service in the United States and salary in Britain—might explain this difference, the number of surgeons in the United States was also proportionately higher.

More recently, Aaron and Schwartz (1984) have examined the use of various technologies in the United States and Great Britain. In the United States the economic incentives of fee-for-service encourage the use of nearly all technologies; in Britain essentially all costs are budgeted directly by the National Health Service. For some technologies British use approximates that in the United States, while in other cases British use is markedly lower. We can reconcile these findings by focusing on the role of direct constraints in the British system. Many of the medical technologies are clearly valuable in improving health status, yet some are more easily constrained than others. One of the characteristics of technology in relatively short supply is that, according to Aaron and Schwartz, it requires major capital investment. CT scanners, which can be centrally controlled, are a good example. Technologies that can be used incrementally at the discretion of individual physicians, such as total parenteral nutrition, have been much more difficult to control in the British system.

The contrast between conventional fee-for-service practice and prepaid care such as in health maintenance organizations (HMOs) should be more telling because the first has incentives to provide more services while the second has incentives to provide fewer services.

In almost all comparisons of persons enrolled in HMOs of the prepaid group practice type (PGPs) and those obtaining care in conventional fee-for-service settings, the hospitalization rate for the HMO enrollees is lower (Luft 1981; Manning et al. 1984). Some evidence shows that people who switch into PGPs from conventional plans have previously been lower utilizers of hospital care than those who do not switch into a PGP (Berki and Ashcraft 1980; Eggers and Prihoda 1982; Luft 1981). Despite these findings, the average PGP enrollee is not noticeably more healthy than enrollees in conventional insurance plans (Blumberg 1980). (This is possible because relatively recent enrollees make up only a relatively small proportion of PGP members at any one point.) Therefore, it is unlikely that differential health status accounts for all the observed differences in hospitalization rates between enrollees in conventional plans and prepaid group practice HMOs (Luft 1981). The Rand Health Insurance Experiment findings from Seattle provide clear evidence that utilization and costs are substantially lower for persons in a large, mature PGP, even when most of the selection effects are eliminated by the experimental design (Manning et al. 1984).

The observed differences in hospitalization rates between HMOs and conventional settings do not necessarily reflect differences in physicians' decisions to treat patients. Some of the changes in utilization rates reflect differences in the ways that treatments are provided. For instance, the design of most PGPs involves comprehensive coverage of diagnostic services in and out of the hospital, incentives to reduce hospital use, and physically convenient ambulatory facilities. Thus, for example, patient stays may be shortened by having the patient arrive the morning of the operation rather than the night before. Kaiser-Portland reports that 35 percent of all its operative procedures were performed on a come-and-go basis, that is, in the operating room but without a hospital admission unless complications occur (Marks et al. 1980). Such practices are becoming increasingly common in the fee-for-service sector, but the different incentives in prepaid and nonprepaid settings may explain why this cost-saving technique was more quickly adopted by HMOs (Lavin 1982). More important, innovations such as ambulatory diagnostic work-ups, same-day (come-and-go) surgery,

and come-and-stay surgery (i.e., the patient is admitted on the day of the operation) really involve minimal changes in clinical practice; they are primarily production process decisions concerning the most efficient way to carry out a specific task.

Another issue to be considered in the HMO studies is the extent to which differences may be attributable to group practice rather than to the economic incentives resulting from prepayment. The relative performance of independent practice associations (IPAs), which involves some financial risk sharing by independent, primarily fee-for-service practitioners, is much less impressive than that of PGPs (Luft 1981). But some fee-for-service groups seem to have hospitalization rates for their patients comparable to those of prepaid groups (Broida et al. 1975; Nobrega et al. 1982; Scitovsky 1981). Why this is the case is not clear, but speculating on the cause may help clarify physicians' and economists' different perspectives on the role of incentives.

One explanation offered for the low hospitalization rate in certain group practices is that the number of specialists relative to the population served is so low that the specialists are occupied with clearly necessary admissions and do not have time for the more discretionary cases. (Most of the practices studied also serve as referral centers for generalists in a wide area, so the specialists see a relatively complex mix of cases.) This explanation implies that different decision criteria are used, that the same patient would be treated differently by the specialist in group practice than by a similar specialist in solo practice. If solo practitioners are less busy (in general this is the case, with surgeons preferring to do more procedures than they actually do), then their patients may have more extensive tests and workups, followed by hospitalization. By contrast, patients in a group setting more likely might be told to monitor the condition over the next few months and, if it does not improve, more aggressive treatment will be undertaken.

Notwithstanding the differences in hospitalization, patient outcomes in both styles of practice may be similar because many medical problems are self-limiting. Practitioners in both settings see their own practice styles as clinically successful. But one may ask, If both the solo and group physicians are in a fee-for-service environment, why do they not develop similar practice patterns? Put another way, What prevents the group practice from adding more specialists who, presumably, would do more discretionary procedures?

We must now move back from the economist's model to something closer to clinical practice. Procedures often seen as discretionary, such as cholecystectomy, hysterectomy, and hemorrhoidectomy, are probably seen as more mundane and less challenging if only because they are so common and the patient is not in a crisis situation. If the specialists can keep busy with interesting cases by limiting the number of physicians in the group, then they probably will do so, rather than expand the group just for the sake of bigness at the cost of diluting the clinical case mix. Although this scenario is plausible, one should note that the empirical base

for these observations is extraordinarily thin, being limited to a handful of studies focusing on large, well-respected multispecialty group practices, often with large numbers of referral patients, such as the Mayo Clinic. Specialists in such settings may well establish stringent criteria for hospitalization because they have more experience with sicker patients and thus feel more comfortable managing less ill patients on an ambulatory basis.

Observational studies suffer from an inability to control for case mix, so a standard retort to the differences between HMO and fee-for-service settings is that in some subtle way HMO enrollees were healthier at the outset. Hlatky et al. (1983) undertook an important, although limited, study that controls for this problem. They sent a series of case histories of patients with various types of heart problems to a sample of board-certified cardiologists. Each physician was asked a series of questions about how he or she would manage the case and, in particular, whether certain diagnostic tests or bypass surgery would be recommended. Physicians in independent fee-for-service practice were significantly more likely than those in a prepaid group practice to recommend the tests and surgery. This finding supports the notion that clinical decision-making patterns in prepaid groups are different. Interestingly, the recommendations of the HMO physicians were similar to those of university cardiologists, making it more difficult to maintain that the PGP practice pattern represents inferior care. It remains impossible to separate the prepayment aspect from the group practice effects. And further, the data do not indicate why or how the difference occurred.

Individual versus Collective Patterns of Practice

Most clinicians develop preferred ways to handle particular clinical situations and, when presented with a case, may not give much thought to alternatives or at least to the role that nonclinical factors, such as price, might have on the selection among alternatives. Medicine abounds with situations in which alternative clinical strategies are available with no scientific evidence indicating which is preferable. Despite this practice, physicians may have strong preferences concerning these alternatives, and a correlation may exist between economic incentives and these preferences.

In a wide range of situations, adequate scientific evidence does not exist to establish one treatment as definitively superior. For instance, Wennberg, Bunker, and Barnes (1980) found substantial controversies surrounding nine common surgical procedures. A great debate continues over whether certain types of coronary diseases are best managed surgically or medically (Carr, Engler, and Ross 1982; McIntosh 1981). Yet in each situation individual physicians tend to prefer and to use one mode of treatment and do not behave as though there is a gray area characterized by uncertainty.

Definitive clinical trials to narrow the gray area are extremely difficult and costly because the patient's outcome in any particular case is dependent on a variety of factors in addition to the one under consideration. Thus, very large samples and sophisticated methods may be required to identify the specific gray-area situations in which treatment *A* is superior to treatment *B*. Individual clinicians cannot undertake such studies in a systematic way. Yet many act as if the evidence were clear. The reason is threefold. First, medical education generally provides little training in research design, epidemiology, and other analytic methods. Case reports and uncontrolled trials abound in the medical literature (McKinlay 1981). Second, reports of new techniques are usually made by their innovators, who are strong advocates of the technique. Although this may not intentionally bias the results, subsequent controlled trials often are far less supportive of the technique. Third, although the medical literature offers little useful guidance, practitioners constantly make ad hoc observations that tend to support and reinforce their initial views.

Suppose the decision concerns a service that, given the available research, is truly in the gray area; bypass surgery for two diseased coronary arteries is a good example. For more severe disease there is clear evidence of improved survival with surgery, but the available studies are less clear for intermediate levels of obstruction. Survival rates for medical and surgical management are roughly comparable. While death rates tend to be low for both treatments, the morbidity (and costs) associated with each method differ. A physician choosing one method will tend to focus on the good outcomes, recalling that the failure rate is really no higher than for the alternative. Because patients' beliefs often are significant factors in improved outcomes (the placebo effect), a physician who strongly recommends one alternative as "superior in my experience" may well be correct because of the attitude communicated to the patient.

Within the often broad gray areas concerning clinical choices, physicians may develop clear preferences for certain practice styles, preferences that have no particular scientific basis yet are self-reinforcing through a combination of placebo effects, patient selection, and the self-limiting nature of many conditions. This process may explain the wide variations in practice patterns seen among physicians, even those practicing in the same type of setting. In various studies, Wennberg and Gittelsohn have identified consistent differences over time in surgical use across small areas in New England (Wennberg and Gittelsohn 1973, 1975, 1982). One area may have a high hysterectomy rate and a low cholecystectomy rate. The differences appear not to be related to specialty mix or population differences but to the presence of particular surgeons who use either broad or stringent indications for certain procedures. Moreover, particular surgeons are not necessarily conservative (or aggressive) across all types of procedures; instead, there seems to be little consistency. These studies also indicate that the wide variations in practice patterns tend to occur for those procedures about which the research literature provides no definitive rules, that is, where the gray area is broad. For instance, there is little variability in the rates of herniorrhaphy, where the research is fairly definitive, in contrast to hysterectomy, where surgery often is more discretionary (Wennberg and Gittelsohn 1982).

Wide differences in practice patterns are not limited to fee-for-service surgeons in rural New England. Studies have shown wide variations in the use of laboratory tests, prescription drugs, X rays, return appointments, and telephone consultations among similarly trained physicians within (not only across) such settings as large prepaid group practices, relatively small single-specialty groups, large fee-for-service multispecialty groups, and university-based HMOs (Freeborn et al. 1972; Lyle et al. 1976; Roney and Estes 1975; Schroeder et al. 1973). Even the study by Hlatky et al. (1983), which controls for case mix by using identical case histories, shows substantial variability in the recommendations of physicians within the same types of settings. Some of the PGP cardiologists were more aggressive in their recommendations than some independent fee-for-service specialists. However, nearly all the cardiologists in all three types of settings recommended surgery for patients with left main artery and triple vessel disease, a recommendation clearly supported by the research literature. The variability was concentrated among the less severe cases where the evidence is most ambiguous.

Although the wide variation in patterns within practice settings may have idiosyncratic origins, such as the teachings of an influential professor or a memorably bad experience with an alternative strategy, there also seem to be consistent patterns of care related to the method of payment and other economic incentives. The reasons for a statistical relationship between economic incentives and practice patterns are not well established. Two explanations may be offered. First, it may be that economics directly shapes the clinical patterns, so, for example, a new physician, even one trained in a conservative, watch-and-wait style, who enters fee-for-service practice, quickly recognizes that the loan will not be paid off unless he or she does more tests and procedures. (One can describe a counter-example for a new partner in an HMO.) This explanation is implicit in much of the rhetoric about fee-for-service and prepaid systems, but physicians rarely explain their behavior in this way.

The second explanation focuses on the selection behavior of patients and physicians. Just as patients select a physician they think will provide the advice they desire and with whom they feel comfortable, physicians select practice patterns. By the time residency is completed, a clinically aggressive physician probably knows an HMO is not the setting most conducive to that style of practice. In many cases choice may not be conscious. Such a physician's mentors are much more likely to be in a fee-for-service setting, and the new physician drifts into a compatible type of practice that seems to work. Similarly, a conservatively oriented physician may find the HMO environment more comfortable. Decisions may also reflect what one's immediate colleagues do; it may be difficult to differ frequently from one's colleagues in one's clinical recommendations. The role of colleagues may also explain the relatively low utilization of hospital services in many multispecialty group practices. These settings were often established by innovative physicians who valued a distinctive practice style and were willing to accept vigorous criticism from mainstream medicine.

The selection hypothesis also helps explain the observed positive correlation between the supply of surgeons and the incidence of surgery, without resorting to a crude demand-generating model (McClure 1982). If physicians have some implicit income target, this income level can be reached by aggressive practitioners with a small but intensively treated population or by conservative practitioners with a larger and less intensively treated population.[3] This could result in a natural sorting process through which areas with conservative practitioners are in equilibrium with low intensity care, while areas with aggressive practitioners reach an equilibrium with high-intensity care. Of course, such a situation requires consumer insensitivity to costs, which may be encouraged by extensive third-party coverage, and lack of knowledge or relative indifference to alternative treatment options. Individual physicians may firmly believe that they are following appropriate practice and that their decisions have little to do with economic incentives. Furthermore, most clinicians appear to be unaware of costs or to believe that a third-party payer, not the patient, will pay, so the patient will not be harmed.

The Aaron and Schwartz study of practices in Great Britain also provides a valuable illustration of how physicians can incorporate constraints into their decision making in a manner that minimizes visibility and awareness. In contrast to the widespread availability in the United States of dialysis for patients with end-stage renal disease, this type of treatment is in short supply in Britain. Instead of having large queues or arbitrary cutoffs, general practitioners only refer the youngest patients without complications for dialysis. The nephrologists see a relatively small number of patients, all of whom can be accommodated, and the general practitioners convince their patients and themselves that all those with a good prognosis are being helped and those with major complications are spared a prolongation of their suffering.

Conclusion

The evidence concerning the adoption and use of medical technology and different practice patterns suggests that economic incentives matter. It may even be sufficient to convince policymakers to alter incentives. However, much of the evidence lacks the power of a randomized controlled trial and does not easily convince skeptical physicians. From the clinician's perspective, the observational studies lack an explanation of how economic incentives alter practice patterns, particularly when they themselves do not see these factors influencing their behavior. Clearly there is often a wide range of acceptable clinical practice, even though each clinician may believe in his or her own way. If clinicians sort themselves into different practice settings whose economic incentives are consistent with aggressive or conservative practice styles, we will observe clinical patterns that appear to be shaped by economics, although the clinicians themselves do not recognize these effects.

The gray area in medical choice is often large, but there has been relatively little exploration thus far of the dimensions of ambiguity. More studies are now being proposed or undertaken to evaluate new technologies (Bunker, Fowles, and Schaffarzick 1982; Greenberg and Derzon 1981; Towery and Perry 1981). Wennberg, McPherson, and Caper (1984) found that the vast majority of diagnoses and surgical procedures show wide variability in admission rates. Simultaneously, the growth and development of HMOs, for-profit hospitals, health care corporations, and other organized systems provide additional incentives to evaluate the cost effectiveness of alternative clinical strategies. Such organizations may increasingly use incentives or pressures to alter clinicians' practice patterns. Some physicians already are beginning to adopt the worldview of the economist and use the language of choice, trade-offs, and financial transactions (Fein 1982). Whether such changes are desirable is a larger question and one important to the future of medical care.

Acknowledgment

Some of the material presented in this chapter appeared under the title "Economic Incentives and Clinical Decisions," in *The New Health Care for Profit: Doctors and Hospitals in a Competitive Environment*, edited by Bradford H. Gray (Washington D.C.: National Academy Press, 1983).

Notes

1. Surgeons often charge a fee that includes pre- and postoperative visits, obstetricians offer prenatal/maternity packages, and pediatricians sometimes have a single fee for the first year of well-baby care. In most of these cases, however, tests and treatments for complications are handled on a standard fee-for-service basis.

2. One could imagine a setting in which the diagnostician-physician-agent merely interpreted results on a fee-for-time basis, with all the diagnostic tests being performed by others and paid for separately. The difficulties in coordinating such an approach and the consequent delays in reaching a diagnosis in the vast majority of cases suggests why it has not occurred in practice. Requests for a second opinion before surgery are a step in this direction, but in most instances the second physician merely reviews the existing diagnostic test results.

3. The target-income hypothesis is hotly debated by economists, who seem unable to reach a definitive conclusion on this issue yet continue to hold strong beliefs about it. Gray areas exist in medical economics as well as in medicine. See Fuchs and Newhouse 1978, Hixon 1980, Richardson 1981, Wilensky and Rossiter 1981.

References

Aaron, Henry J., and William B. Schwartz. 1984. *The painful prescription: Rationing hospital care.* Washington D.C: Brookings Institution.

Berki, S. E., and Marie L. F. Ashcraft. 1980. HMO enrollment: Who joins and why: A review of the literature. *Milbank Memorial Fund Quarterly: Health and Society* 58(4):558–632.

Blumberg, Mark S. 1979. Provider price charges for improved health care use. In *Health handbook*, ed. George K. Chako. Amsterdam: North-Holland.

————. 1980. Health status and health care use by type of private health coverage. *Milbank Memorial Fund Quarterly: Health and Society.* 58(4): 633–655.

Broida, Joel, Monroe Lerner, F. N. Lohrenz, et al. 1975. Impact on membership in an enrolled prepaid population on utilization of health services in a group practice. *New England Journal of Medicine* 292(15):780–783.

Bunker, John P. 1970. A comparison of operations and surgeons in the United States and in England and Wales. *New England Journal of Medicine* 282(3):135–144.

Bunker, John P., Jinnet Fowles, and Ralph Schaffarzick. 1982. Evaluation of medical technology strategies. *New England Journal of Medicine* 306(10–11):620–624, 687–692.

California Medical Association. 1975. *1974 revision of the 1969 California Relative Value Studies.* San Francisco: Sutter Publications.

Carr, Kenneth W., Robert L. Engler, and John Ross, Jr. 1982. Do coronary artery bypass operations prolong life? *Western Journal of Medicine* 136(4):295–308.

Childs, Alfred W., and E. Diane Hunter. 1972. Non-medical factors influencing the use of diagnostic X-ray by physicians. *Medical Care* 10(4):323–335.

Cook, Wallace H. 1971. Profile of the permanente physician. In *The Kaiser-Permanente medical care program: A symposium,* ed. Anne R. Somers. New York: Commonwealth Fund.

Danzon, Patricia M., Willard G. Manning, Jr., and M. Susan Marquis. 1984. Factors affecting laboratory test use and prices. *Health Care Financing Review* 5(4):23–32.

Eddy, David M. 1982. Clinical policies and the quality of clinical practice. *New England Journal of Medicine* 307(6):343–347.

Eggers, Paul W., and Ronald Prihoda. 1982. Pre-enrollment reimbursement patterns of Medicare beneficiaries enrolled in "at-risk" HMOs. *Health Care Financing Review* 4(1):55–74.

Fein, Rashi. 1982. What is wrong with the language of medicine? *New England Journal of Medicine* 306(14):863–864.

Feldstein, Martin. 1974. Econometric studies of health economics. In *Frontiers in quantitative economics,* vol. 2, ed. M. D. Intriligator and D. A. Kendrick. Amsterdam: North-Holland.

Fineberg, Harvey V. 1979. Clinical chemistries: The high cost of low-cost diagnostic tests. In *Medical technology: The culprit behind health care costs?* Proceedings of the 1977 Sun Valley Forum on National Health. National Center for Health Services Research. DHEW Publishing No. (PHS) 79-3216. Washington, D.C.: Government Printing Office.

Foltz, Anne-Marie. 1984. Diffusion of technology: Roles of physicians and consumers. Presented at the American Public Health Association meetings, Anaheim, Calif.

Freeborn, Donald K., et al. 1972. Determinants of medical care utilization: Physicians' use of laboratory services. *American Journal of Public Health* 62(6):846–853.

Fuchs, Victor R., and Joseph P. Newhouse. 1978. The conference and unresolved problems. *Journal of Human Resources* 13 (supp.):5–20.

Greenberg, Barbara, and Robert A. Derzon. 1981. Determining health insurance coverage of technology: Problems and options. *Medical Care* 19(10): 967–978.

Griner, Paul F., et al. 1981. Selection and interpretation of diagnostic tests and procedures. *Annals of Internal Medicine* 94(5):553–600.

Grossman, Michael. 1972. *The demand for health: A theoretical and empirical investigation.* New York: Columbia University Press for the National Bureau of Economic Research.

———. 1982. The demand for health after a decade. *Journal of Health Economics* 1(1):1–3.

Hixon, Jesse S., ed. 1980. *The target income hypothesis.* Bureau of Health Manpower. DHEW Publishing No. (HRA) 80-27. Washington, D.C.: Government Printing Office.

Hlatky, Mark A., et al. 1983. Diagnostic test use in different practice settings: A controlled comparison. *Archives of Internal Medicine* 143(10):1886–1889.

Kuhn, Thomas S. 1970. *The structure of scientific revolutions.* 2d ed. Chicago: University of Chicago Press.

Lavin, John H. 1982. Same-day surgery: Why everyone is learning to love it. *Medical Economics* 59(12):110.

Lewin, Lawrence S., Robert A. Derzon, and Rhea Margulies. 1981. Investor-owneds and nonprofits differ in economic performance. *Hospitals* 55.

Luft, Harold S. 1981. *Health maintenance organizations: Dimensions of performance.* New York: Wiley-Interscience.

Lyle, Carl B., et al. 1976. Practice habits in a group of eight internists. *Annals of Internal Medicine* 84(5):594–601.

McClure, Walter. 1982. Toward development and application of a qualitative theory of hospital utilization. *Inquiry* 19(2):117–135.

McIntosh, H. D. 1981. *Overview of aortocoronary bypass grafting for the treatment of coronary artery disease: An internist's perspective.* Washington, D.C.: National Center for Health Care Technology.

McKinlay, John B. 1981. From "promising report" to "standard procedure": Seven stages in the career of a medical innovation. *Milbank Memorial Fund Quarterly: Health and Society* 59(3):374–411.

McNeil, Barbara J., and S. James Adelstein. 1975. The value of case finding in hypertensive renovascular disease. *New England Journal of Medicine* 293(5):221–26.

McNeil, Barbara J., et al. 1982. On the elicitation of preferences for alternative therapies. *New England Journal of Medicine* 306(21):1259–1262.

Manning, Willard G., Arleen Liebowitz, George A. Goldberg, et al. 1984. A controlled trial of the effect of a prepaid group practice on use of services. *New England Journal of Medicine* 310(23):1505.

Marks, Sylvia D., et al. 1980. Ambulatory surgery in an HMO: A study of costs, quality of care, and satisfaction. *Medical Care* 18(2):127–146.

Martin, Albert R. 1982. Common and correctable errors in diagnostic test ordering. *Western Journal of Medicine* 136(5):456–461.

Moloney, Thomas W., and David E. Rogers. 1979. Medical technology: A different view of the contentious debate over costs. *New England Journal of Medicine* 301(26):1413–1419.

Nobrega, Fred T., et al. 1982. Hospital use in a fee-for-service system. *Journal of the American Medical Association* 247(6):806–810.

O'Donnell, Walter E. 1982. Let's stop ducking decisions on patient care. *Medical Economics* 59(14):32.

Pattison, Robert V., and Hallie M. Katz. 1983. Investor-owned and not-for-profit hospitals: A comparison based on California data. *New England Journal of Medicine* 309(6):347–353.

Pauker, Stephen G., and Jerome P. Kassirer. 1975. Therapeutic decision making: A cost-benefit analysis. *New England Journal of Medicine* 293(5): 229–234.

Pauly, Mark V. 1980. *Doctors and their workshops: Economic models of physician behavior.* Chicago: University of Chicago Press.

Richardson, J. 1981. The inducement hypothesis: That doctors generate demand for their own services. In *Health, economics, and health economics,* ed. Jacques van der Gaag and Mark Perlman. Amsterdam: North-Holland.

Roney, James G., and Hilliard D. Estes. 1975. Automated health testing in a medical group practice. *Public Health Reports* 90(2):126–132.

Schroeder, Steven A., et al. 1973. Use of laboratory tests and pharmaceuticals: Variation among physicians and effects of cost audit on subsequent use. *Journal of the American Medical Association* 225(8):969–973.

Schroeder, Steven A., and Jonathan A. Showstack. 1978. Financial incentives to perform medical procedures and laboratory tests: Illustrative models of office practice. *Medical Care* 16(4):289–298.

Scitovsky, Anne A. 1981. The use of medical services under prepaid and fee-for service group practice. *Social Science and Medicine* 15C:107–116.

Showstack, Jonathan A., et al. 1979. Fee-for-service physician payment: Analysis of current methods and their development. *Inquiry* 16(3):230–246.

Showstack, Jonathan A., and Steven A. Schroeder. 1981. The cost effectiveness of upper gastrointestinal endoscopy. Background Paper No. 2, Case Studies of Medical Technologies—Case Study 8: Implications of Cost-Effectiveness Analysis of Medical Technology. Office of Technology Assessment, U.S. Congress. Washington, D.C.: Government Printing Office.

Towery, O. B., and Seymour Perry. 1981. The scientific basis for coverage decisions by third-party payers. *Journal of the American Medical Association* 245(1):59–61.

Wennberg, John E., John P. Bunker, and Benjamin Barnes. 1980. The need for assessing the outcome of common clinical practices. *Annual Review of Public Health* 1:277–295.

Wennberg, John E., and Alan Gittelsohn. 1973. Small variations in health care delivery. *Science* 182(4117):1102–1108.

————. 1975. Health care delivery in Maine, 1: Patterns of use of common surgical procedures. *Journal of Maine Medical Association* 66(5):123–130, 49.

———. 1982. Variations in medical care among small areas. *Scientific American* 246(4):120ff.

Wennberg, John E., Klim McPherson, and Philip Caper. 1984. Will payment based on diagnosis-related groups control hospital costs? *New England Journal of Medicine* 311(5):293–300.

Wilensky, Gail Roggin, and Louis F. Rossiter. 1981. The magnitude and determinants of physician initiated visits in the United States. In *Health, economics, and health economics,* ed. Jacques van der Gaag and Mark Perlman. Amsterdam: North-Holland.

Wilson, Edward O. 1978. The ergonomics of caste in the social insects. *American Economic Review* 68(6):25–36.

Chapter 24

Surplus versus Cost Containment
The Changing Context for Health Providers

Donald W. Light

The American health care system is undergoing revolutionary changes in its organization and financing. Efforts at cost containment are imposing fundamentally new ways of defining health care and new relationships between providers, patients, and payers. At the same time, the number of providers has been increasing dramatically. The thesis of this chapter is that important dangers and opportunities, unknown before in this century, are impending for physicians and other providers. Those who understand these opportunities and embrace them will thrive while others will not because, overall, a significant surplus of health professionals is likely to develop. To understand the organizational and economic forces that are shaping this surplus and its consequences, one must understand their origins.

Prosperity and the Provider Boom

If one thinks of the baby boom's consequences for American life over the past forty years—the creation of new markets, the restructuring of institutions, the changes in the job market, and the basic shifts in values (Jones 1981)—one grasps the significance of about 200,000 doctors (M.D.s and D.O.s) being added to the physician population between 1960 and 1980 (see table 24.1). The organizational, economic, and cultural impact of still another 200,000 physicians by the year 2000 will be greater yet. This expansion had its origins, as did the baby boom, in the postwar prosperity following World War II.

It is widely believed that medical school enrollments expanded in the 1960s to meet a physician shortage. While a shortage was declared in the political sense, an organizational and cultural analysis of physician manpower policy puts the current growth of physicians in another perspective. After World War II, hospitals pressed for and Congress passed the Hill-Burton Act, which provided funds for the construction of hospitals, particularly in states that had low bed/population ratios. The target was set at 4.5 beds per 1,000 people, "a figure suggested by [hospital] industry experts that was far above the levels of any state" (Starr 1982, 349). By the time it was phased out, the Hill-Burton program had disbursed $3.7 billion and generated another $9.1 billion from state and local sources for hospital construction. This massive expansion created an organizational demand for more physicians. The increase in medical school enrollments during the 1950s, however, did not even keep up with the population increase caused by the baby boom (table 24.1). As for the distribution, while Hill-Burton equalized hospital beds between low-income and high-income states, the funds went disproportionately to middle-income communities *within* states. On the whole, doctors practice where hospitals are built; so this pattern laid the organizational ground for the geographic maldistribution of physicians. In addition, this bias toward hospitals, rather than em-

TABLE 24.1
Number of Physicians, 1950 to 1980, with Projections to the Year 2000

	Number of Graduates		Number of Active Physicians		Total Active Physicians	Patients per Active Physician
	M.D.	D.O.	M.D.	D.O.		
1950	5,553	373	209,000	10,900	219,900	706
1960	7,081	427	239,700	12,200	251,200	735
1970	8,367	432	314,200	12,300	326,500	641
1980	15,135	1,033	440,400	17,100	457,500	508
1990	16,695	1,502	563,300	27,900	591,200	411
2000	16,523	1,486	665,700	39,000	704,700	369

Source: U.S. Department of Health and Human Services 1982.

phasizing the comprehensive care called for in the landmark 1932 report of the Committee on the Costs of Medical Care, set the stage for training mostly hospital-based specialists.

Meanwhile, research in medical schools received comparable support. In the 1940s, national expenditures for research rose from $18 million to $181 million, and federal contributions rose from $3 million to $76 million. The average annual income of medical schools tripled, from $0.5 million to $1.5 million. It more than doubled to $3.7 million during the 1950s, as did the number of full-time faculty (Starr 1982, chap. 3). With no comparable increase in students, this research expansion created a second source of demand for training more doctors, particularly specialists.

At the consumer level, general prosperity after World War II produced more disposable income. In addition, hospital-based insurance insulated patients as well as doctors from feeling the cost of specialized procedures performed in hospitals. Prosperity and insurance combined with a cultural fascination for medical "breakthroughs" to spur demand for services. Thus, the push for more care joined the demand of medical faculty for students and of hospitals for housestaff. Paul Starr (1982, 360) observes, "By 1957 hospitals were looking for more than 12,000 interns annually, but American medical schools were graduating fewer than 7,000 students a year." Hospital residency places shot up from 12,000 in 1947 to 25,000 in 1955. These inexpensive yet highly skilled apprentices not only increased services but contributed to hospital profits. Many hospitals had to search abroad for foreign medical graduates to fill these positions.

Thus, the physician shortage declared in the early 1960s, given the tremendous expansion of hospitals and medical school faculties along with generous reimbursement for hospital services, seems an almost foregone conclusion. Put another way, the president of the AMA in 1933 announced that careful studies showed there to be a surplus of 25,000; by 1961 the AMA was calling for federal funds to build and support new medical schools to alleviate the physician shortage (Lewis 1933; Lewis 1982). The shortage, however, depended on the economic and political demand for more hospitals, more medical research, and more insurance to cover the resulting costs.

Shortage and surplus cannot be calculated apart from their institutional context. In 1960, there were about 148 physicians per 100,000 population; almost 50 percent more doctors than health maintenance organizations (HMOs) found they needed to provide comprehensive care to all subscribers (Stevens 1971; California Auditor General 1983). Yet a shortage was declared. In 1980 the Graduate Medical Education National Advisory Committee concluded that there would be a surplus of 70,000 physicians by 1990 and a surplus of 144,700 by the year 2000. These calculations assumed that the postwar structure of generous, hospital-based insurance would continue. Were this structure to change toward cost containment and prospective payment, however, the surplus could become much larger. Today, the physician/population ratio is twice that of HMOs and still rising (U.S. Department of Health and Human Services 1980).

Of equal concern in the 1960s was the maldistribution of physicians both geographically and among specialties. For example, 65 counties had no practicing physician in 1950, but in 1963 there were 100 such counties. The number peaked at about 130 in 1971 but began to decline in the late 1970s, as primary care programs and increased supply took effect (Perry and Breitner 1982, 60). Solving the problem of underserved rural and inner-city areas by producing a surplus of physicians is an extremely expensive and inefficient policy because only about one in ten physicians settles in these areas (California Auditor General 1983). More focused programs such as the National Health Service Corps, which locates physicians in underserved areas, have met with limited success.

The rapid growth of specialists and subspecialists was to be expected with the massive construction of hospitals, expansion of hospital insurance, and infusion of medical schools with clinical research faculty who wanted to train medical students in their own image. By the 1960s, however, a crisis in primary care was perceived because physicians in general practice had declined from about 90 percent in 1923 to about 35 percent in 1960 and would continue to decline into the 1970s (Perry and Breitner 1982). To offset the decline in general practitioners, the new specialty of

family medicine was created in 1969. Federal subsidies to family practice programs were soon followed by support for primary-care residencies in pediatrics and internal medicine. These policies appear to have reversed the decline of primary-care general practitioners, but redefining primary care to include all internists, obstetricians-gynecologists, pediatricians, and family practitioners is somewhat misleading. Given that over 80 percent of all physicians by the 1970s were specialists, while fewer than 20 percent of the population had medical problems that demanded the services of a specialist, most primary care was necessarily performed by specialists. Large numbers of physicians rushed in to fill the vacuum in primary care during the 1970s (Aiken et al. 1979), at the same time that physician assistants (PAs) and nurse-practitioners (NPs) were introduced to replenish the depleted ranks of general practitioners (GPs). Thus, the once depleted area of primary care has become overcrowded.

The Increasing Supply of Nurses

The same postwar developments that greatly expanded and emphasized hospital-based specialty care, and thus increased the demand for physicians, also increased the demand for nurses. Clinical nursing shortages have been declared since World War II, even though the number of nurses has grown significantly. While there were about 600,000 RNs in 1960 (U.S. Department of Commerce 1975), their ranks have swelled to nearly 1.3 million in 1980 and were recently projected to grow to 1.9 million by the year 2000 (U.S. Department of Health and Human Services 1984). The number of licensed practical nurses likewise more than doubled, from 217,000 in 1960 to about 550,000 in 1980, but are expected to grow more slowly to about 750,000 by the year 2000 (see table 24.2). Unlike physicians, however, the rapid expansion in the 1960s and 1970s was not enough to meet the demand for nurses in hospitals, where about two-thirds of all nurses work. Despite a dramatic increase in the supply of nurses, an estimated 100,000 unfilled positions were reported by hospitals in the late 1970s (Levine and Moses 1982). As recently as 1982, an important book on nursing in the 1980s devoted many chapters to the nursing shortage and how to alleviate it by making the work of nurses financially and organizationally more attractive (Aiken 1982). However, programs to contain hospital costs in the past few years have reversed the picture. Since nurses make up more than a third of hospital personnel, reductions in admissions and length of stay are translated into a reduced demand for hospital nurses.

Nursing is the center of hospital care. "If patients do not need *nursing* care, they have no need to be admitted to a hospital; all [other] health

TABLE 24.2
Proliferation of Providers

Practitioners	1960	1980	2000
Physicians (MDs, DOs)	251,900	457,500	704,700
Chiropractors	unknown	24,400	88,100
Registered nurses[a]	592,000	1,272,900	1,900,000
Licensed practical nurses[a]	217,000	549,300	724,500
Nurse-midwives[b]	500(?)	2,000	4,800
Physician assistants[c]	0	11,000	32,800
Nurse-practitioners[d]	0	14,700	36,400

Sources: U.S. Department of Health and Human Services 1980, vol. 1; 1982; 1984; U.S. Department of Commerce 1975; *Chiropractic Demography* 1983; *Chiropractic* 1983; Adams 1984.
a. The figure for 2000 was an interpolation between high and low estimates.
b. The figure for 2000 was calculated by assuming 200 graduates per year, with gross attrition rate of 20 percent.
c. The figure for 1980 was based on the figure for 1983 minus attrition projected back to 1980; the figure for 2000 was calculated by assuming 1,500 graduates per year, with gross attrition rate of 20 percent.
d. The figure for 2000 was calculated by assuming 2,100 graduates per year, with gross attrition rate of 20 percent.

care can be provided on an outpatient basis" (McClure and Nelson 1982, 59). It is nurses who provide continuous care for patients, with physicians coming in from time to time as consultants. As the procedures used on patients have become more sophisticated and have required sensitive monitoring, the technical demands of nursing have increased. Hospitalized patients are, on average, more ill than in previous decades, because advances in pharmacology and medicine have enabled more patients to be treated on an outpatient basis. This trend will accelerate as cost-containment efforts keep all but the sickest patients out of the hospital.

The increasing demands of nursing are reflected in the decline of diploma nurses, the growth of baccalaureate nurses, and the rapid increase of clinical nurse specialists, nurse-clinicians, nurse-practitioners, and nurses with master's degrees (Aiken 1982; Levine and Moses 1982). The ranks of nurses, like those of physicians, have increased rapidly since World War II, with a strong bias toward specialized, hospital care. An era of cost containment will limit the use of hospitals even as it intensifies the need for skilled nursing among those who are hospitalized.

The Creation and Growth of Nurse-Practitioners

Nurse-practitioners (NPs) were created as a new kind of nurse professional during the era of declared physician shortages. In reviewing the development of NPs, Charles Lewis notes that between 1965 and 1970 the primary goals were to increase nurses' professional skills so that patient care could be improved and to alleviate the shortage of physicians (Lewis 1982). In response to specialty medicine, the NP curriculum focused on producing a practitioner who assessed patients' problems wholistically in terms of their history, family, and living patterns so as to promote maximum health and functioning (Ford 1982). The emphasis on independent practice, Lewis maintains, came from the sexism and arrogance of physicians, who inflicted on early NPs such recorded remarks as "'Better watch out fellows (to medical students standing near), you may have to pick up the pieces'" (Lewis 1982, 255–256). During the 1970s NPs lobbied hard to gain as much independent status as they could. Federal funds for NP programs expanded rapidly, from a few hundred thousand dollars in 1971 to several million a year (Lewis 1982). Nurse-practitioners increased from less than 1,000 in 1970 to 14,700 in 1980 and are projected to reach 36,400 by the year 2000 (U.S. Department of Health and Human Services 1980, vol. 6). Evaluation data sketch a profile of practice: 90 percent of NPs are employed, largely in roles for which they were trained; almost half the patients served by NPs are in the lowest income bracket; employers as well as patients are almost universally satisfied with the quality of the NPs' work; and 93 percent of NP employers consider them cost beneficial (Sultz, Zielezny, and Gentry 1980; Ford 1982).

The Creation and Growth of Physician Assistants

In 1961 Dr. Charles Hudson suggested at an AMA conference that assistants to physicians be trained to serve as medical technicians for suturing, intubation, catheterization, and similar procedures so that physicians could have more time for community office practice (Carter and Gifford 1982). When Duke University developed a program to train nurses to be PAs, the National League of Nursing opposed it. The program shifted in 1965 to training non-nurses for two roles: one for specialized service in hospitals and one for assisting general practitioners. The overall emphasis, however, was on a technician who "would relieve the doctor of direct responsibility for many procedures" and "would conserve the costly talents of other health professionals" (Carter and Gifford 1982, 26). The Duke model was adopted at a number of schools over the next several years. Another approach was developed in 1969 at the University of Washington School of Medicine to certify former military corpsmen for work in medically underserved rural areas. This Medex program emphasized a twelve-month preceptorship with a physician who tentatively agreed to employ the student after graduation. Variations of these two approaches proliferated in the next few years. Meanwhile, the accreditation of training programs for PAs was worked out under the auspices of the AMA, and fourteen national organizations joined to form a National Com-

mission on Certification of Physicians Assistants. By 1974 there were over fifty programs graduating a total of more than one thousand PAs a year.

Several federal agencies became interested in the PA concept and funded the training of PAs to serve in the merchant marine, federal prisons, Indian reservations, and the Public Health Service (Carter and Gifford 1982). In 1977 legislation was passed to reimburse PAs and NPs directly from Medicare and Medicaid for services rendered in rural health clinics. PAs also gained early, wide acceptance among physicians. Sadler, Sadler, and Bliss noted in 1972 that "physician assistants are quickly surpassing other supporting health professionals in direct patient management and in financial reward" (pp. 33–34). This aroused alarm in the nursing profession, where half its members were not working and where turnover of nurses in hospitals was high because of inadequate pay and recognition. The success of the PA movement was a spur to NPs, who emphasized their broader, psychosocial training for total patient care in contrast to the more narrow and technical role of PAs (Bullough 1976). A systematic comparison of the two new health practitioners confirmed this difference (System Science Inc. 1976). It is revealing that early directors of NP programs emphasized the goals of increasing the overall quality of medical care and reducing physician dominance, while directors of PA programs emphasized increasing physicians' productivity and decreasing costs. Clearly the NP focus has been more competitive with physicians, while the PA focus has emphasized the two key central concerns of the present health care system.

The supply of physician assistants has grown to about 11,000 in 1980 and is projected to reach 32,800 by the year 2000 (Department of Health and Human Services 1984). A majority of PAs work in primary care, with more in private practice than NPs. About a quarter work in hospitals (as do NPs), but PAs work under the medical department while NPs work under the nursing department. On the one hand, this placement enables PAs to show their relevance to doctors more directly and puts them on the physician team. On the other hand, it makes PAs more dependent on physicians. Increasingly, PAs seem to be working for clinics and other institutions rather than for individual physicians, and they seem to be diversifying into a wide range of roles (Reisz, Cawley, and Barry 1984; Cawley, Ott, and DeAtley 1983; Cawley et al. 1984).

In conclusion, the proliferation of providers illustrated in table 24.2 had its origins in the rapid expansion of hospital beds and medical research after World War II. General prosperity, rising expectations, and expanding health insurance also contributed to the demand for more providers. The figures in table 24.2 indicate that all provider groups are projected to increase significantly by the year 2000 simply by training as many graduates each year as they do now. No growth in training programs in fact means rapid growth because the graduating classes are so much larger than the annual number of providers who die

or retire. This swelling population of providers has contributed in part to its greatest problem—how to contain health care costs.

Cost Containment and Competition

As early as 1969, President Richard Nixon announced that a "massive crisis" of escalating health costs needed immediate attention, only a few years after the "crisis" of insufficient services and physician shortages had been declared. The next decade was filled with efforts to contain costs through regulation. President Nixon imposed wage and price controls. States enacted laws to control capital expenditures and to regulate hospital rates. Professional standard review organizations were established, as were health systems agencies. President Nixon advocated HMOs (health maintenance organizations) as the cost-effective way to deliver comprehensive care, and a federal program was established both to provide start-up funds and to regulate HMOs. While some of these policies temporarily contained health costs, all of them together challenged the long-held assumption that decisions about the delivery of health care should be left in the hands of physicians and hospitals.

In the meantime, health care corporations began to form during the 1960s to take advantage of the seemingly endless reimbursements provided by health insurance policies, Medicare, and Medicaid (Relman 1980; Starr 1982; Tarlov 1983). Private corporations assumed early domination in certain sectors, such as nursing homes and renal dialysis centers. Hospital corporations were much less dominant but gained momentum in the 1970s. Consolidation through buy-outs and mergers began to transform hundreds of local hospitals into multihospital systems. The health care system was experiencing its most significant restructuring since the turn of the century, and the driving forces were capital and finance. Bent on increasing gross sales and profits, these corporations exacerbated the problems of the rising costs of medicine. So also did the rapidly growing number of providers, especially hospital-based specialists. The organization of the lucrative practice of medicine into larger corporate bodies expanded to office practices and other sectors through the 1970s and into the 1980s.

Of equal importance to the corporate restructuring of providers has been the awakening and restructuring of purchasers, for they hold the key to cost containment and to competition (Tell, Falik, and Fox 1984). In an unrestrained and expanding market, providers have no incentive to contain costs and experience only modest competition. Traditionally, purchasers are patients, millions of individuals who know little about medicine and who come to providers when they are most vulnerable. Corporate or organized buyers, by contrast, can negotiate price, method of payment, scope of services, and guarantees to render all services for a preestablished price per patient. Corporate or organized buyers, such as Chrysler Corporation, Medicare, John Deere, or

Medicaid, can limit the market for providers and foster competition in a number of ways. They can create incentives for prevention and self-care, design disincentives for hospital care and costly procedures, and alter the traditional division of labor among health providers.

The awakening of corporate purchasers began in the 1970s when high inflation pushed health insurance premiums up by more than 20 percent a year and an economic recession drew attention to this relatively small item on corporate balance sheets (Starr 1982). A few presidents and board chairmen started asking questions and quickly found that health insurance was the most rapidly escalating cost-item in their budget. U.S. automobile manufacturers, for example, pay more per car for health insurance than for steel. Corporations also realized that by sending premiums to Blue Cross, Prudential, and other insurance carriers, they were losing interest on a large pool of money. Some companies began to insure themselves. As a result, they gathered detailed data on medical expenditures and had a direct financial incentive for minimizing medical bills charged against their premium pool. The number of corporations that convert from passive payers of health insurance benefits to active purchasers of health services is likely to grow throughout the 1980s (Goldsmith 1984).

The actions taken by corporate purchasers are diverse, but one can distinguish two major program areas. Internally, a growing number are developing wellness, or health promotion, programs. Externally, they are entering the medical marketplace to obtain competitive prices for medical care or to restructure the market (Wack and Horwitz 1985; MacKay 1984). In a few cases, for example, companies first tried to negotiate with the local medical community; when they met resistance, they formed their own HMO. This kind of forceful restructuring was unthinkable only a few years ago. To increase their economic clout, corporations are also forming local and regional health care coalitions (Herzlinger 1984). Most coalitions share information about the concerns of their members, but several have become active in lobbying for legislation that reduces barriers to competition, and several have negotiated in concert for most cost-effective services.

Among the largest purchasers of health care are state and federal governments. Their transformation from passive to active buyers is still in process, but already their impact has been profound. Some states, as employers, have vigorously promoted HMOs and capitation premiums for their employees in order to promote health and control costs. Others have promoted or required prepaid systems to contain hospital costs. But most influential have been the demonstrations, experiments, and programs of Medicare and Medicaid. The fear that the Medicare trust fund might soon be depleted has led the Health Care Financing Authority (HCFA) and Congress to promote new programs to change the behavior of physicians and patients. These programs include the national restructuring of Medicare hospital reimbursements to a prepayment system based on diagnostic-related groups (DRGs) and experiments with capitation. State Medicaid programs have not been far behind in efforts to restructure health behavior, medical markets, and therefore the socioeconomic context in which the growing supply of providers will work.

Cost-Containment Strategies and Their Consequences for Health Care Providers

Each cost-containment strategy affects the incentives and organization of health care; thus, the use of different provider groups is altered. Here, we shall consider three strategies: capitation and HMOs; hospital prepayment systems and DRGs; and corporate health programs. While some research exists on these initiatives and how they affect providers, policy implications will necessarily be speculative.

Capitation and HMOs

Capitation refers to a family of methods for limiting the costs of care to a fixed price per person per year. The best known system of capitation in the United States is the health maintenance organization (HMO), in which the functions of insurer and provider are united. As a comprehensive payment for all services, capitation leads to rationing by some mixture of central administrative decisions and individual clinical decisions (Mechanic 1984). Because capitated services are complex and can be organized in several ways, this brief discussion will focus on only the more general implications for provider groups.

The principal way in which capitated systems save money is by minimizing hospital bed days. Well-run HMOs have an admission rate that is 20 to 40 percent lower than comparable patient populations under fee-for-service (Luft 1981; Brown 1983). Thus, HMOs and other delivery systems under capitation seek providers with the skills and outlook that will enable them to treat as many patients as possible on an ambulatory basis. Although the number of patients under capitation is growing steadily (Masso 1985), most physicians and nurses continue to be trained in hospital-based skills and values. As David Mechanic wrote a decade ago, "The work of primary care physicians differs considerably from the model of practice students observe in caring for seriously ill patients in teaching hospitals" (1976, 109). Many of the problems physicians will encounter in primary care do not fit easily into the categories learned in the hospital. Moreover, the attitudes and habits learned in training do not fit the needs of an HMO or other health care organization based on capitation.

Besides seeking providers who will minimize hospitalization, delivery systems under capitation want doctors, nurses, NPs, and PAs with the ability to ration care within a limited budget. The dilemma that capitated systems face is offering comprehensive care to patients while keeping within a fixed budget. This dilemma necessitates making some hard choices. How many problems can one ignore or postpone treating, given that so many presenting problems are self-limiting or medically trivial, without alienating subscribers or missing a serious problem? The economic incentive under capitation is to underserve patients; yet underservice can be its own undoing. Such clinical rationing takes place in the context of explicit rationing by administrators of the resources available to the providers and patients in the system. Thus, effective providers must balance what the organization needs against what they judge the patient to need, and both against what the patient wants. As Mechanic points out (1976; chap. 6; 1979a; chap. 2), medical work involves a considerable amount of uncertainty and discretionary judgment within which this balancing can take place.

Of central importance to reconciling these competing interests is changing patient behavior. Capitated systems may seek providers who can help patients learn to manage more of their problems and thus require fewer services. For example, some evidence shows that nurse-practitioners are more skilled than physicians and PAs in meeting patients' felt needs and teaching them how to manage their problems so that they have fewer return visits, greater "compliance" with the treatment plan, and less hospitalization (Ramsey, McKenzie, and Fish 1982; Sullivan 1982; Prescott and Driscoll 1979). Prevention is also a logical part of reducing patients' need for services, but it is not clear that HMOs and similar organizations devote a significant amount of time to prevention. One would therefore expect only limited and highly focused efforts at prevention.

In holding down costs, capitated delivery systems logically seek to delegate as much work as possible to less expensive personnel and to substitute less costly providers for more expensive ones (Record 1981). Thus, one can expect that with the steadily accelerating growth of patients under capitation, there will be a relatively greater demand for nonphysicians and less demand for physicians than under fee-for-service. In reality, the amount of delegation and substitution varies considerably from plan to plan becaues of local customs, staff attitudes, client base, and other factors (Steinwachs, Shapiro, and Weiner 1983). However, the pressures to hold down costs are increasing, and the potential for delegation is much greater than many people imagine. Scores of studies over twenty years indicate that about 75 to 80 percent of ambulatory care can be delegated by strategically smart physicians in primary care (Light 1985; Crandall et al. 1984; Light 1983; Yankauer and Sullivan 1982; Repicky, Mendenhall, and Neville 1982; Abdellah 1982; Record 1981; Rivlin 1979; Mechanic 1979b; Lawrence 1978). The more detailed of these studies show no functional differences between these nonphysicians and physicians in accuracy of diagnosis, treatment plans, referrals to specialists, and a number of other dimensions of clinical care. On the other hand, patient satisfaction and so-called patient compliance with NPs is higher.

The other important group which can be used extensively to reduce costs is nurse-midwives (NMWs). Roemer (1978, 1979) points out that nurse-midwives are widely used in some countries with no ill effects and with high patient satisfaction. Even the physician-dominated panel in obstetrics and gynecology for the Graduate Medical Education National Advisory Committee (U.S. Department of Health and Human Services 1980, vol. 2) concluded that only 20 percent of all births were high risk and needed the care of a specialist.

The more independent nonphysicians, such as NMWs and NPs, have the cost-effective advantage of practicing a more wholistic, health-promoting type of medicine; thus they tend to use fewer high-cost procedures and less hospitalization than do physicians (Ramsey, McKenzie, and Fish 1982; Sullivan 1982; Prescott and Driscoll 1979; Aiken 1981; Tom 1982). From the perspective of HMOs and large-scale buyers interested in controlling the cost of total care, their kind of practice is preferable to the hi-tech, cost-intensive style of specialists.

The effective use of nonphysician providers depends on good managerial skills so that the providers do not duplicate the work of physicians (Record 1981; Steinwachs, Shapiro, and Weiner 1983). Rationing services within a capitated system is difficult to do well (Mechanic 1979a, chap. 8), and therefore the growing number of prepaid practices will be seeking providers with the ability to manage clinical teams in a cost-effective way. Providers familiar with the use of clinical protocols, triage systems, and forms of effective delegation will be valued.

In conclusion, capitation is the most complete strategy for containing health care costs. Drawing out the consequences implicit for providers in prepaid capitation is therefore an important policy exercise. As mentioned earlier in this chapter, HMOs use significantly fewer physicians per thousand people than do the fee-for-service arrangements that have characterized the American system for many decades. This discussion has identified five other trends. Capitated systems will use NPs and PAs more heavily than fee-for-service physicians now use them, and the increasing pressures to contain costs may accelerate this trend. The other four trends pertain to certain skills and attitudes or practice styles of providers. Capitated systems will seek clinicians with the ability to minimize hospitalization, to ration ambulatory care wisely, to teach patients how to manage their problems themselves and how to use fewer services, and to know how to manage a clinical team effectively. These capacities imply major changes in how all four provider groups are trained. Educational programs that respond to meet this new cluster of needs should be well rewarded for their efforts. Young physicians particularly need to acquire these four skills if they wish to be in demand. As surpluses grow, older and established physicians are likely to shut younger ones out of practice settings and hospital staffs (Light 1984). A generation gap is likely to arise, and young physicians may have difficulty finding work in their chosen profession. However, if younger doctors can learn the skills of minimizing hospitalization, practicing cost-effective medicine, making patients more capable of self-care, and managing teams of nonphysician providers, they can compete successfully against established physicians by delivering more cost-effective care.

Hospital Case-Based Prepayment and DRGs

A major strategy for containing the costs of expensive hospital care is to pay hospitals a fixed sum for treating patients with similar diagnoses that have similar treatment costs. At present, the system for employing this strategy is called diagnosis-related groups (DRGs). Using hospital records, a team at Yale University has identified 470 groups and calculated the average charges for each. Under a DRG prepayment system, hospitals are paid according to the case mix of DRGs they treat. This approach has certain advantages in containing costs. First, it pays a hospital a fixed sum for treating a problem instead of reimbursing a hospital for any services ordered to treat a problem. Second, the system can be tightened more easily than before by freezing or reducing the payments for DRGs. Medicare has adopted DRGs as a way to control hospital costs, and a number of states are likely to apply DRGs to all payers of hospital care.

Certain aspects of case-based prepayment are relevant to our focus on how this strategy will affect providers. First, there is no single DRG payment system because one can embellish basic DRGs with other financial items. In New Jersey, for example, hospitals receive different payments depending on how much indigent and uncompensated care they provide, how much capital debt they have, how variable each DRG is, and so on (May and Wasserman 1984). The Medicare DRG system includes none of these additional provisions, which significantly affect the calculus of care. For example, New Jersey's decision to pay for uninsured patients and to use more of a hospital's historic costs in paying for more variable DRGs mean that few patients are deemed economically undesirable. Second, DRG rates are based on historical *charges*, which may be quite discrepant from actual costs. As hospitals learn their true costs, they are discovering that some DRGs are quite profitable while others lose them money. As a result, they may change how certain DRGs are treated or they may try *not* to admit certain DRGs. Third, there may be other, more accurate systems for paying hospitals by case mix, such as the intensity system developed by Susan Horn (1983; Horn and Sharkey 1983; Horn, Sharkey and Bertram 1983). But any system will create its own clinical distortions and therefore affect providers. Finally, DRGs address health care costs only while patients are hospitalized. Conceivably, DRGs could be developed for ambulatory care, long-term care, and physicians' fees; but there are many problems in designing them for these areas.

Given these features of case-based prepayment systems for hospitals, one can turn to their consequences for providers. These consequences are clearest in the all-payer DRG system in New Jersey because it is the oldest and was the subject of a study comparing matched samples of DRG and non-DRG hospitals (Boerma 1983; May and Wasserman 1984). A major consequence, with implications for providers, is the transformation of clinical and medical records from minor documents required by the law and the hospital to central documents for determining how much money is received and how much money is spent. May and Wasserman (1984) found that the accuracy and detail of these records increased considerably after the DRG system was implemented.

The central role of records changes the power structure of the hospital. From relative obscurity, the head of medical records becomes a central figure, and some New Jersey hospitals have redefined these administrators as senior officers. The implication of this change for providers is that bills no longer reflect the medical decisions made by physicians and are no longer sent out to reimburse the costs of whatever medical decisions are made. Instead, medical decisions are made within the context of a fixed prepayment for the case.

A related consequence for providers is that more complete and accurate records contain a profile of how each physician and nursing team practices medicine. Any case-mix prepaid system leads to administrators sending printouts to physician groups and nursing teams, which indicate who is ordering significantly more tests or using significantly more expensive procedures to treat patients with the same DRG (Keane, Solnick, and Cohen 1985). The question is whether the extra expense is justified or whether it reflects a costly style of practice.

Practice styles vary widely from hospital to hospital and from region to region, and raising the question of unnecessary cost is changing many medical habits. For example, the widely held norm that patients with a myocardial infarction would be kept in the hospital for twenty-one days has been found to be based on professional custom. The norm is now ten to fourteen days, and in England many of these cases are treated as effectively without any hospitalization (Young 1985). In sum, prepayment systems give financial officers of a hospital considerably more power and lead clinicians to question their old treatment habits.

If one moves from the level of making decisions about cases to the question of what kind of personnel a hospital should have to be efficient, then the need for each provider group to show that they are cost-effective emerges as another implication of prepayment systems. The principal issue at this level is how much of physicians' work can be delegated to less costly personnel such as nurses, nurse-practitioners, nurse-midwives, and physician assistants. Although the medical profession has erected significant legal and regulatory barriers to cost-effective delegation (Lazarus et al. 1981), hospital administrators and their medical staff may become increasingly motivated to join payers and insurers in lowering those barriers. Throughout this cen-

tury, more and more procedures have been passed on from physicians to nurses and technicians, but delegation or substitution can be extended much further. A particularly interesting example is the substitution of NPs and PAs for physician-residents. Not only do the supervising physicians report that nonphysicians can do the sophisticated clinical work of residents well, but their substitution solves the problem of residency training programs graduating specialists who then compete against their mentors (Silver and McAtee 1984; Detmer and Perry 1982; Cawley et al. 1984; Light 1985).

Although realigning the division of labor and its consequent ratios of different staff in hospitals is a long-range implication of hospital prepayment systems, provider groups should appreciate the importance of having financial records reflect their contributions to cost-effective care. Two examples will illustrate the issues. A recent study claimed that the intervention of child psychiatrists on pediatric wards could save 9.2 percent of the costs for treating certain classes of hospitalized cases (Houts et al. 1985). For such a claim to be documented on a continuing basis, however, medical records would have to be organized so that the cost-effectiveness of psychiatric intervention could be measured. To put the matter more broadly, the well-established observation that mental health problems lead to more medical problems and to slower recovery is a promising basis for psychologically trained clinicians to contribute to limiting medical costs; but such services are more likely to be cut than added if medical

and financial records are not organized to document their contributions.

The second example concerns
nurses. Their central political and
economic problem under the new
DRG systems is that their contributions to cost containment (whether
large or small) are not part of hospital
records (Joel 1983). Instead, hospitals
continue to use a bed-day rate for cal-
culating the cost of length of stay under the DRG system, and nurses'
salaries are thrown in with housekeeping expenses, heat, laundry, elec-
tricity, and maintenances costs as
part of that rate. Nurses want their
own cost and revenue center, and
considerable effort is going into finding acceptable cost-accounting systems that will fulfill this goal (Joel
1983). In a prepaid system, one's contribution must be measured or it does
not exist.

Another consequence of hospital
prepaid systems is that some DRGs
lose money for given hospitals, and
within DRGs some kinds of patients
lose money. There is thus a natural
tendency for hospitals to avoid both
groups of patients. In the former case,
neighboring hospitals may find that
each can do some DRGs more cost-
effectively than others and therefore
trade or regionalize certain DRGs. In
the latter case, the more costly patients within DRGs are probably
older or poorer patients as well as patients with other, ongoing medical
problems besides the one for which
they are admitted. The ethical problems are the subject for another paper,
but the implications of DRG selectiv-
ity for providers is that certain kinds
of specialists may be in greater or less

demand at a given hospital. Providers
should look into how remunerative
are the DRGs around which their
work focuses.

At the same time that hospitals
may be selecting certain DRGs, or patients within them, while attempting
to avoid others, hospitals will also be
motivated by any hospital prepayment system to "unbundle" or remove as many services as they can
from the hospital. Unbundled services, such as EKGs and radiology,
reduce hospital costs for treating a
patient and therefore increase net revenues from DRG payments. At the
same time, these services often benefit physicians affiliated with the
hospital because they can bill for
these unbundled services separately.
The loopholes provided by a system
that covers only hospital costs is the
major way in which the present DRG
systems differ from comprehensive
capitation systems.

Taking advantage of the extensive
terrain that the present DRG systems
do not regulate, hospitals are creating group practices, nursing homes,
health promotion programs, same-
day surgicenters, cataract and cardiac
programs, home health care divisions, and numerous other "revenue
centers" (Ermann and Gabel 1984;
Mundinger 1983). These actions are
creating important prehospital and
posthospital services that have not
existed before. At the same time,
however, their use seems driven by
the profit motive. Hospitals are using
nursing homes, for example, as places
where they can discharge patients
early before they have fully recovered
(Aiken et al. 1985; U.S. General Accounting Office 1985). Same-day sur-

gery enables some hospitals in New Jersey's all-payer DRG system to charge $300 to $400 an hour for their operating rooms. Ginzberg, Balinsky, and Ostow (1984) found that hospital-run home health care services charge twice as much as those run by community agencies, even though their costs are not much higher. In mental health care, some New Jersey hospitals have arranged better follow-up care with community agencies so that they can treat in seventy-two hours many of the psychiatric patients they used to keep for ten to twelve days. Since the hospital continues to receive the full DRG payment, which covers ten to twelve days, the seventy-two-hour service is highly profitable.

These activities have a number of consequences for providers. First, within the hospital, patient care becomes more intensive because of early discharge. This practice implies a different nursing mix oriented to fewer, more highly skilled nurse-specialists (Institute of Medicine 1983). Second, the number of bed-days and the overall demand for nurses in hospitals are declining as the historic predominance of the hospital declines. While this major structural change applies to physicians and other providers as well, it has its greatest impact on nurses because of their deep professional identification with hospital care. Yet the hospital-related opportunities for nurses are greatest in the growth and restructuring of rehabilitative and follow-up care. Clinically, nurses have been strong in this area, and their professional orientation is more suited to them than is the medical orientation

of physicians (Aiken et al. 1985). In an era of provider surplus and selected cost-containment, the nursing profession's best strategy is to refocus its energies toward the much-needed services and expanding opportunities to professionalize postdischarge, rehabilitative, and long-term care (Reif and Estes 1982; Aiken et al. 1985; Rubenstein et al. 1984; Ebersole 1983; Lynaugh 1984).

Corporate Health Programs

Besides direct efforts to contain medical expenses, one group of payers— major corporations—is developing programs to reduce risk factors and to promote "wellness." The most recent survey of these corporations showed that about 12 percent had alcohol and drug programs, 9 percent had programs to stop employees from smoking, 8 percent offered various kinds of preventive'care, and 7 percent gave courses in stress management (Herzlinger 1984). These numbers are significantly larger than a few years ago and appear to be rising. From the descriptions and testimonials that fill the pages of Business and Health, one gathers that these programs are driven by a combination of almost religious conviction and hard-headed cost accounting. Most corporations that have developed comprehensive health programs have a president or chairman of the board who became converted to the belief that wellness (however defined) was essential for high productivity, happy employees, and decreased medical costs. The most elaborate programs include extensive diagnostic screening, numerous classes on subjects ranging from aerobics to stress management, an elaborate gym supervised by a professionally trained expert, free personal and family counseling, and dietary advice. Supporters claim that employees appreciate the care and attention, leading to fewer absentee days and lower turnover. They claim that accidents and sick days also decrease. However, few corporations keep systematic records, and virtually none uses control samples to measure accurately the impact of these programs (Akabas 1984).

At the same time, corporate health programs aimed at selected groups of employees with costly problems are likely to save many times their cost (Rosenbloom and Gertman 1984). Employees who abuse alcohol and drugs are much more likely to make errors, be less productive, have accidents, disrupt the workplace, and have high medical bills for themselves and members of their family. Employees with disabilities are also very costly, not only because of their medical bills but because of their disability payments. Any program that gets them back to work and teaches them how to manage their disabilities will save thousands of dollars. Finally, a certain number of employees have high blood pressure, smoke heavily, or have other high risk factors amenable to change. As the initial enthusiasm for wellness settles down to cost-effective efforts, corporations are likely to focus their energies on selected groups of employees such as those with high-risk factors. Physicians, nurses, NPs, and PAs who acquire the education and ad-

ministrative skills to run such programs will be in demand.

Conclusion

The rapidly growing supply of physicians, nurses, and other providers is on a collision course with cost containment. On one hand, more physicians means more bills, unless strict measures such as capitation are in force. On the other hand, serious efforts at containing costs means a demand for fewer providers. The provider growth rate needs to be slowed down, but by how much and in what configuration are complex questions. For example, cardiac surgeons are projected to be in surplus by 1990 (U.S. Department of Health and Human Services 1980); but developments in the field suggest a surge in demand that will be morally and emotionally difficult to deny. In nursing, one might expect DRG systems to reduce the demand for general nurses in hospitals but perhaps increase the demand for nurse-specialists and nurse-administrators. Outside the hospital, nurses can now find major new opportunities in nursing homes, home health care, rehabilitation, and corporate health programs. From such observations one might conclude that the restructuring of the marketplace and the organization of medical services are as important pressures on the growing supply of providers as cost containment. Providers who recognize the opportunities and capitalize on them will have much to gain because cardinal rules of market strategy are getting there first and becoming dominant in the market

(Porter 1980; Lamb 1984). An important decision for any group of providers is which emerging markets does it wish to enter and in which markets is reduction of emphasis prudent. Thus, in an era of possible contraction, both dislocations and opportunities abound.

References

Abdellah, F. G. 1982. The nurse practitioners 17 years later: Present and emerging issues. *Inquiry* 19:105–116.

Adams, C. 1984. *Nurse-midwifery in the United States, 1982.* Washington, D.C.. American College of Nurse-Midwifery.

Aiken, L. H. 1981. Nursing priorities for the 1980s: Hospitals and nursing homes. *American Journal of Nursing* 81:324–330.

Aiken, L. H., ed. 1982. *Nursing in the 1980s: Crises, opportunities, challenges.* Philadelphia: J. B. Lippincott.

Aiken, L. H., C. E. Lewis, J. Craig, R. C. Mendenhall, R. J. Blendon, and D. E. Rogers. 1979. The contribution of specialists to the delivery of primary care: A new perspective. *New England Journal of Medicine* 300:1363–1370.

Aiken, L. H., M. D. Mezey, J. E. Laynaugh, and C. R. Buck, Jr. 1985. Teaching nursing homes: Prospects for improving long-term care. *Journal of the American Geriatric Society.*

Akabas, S. H. 1984. Expanded view of worksite counseling. *Business and Health* 2(2):24–28.

Boerma, H. 1983. *DRG evaluation, vol IV-B: Organizational impact.* Princeton: Health Research and Education Trust of New Jersey.

Brown, L. D. 1983. *Politics and health care organization: HMOs as federal policy.* Washington, D.C.: Brookings Institution.

Bullough, B. 1976. Influences on role expansion. *American Journal of Nursing* 75:1476–1981.

California Auditor General. 1983. *California has more physicians than it needs.* Sacramento: Office of Statewide Health Planning and Development.

Carter, R. D., and J. F. Gifford, Jr. 1982. The emergence of the physician assistant profession. In *Physician assistants: Their contribution to health care,* ed. H. B. Perry and B. Breitner, pp. 19–50. New York: Human Sciences Press.

Cawley, J. F., et al. 1984. Diagnosis related groups (DRGs) and non-physician providers: Hospital staffing strategies and the future. George Washington University Medical Center, Washington, D.C. Typescript.

Cawley, J. F., J. F. Ott, and C. A. DeAtley. 1983. The future for physician assistants. *Annals of Internal Medicine* 98:993–997.

Chiropractic demography: Distribution of doctors in the United States. 1983. Arlington, Va.: American Chiropractic Association.

Chiropractic, state of the art, 1983. 1983. Arlington, Va.: American Chiropractic Association.

Clifford, J. C. 1982. Professional nursing practice in a hospital setting. In Aiken 1982, pp. 101–120.

Committee on the Costs of Medical Care. 1932. *Medical care for the American people.* Chicago: University of Chicago Press.

Crandall, L. A., W. P. Spantulli, M. L. Radelet, K. E. Kilpatrick, and D. E. Lewis. 1984. Physician assistants in primary care. *Medical Care* 22:268–282.

Detmer, E. E., and H. B. Perry. 1982. The utilization of surgical physician assistants: Policy implications for the future. *Surgical Clinics of North America* 62:669–675.

Ebersole, P. P. 1983. Geriatric nurse practitioners. *Long-Term Care Currents* 6(3):11–14.

Ermann D., and J. Gabel. 1984. Multihospital systems: Issues and empirical findings. *Health Affairs* 3(1):50–64.

Ford, L. C. 1982. Nurse practitioners: History of a new idea and predictions for the future. In Aiken 1982, pp. 231–248.

Ginzberg, E., W. Balinsky, and M. Ostow. 1984. *Home health care: Its role in the changing health services market.* Totowa, N.J.: Rowman and Allanheld.

Goldsmith, J. 1984. Death of a paradigm: The challenge of competition. *Health Affairs* 3(3):5–19.

Herzlinger, R. 1984. Corporate experiences in controlling health care expenses. Part 3. Harvard Business School. Typescript.

Horn, S. D. 1983. Measuring severity of illness: Comparisons across institutions. *American Journal of Public Health* 73:25–31.

Horn, S. D., and P. D. Sharkey. 1983. Measuring severity of illness to predict patient resource use within DRGs. *Inquiry* 20:314–321.

Horn, S. D., M. S. Sharkey, and D. A. Bertram. 1983. Measuring severity of illness: Homogenous case mix groups. *Medical Care* 21:14–30.

Houts, C. B., J. A. Turbett, L. E. Arnold, and E. Kruse. 1985. Cost of medical/surgical pediatric hospital days preventable by psychiatric treatment. *Journal of the American Academy of Child Psychiatry* 24:227–230.

Inglehart, J. K. 1984. Cutting costs of health care for the poor in California. *New England Journal of Medicine* 311:745–748.

———. 1985. Medicare turns to HMOs. *New England Journal of Medicine* 312:132–136.

Institute of Medicine. 1983. *Nursing and nursing education: Public policies and private action.* Washington, D.C.: National Academy Press.

Joel, L. A. 1983. DRGs: The state of the art of reimbursement for nursing services. *Nursing and Health Care* 4:450–563.

Jones, L. Y. 1981. *Great expectations: America and the baby boom generation.* New York: Ballantine.

Keane, J. C., M. F. Solnick, and H. A. Cohen. 1985. Hospital data use in Maryland. *Business and Health* 2(4):7–10.

Kenny, J. B. 1984. Coalition, Minnesota style. *Business and Health* 1(3):35–38.

Lamb, R. B., ed. 1984. *Competitive strategic management*. Englewood Cliffs, N.J.: Prentice-Hall.

Lawrence, D. 1978. Physician assistants and nurse practitioners: Their impact on health care access, costs, and quality. *Health and Medical Care Service Review* 1:1–12.

Lazarus, W., E. S. Levine, L. S. Lewin, and Lewin and Associates, Inc. 1981. *Competition among health practitioners: The influence of the medical profession on the health manpower market*. Washington, D.C.: Federal Trade Commission.

Levine, E., and Moses E. B. 1982. Registered nurses today: A statistical profile. In Aiken 1982, pp. 475–494.

Lewis, C. E. 1982. *Nurse practitioners and the physician surplus*. In Aiken 1982, pp. 249–266.

Lewis, D. 1933. The place of the clinic in medical practice. *Journal of the American Medical Association* 100:1905–1910.

Light, D. W. 1983. Is competition bad? *New England Journal of Medicine* 309:1315–1319.

————. 1984. Growing physician supply: Implications for hospitals and doctors. Leonard Davis Institute of Health Economics, Philadelphia. Typescript.

————. 1985. Physician surplus and the future of physician extenders: GMENAC in an era of cost-containment. Policy Paper No. 4. Philadelphia: Leonard Davis Institute of Health Economics.

Luft, H. S. 1981. *Health maintenance organizations: Dimensions of performance*. New York: Wiley-Interscience.

Lynaugh, J. E. 1984. The teaching nursing home: Bringing together the best. *American Health Care Association Journal*, pp. 24–28.

McClure, M. L., and M. J. Nelson. 1982. *Trends in hospital nursing*. In Aiken 1982, pp. 59–74.

MacKay, C. 1984. CEOs balance corporate, community needs. *Business and Health* 2(2):34–37.

Masso, A. R. 1985. HMOs in transition: What the future holds. *Business and Health* 2(3):21–224.

May, J. J., and J. Wasserman. 1984. Selected results from an evaluation of the New Jersey diagnosis-related group system. *Health Services Research* 19:547–559.

Mechanic, D. 1976. The growth of bureaucratic medicine. New York: John Wiley and Sons.

————. 1979a. *Future issues in health care: Social policy and the rationing of medical services*. New York: Free Press.

————. 1979b. *Mental health and social policy*. 2d ed. Englewood Cliffs, N.J.: Prentice-Hall.

_____. 1984. The transformation of health providers. *Health Affairs* 3(1): 63–72.

Meyerhoff, A. S., and D. A. Crozier. 1984. Health care coalitions: The evolution of a movement. *Health Affairs* 3(1):120–127.

Mundinger, M. O. 1983. *Home care controversy.. Too little, too late, too costly.* Rockville, Md.: Aspen.

Musser, M. J., and S. Bognanni. 1984. Coalition spirit in Iowa. *Business and Health* 1(5):9–13.

Perry, H. B., and B. Breitner. 1982. *Physician assistants: Their contributions to health care.* New York: Human Sciences Press.

Perry, H. B., D. E. Detmer, and E. L. Redmond. 1981. The current and future role of surgical physician assistants: Report of a national survey of surgical chairmen in large U.S. hospitals. *American Surgeon* 193:132–137.

Placek, P. J., S. Taffel, and M. Moien. 1983. Cesarian section delivery rates: United States, 1981. *American Journal of Public Health* 73:861–862.

Porter, M. E. 1980. *Competitive strategy: Techniques for analyzing industries and competitors.* New York: Free Press.

Prescott, P. A., and L. Driscoll. 1979. Nurse practitioner effectiveness: A review of physician-nurse comparison studies. *Evaluation and the Health Professionals* 2:387–418.

Ramsey, J. A., J. K. McKenzie, and D. G. Fish. 1982. Physicians and nurse practitioners: Do they provide equivalent health care? *American Journal of Public Health* 72:55–57.

Record, J. C., ed. 1981. *Staffing primary care in 1980: Physician replacement and cost savings.* New York: Springer-Verlag.

Reif, L., and C. L. Estes. 1982. Long-term care: New opportunities for professional nursing. In Aiken 1982, pp. 147–182.

Reisz, W. G., J. F. Cawley, and W. S. Barry. 1984. The current status of physician assistants. *Maryland State Medical Journal* 33:288–291.

Relman, A. S. 1980. The new medical-industrial complex. *New England Journal of Medicine* 303:963–970.

Repicky, P. A., R. C. Mendenhall, and R. E. Neville. 1982. The professional role of physician's assistants in adult ambulatory care practices. *Evaluation and the Health Professions* 5:283–301.

Rivlin, A. 1979. *Physician extenders: Their current and future roles in medical care delivery.* Congressional Budget Office. Washington, D.C.: Government Printing Office.

Roemer, M. I. 1979. Innovative functions of health personnel in other countries: Lessons for U.S. health planners. *Inquiry* 16:259–263.

Roemer, M. I., and R. Roemer. 1978. Health manpower policies under five national health care systems: Insights for the United States from the experience of Australia, Belgium, Canada, Norway, and Poland. Health Resources Administration. Washington, D.C.: Government Printing Office.

Rosenbloom, D. L., and P. M. Gertman. 1984. An intervention strategy for controlling costly care. *Business and Health* (July/August), pp. 17–21.

Rubenstein, L. Z., et al. 1984. Effectiveness of a geriatric evaluation unit. *New England Journal of Medicine* 311:1664–1670.

Sadler, A. M., B. L. Sadler, and A. Bliss. 1972. *The physician's assistant: Today and tomorrow.* New Haven: Yale University Press.

Silver, H. K., and P. A. McAtee. 1984. On the use of nonphysician "associate residents" in overcrowded specialty-training programs. *New England Journal of Medicine* 311:326–328.

Silver, H. K., J. E. Ott, C. I. Dungy, L. L. Eine, V. M. Moore, and R. D. Krugman. 1981. Assessment and evaluation of child health associates. *Pediatrics* 67:47–52.

Somers, A., and D. R. Fabian. 1981. *The geriatric imperative.* Norwalk, Conn.: Appleton-Century-Crofts.

Starr, P. 1982. *The social transformation of American medicine.* New York: Basic Books.

Steinwachs, D., S. Shapiro, and J. Weiner. 1983. An application of the GMENAC physician requirement model to empirical data derived from three HMOs: Final report. Johns Hopkins University Health Services Research and Development Center, Baltimore, Md. Mimeographed.

Stevens, C. M. 1971. Physician supply and national health care goals. *Industrial Relations* 10:119–144.

Stowe, J. B. 1984. The Massachusetts all-payer model. *Business and Health* 1(5):9–13.

Sullivan, J. A. 1982. Research on nurse practitioners: Process behind the outcome? *American Journal of Public Health* 72:8–9.

Sultz, H. A., M. Zielezny, and J. M. Gentry. 1980. *A longitudinal study of nurse practitioners.* Phase 2. Washington, D.C.: Government Printing Office.

System Science Inc. 1976. *Nurse practitioner and physician assistant training and deployment study.* Department of Health, Education, and Welfare. Washington, D.C.: Government Printing Office.

Tarlov, A. R. 1983. Shattuck lecture: The increasing supply of physicians, the changing structure of the health-services system, and the future practice of medicine. *New England Journal of Medicine* 308:1235–1244.

Tell, E. J., M. Falik, and P. D. Fox. 1984. Private-sector health care initiatives: A comparative perspective from four communities. *Milbank Memorial Fund Quarterly* 62:357–379.

Tom, S. 1982. Nurse-midwifery: A developing profession. *Law, Medicine, and Health Care*, Dec., pp. 262–282.

U.S. Department of Commerce. 1975. *Historical statistics of the United States.* Washington, D.C.: Government Printing Office.

U.S. Department of Health and Human Services. 1982. *Health United States, 1982.* Hyattsville, Md.: Government Printing Office.

⸻. 1983. *Health United States, 1983.* Hyattsville, Md.: Government Printing Office.

⸻. 1984. *Report to the president and Congress on the state of health personnel in the United States.* Vols. 1, 2. Washington, D.C.: Government Printing Office.

––––––. Graduate Medical Education National Advisory Committee. 1980. *Report to the secretary.* Vols. 1–7. Washington, D.C.: Government Printing Office.

U.S. General Accounting Office. 1985. Information requirements for evaluating the impacts of Medicare prospective payments on post-hospital long-term-care services: Preliminary report. GAO/PEMD-858, pp. 1–9. Washington, D.C.: Government Printing Office.

Wack, R. L., and L. Horwitz. 1985. An alliance for economic revitalization. *Business and Health* 2(3):34–37.

Yankauer, A., and J. Sullivan. 1982. The new health professionals: Three examples. *Annual Review of Public Health* 3:249–276.

Young, D. 1985. Evaluating the medicare prospective payment system. Lecture delivered at the Leonard Davis Institute of Health Economics, Philadelphia.

Chapter 25

Ethical Issues in a Social Context

Bradford H. Gray and Marian Osterweis

The past thirty years of rapid change in the development and application of biomedical knowledge and technology and in the organization and financing of health services have produced an increased awareness of ethical issues and dilemmas. A wide variety of ethical problems exist in medicine (*Encyclopedia of Bioethics* 1978). In this chapter we will focus on three disparate topics that pertain to the responsibilities of professionals or institutions: research involving human subjects, decisions to forego life-sustaining therapy in the care of the terminally ill, and the rise of for-profit health care companies. One of these topics —decisions at the end of life—was created by medical progress, by medicine's growing ability to control or influence life and death

matters that were once beyond human intervention. Another—the ethics of human experimentation—is raised in the very process of innovation and change. The third issue— the emergence of new types of for-profit, investor-owned health care organizations—raises new incarnations of old ethical problems about the reconciliation of the commercial and professional sides of medicine (Veatch 1983).

These examples illustrate two basic ethical tensions in professional responsibilities. The first is the tension between altruism and self-interest, two basic principles of morality that ethicist Albert Jonsen sees in "incessant conflict" in medicine (Jonsen 1983). Medicine is treated by physicians and by society as both a way to earn a living and a way to benefit others. Most physicians, Jonsen believes, "attempt to maintain a precarious balance" between self-interest and altruism. The second tension is between what Beauchamp and McCullough (1984) call the beneficence model and the autonomy model. The beneficence model defines the physician's responsibilities in terms of determining and doing what is best for the patient. This model has deep historical roots in the medical profession. The autonomy model, more recent and imposed to a significant degree from outside the profession by the law, defines the physician's responsibility much more as enhancing and respecting the patient's right of self-determination. Many ethical dilemmas in medicine occur in situations in which the actions judged to be in the patient's best interests may not be the actions that the patient would choose.

In examining human experimentation, decision making about life and death, and the growth of for-profit enterprise in health care, we will attempt to describe the current status of the issues and to show how they have been illuminated by theoretical, empirical, and methodological traditions of the social sciences applied to health.

The Ethics and Regulation of Research Involving Human Subjects

Although legal cases about "human experimentation" go back a couple of centuries (Katz 1972), serious modern concern began with the revelations at Nuremburg of the Nazi medical experiments. In the United States, the ethics of research involving human subjects emerged as a public policy issue in the early 1960s, with revelations in the mass media of experiments in which live cancer cells were injected beneath the skin of terminally ill patients at a leading research institution; the subjects had not been informed of the nature of the substance being implanted because the researchers believed that they would be unduly alarmed by this information. These revelations were followed by the publication in the *New England Journal of Medicine* of an article by a distinguished physician-researcher, Henry K. Beecher (1966), describing a number of apparently unethical experiments that had been published in recent years in major biomedical journals. The nature of the experiments were such that it was difficult to believe that subjects would have agreed to participate if they had understood the risks and alternatives. Thus, research involving human subjects became a public policy problem.

In 1966 the surgeon general of the United States initiated a policy requiring research supported by the Public Health Service (primarily through the National Institutes of Health) to be approved by a local review committee at the sponsoring institution, with written informed consent to be obtained from subjects prior to their participation. The basic elements of the 1966 policy—the use of institutional committees to review risk/benefit and provisions for obtaining informed consent from subjects—are still central to the structure for studies that are regulated by the Food and Drug Administration or that are supported by the federal government or conducted at institutions that receive federal support for such research.

In the mid-1970s, after further examples of ethically problematic research gained public attention (U.S. Congress, Senate 1973), Congress created the National Commission for the Protection of Human Subjects of Biomedical and Behavioral Research. Much of the Senate hearing was devoted to examples of ethically dubious research. Systematic data that confirmed the existence of a problem was presented by sociologist Bernard Barber (1973), who reported on studies his group had conducted (Barber et al. 1973) that showed great variation in the ethical standards of researchers and inadequacies in existing review procedures. Barber also reported a study at one major medical center in which research with unfavorable risk/benefit ratios made disproportionate use of poorly educated and minority patients as subjects. (This finding was not confirmed in a later study based on national data; Gray, Cooke, and Tannenbaum 1978.)

The National Commission was directed to identify the ethical principles that should govern such research, to make recommendations regarding the ethical circumstances under which the federal government could support research involving several special categories of subjects where informed consent was problematic (human fetuses and pregnant women, children, the "institutional-ized mentally infirm," and prisoners), and to investigate the adequacy of the institutional review system and regulations for protecting human research subjects. Recommendations from a series of National Commission reports were substantially incorporated into federal regulations (see particularly, National Commission 1978b). A subsequent body, the President's Commission for the Study of Ethical Problems in Medicine and Biomedical and Behavioral Research, was given a legislative mandate to study the adequacy and uniformity of federal rules for protection of human subjects and to report biennially to Congress and the president. Two such reports were made before the President's Commission's statutory life ended in 1983 (President's Commission 1981, 1983b).

Three basic ethical principles have been identified that should govern such research: beneficence (i.e., to do good rather than harm), respect for persons (usually embodied in the requirement of informed consent), and justice (e.g., not taking advantage of vulnerable subjects even if they are readily available) (National Commission 1978b). The most interesting problems arise when a conflict is seen between principles—when the obligation to do good research is seen as conflicting with the obligation to inform subjects—or when the vulnerability of subjects or their inability to give informed consent raises questions about how to apply the respect-for-persons doctrine, which usually begins with the informed consent requirement.

How to conduct morally sound research involving human subjects is not the province of any one discipline. Contributions have been made by biomedical, behavioral, and social scientists from virtually all disciplines, from philosophers and legal scholars, and from the courts, legislatures, and governmental agencies that support research. This discussion will focus on contributions of the social sciences in three areas: describing the ways that research settings and researcher-subject relationships can vary; understanding the empirical complexities of informed consent; and understanding the functioning of the institutional review process established by federal regulations to protect the interests of subjects.

From the relatively few sociological studies of research involving human subjects it is clear that the nature of researcher-subject relationships varies in important ways. In *Experiment Perilous*, Fox (1959) analyzed the complex and somewhat collaborative relationship that existed between physician-researchers and their chronically ill patients on a metabolic ward of a research hospital in the 1950s. Some of the research involved extended periods of hospitalization, and many subjects had participated in several studies over a period of years. Many of the subjects had acquired a great deal of knowledge about their diseases and could understand well the logic of the researchers' efforts. And the researchers came to know the subjects well as human beings. Thus, a major part of Fox's analysis concerns the researchers' adaptations to doing risky studies on people whom they have come to know as individuals and whose prognosis for survival is poor.

An important aspect of this problem was the physicians' knowledge that they had mixed obligations— their efforts were not just to take care of patients but to learn from research subjects. As clinical researchers they responded not only to the attitudes, norms, and values of medicine but also to those of science, which may be in conflict in some circumstances.

For example, the Hippocratic oath includes the admonition to do no harm; yet the hallmark of research is uncertainty. Fox describes experimental surgery that was carried out on patients who had exhausted conventional treatment options and who were not expected to live. Although there was a remote chance the innovative treatment would result in some benefit to the patient, the goal of such research was not to help the patient but to advance scientific knowledge. In such instances there were few guidelines for deciding "whether the particular experiments . . . fell within the limits of the physicians' rights as investigators, or whether they were overstepping those rights by subjecting the patients involved to more inconvenience and danger than the possible significance of those experiments for the 'advancement of health, science, and human welfare' seemed to warrant" (Fox 1959, 48). Experimental drug trials were another area in which this question arose. And in some drug trials the research protocol called for withholding a drug with some known potential benefit and giving a new one whose potential benefits and risks were greater but whose effects were more uncertain. Thus, the physician-researchers were constantly faced with the dilemma of having to make responsible decisions about the appropriate limits of their research endeavors in the face of great uncertainty and in the context of their obligation to do no harm to their patients.

A far different research (and regulatory) context was studied by Gray (1975), who described how pregnant women became involved as research subjects in a study of drugs for inducing labor. Women were referred into the research project by resident physicians in the hospital clinic or by private physicians. Consent forms were presented to the women by the nurses who prepared them for labor and who initiated the infusion of the drug. The relationship of the subjects to the physician-researchers was limited to occasional (if intensive) contacts during the process of labor and delivery. Within this single study there were important variations in subjects' reasons for participation. Among the better-educated women who saw private physicians, the research was used as a tool for manipulating the system: space in the hospital was tight, and these women, for one reason or another, wanted to control the timing of their delivery and saw in the research a way to do so. At the other extreme were many women, mostly with low levels of education and no private physicians, who did not even realize that they had been entered into a research project, notwithstanding their having signed a consent form. Few women gave altru-

istic reasons for volunteering; a few felt coerced into participating. Many did not recognize that the researchers, who were obstetricians, might ask them to take a drug (or in this case one of two drugs in a double-blind design) for reasons other than their own individual medical condition despite explanations about the experiment.

This brief description of two sociological studies of human experimentation suggests something of the complexities of informed consent, a key element in distinguishing the ethical from the unethical in research. Fox described research in which researchers and subjects found themselves in a complex web of dependence and obligation; while her research predated the major growth of interest in the concept of informed consent, it is clear that many of the subjects she studied were very well informed (indeed, she found this was one way in which they coped), but they were also constrained by their disease and by their relationship with the medical group that was their only source of hope. Gray's work emphasized the difference between informed consent and a signature on a consent form by describing a situation in which the informed consent transaction was little more than a bureaucratic detail, in which key information was not understood by many subjects, and in which many subjects understood the request to participate to be advice to participate.

Similar reliance on physician-researchers as providers of professional advice was reported in the detailed observational studies of informed consent by Lidz et al. (1984). In their studies of a psychiatric research ward, they found several different types of decisions being made: those made by the staff for the patients, those implied by the decision to enter the ward (this included the decision to enter into research studies), the collective decisions made in the "therapeutic community" environment by staff and a formal advisory body of patients, and decisions made through "mutual participation" of staff and patients. The Lidz study is particularly valuable because of its empirical distinctions among the key elements of informed consent—disclosure of information, understanding of information, and decision making. By observing the making of various types of decisions within one psychiatric institution, they found that the ideals of informed consent are rarely even approached—partly because of the pressure of institutional imperatives, partly because patients often wanted decisions made for them, and partly because the staff was more committed to getting patients to agree to what was seen as in their best interests than to getting patients to exercise their autonomy. The two conceptions of the professional's responsibility that this implies—doing what is seen as best for the patient (even if this must be done manipulatively) versus providing the patient with the tools needed to act autonomously—constitute a fundamental ethical conflict in medicine.

The above discussion suggests some of the complexities of risk/benefit decisions in human experimentation and of pursuing the ideal of informed consent. Research is carried out in more than seven hundred universities, medical schools, hospitals, psychiatric institutions, research centers, and other institutions around the country. The response to past scandals shows the power of the values that are at stake when gross ethical violations occur. The ethical filter through which proposals for all but the most risk-free studies must now pass are hundreds of institutional review boards (IRBs) located at the institution where research is conducted. IRBs, which must meet certain regulatory requirements regarding size, composition, and procedures, must judge the acceptability of research from the standpoint of regulatory criteria regarding risk, informed consent, confidentiality, and so forth.

IRBs themselves have been the object of social research, both by independent researchers and in a major study conducted for the National Commission for the Protection of Human Subjects (Cooke, Tannenbaum, and Gray 1977; Gray, Cooke, and Tannenbaum 1978). By and large, this research has supported the continuation of the system of institutional review. Insofar as survey research methods allowed measurement of risks and benefits of research that had been approved by IRBs (measurement was done by asking researchers for their assessments), it appeared that only very small numbers of projects approved by IRBs were questionable on risk/benefit grounds alone. However, IRBs did not appear to be effective in improving informed consent forms; approved forms tended to have important information omitted and tended to be unrealistically difficult to read. Although the system was clearly not perfect at the time of the National Commission's survey, widespread support for the IRB system was found among both IRB members and researchers. The tendency of IRBs to spend inordinate amounts of time on innocuous research was identified in the National Commission's survey, which made recommendations (which were accepted) to exempt some types of very-low-risk research from IRB review and allow the use of "expedited" procedures for other types.

The National Commission's survey also documented the wide variety of circumstances in which IRBs operate; the IRBs studied were in many different types of institutions, had as few as five and as many as fifty-five members, reviewed as few as no proposals and as many as several hundred, reviewed studies that involved no perceptible risk and studies that presented a real risk of death. While the regulations specify the judgments that IRBs are to make, institutions have great latitude in the operation of their review committees. On the basis of its own site-visit project, the President's Commission (1983b) concluded that too much variation exists in the operation, procedures, level of effort, and so forth of IRBs. It recommended that more active educational programs be instituted by the federal government.

While the IRB system is clearly not perfect, it has been unusually successful as a regulatory device. Because IRBs are located at institutions that have a vested interest in research and because researchers constitute substantial majorities on most IRBs

(even if they cannot vote on projects in which they are involved), they can be seen as an example of the capture of a regulatory process by the regulated entity. A further problem with IRBs as a mechanism is that their operation can become routinized and uninteresting to members; a key to the operation of good IRBs has probably always been the presence of at least one highly committed individual, although that has never been documented. However, despite its problems the IRB mechanism appears to be working; its main effects may be less in what it does than in its presence.

Extending Life or Foregoing Life-Sustaining Treatment

It was not until 1976 that the general public became aware of the issues surrounding decisions to forego life-sustaining treatment. In that year the New Jersey Supreme Court granted Joseph Quinlan's request (*In re Quinlan* 70 N.J. 10 355 A.2d 647, *cert. denied* 429 U.S. 922 (1976)) to be appointed guardian of his comatose daughter for the express purpose of authorizing the removal of her respirator, knowing that such an act was likely to result in her death. (In fact, Karen Ann Quinlan lived for nine years, breathing on her own but unconscious.) Prior to this 1976 court decision that overruled Karen Quinlan's physicians and overturned the rulings of the local prosecutor and the state attorney general, most such decisions were made quietly and privately by patients, their families, and their doctors. Although the ethical issues had long been debated by philosophers, theologians, and occasionally by the courts, never before had a case received such extensive media coverage and never before had the issues been so hotly debated in the public arena.

Since that time numerous cases involving withholding or discontinuing treatment for seriously ill patients have come to the public's attention. Not only have the courts increasingly been called upon to adjudicate, but the federal government has issued regulations in this very complex area and the issues have become politicized. Ethical and legal discussions of the complex set of issues involved in decisions to extend life or forego life-sustaining treatment have been informed by a wealth of social research —analyses of the shifting historical and sociocultural context, attitudinal surveys of patients, the public, and health professionals, observational studies, and hospital record reviews.

The Changing Social Context

Until the middle of this century, death was accepted as inevitable and medicine could do relatively little to forestall it. People died at home surrounded by friends and relatives and, insofar as possible, orchestrated events surrounding their dying as they wished (Aries 1974). As medicine's capabilities increased dramatically, radical changes have taken place in the process of dying and in

our attitudes toward death. Now the vast majority of people who die are elderly and have chronic illness; they die in institutions where physicians play a key role in directing treatment and in determining when death has occurred (Fox 1979, 1980). With the increased capability of medical science came the implicit assumption that everything that could be done to delay death should be done. Death came to be viewed as failure—failure of the "omnipotent" physician to effect a cure and failure of the patient to resist sickness and death (Glaser and Strauss 1965; Thomas 1980).

Observational studies conducted in the 1960s described the way terminally ill patients were cared for in hospitals. These studies noted the physical and social isolation of patients and the lack of communication about treatment procedures, options, and impending death, behaviors that appeared to stem from discomfort on the part of physicians for having failed and from their own fears of death (Glaser and Strauss 1965; Sudnow 1967). Health professionals and families seemed to share the expectation that an "acceptable" death was one that was not discussed (Aries 1974). A "conspiracy of silence" surrounded the death bed. This was all deemed to be in the patients' best interests.

In the last two decades attitudes have changed again, and new questions are being raised. Should everything that can be done to extend life always be done? Who should decide? And on what basis should such decisions be made? Many of the questions that are now being asked about whether and how to treat seriously ill patients could not have been asked before because medicine was simply not capable of forestalling death until recently. But the fact that these questions are being raised in the public arena and the way in which they are being framed are not merely reactions to increased technology; they are reflections of our changing society and our values (Fox 1979, 1980; Aries 1974).

One indication of the shift in attitudes is the recent growth of hospice programs for the terminally ill. By electing hospice care, patients effectively make the decision to forego life-sustaining treatment and enter a program in which the health professionals know and accept the fact that death is close at hand. The extent to which this is made explicit to patients when they enter hospices is evidently quite limited, thus raising a serious informed consent issue (Lynn and Osterweis 1984).

Another indication of changing attitudes comes from survey data that have documented the public's wish for information and a remarkable shift in physicians' willingness to disclose information about "bad news." In 1961 Oken found that 90 percent of physicians preferred not to inform patients of a diagnosis of cancer, whereas a survey in 1977 (Novak et al. 1979) found that 97 percent of doctors routinely disclosed such information. In a survey conducted by the President's Commission on Medical Ethics (President's Commission 1982), 94 percent of the public reported they would "want to know everything," and 86 percent of physicians believed that all or most of their patients wanted candid assessments

of their diagnosis and prognosis. Such information is vital if patients are to participate in a meaningful way in decision making about their care. The values promoted by informed consent—self-determination and individual well-being—cannot be served if the patient is uninformed about his or her condition and the treatment options.

In all spheres of life the public is demanding more information, more control over decisions that affect them, and greater professional accountability. There is a growing recognition that our resources are not infinite and that hard choices about their allocation must be made. The rights and responsibilities of patients, families, the public, health professionals, and society are being reanalyzed, more clearly articulated, and in some instances, realigned. Concerns about the appropriateness of clinical decision making occur at both the microlevel of the individual patient and at the macrolevel of allocation of resources, particularly the proportion of health care expenditures devoted to the very end of patients' lives.

Underlying Values and Their Potential Conflicts

Good medical care decision-making promotes four basic values: preservation of life, respect for patient self-determination (autonomy), promotion of individual well-being, and equitable access to health care for all people (President's Commission 1983a). Ethical dilemmas arise when these values are in conflict with one another. Such conflicts are especially likely to arise in making treatment decisions for seriously ill patients. Examples of such conflicts are numerous—a patient may ask that no further attempts be made to preserve his life because he is in pain, because treatment results in additional discomfort or in expenditures he and his family can ill-afford, because further treatment is not sure to extend his life for very long. Trade-offs between the quality and quantity of life are a very real issue for many sick elderly patients and for some younger people as well.

In one of the most ambitious studies ever undertaken on the subject of decision making for critically ill patients, Diana Crane (1975) combined surveys, observation, and record reviews to determine what physicians thought they would do in various hypothetical case study circumstances, what they actually did when faced with such questions, and the basis for their choices. Somewhat surprisingly, results of the hypothetical survey questions and actual behavior coincided well. This study showed that physicians were, in fact, willing to make decisions about when it is (and is not) appropriate to intervene in the interest of preserving the sanctity of life, and it elucidated some of the explicit and implicit criteria used to make such decisions and the conflicts between them. For example, in addition to patients' physiological status, most physicians, when making treatment decisions, take account of the patient's capacity for social interaction. Seriously ill adults and severely handicapped infants who lacked the potential for meaningful social interaction were likely to be seen as un-treatable. Although Crane found that active euthanasia was rare, it was not uncommon for physicians to administer large doses of narcotics to terminally ill cancer patients for the express purpose of alleviating pain or to remove severely brain damaged patients from respirators, knowing that such actions might lead to respiratory arrest.

Legal and Procedural Mechanisms to Assist with Decision Making

Special problems arise when the patient lacks the capacity to participate in decision making, as is discussed in detail by the President's Commission on Medical Ethics (President's Commission 1983a). For infants, young children, and some adults who because of their illness or medications may no longer be able to exercise clear judgment, someone else must decide what should be done. Usually the family is designated to make these determinations—to try to decide what is in the patient's best interest or what the patient would have wanted. However, family members may disagree with one another or with the physician, and their own values and preferences may interfere with their objective assessment of what is in the patient's interest. Even when a patient is fully capable of making his or her own decisions, conflicts among the various parties may arise.

There are a number of legally recognized ways for people to make advance directives about their care as a way of planning for a time when they may be too ill and incapacitated to direct their care. Living wills are written instructions about care at the end of life, usually directing that no "heroic" or "extraordinary" measures be used to prolong life. Because the legal status of living wills was frequently questioned, beginning in 1976 states began to enact Natural Death Acts. Most states now have such acts. Their intent is to make advance directives legally binding, but individual state laws vary considerably in scope and in their specific provisions. For example, many do not deal at all with the issue of what happens if a physician refuses to go along with the patient's directive.

Powers of attorney are another legally recognized way to make advance directives. Although often thought of as instruments for making property decisions, these documents can also specify who is to be empowered to make health care decisions and how they are to be made. Each type of directive has some benefits and some potential pitfalls. Like the Natural Death Acts, they also vary substantially from state to state. Several groups are working toward the creation of uniform laws regarding directives about medical care at the end of life.

In addition to legal documents, there are mechanisms being developed to assist health care institutions to determine what should be done when the patient lacks the capacity to participate in decision making and the family does not favor life-sustaining treatment. Beginning in the 1970s a few hospitals established ethics committees. The American Hospital Association now estimates that about 26 percent of hospitals have such committees (Tames 1984). Many deal only with issues regarding the treatment of newborns, but some are more general committees. The role of these committees is not yet fully clear, and there are differences of opinion regarding what their role should be. Some see these committees as ways to help institutions formulate policies on a wide range of issues, such as when to use orders not to resuscitate patients and how decisions to forego treatment should be made. Others see their role more as assisting with particular cases—helping to sort out issues, sometimes making recommendations about particular cases; a few actually were designed to be the collective decision maker. In addition to variations in their roles, ethics committees vary widely in their composition and in their rules about the participation of the patient, family, and health professionals directly involved in a particular decision.

The Role of Government

The role of the federal government has generally been very limited and indirect except in the case of what Annas terms "neonatal rescue medicine" (Annas 1984a). In 1982 the Department of Health and Human Services (HHS), at the specific request of the White House, put hospitals on notice that it was "unlawful for a recipient of Federal financial assistance to withhold from a handicapped infant nutritional sustenance or medical or surgical treatment required to correct a life-threatening condition if (1) the withholding is based on the fact that the infant is handicapped; and (2) the handicap does not render treatment or nutritional sustenance contraindicated" (48 *Federal Register* 9630–9632, March 7, 1983). Notices had to be posted and a hotline was set up to report suspected offenders. HHS subsequently issued the formal Baby Doe regulations as part of the Rehabilitation Act of 1983 (sec. 504). These regulations have been hotly contested in court by physician groups and others and have been publically debated in the mass media. The regulations were revised in minor ways several times, with the final version suggesting (but not requiring) that Infant Care Review Committees (ICRCs) be established to develop treatment guidelines, to review particular cases, and "to ensure that all considerations in favor of the provision of life-sustaining treatment are fully evaluated and considered by the ICRC" (49 *Federal Register* 1622–1654, Jan. 12, 1984). As noted earlier, it is still the minority of hospitals that have such committees. And there is still tremendous controversy about the legality of the regulations and about the appropriateness of the direct involvement of the federal government in determining medical practice, in intervening in what were once (and many believe should remain) private decisions, and in promulgating treatment guidelines that are too uniform given the diversity in the medical status of the patients (Shapiro and Rosenberg 1984; Annas 1984a, 1984b, 1984c).

The more usual way for the government to be involved in medical care decision-making is through policies that define reimbursable services. Such policies may effectively limit the scope of individual choice and raise ethical questions about the equitable allocation of resources. Commitments to certain technologies and their costs constrain other types of commitments that may be equally or more valuable for the same group of patients or for other populations. For example, the question of whether to concentrate resources at the beginning or at the end of life is looming ever larger on the horizon.

There was outrage when Colorado's governor Richard Lamm said bluntly that society cannot afford to "keep people alive . . . far beyond the time when any kind of quality of life is left at all" and suggested that terminally ill elderly patients have a "duty to die" ("Governor Asserts Elderly, if Very Ill, Have 'Duty to Die'" 1984). Although not felicitously stated by the governor, the issue is a real one. The Health Care Financing Administration (HCFA) now estimates that 28 percent of all Medicare expenditures are for the 6 percent of beneficiaries who are in their last year of life (Lubitz and Prihoda 1984). There is no question that this is a period in which people are ill and in need of care. In the HCFA study only 6 percent of persons who died had Medicare expenses in excess of $15,000 in their last year of life. Still, the question arises whether available resources, which are increasingly recognized to be limited, should be concentrated more on younger patients than on the elderly, as is done in England (Aaron and Schwartz 1984; Schwartz and Aaron 1984). Is it ethical to base rationing on age considerations? By.what devices might this be done? These are questions that are just beginning to be discussed (Mechanic 1979). How much they are discussed in the future will be a function of the cumulative impact of patient care decisions for millions of patients and of the public's willingness to devote ever increasing proportions of the nation's wealth to health care. Some decisions may be made by government — for example, whether and for what types of patients Medicare will pay for artificial heart implantation. Others will be made locally in medical institutions whose economic survival may be at stake.

For-Profit Health Care Companies

Few changes in our health care system have sparked as much interest as the emergence of investor ownership of health care institutions. Although there have long been entrepreneurial elements in health care—in the manufacture and sale of pharmaceuticals, equipment, and supplies, in physicians' and dentists' practices, and even in physician-owned hospitals— the creation of publicly traded, investor-owned companies that own multiple health care institutions is a phenomenon of the past fifteen to twenty years. In this major sector of the economy (11 percent of the gross national product), which has long been thought of as the bailiwick of professionals and of nonprofit and public institutions, investor ownership now constitutes a significant and

growing portion of virtually all traditional types of health care providers (hospitals, nursing homes, psychiatric hospitals, home health agencies, and even health maintenance organizations, which have been some of the hottest stocks on Wall Street), as well as a variety of new types of providers (alcoholism and drug abuse treatment centers, freestanding diagnostic and surgical centers) (Gray 1985). Some of these are owned privately by local investors, many of whom are physicians, but the stock of at least thirty-five investor-owned health care companies is publicly traded ("Financial and Stock Report" 1984). Some of these companies concentrate on one line of business. The Hospital Corporation of America, for example, now owns or manages almost 400 hospitals, approximately 7 percent of the hospitals in the United States. Other companies are more diversified. National Medical Enterprises and its subsidiaries own or manage more than 100 hospitals, 30 psychiatric hospitals, and 330 nursing homes. Some companies that are primarily in other lines of business now have health care subsidiaries or divisions (e.g., American Hospital Supply Corporation with home care, W. R. Grace and Company with hemodialysis centers). Several companies, not all of which own HMOs, are combining elements of the insurance function with the provision of services.

Health care institutions generally have been affected by several major changes in the past twenty years— particularly the continued and escalating capital intensity of health care resulting from ever more sophisticated medical technologies, the decline both in charity and governmental grants as sources of capital for health care, and the monetarization of health care as various forms of third-party payment (particularly Medicare and Medicaid) led institutions and professionals to expect payment for services provided (Ginzberg 1984). These changes have led, among other things, to behavioral patterns in many nonprofit institutions that the unwary could assume are characteristic of for-profit institutions—aggressive marketing and recruitment of physicians, "de-marketing" and "dumping" economically unattractive patients (particularly when a public hospital is available), formation of multi-institutional systems (which have been growing faster among nonprofit hospitals than among for-profit hospitals), achieving and retaining surpluses (profits) for future expansion and other capital needs, borrowing millions of dollars, and integrating vertically through ownership of ambulatory care centers and nursing facilities. Various forms of nonprofit/for-profit hybrids have sprung up. Nonprofit hospitals have been "restructured" to establish for-profit subsidiaries; nonprofit (and public) hospitals have been contracting with for-profit companies for management of the entire institution or of particular departments (e.g., emergency services, respiratory therapy); for-profit "affiliation" organizations are being created, such as Voluntary Hospitals of America, which is wholly owned by a group of large nonprofit hospitals that are seeking to gain the advantages of multi-institutional arrangements (Gray 1985).

This chapter is not the place, however, for a detailed review and critique of the existing literature on how investor-ownership type affects institutional behavior. Several literature reviews have recently been written and an Institute of Medicine study will review these matters in 1986 (Ermann and Gabel 1984; Gray 1983b; Schlesinger 1985). Most of the limited empirical literature has focused on relative quality and efficiency or costliness of health care institutions with different types of ownership, what types of patients they serve, and what types of services they provide (Pattison and Katz 1983; Lewin and Associates, Inc. 1981; Sloan and Vraciu, 1983). The data to date suffer from methodological problems (e.g., the measurement of quality and the specification of appropriate control groups in any particular study), and major changes are taking place in the environment which cast doubt on past research results. (For example, Medicare's prospective rate setting provides efficiency incentives, lacking when the studies were conducted, that show that investor-owned chain hospitals are not less costly than nonprofit hospitals.)

While questions of cost, quality, and access (particularly for poor people) are important, only the latter is commonly defined in ethical terms. Most studies thus far have shown relatively small differences between investor-owned and nonprofit hospitals regarding service to Medicaid patients and the combined amount of bad debt and charity dollars. It is important to be wary of easy assumptions that the ethical superiority of the nonprofit form is readily demonstrable.

Still, the sense remains that there are important ethical issues here that should be identified and clarified. While it is often stated that these various corporate trends raise ethical issues in health care, there is much less consensus on just what these issues are than around the two topics considered earlier in this essay (Relman 1980; Gray 1983a; Wikler 1985). Is it unethical to make money by caring for the sick? Physicians have been businessmen as well as healers for years and remain at the top of most polls of occupational prestige and trust. Is it unethical for large-scale organizations to control operations from a home office far from the community? Although not on the scale of the large investor-owned hospital companies, multi-institutional systems have long existed in both the nonprofit and public sectors and have never been viewed as an ethical problem. Is it unethical for investors to make money from health services? Most of the capital financing for nonprofit hospitals comes from debt and the sale of bonds, all of whose dollars come from investors. Is it because of the lack of physician control? Nonprofit hospitals have in the past alternatively been accused of indifference to their medical staffs (few of whom were on the hospital boards) and of giving in to every physician demand because of cost-based reimbursement and the nonprofit form's perceived lack of economic discipline. In any case, AHA data show governing boards in investor-owned hospitals to have much heavier physician representation than in nonprofit hospitals (Sloan 1980). Whether this is for marketing purposes (with physicians viewed as customers) or communication purposes, it does not indicate indifference to physicians.

The rise to prominence of for-profit health care organizations highlights the conflicting principles of self-interest and altruism in health care. Since trust has long been viewed as an essential part of the doctor-patient relationship, professionals and institutions have always had to strike a balance in which it was expected that patients' interests would be put first. Hence, Parsons (1951) could identify a "collective" rather than "self" orientation as a basic characteristic of professions, and the major hospital trade association, the American Hospital Association (1981), could identify service to the "community" as an ethical obligation of hospitals, although the AHA statement also acknowledges the "limits of available resources." One concern about explicitly for-profit institutions, with the responsibilities to stockholders that this entails, is that the balance between self-interest and altruism will be changed—that institutions will feel less obligation to provide care for people who cannot pay or to offer services that are "needed" in the community but that are not economically viable, and that the service orientation of the medical profession will be debased either because physicians will come under the control of people with a strong bottom-line orientation or because physicians will compromise themselves and enmesh themselves in conflicts of interests by investing (or participating in profit-sharing arrangements) in organizations whose profitability is affected by the physicians' patient care decisions (Gray 1983b; Miller 1983).

These concerns should all be taken seriously. Officials of investor-owned hospital companies have sometimes rejected the idea that their hospitals should be willing to provide services to people who need care but cannot pay. This sentiment comes from the fact that a "for-profit" institution is also a "tax-paying" institution; taxes are seen by some as discharging much of the institution's social responsibilities. However, the data to date do not show investor-owned hospitals to be doing consistently or significantly less charity care than do nonprofits, a fact that may lead to questions about the continuing justification of some nonprofit institutions' tax exemptions. (Cream skimming by some of the other types of for-profit organizations, such as freestanding urgent care centers, is fundamental to their way of doing business.) The problem remains that dollars are required to provide care—dollars that must come from taxes, charity, or from elevated charges to paying patients (cross subsidization). Whether one or another of these methods is ethically superior to the others is a question that may be muted by events—economic constraints (pressure from payers) are making it increasingly difficult for even those institutions that are inclined to use the latter method to be able to do so.

What about the impact of the for-profit orientation on the ethical position and standards of physicians? This aspect may ultimately be the most troublesome, as Starr (1983), Relman (1980, 1983), and others have noted, although one of the many paradoxes of growth of the for-profit hospital corporations is that it has come substantially through acquisition of independent, doctor-owned hospitals, thereby reducing the con-

flict of interest apparent in that form of ownership. A spirited debate has begun about whether physicians should keep apart from ownership of for-profit health care organizations (other than their own practices) to preserve their moral position of patient advocate, or whether they should become involved in ownership so as not to give up their control and influence (Relman 1983; Guidotti 1984). Furthermore, broader changes are taking place in the autonomy of the medical profession (Mechanic 1984; Freidson 1986). Policymakers and payers for medical care increasingly perceive physicians as responsive to economic incentives and are increasingly trying to arrange incentives so as to reduce the number of services provided. Physicians' behavior is also increasingly amenable to monitoring through techniques developed in research and in the professional standards review organization (PSRO) program. Hospitals and payers are putting data systems into place that will reveal which physicians are "efficient providers" and which are money losers (because of long lengths of stay, high use of ancillary services, etc.); physicians' admitting privileges may be at stake. It is increasingly clear that physicians will be monitored as never before; the question is by whom and for what purpose.

A final ethical issue in the growth of for-profit health care has to do with the role of the patient and the extent to which patients need to look out for their own interests. Theorists suggest that one explanation for the prominence of nonprofit organizations in fields in which the customer finds it difficult to monitor performance is that the nonprofit itself provides a crude sort of consumer protection (Weisbrod 1977; Hansmann 1980). Yet the success of many of the profit-oriented health care companies has apparently come in part from their attention to patient preferences and desires—for convenience, courtesy, gourmet hospital food, and so forth. Does more attention to the patient's view mean that the caveat emptor ethic of the marketplace will become the ethic of health care? Although patient autonomy has gained a high place in the pantheon of values in medical ethics, there are still serious reasons to doubt whether the average patient, particularly in times of vulnerability and stress, can adequately protect his or her best interests (Arrow 1963). Thus, there appears to be reason for concern about changes that might weaken the sense among professionals that their first responsibility is to think of the interests of their patients. Whether the for-profit health care companies will increase or decrease this aspect of professionalism remains to be seen, although it is apparent that traditional fee-for-service medical practice contains many of the same pressures.

Conclusion

In this brief examination of three diverse topics, some consistent ethical themes appear. All involve issues of physician and institutional responsibilities in circumstances where there are possible conflicts of interests or of values—trying to advance knowledge while providing patient care, weighing quality of life against the imperative to try to preserve life, providing care when profit is the purpose of the organization. In all three cases, the patient's right to choose is a major part of the issue. However, in the cases of human experimentation and decisions to forego life-sustaining treatment, the exercise of patient autonomy is seen as a major part of the solution to the problem. In the case of for-profit health care, the exercise of patient autonomy has, at least for some observers, become part of the problem.

Virtually all ethical analyses of research with human subjects hold that research in which there are significant risks that are not compensated by expected benefits to subjects (in distinction to benefits to science) is ethically acceptable only if done with subjects' informed consent. Similarly, many of the most difficult problems concerning decisions to forego life-sustaining therapy arise when the patient's ability to make a sound decision is clearly (or possibly) impaired; clear evidence (e.g., in the form of advance directives) about what the patient's preferences are can be very helpful in resolving problems.

By contrast, some of the concern about the growth of for-profit enterprise in health care is a result of patient decision-making, particularly decisions to use for-profit facilities. (Of course, the decision of which facility to use does not always rest entirely with patients.) One concern is that the cumulative choices of paying patients not to use institutions where large numbers of poor and uninsured patients are treated may jeopardize the economic status of those institutions, which have long cross-subsidized indigent care from revenues from paying patients. A second concern is that patients' inability to judge quality will preclude their protecting their own interests in settings where the profit motive weighs too heavily. Thus, while a major thrust of ethical concern about the research and terminal illness topics is to restrain or balance the excesses of medical hegemony, even if based on the goal of serving patients' interests, a source of concern about the coming of investor-owned companies is whether the medical values that protect the interests of patients are sufficiently present.

Not only in the for-profit health care context does concern exist that patients might be exploited or that their interests may not be served by following their expressed preferences rather than by trying to meet their "true" needs. Despite the emphasis given to the importance of patient autonomy in bioethics, a significant source of concern about both research involving human subjects and decisions to forego life-sustaining treatment is the suspicion or certainty that in the ordinary course of things, people would not be able to protect their own interests—that they would unknowingly end up as guinea pigs, or that they would give up on life too soon.

With the dramatic advances in medical technology and changes in the delivery of health care have come increasingly explicit safeguards for the public in the form of government regulations and state laws. The doctor-patient relationship is no longer an entirely private matter in which the parties feel free or are free to act only in accord with their own personal preferences. Strong outside forces impinge on that relationship because the entire social context has changed and the public is increasingly aware of the issues. New ethical codes are also evolving in response to these changes. Dozens of ethical codes governing research involving human subjects have existed over the years, and a fine-grained regulatory apparatus has been put in place to be sure that the rights of subjects are protected. There is movement in a similar direction in decisions to forego life-sustaining treatment, although the problem is still relatively new and evolving. Regarding for-profit health care, however, the direction of movement is quite different. The provisions of older ethical codes that restrict or prohibit commercial activities by physicians have given way to weaker and more general exhortations that physicians not allow their economic interests and investments to sway their patient care decisions (Veatch 1983). Whether this weakening is a problem depends upon one's view of the importance of codes of ethics. Health policy appears to be relying less and less on ethical codes and more on regulatory mechanisms by which medical decision making is reviewed and on explicit attention to the economic incentives that are presented to medical decision makers.

References

Aaron, Henry J., and William Schwartz. 1984. *The painful prescription: Rationing hospital care.* Washington, D.C.: Brookings Institution.

American Hospital Association. 1981. Guidelines on ethical conduct and relationships of health care institutions. Chicago: American Hospital Association.

Annas, George. 1984a. The Baby Doe regulations: Governmental intervention in neonatal rescue medicine. *American Journal of Public Health* 74: 618–620.

―――. 1984b. The case of Baby Jane Doe: Child abuse or unlawful federal intervention? *American Journal of Public Health* 74:727–729.

―――. 1984c. Ethics committees in neonatal care: Substantive protection or procedural diversion? *American Journal of Public Health* 74:843–845.

Aries, Philippe. 1974. Death inside out. *Hastings Center Studies* 2(2):3–18.

Arrow, Kenneth. 1963. Uncertainty and the welfare economics of medical care. *American Economic Review* 53(2):941–973.

Barber, Bernard. 1973. Testimony before Subcommittee on Health, Committee on Labor and Public Welfare, U.S. Senate, March 8. *Quality of health care: Human experimentation, 1973* 3:1043–1049. Washington, D.C.: Government Printing Office.

Barber, Bernard et al., 1973. *Research on human subjects.* New York: Russell Sage.

Beauchamp, Tom L., and Lawrence B. McCullough. 1984. *Medical ethics. The moral responsibilities of physicians.* Englewood Cliffs, N.J.: Prentice-Hall.

Beecher, Henry K. 1966. Ethics and clinical research. *New England Journal of Medicine* 174:1354–1360.

Cassell, Eric. 1974. Dying in a technological society. *Hastings Center Studies* 2(2):31–36.

Cooke, Robert A., Arnold S. Tannenbaum, and Bradford H. Gray. 1977. A survey of institutional review boards and research involving human subjects. In *Report and recommendations: Institutional review boards*, National Commission for the Protection of Human Subjects, appendix. Washington, D.C.: Government Printing Office.

Crane, Diana. 1975. *The sanctity of social life: Physicians' treatment of critically ill patients.* New York: Russell Sage Foundation.

Encyclopedia of bioethics. 1978. 4 vols. New York: Free Press.

Ermann, Dan, and Jon Gabel. 1984. Multi-hospital systems: Issues and empirical findings. *Health Affairs* 3:50–64.

Financial and Stock report. 1984. *Modern Health Care*, Oct., p. 174.

Fox, Renée C. 1959. *Experiment perilous.* Glencoe, Ill.: Free Press.

―――. 1979. *Essays in medical sociology.* New York: John Wiley and Sons.

_____. 1980. The social meaning of death: Preface. *Annals of the American Academy of Political and Social Science* 447:VII–XI.

Freidson, Eliot 1986. The Medical Profession in Transition. In *Application of Social Science to Clinical Medicine and Health Policy*, ed. L. H. Aiken and D. Mechanic. New Bruswick: Rutgers University Press.

Glaser, Barney, and Anselm Strauss. 1965. *Awareness of dying*. Chicago: Aldine.

Ginzberg, Eli. 1984. The monetarization of medical care. *New England Journal of Medicine* 310:1162–1165.

Governor asserts elderly, if very ill, have "duty to die." 1984. *New York Times* 133 (March 29):12.

Gray, Bradford H. 1975. *Human subjects in medical experimentation*. New York: Wiley-Interscience.

_____, ed. 1983a. *The new health care for profit*. Washington, D.C.: National Academy Press.

_____. 1983b. An introduction to the new health care for profit. In *The new health care for profit*, ed. B. H. Gray. Washington, D.C.: National Academy Press.

_____. 1985. The new entrepreneurialism in health care: Overview of developments and trends. *Bulletin of the New York Academy of Medicine* 61(1):7–22.

Gray, Bradford H., Robert A. Cooke, and Arnold S. Tannenbaum. 1978. Research involving human subjects. *Science* 201:1094–1101.

Guidotti, Tee L. 1984. Limiting MD investment in health field ill-advised. *American Medical News*, Sept. 14, p. 31.

Hansmann, Henry B. 1980. The role of nonprofit enterprise. *Yale Law Journal* 89:835–901.

Institute of Medicine. 1986. *For Profit Enterprise in Health Care*. Washington D.C.: National Academy Press.

Jonsen, Albert. 1983. Watching the doctor. *New England Journal of Medicine* 308:1531–1535.

Katz, Jay. 1972. *Experimentation with human beings*. New York: Russell Sage Foundation.

Lewin and Associates, Inc. 1981. *Studies in the comparative performance of investor-owned and not-for-profit hospitals*. 4 vols. Washington, D.C.: Lewin and Associates.

Lubitz, James, and Ronald Prihoda. 1984. The use and cost of Medicare services in the last two years of life. *Health Care Financing Review* 5:117–131.

Lidz, Charles et al., 1984. *Informed consent: A study of decisionmaking in psychiatry*. New York: Guilford.

Lynn, Joanne, and Marian Osterweis. 1984. Ethical issues arising in hospice care. In *Hospice programs and public policy*, ed. Paul Torrens. Chicago: American Hospital Publishing.

Mechanic, David. 1979. *Future issues in health care: Social policy and the rationing of medical services.* New York: Free Press.

———. 1984. The transformation of health providers. *Health Affairs* (Spring):65–72.

Miller, Frances H. 1983. Secondary income from recommended treatment: Should fiduciary principles constrain physician behavior? In *The new health care for profit,* ed. Bradford H. Gray. Washington, D.C.: National Academy Press.

National Commission for the Protection of Human Subjects of Biomedical and Behavioral Research. 1978a. *The Belmont report: Ethical principles and guidelines for protection of human subjects.* Washington, D.C.: Government Printing Office.

———. 1978b. *Report and recommendations: Institutional review boards.* Washington, D.C.: Government Printing Office.

Novak, David, et al. 1979. Changes in physicians' attitudes towards telling the cancer patient. *Journal of the American Medical Association* 241:897–900.

Oken, D. 1961. What to tell cancer patients: A study of medical attitudes. *Journal of the American Medical Association* 175:1120–1128.

Parsons, Talcott. 1951. *The social system.* New York: Free Press.

Pattison, Robert, and Hallie Katz. Investor owned and not-for-profit hospitals: A comparison based on California data. *New England Journal of Medicine* 309:347–353.

President's Commission for the Study of Ethical Problems in Medicine and Biomedical and Behavioral Research. 1981. *Protecting human subjects: The adequacy and uniformity of federal rules and their implementation.* Washington, D.C.: Government Printing Office.

———. 1982. *Making health care decisions: The ethical and legal implications of informed consent in the patient-practitioner relationship.* Washington, D.C.: Government Printing Office.

———. 1983a. *Deciding to forego life-sustaining treatment: Ethical, medical, and legal issues in treatment decisions.* Washington, D.C.: Government Printing Office.

———. 1983b. *Implementing human subjects regulations.* Washington, D.C.: Government Printing Office.

Relman, Arnold S. 1980. The new medical-industrial complex. *New England Journal of Medicine* 303:963–970.

———. 1983. The future of medical practice. *Health Affairs* (Summer): 5–19.

Schlesinger, M. 1985. Multi-facility corporations, the delivery of health care, and health policy: A review and appraisal. Paper presented at the annual meeting of the American Public Health Association.

Schwartz, William, and Henry Aaron. 1984. Rationing hospital care: Lessons from Britain. *New England Journal of Medicine* 310:52–56.

Shapiro, Donald, and Paul Rosenberg. 1984. The effect of federal regulations regarding handicapped newborns. *Journal of the American Medical Association* 252:2031–2033.

Sloan, Frank A. 1980. The internal organization of hospitals: A descriptive study. *Health Services Research* 15:224–230.

Sloan, Frank A., and Robert Vraciu. 1983. Investor-owned and not-for-profit hospitals: Addressing some issues. *Health Affairs* 2:23–37.

Starr, Paul. 1983. *The social transformation of American medicine.* New York: Basic Books.

Sudnow, David. 1967. *Passing on: The social organization of dying.* Englewood Cliffs, N.J.: Prentice-Hall.

Tames, Stephanie. 1984. Withholding treatment: Who should decide? *Washington Report on Medicine and Health* 38(supp.):1–4.

Thomas, Lewis. 1980. Dying as failure. *Annals of the American Academy of Political and Social Science* 447:1–4.

U.S. Senate. 1973. *Quality of health care: Human experimentation, 1973.* Hearings before the Subcommittee on Health, Committee on Labor and Public Welfare. 4 vols. Washington, D.C.: Government Printing Office.

Veatch, Robert. 1983. Ethical dilemmas of for-profit enterprise in health care. In *The new health care for profit*, ed. Bradford H. Gray. Washington, D.C.: National Academy Press.

Weisbrod, Burton. 1977. *The voluntary nonprofit sector.* Lexington, Mass.: D.C. Heath.

Wikler, Daniel. 1985. Health care for profit: Some ethical issues. *Business and Health* 2(1):25–29.

Index

HBP (high blood pressure). *See* Hypertension

Health: medical services and social class and, 44–46; neighborhood centers and, 46–49, 52–53; perception of general, 217–218; poverty and, 37–44; social class and, 32–37; stress and seeking assistance for, 428–429

Health Care Financing Administration (HCFA), 554–555

Health care services. *See* Services

Health care system: access to, 31, 52, 101, 107–109; costs and, 101, 103–107; elderly and, 341, 342; health policy and, 102–103; health status and, 101, 109–110; pace of policy change (in U.S.) and, 102

Health habits, 371–374, 377

Health insurance. *See* Insurance

Health Insurance Plan of New York, 45

Health maintenance organizations (HMOs), 107; cost containment and, 528–531; doctor shortage and surplus and, 521; economic incentives analysis and, 503, 507, 511, 512, 513; the elderly and, 345–346; for-profit health care and, 555; health insurance and, 230, 241–242; medical errors and, 469, 471; occupation-based, 394; payment incentives and, 507–508, 509, 511, 512, 513; payment systems and, 488, 489; physicians and, 67, 68

Health monitoring system, 408

Health policy: Cardiovascular disease and, 139–141; contribution of social science to, 2–3, 4–5; the elderly and, 348–349; health care system and, 102–103; the poor and, 49–52; research and, 113–125; teenage pregnancy and, 326–328

Health professionals, coping and social support and, 417–418

Health promotion, 359–360, 377; work environment and, 394–395, 408–409

Health Services Research, 222

Health status: conceptualizing, 205–206; defining measures of, 206–207; health care system and, 101, 109–110; instruments for and standards of, 220–222; mental health and, 205, 212–214; perception of general health and, 217–218; physical functioning and, 205, 207–212, 216; physiologic status concept and, 219–220; role functioning and, 216–217; self-reported (chronic illness), 37; social well-being and, 206, 214–216; symptoms and, 218–219

Hearing loss, 429

Heart disease, 109, 363, 397. *See also* Cardiovascular disease (CD)

Height, death rate and, 42

Hicks, L. E., 46

High blood pressure. *See* Hypertension

Hill-Burton legislation, 520

Hippocratic standards, 546; managers and, 473

HMOs. *See* Health maintenance organizations (HMOs)

Hogarty, Gerry, 180

Holroyd, K. A., 426

Home care, 80, 107

Home visits, compliance and, 447

Homosexuality, 7, 170

Honolulu Heart Project, 370

Hospice services: hospital-based, 9; insurance study and, 234–235

Hospital Corporation of America, 555

Hospitalization: infant mortality and, 289; poverty and utilization rates and, 42–43; social class and, 34; technological and medical advances and, 23–24

Hospitals: ambiguous values and, 92; chain, 96, 108; community concept of, 80–81, 87–92; cost containment and, 116, 527; cultural specific characteristics of, 92; DRGs and, 93; elderly and, 343, 345; finance and, 80–82; government and, 88–89, 95, 96; health care system analysis and, 100–111; historical overview of, 84–87; infant mortality and, 286–287; investor-owned, 94, 95–96, 493–494; management of,

Services (*continued*)
301–303; mothers and childbirth, 273–274; payments to doctors and distribution of 484–485; rationing of, 530; social class and effectiveness of medical, 44–46; unbundled, 534
Sex education, 322
Sexual activity: cancer and, 170–171; cardiovascular disease (CD) and, 135; changing patterns of, 308–313; postponement of (during adolescence), 321–322; premarital, 260
Sexual harrassment, 473
Sexually transmitted disease (STD), 313
Shekelle, R. B., 132
Shipley, M. J., 41, 42
Sickness Impact Profile (SIP), 215
Siegmann, A. E., 222
Singer, J. L., 426
Single-parent households, 9, 312
Smoking, 322; cancer and, 159, 165, 169, 171–172; Cardiovascular disease and, 130, 131, 132, 133, 138, 139; as risk factor, 374–375; stress and, 426; stress analysis and, 41, 53; tobacco industry and, 146; work environment and, 394, 397, 403
Social class: attitudes toward, 31; effectiveness of medical services and, 44–46; health and, 32–37; health care system change and lower, 108, 110, 111; health policy (current) and the poor, 49–52; mental illness and, 177; neighborhood health centers and, 46–49, 52–53; poverty and illness and, 37–44
Social control, birth control and, 260–262
Social experiments in health. *See* Randomized controlled trials (health insurance)
Social health maintenance organizations (SHMOs), 345
Social isolation, 40–41
Social science: cancer study and, 157; contribution to health policy and, 2–3, 4–5; health services research and study and, 1–2, 4; medicine (his-

torical background) and, 1; study organization and, 3–4; technology and illness and study and, 5, 6–7, 8; teenage pregnancy programs and, 328; values and prevention and health care study and, 9; Social Security, 336, 338, 339, 340, 348
Social service departments (hospitals), 86–87
Social support, 369–371; coping and, 417–435; work environment and, 400–402, 403, 409
Social well-being, 206, 214–216
Socioeconomic status: Cardiovascular disease and, 132, 133–134; Coronary heart disease and, 132–133
Special care units, 506
Specialization, 72, 76, 86
Spiegel, J. S., 213
Spinal cord injury, 429
Standards, 66–67, 69, 72, 76; health status, 220–222
Stanford three community risk factor study (health insurance), 239–240, 241
Starfield, B., 37
Starr, A. S., 558
Starr, Paul, 521
Stein, Leonard, 181
Sterilization, 315
Stingfellow Acid Pits (California), 165
Stone, Martin, 264
Strauss, A. L., 92
Streptococcal infections, 48
Stress: cancer and, 171; control of symptoms of, 423–424; infant mortality and financial, 291; multiple conditions as cause of, 430–433; paradigm of support in, 417, 418–424; psychological, 40, 41; risk factors and, 367–369, 371; work and, 400, 401. *See also* Coping
Stressful life events (SLEs), 368–369, 418–419, 430–433
Stress and Human Health (Institute of Medicine), 365
Stroke, 109; diagnosis and, 137; morbidity and mortality from Cardiovascular disease and, 129; morbidity and

Notes on Contributors

Linda H. Aiken, Ph.D., is vice president of the Robert Wood Johnson Foundation, Princeton, New Jersey, a private philanthropy devoted to improving health care in the United States. Aiken is a medical sociologist and nurse whose research interests include health policy and evaluation research. She is a member of the Institute of Medicine of the National Academy of Sciences, past chair of the American Sociological Association's Medical Sociology Section, and past president of the American Academy of Nursing. Aiken was a member of the 1982–1983 National Advisory Council on Social Security. She is author of numerous articles and is editor of *Evaluation Studies Review Annual 1985* (with Barbara H. Kehrer), *Health Policy and Nursing Practice*, and *Nursing in the 1980s: Crises, Opportunities, Challenges.*

David Mechanic, Ph.D., is university professor and René Dubos Professor of Behavioral Sciences at Rutgers University, New Jersey. A leading specialist in the field of medical sociology and health care organization, Mechanic is the author of numerous articles and books including *From Advocacy to Allocation: The Changing Health Care System, Medical Sociology, Mental Health and Social Policy, The Growth of Bureaucratic Medicine*, and *Future Issues in Health Care.* He is a member of the Institute of Medicine of the National Academy of Sciences and the National Advisory Council of the National Institute on Aging, and has served as chairperson of a panel of the President's Commission on Mental Health and as a member of the Panel on Health Services Research and Development of the President's Science Advisory Committee.

Drew E. Altman, Ph.D., is vice president of the Robert Wood Johnson Foundation. He came to the foundation from the federal Health Care Financing Administration in Washington, D.C. Altman earned his Ph.D. in political science at the Massachusetts Institute of Technology. Among his publications is *Health Planning and Regulation: The Decision-Making Process.*

Carol S. Aneshensel, Ph.D., is acting associate professor in the Division of Population and Family Health, School of Public Health, University of California, Los Angeles. Aneshensel received her Ph.D. in sociology from Cornell University in 1976. She has published on the antecedents and consequences of depression in the general population. Her research interests include psychiatric epidemiology, stress, adolescent health, and research methods.

Charles L. Bosk, Ph.D., is associate professor of sociology at the University of Pennsylvania. Bosk's primary research interests are the regulation of medical practice, decision making in critical care medicine, the applications of genetic technology, and the impact of law on medical practice. *Forgive and Remember: Managing Medical Failure* and numerous articles on health care are among his publications.

Jeanne Brooks-Gunn, Ph.D., is a senior research scientist in the Division of Education Policy Research, and Services at Educational Testing Service. In addition, Brooks-Gunn is director of the Adolescent Study Program at St. Luke's–Roosevelt Hospital Center and ETS. She holds clinical appointments in pediatrics at Col-

umbia University, College of Physicians and Surgeons, and University of Pennsylvania Medical School. A developmental psychologist, she received her M.A. from Harvard University and her Ph.D. from the University of Pennsylvania. Her current research is on the psychosocial and physical development of adolescent females. Within this area she is involved in two projects that concern young teenagers from disadvantaged families: she is evaluating an intervention program for pregnant women and mothers of young infants in Harlem and is conducting an intergenerational study of teenage pregnancy across three generations in Baltimore.

George W. Brown, Ph.D., is professor of sociology at the University of London and member of the External Scientific Staff of the Medical Research Council. Brown has worked mainly in the area of psychiatry. His early research concerned the impact of social factors on the course of schizophrenic disorders. Since 1969 he has been largely concerned with the role of psychosocial factors in the etiology and course of depressive disorders. He has published widely, including *Institutionalism and Schizophrenia* (with J. K. Wing) and *Social Origins of Depression* (with Tirril Harris).

Eric M. Cottington, Ph.D., is an epidemiologist at Allegheny-Singer Research Institute, Allegheny General Hospital, Pittsburgh, Pennsylvania, and an adjunct instructor in the Department of Epidemiology, University of Pittsburgh. His research interests include the psychosocial aspects of chronic disease etiology, specifically the health effects of occupational stress and anger.

Karen Davis, Ph.D., is chairperson of the Department of Health Policy and Management in the School of Hygiene and Public Health and has a joint appointment as professor of political economy at Johns Hopkins University. Davis served in the Carter administration as deputy assistant secretary of Planning and Evaluation/Health, Department of Health and Human Services. She is a health economist specializing in issues in health policy analysis and legislation. Her current research interests include acute and long-term care for the elderly, physician supply and distribution, access to health care, child health, health care costs, and design of innovative provider reimbursement methods. She is the author of numerous books and articles on health economics and policy analysis, including *Health and the War on Poverty: A Ten-Year Appraisal* (with Cathy Schoen).

Diana B. Dutton, Ph.D., is senior research associate at the Stanford University School of Medicine. Dutton received an interdisciplinary Ph.D. in health policy analysis from M.I.T., and has taught in the School of Public Health at the University of California at Berkeley and at Stanford University in the Department of Family, Community, and Preventive Medicine. She served as a consultant to the 1981 Congressional Select Panel for the Promotion of Child Health, analyzing problems of medical care access among disadvantaged children. Her publications have focused on the nature of ambulatory care in different practice settings and the relation between socioeconomic status and health. She has also done qualitative research on the policy-making process in biomedical innovation, which will appear in her forthcoming book, *Dilemmas of Medical Progress*.

Carroll L. Estes, Ph.D., professor of sociology, is chairperson of the Department of Social and Behavioral Sciences and director of the Institute for Health and Aging, School of Nursing, University of California, San Francisco. Estes conducts research and writes about policy issues in long-term care for the elderly. She is author of *The Aging Enterprise* and coauthor of *Long Term Care of the Elderly: Public Policy Issues, Political Economy, Health and Aging*, and *Fiscal Austerity and Aging* and coeditor of *Readings in Political Economy of Aging*. Estes is a member of the Institute of Medicine of the National Academy of Sciences and past president of the Western Gerontological Society and of the Association for Gerontology in Higher Education.

Renée C. Fox, Ph.D., is professor of sociology at the University of Pennsylvania, where she has joint appointments in the Department of Sociology, the Department of Psychiatry, the Department of Medicine, and the School of Nursing. Fox also holds an interdisciplinary chair—the Annenberg Professor of the Social Sciences —at the University of Pennsylvania. Her major teaching and research interests—sociology of medicine, medical research, medical education, and medical ethics—have involved her in first-hand studies in Europe, Africa, and China as well as in the United States. She is the author of numerous articles and four books —*Experiment Perilous, The Emerging Physician* (with Willy De Craemer), *The Courage to Fail* (with Judith P. Swazey), and *Essays in Medical Sociology.* Fox is an elected member of the American Academy of Arts and Sciences and of the Institute of Medicine of the National Academy of Sciences.

Eliot Freidson, Ph.D., is professor of sociology in the Faculty of Arts and Sciences of New York University and a member of the Institute of Medicine of the National Academy of Sciences. Freidson is past chair of the Medical Sociology Section of the American Sociological Association. He has written a number of articles and books, including *Profession of Medicine, Professional Dominance: The Social Structure of Medical Care, Patients' Views of Medical Practice,* and *Doctoring Together.* His latest book, *Professional Powers: A Study of the Institutionalization of Formal Knowledge,* will be published by the University of Chicago Press in 1986.

Frank F. Furstenberg, Jr., Ph.D., is professor of sociology at the University of Pennsylvania. Furstenberg's interest in the changing American family life began at Columbia University where he researched family life in the nineteenth century, studied intergenerational transmission of values, and initiated a longitudinal investigation described in *Unplanned*

Parenthood: The Social Consequences of Teenage Childbearing. Furstenberg's recent work, *Recycling the Family: Remarriage after Divorce* with Graham Spanier, and a forthcoming book on *American Grandparents* with Andrew Cherlin examine the consequences of divorce and remarriage on the American kinship system.

William A. Glaser, Ph.D., is professor of health services administration, Graduate School of Management, New School for Social Research, New York. Trained as a political scientist and sociologist, Glaser has specialized in cross-national research about health services, government, industry, and other topics. In the area of reimbursement of health care providers, he has written two books about the payment of doctors abroad, *Paying the Doctor* and *Health Insurance Bargaining.* He is completing a book about the payment of hospitals in Europe and North America, and earlier he published a book about the social structure of hospitals in many countries, *Social Settings and Medical Organization.* From his other comparative research, he wrote *The Brain Drain.* From his research about American government, he wrote *Public Opinion and Congressional Elections* and *Pretrial Discovery and the Adversary System.*

Saxon Graham, Ph.D., is chairperson of the Department of Social and Preventive Medicine, School of Medicine, State University of New York at Buffalo. After receiving his Ph.D. from Yale University, Graham worked in biostatistics, medical sociology, and epidemiology at the School of

Public Health, University of Pittsburgh, before moving to his current location in 1957. He has been interested in the study of behavior change to enhance public health and particularly to reduce the incidence of cancer. Most of his publications have been in the social epidemiology of cancer at various sites.

Bradford H. Gray, Ph.D., a sociologist, is senior professional associate at the Institute of Medicine at the National Academy of Sciences in Washington. He is director of the institute's study of the implications of the growth of for-profit enterprise in health care and edited *The New Health Care for Profit*. Gray was also principal staff member and primary author of three Institute of Medicine reports as well as two federal commission reports: the President's Commission for the Study of Ethical Problems in Medicine and Research report, *Implementing Human Research Regulations*, and the National Commission for the Protection of Human Subjects' report, *Institutional Review Boards*. Gray is also the author of *Human Subjects in Medical Experimentation*. His interests are in bioethical issues and in the changing power relationships in health care.

James S. House, Ph.D., is research scientist in the Survey Research Center and Department of Epidemiology and professor of sociology at the University of Michigan. He has been involved in research on occupational stress and health for over a decade, has written many research and review articles in professional journals and books, and is author of *Work*

Stress and Social Support. House served as a consultant on occupational stress and health to both the Health, Education, and Welfare Committee on Work in America and the President's Commission on Mental Health. He has held major elected and appointed positions in the American Sociological Association and is also a member of the Academy for Behavioral Medicine Research, Society of Behavioral Medicine, Society for Epidemiological Research, and the American Psychological Association, among others.

Stanislav V. Kasl, Ph.D., is professor of epidemiology in Department of Epidemiology and Public Health, Yale University School of Medicine. He received his Ph.D. in psychology from the University of Michigan in 1962 and worked at the Institute for Social Research before coming to Yale in 1969. His primary research interest is in social and psychological influences on health status, with a special emphasis on "stress and disease" issues.

Philip R. Lee, M.D., is professor of social medicine at the University of California, San Fransisco, School of Medicine, where he has served as director of the Institute for Health Policy Studies since 1972. Lee served as chancellor of the University of California, San Francisco, from 1969 to 1972 and as assistant secretary for health and scientific affairs in the Department of Health, Education, and Welfare from 1965 to 1969. He is the author of over one hundred articles in the health field and has coauthored numerous books, including *Pills,*

Profits, and Politics, *Primary Care in a Specialized World, Exercise and Health, Pills and the Public Purse,* and *Prescriptions for Death: The Drugging of the Third World*; he is also coeditor of *The Nation's Health.*

Donald W. Light, Ph.D., is professor of social medicine and psychiatry at the University of Medicine and Dentistry of New Jersey, School of Osteopathic Medicine, and serves on the graduate faculty of sociology at Rutgers University. His research interests include the restructuring of the U.S. health care system and the growing supply of health providers. Light has received an award from the Twentieth Century Fund to write a book on these topics, and he is senior fellow at the Leonard Davis Institute of Health Economics. His most recent book, edited with Alexander Schuller, is *Political Values and Health Care: The German Experience.*

Harold S. Luft, Ph.D., is professor of health economics at the Institute for Health Policy Studies, University of California, San Francisco. Luft received his undergraduate and graduate training in economics at Harvard University. His research has covered a wide range of areas, including applications of benefit cost analysis and studies of medical care utilization, the relationship between volume of surgery in hospitals and postoperative mortality, regionalization of hospital services, duplication of health insurance coverage, competition in the medical care market, and health maintenance organizations. In addition to numerous articles in scientific journals, he authored *Health Mainte-*

nance *Organizations: Dimensions of Performance.*

James Marshall, Ph.D., is associate professor of social and preventive medicine in the School of Medicine and associate professor of sociology at the State University of New York at Buffalo. Marshall received his Ph.D. in sociology from the University of California, Los Angeles, in 1977. His publications include studies of suicide, mental health, and the epidemiology of cancer at various sites. He is currently involved in a series of studies of epidemiology of gastrointestinal cancer.

Marie C. McCormick, M.D., Sc.D., is assistant professor of pediatrics at the University of Pennsylvania School of Medicine, with appointments in the Division of General Pediatrics, Children's Hospital of Philadelphia, and the Clinical Epidemiology Unit of the Section of General Medicine. McCormick received her doctoral degrees at Johns Hopkins University (Schools of Medicine, and Hygiene and Public Health) where she was a Robert Wood Johnson Clinical Scholar. Her major research is in the evaluation of child health services, with a special interest in infant mortality and the health outcomes of very-low-birth-weight and other high-risk infants.

Constance A. Nathanson, Ph.D., has recently completed a year as visiting professor in the Department of Sociology at the University of Pennsylvania and has returned to the Department of Population Dynamics, Johns Hopkins University, School of

Hygiene and Public Health. Nathanson's research interests include the effects of health care organization on professional practice and client outcomes, sex differences in health, illness, and mortality, and reproductive behavior. For the past several years, she has been studying teenage contraception and is writing a book based on this work, *Social Control of Private Behavior: The Case of Teenage Pregnancy.*

Joseph P. Newhouse, Ph.D., is head of the economics department at the Rand Corporation. Most of his research efforts have focused on the economics of health and medical care. Newhouse is principal investigator and project director of the Health Insurance Study, a decade-long project to study the consequences of different ways of financing medical care services. He is also director of the Rand/UCLA Center on Health Care Financing Policy. He is the founding editor of the *Journal of Health Economics.*

Marian Osterweis, Ph.D., is senior professional associate at the Institute of Medicine, National Academy of Sciences. She received her Ph.D. in social relations and public health from Johns Hopkins University in 1972. Osterweis was a member of the faculty of Georgetown University Medical School for ten years before serving as staff sociologist for the President's Commission for Ethical Problems in Medicine and Biomedical and Behavioral Research, where she had primary responsibility for the commission's report on informed consent and contributed to the reports on decisions to forego life-sustaining treatment and on compensation for research injuries. She was study director for the Institute of Medicine study of bereavement and edited the book *Bereavement: Reactions, Consequences, and Care.* Currently she is directing a project on pain, disability, and chronic illness behavior.

Adrian M. Ostfeld, M.D., is the Anna M. R. Lauder Professor of Epidemiology and Public Health and head of the Division of Chronic Disease Epidemiology, Yale University School of Medicine. His publications deal principally with the effect of psychosocial variables on human health and disease and longitudinal studies of the health of older people and of cardiovascular disease. Ostfeld is editor of *American Journal of Epidemiology* and is on the editorial board of four other journals. He also served on the National Advisory Council on Aging. His current interests are the old old, the epidemiology of senile dementia, and longitudinal studies of populations in nursing homes.

Leonard I. Pearlin, Ph.D., is professor of medical sociology in the Department of Psychiatry, University of California, San Francisco. Prior to his present post, Pearlin had been a research sociologist in the Intramural Research Program of the National Institute of Mental Health since 1957. His research in recent years has been in the general area of stress, and he has written extensively on the social origins of stress, its mediation by coping and social supports, and its variations and changes across the life course.

Catherine Kohler Riessman, Ph.D., is visiting associate professor of sociology in the Department of Psychiatry, Massachusetts Mental Health Center, Harvard Medical School. A medical sociologist with a background in social work, Riessman is currently on leave from Smith College School for Social Work, where she chairs the Social Policy Sequence. Riessman's research interests are women and the health care system, social class and health service use, and health risks associated with marital dissolution for women compared to men. She is currently writing a book based on an empirical study of gender differences in the experience of marital separation, with special emphasis on mental health.

Rosemary Stevens, Ph.D., is professor of history and sociology of science at the University of Pennsylvania and a longtime analyst of health policy, health services history, and hospital affairs. Stevens was trained and worked as a hospital administrator in England before coming to the United States and has taught hospital and health systems management at Yale and at Tulane. Among her books are *American Medicine and the Public Interest* and *The Alien Doctors: Foreign Medical Graduates in American Hospitals.* She is now working on a book about the development of the U.S. hospital system in the twentieth century, from 1900 to the present.

Bonnie L. Svarstad, Ph.D., is associate dean for academic affairs and associate professor of social studies of pharmacy, School of Pharmacy, University of Wisconsin–Madison. Svarstad received her Ph.D. in sociology from the University of Wisconsin–Madison in 1974. Her research interests include the epidemiology of prescription and nonprescription drug use, patient compliance with drug regimens, the dynamics of physician-patient and pharmacist-patient communication, social factors affecting the use of psychoactive drugs in institutional settings, and the sociology of pharmacy.

John E. Ware, Jr., Ph.D., is a research psychologist at the Rand Corporation. His research has focused on the development and validation of measures of health status and patient satisfaction and on the application of these measures in clinical and health policy research. In Rand's Health Insurance Experiment, Ware examined the effects of different health care financing and organizational arrangements on health status. He is currently directing a study of differences in patient functional outcomes related to system of care, provider specialty, and other factors.